Principles of
Sensory Evaluation of Food

FOOD SCIENCE AND TECHNOLOGY

A Series of Monographs

PRINCIPLES OF
SENSORY EVALUATION
OF FOOD

by

Maynard A. Amerine
Rose Marie Pangborn
Edward B. Roessler

DEPARTMENTS OF VITICULTURE AND ENOLOGY,
FOOD SCIENCE AND TECHNOLOGY, AND MATHEMATICS,
UNIVERSITY OF CALIFORNIA,
DAVIS, CALIFORNIA

1965

ACADEMIC PRESS   New York and London

ACADEMIC PRESS INC.
111 Fifth Avenue, New York, New York 10003

United Kingdom Edition published by
ACADEMIC PRESS INC. (LONDON) LTD.
Berkeley Square House, London W.1

LIBRARY OF CONGRESS CATALOG CARD NUMBER: 65-22766

Second Printing, 1968

PRINTED IN THE UNITED STATES OF AMERICA.

Preface

Food science deals with the multitude of problems involved in providing food for human consumption. It includes the entire process from harvesting to serving. Investigations on the problems of food science involve biochemistry, microbiology, genetics, plant physiology, and other basic sciences, as well as engineering, horticulture, animal science, and other applied sciences. The research emphasis in the food industry has been primarily on economical preparation and distribution of safe and nutritious foods. Universities and experiment stations throughout the world have concerned themselves mainly with studies on chemical and nutritive composition, microbiological control, processing, and the functional properties of foodstuffs.

World War II focused attention upon another aspect of food science: that foods were sometimes rejected by the potential consumer, no matter how sound and nutritious they were. Furthermore, modern technology gradually changed the traditional methods of food preparation, and new and cheaper methods of production, storage, and distribution frequently altered the sensory appeal of foods. These developments emphasized the growing need for research in a previously neglected area —the sensory analysis of food. A review of food literature since 1940 reveals the rapid growth of this aspect of food science. It was thus natural that, in 1957, the University of California at Davis instituted an upper-division course intended for food majors in the analysis of foods by sensory methods. The present text is an outgrowth of that course.

Our philosophy has been that sound methodology for the sensory analysis of foods rests on a thorough knowledge of sensory physiology and an understanding of the psychology of perception. Essential in addition is careful statistical design and analyses of the data. Finally, new understanding of sensory judgment is to be sought through correlation with physical and chemical data.

This text therefore includes chapters on the physiology and psychology of the senses, a consideration of the present status of methodology, and appropriate statistical analyses of the results. The problems of measuring consumer acceptance are also discussed. Finally, we include a brief treatment of the relationship between sensory characteristics and various physical and chemical properties of foods. It is our belief that objective tests will someday replace many of the present subjective methods used in food science. In the final analysis, however, food acceptance and preference depend on human sensory responses, so it is imperative that tests employing human subjects continue.

We wish to thank, especially, Mrs. Elly Hinreiner Platou and Mrs.

Marion Simone Kunze for their help in organizing the course and in reviewing the literature for this text. Appreciation is extended to Professor F. N. Jones, University of California, Los Angeles; Dr. B. P. Halpern, State University of New York; Dr. Herbert Stone, Stanford Research Institute; Dr. Mildred Boggs, Western Regional Research Laboratory; and Professors H. W. Berg, W. F. Dukes, P. W. M. John, G. F. Stewart, and J. R. Whitaker, University of California, Davis, for advice on particular chapters. The helpful suggestions of our colleagues, Dr. M. H. Woskow, Mr. C. S. Ough, and Mr. Frank Winter, are gratefully acknowledged. Needless to say, any errors are the responsibility of the authors. We shall, of course, welcome any suggestions and corrections from the readers of the text. We hope this book will be of use in the training of food technologists in colleges and universities and for those engaged in research on problems of the sensory evaluation of food in university, government, and industrial laboratories. In view of the many unsolved problems, many of which we have indicated, we also hope that it will stimulate further research.

MAYNARD A. AMERINE
ROSE MARIE PANGBORN
EDWARD B. ROESSLER

Davis, California
August, 1965

Contents

CHAPTER 4
Visual, Auditory, Tactile, and Other Senses

CHAPTER 5
Factors Influencing Sensory Measurements

CHAPTER 6
Laboratory Studies: Types and Principles

CHAPTER 7
Laboratory Studies: Difference and Directional
Difference Tests

CHAPTER 8
Laboratory Studies: Quantity-Quality Evaluation

CHAPTER 9
Consumer Studies

CHAPTER 10
Statistical Procedures

CHAPTER 11
Physical and Chemical Tests Related to Sensory Properties of Foods

Chapter 1

Sensory Evaluation Problems of the Food Industry

The most primitive animals develop likes and dislikes for food, with many species displaying well-known predilections for one food over another. Although Paleolithic man, in his never-ending quest for food, had little opportunity to make fine quality distinctions, he obviously rejected certain foods altogether and consumed others only in time of dire need. The idea of improving flavor probably did not occur to early man until he accidentally discovered the art of roasting. Further changes in eating habits were brought about when Neolithic man planted cereals, domesticated animals, irrigated fertile land, and settled in villages. As food became abundant, society differentiated itself into producers, artisans, rulers, warriors, priests, etc. All had some leisure time and some had a good deal. Flavor distinctions and food preferences developed rapidly, especially along class or status lines (see Stewart *et al.*, 1965).

Many of our present-day food taboos and food habits undoubtedly developed during the Neolithic period (Simoons, 1961). Some were based on clan distinctions whereas others probably arose from conflicts between the nomadic way of life as compared to that of settled communities. The prejudice of nomadic peoples against pork is one example. Although the prophet Mohammed preached that pork was dangerous to eat, Simoons believes there was an economic basis also: the conflict between nomadic tribes, which could not raise pork, and settled communities, which could. A few of the taboos may have had a cultural or religious origin as a basis for separating the tribe or social unit from the neighbors. According to Simoons, the Moslem prohibition of alcoholic beverages was most likely due to a desire to distinguish the new religion from the alcohol-drinking Christians.

I. Early History

It is not fully realized how often the senses of taste and smell have influenced the history of human behavior. Henning (1924) listed a wide variety of odorous materials that were important to the Egyptians, including myrrh, cedar oil, asphalt, resin, cardamon, balsam, iris, and turpentine. That the Jews were very conscious of odor is indicated by the number of references to odorous materials in the Bible. Incense was common, and Moses was given a recipe for one (*Exodus* 30, 34): equal parts of stacte, sweet spices, galbanum, onycha, and frankincense. Arabians and Persians also used large amounts of odorous materials for incense and perfumes. Association of odorous materials with religious and sexual practices was undoubtedly important, as was propitiation of the gods with expensive, rare, and pleasant things. Even today, religious use of incense to engender a worshipful frame of mind is not unknown. Flowers at funerals may have a similar olfactory-religious origin.

In India, sandalwood oil was used as an odorous substance in the 9th century. Spices, butter, oil, lemon, and other materials were used in cooking. When the Portuguese and British came to India they found a well-developed spice industry. The discovery of America was indirectly related to Europe's demand for oriental odorous material for food flavoring and for cosmetics. Chinese emperors had such a fondness for aromatic foods that the Sung Dynasty (960–1279) exacted tribute of odorous foods from south China. A whole cult of floral esthetics developed in Japan, and the formal tea-drinking ceremony which developed from this has sensory as well as esthetic aspects. Greek mythology is filled with the religious use of spices, incense, and perfumes. Roses, violets, and other flowers were assiduously cultivated for the esthetic olfactory pleasures which they engendered. The Romans made perfumes a world-wide industry. This industry reached its heyday during the Renaissance, when Italian and Spanish perfumes were imported to France. Bienfang (1946) and Bedichek (1960) described how the sense of smell has been used in literature.

II. Modern Sensory Problems

A. Odor

Because of the greater range of olfactory responses, there are probably more odor than taste problems in the food industry. Some modern industrial odor problems are of great concern, such as control of waste-disposal odors in food plants that process protein products. The development of desirable odors in fruits, wines, and cheeses with age is well known, but a wide variety of undesirable odors are also associated with the storage of food. Undesirable odors and textures may develop in food when inadequate packaging material or improper storage temperatures are used. There are also persistent odor problems associated with the use of preservatives in foods (sulfur dioxide, benzoic acid, sorbates, etc.) and with the field use of various insecticides and fungicides. Fortification of foods with vitamins and other food accessories may create direct and indirect odor problems of concern not only as possible contaminants of the product but also as esthetic nuisances.

McCord and Witheridge (1949) discussed practical odor problems in the food industry, in ventilation, and in the water supply. Cartwright and Kelley (1954) gave pertinent examples of the problems of identifying foreign odors in foods. The food scientist's problem in this area is an industrial one, including deodorization, evaluation of quality, preferences, acceptance, and rejection (see Dove, 1947). The production of masking agents is now an important business. The use of chlorophyll is an example of the importance the public attaches to the field, even if the odor modifier in this case may not be effective. Harrison *et al.* (1953) maintained that a piece of flavored gum containing 4 mg of soluble sodium or potassium copper chlorophyllin effectively reduced breath odor following ingestion of onions or beer or after cigarette smoking. Other tests have not been so positive. Odors can also serve as danger signals, i.e., the odors of spoiled meat, rancid fat, and moldy foods.

Although little is known of the exact nature of the causal agent of many natural odors, through olfaction we can recognize odors that still elude chemical identification. By smelling we can identify compounds in mixtures. Furthermore, we *expect* some things to smell: leather, tobacco, fish, flowers, hospitals, garages, drug stores, shoestores, creameries, gymnasiums, bakeries, dairies, wineries, and breweries.

B. FLAVOR

The flavors of food products (probably largely odors) are also much stressed in the food industry. As Brožek (1957) noted "Flavor is a complex sensation, with taste, aroma and feeling as the three categories of components." This is recognized in the flavor profile procedure (Chapter 8, Section V), where five characteristics of flavor are measured: over-all impression ("amplitude") of aroma and flavor, perceptible aroma and flavor factors, intensity of each factor, the order in which the factors are perceived, and aftertaste (see Caul, 1956).

The growth of the spice industry is one indication of how important flavor has become in our diet. Advertising readily emphasizes flavor properties—real or imagined. Consider "purity, body, flavor" (Ballantine Ale), "brisk flavor" (Lipton's tea), "fascinating artificial flavor" (Wrigley's Juicy Fruit gum), "famous for its flavor" (Pride of the Farm catsup), etc. The effect on flavor of added salt, sugar, acid, spices, monosodium glutamate, meat tenderizer, etc., is receiving much current interest. The use of gas-liquid partition chromatography has greatly increased our knowledge of the distribution of volatile materials in various foods, but few studies on identification of volatile compounds have indicated their relationship to the sensory properties of flavor (see Chapter 11, Section II).

The food scientist must advise the producer on how production practices affect the composition and quality of the raw material and the processed end product. He must advise the breeder on the desirable color, odor, taste, and textural components of the new plant or animal, and the relation of these to processed quality and consumer acceptability and preference. Finally, within the food processing plant there are innumerable problems relating to processing variables, new-product development, quality control, and consumer acceptability and preference. Even when the product enters the channels of trade, the food scientist must be conscious of the potential changes in the sensory quality of the food.

III. The Senses

Since the senses, particularly taste and smell, are intimately associated with food appreciation, and hence with consumption, the study of their physiology and reaction to stimuli is fundamental to food science.

A. SENSORY RECEPTORS

The sensory receptors are the detectors which inform us of physical and chemical changes in our environment. These specialized cells are usually sensitive to a single stimulus, but under certain circumstances may react to other stimuli. The classification of sense organs in terms of the sensations they mediate is a tenuous one since there is no basis for the opinion that the nature of the sensation is determined by the receptor organ. Actually the sense organs convey, not the true properties of the world, but only a spatial or chronological picture.

The sense organs of animals consist of sensory cells or groups of cells which respond to stimuli and transmit an impulse via the nerves to the brain. The essential property of the sense organ is irritability—to either chemical or physical changes in the environment or within the organism. The receptor may be a neuro-sensory cell or it may be a secondary sensory cell which transmits a stimulus to the nerve and thence to higher brain centers. Definite areas in the brain are stimulated by the sensory input from the receptors. In higher animals the sense organs, in addition to receptor cells, have various mechanisms for protecting, supporting, or conveying stimuli to the receptor cells. Thus there is a great diversity of receptor cells and of sensory nerve terminations, which accounts for the large number of special senses. The response of the sensory cells increases as the stimulus increases—up to a point. The response of the nerve depends on the frequency of the electrical discharge of the nerve; the higher the frequency the stronger the sensation. Sensory receptors also vary in sensitivity.

Even quite primitive animals have highly specialized neuro-muscular systems. Prosser (1954) summarized recent investigations on new types of receptors. Receptors sensitive to carbon dioxide or to oxygen are found in many animals. The tongue of the frog has specific water receptors. Hygroreceptors have been found in the antennae of several insects. *Tribolium* adults, for example, showed a preference for lower humidity in the range 30 to 100% relative humidity, distinguishing differences of 5%. Water receptors have also been postulated for man, based on certain contrast taste reactions. This research is now being pursued very actively in Sweden (Zotterman, 1957, 1961; Zotterman and Diamant, 1959).

Based on Aristotle's authority, man is said to possess five primary, or major, senses: sight, hearing, touch, smell, and taste. Of these, the last two are the most primitive. For the lower animals these senses are of the utmost importance. Fish, for example, have chemoreceptors over much of their exterior surface. In the higher animals these specialized chemoreceptors are so localized as to sample the intake of food. In man, location of the taste receptors in the mouth, and the olfactory receptors in the nose, makes it possible to taste and smell ingested foods simultaneously. Other senses now generally recognized include muscular and visceral, heat, cold, pain, hunger, thirst, fatigue, sex, and equilibrium. As many as 22 special senses or subdivisions of these have been recognized by psychologists.

Many animals cannot hear, and some have no perception of light, but all forms of animal life react to chemical stimuli. In man, at least three different senses respond to certain chemical stimuli: taste, smell, and the so-called common chemical or pain sense (Chapter 4, Section III,E). The chemical senses aid animals in their search for and recognition of food, serve as danger signs, and in some cases function in propagation. Man is primarily sight-guided in his search for food, but pigs, dogs, and other animals are scent-guided.

There are many known facts about the senses, but few unifying theories. Experimentation in this field is difficult, and the gaps in our knowledge are large. Some say that the senses of smell and taste are too simple for elaborate description. Vision and hearing, with their analytical receptor systems, may appear to be more complex, though McIndoo (1927) and Boring (1942) do not think so. Smell, at least, has a great complexity of qualities, and the olfactory membrane, even though its differential sensitivity is less, compares well in absolute sensitivity with the retina (sight) and the organ of Corti (hearing).

One of the few unifying aspects of the senses is that they are unifunctional in nature. Thus sight is dependent on alterations in radiant energy, touch and hearing to pressure changes, and taste and smell to chemical changes (Table 1). There is no proof, however, that the

TABLE 1
Sensory Reactions with Corresponding Stimuli and Receptors

Sensory modality	Type of stimulus	Receptor	Experience
	I. Distance receptors		
Visual	Radiant energy of wavelength 10^{-4} to 10^{-5} cm (light waves)	Rods and cones of retina	Hue, brightness
Auditory	Mechanical vibrations of frequency of 20–20,000 cps (sound waves)	Hair cells of the Organ of Corti	Pitch, loudness
	II. Chemical receptors		
Gustatory	Chemicals in liquid solution	Taste buds	Tastes
Olfactory	Chemicals in gaseous solution	Olfactory cells in uppermost part of nasal cavity	Odors
	III. Somesthetic receptors		
Cutaneous	(1) Temperature changes	Cells in skin	Warmth, cold
	(2) Mechanical pressures	Cells in skin	Contact (light pressure)
	(3) Extreme energy of any class	Free nerve endings	Pain
Kinesthetic	Mechanical pressures	Cells in tendons, muscles, joints	Active movement, weight (deep pressure)
Vestibular (static)	Movement of head (rectilinear or rotary)	Cells in semicircular canals and vestibule	Equilibrium
Organic	Chemical or mechanical action	Cells in viscera	Pressure, visceral disturbance (e.g., hunger, nausea)

stimulation depends on a chemical reaction per se. In each case the sense is due to a group of specialized cells, so specialized that they normally respond only to a particular category of external environmental changes.

Hollingworth and Poffenberger (1917) have compared the senses as shown in Table 2.

It has been said that smell and taste are so unimportant to civilization that men lack interest in them. Interest does excite intellectual activity, but activity depends on systematic knowledge. One reason for the lack of work in this field is that we do not yet know what the stimuli for taste and smell are. We know the stimulus results: acids taste sour, roses smell like roses. Even so, what is it that makes acids taste sour

TABLE 2
Comparison of the Senses

	No. discernible stimuli	Sharpness of discrimination (%)	Av. speed of reaction (sec)	Duration of sensation, degree inertia (sec)
Sight	40,000	1	0.189	0.03
Hearing	15,000	33	0.146	0.002
Smell	?	25	?	?
Touch	3–4 (?)	33	0.149	0.001–0.002
Taste	4 (+, ?)	5	0.300–1.000	?
Kinesthetic	4–5 (+, ?)	5	?	?
Temperature	2 (?)	?	0.150–0.180	?

Source: Hollingworth and Poffenberger (1917).

or roses smell like roses? What is the common property of all sour substances, and of all roselike objects? A "theory" of olfaction and gustation is needed to unify the mass of information which is available. As Prosser (1954) said, "There is still no unifying theory for the chemical senses as to mechanism." The "missing link" lies somewhere in biochemistry, awaiting discovery. Pfaffmann (1956), in a review of recent progress on taste and smell, pointed out that our information comes from such diverse fields as chemistry, physiology, psychology, food technology, and industry.

B. Texts

Boring (1942) believed that a single good textbook can give all the known facts on taste and smell and serve as a history, because there has not been enough time for facts to go out of style or theories to be proven incorrect. Boring reviewed most of the early texts: Haller (1763), Cloquet (1815), Zwaardemaker (1895, 1925), Marchand (1903), Sternberg (1906), Cohn (1914), Henning (1916, 1924), Hollingworth and Poffenberger (1917), Parker (1922), Skramlik (1926), and Parker and Crozier (1929). Of these, the standard text is that of Skramlik. For comprehensive details on taste, Henning (1924) should be consulted; and for odor, Zwaardemaker (1925). See also the excellent reviews in the American Physiological Society handbook (1959). Cohn (1914) has much useful data on the taste of organic compounds.

More recently, Le Magnen (1949) wrote a short but sensitive review of odors, particularly as applied to the perfume industry. The physiological aspects of taste and/or odor are the primary concerns of the texts by Bronshtein (1950), Piéron (1952), Beythien (1949), Geldard (1950, 1953), and Wenger et al. (1956). The several reviews in American Physiological Society (1959) probably make it the best current summary, but Patton's (1960) is a briefer modern account. The books by Kare and Halpern (1961) and Zotterman (1963) contain articles by several authors on behavioral and physiological aspects of taste, primarily in experimental animals. Buddenbrock (1953, 1958) is less satisfactory. The articles in Rosenblith's (1961) text cover sensory systems in general in addition to taste and olfaction.

Reviews of current literature have been given by Dethier and Chadwick (1948), Geldard (1950), Wenzel (1954), Weddell (1955), Pfaffmann (1956), and Beidler (1961). Paschal (1952) and Michels et al. (1961) give useful bibliographies on olfaction. Moncrieff (1946, 1951) presents much material which is primarily of interest for reference. Kalmus and Hubbard (1960) presented a somewhat superficial description of the reaction of the chemical senses in health and disease.

As specifically applied to foods, the books by Dawson and Harris (1951), Marcuse (1954), Tilgner (1957), and Masuyama and Miura (1962) should be consulted. Dawson and Harris have listed considerable data on sensory tests. Marcuse (in Swedish), Tilgner (in Polish), and Masuyama and Miura (in Japanese) gave practical details for conducting sensory tests. Peryam et al. (1960) comprehensively described practice relative to determination of food acceptance by members of the U. S. Armed Forces. Dawson et al. (1963) gave a useful summary of U. S. practice. Pangborn (1964) reviewed the development of research in this field and pointed out the many unresolved problems. A review of the French work on laboratory sensory tasting of foods was given by Renou (1962). A summary of quality control by the use of sensory testing is given by Juran (1962). A series of papers in Laboratory Practice (1964) described theoretical and practical aspects in many laboratories.

Throughout this text, it will be noted that the data are inadequate and often difficult to evaluate critically. Many experiments have been conducted with inadequate numbers of observers and few sensory replications, using methods that were biased or inappropriate. For years, for example, textbooks stated that there was a relation between albinism and anosmia (impaired sense of smell). After this was finally challenged, a search of the literature revealed that the observation was based mainly on anecdotal material. Moulton (1960) has shown that this relation is not true for pigmented versus albino rats, and it is doubtful that it is true for man.

IV. Relation of the Senses to Food Habits

Pfaffmann (1961) has noted that the senses of taste and smell have one unique property: they can and do instigate strong acceptance or rejection responses. When pleasant taste solutions are used as reinforcers in a learning situation, the acquisition of behavior is rapid and dramatic. Certain solutions also elicit strong reactions of disgust. Obviously, the senses of taste and smell are intimately associated with our eating habits.

Tepperman (1961) classifies metabolic and taste interactions into three categories:

The first includes cases in which there is a modification of the metabolic state and the animal ingests larger quantities of some substance to achieve nutritional adaptation. The classical example is the increase in salt consumption following adrenalectomy. That taste is involved seems evident from the fact that when the glossopharyngeal, chorda tympani, and lingual nerves are cut the animal is unable to increase salt intake.

In the second type a nutritional deficiency results in a metabolic defect which leads to nutritional adaptation to rectify the imbalance. An example is the preference of vitamin B-deficient animals for oil and their rejection of sugar.

In the third type, taste modifies the metabolic mixture and thus leads to metabolic adaptation or to a predisposition to disease. Tepperman suggested that in some cases the hedonistic aspects of taste play a role in the development of obesity. See also Carlson (1916).

Beidler (1962) does not exclude the possibility of a peripheral influence upon food selection. He visualizes three methods by which the taste receptors could obtain information about the general conditions of the body: (1) a chemical deficiency may be reflected in the blood bathing the taste receptor and thus change the receptor's environment; (2) reflexes from other tissues to the central nervous system might come back to the peripheral sense organ and thus influence the excitability of a taste cell to a given stimulus; and (3) the molecular structure may change when a deficiency develops. The last is possible since new cells are constantly being formed (Chapter 2, Section I); thus, the surface of the receptor might be changed slightly so that its response to a given stimulus is altered.

Lepkovsky (1963) believes that sensory stimuli: (1) make possible the recognition of food; (2) make it possible for the animal to choose its food in accordance with its need; (3) initiate appropriate responses in the viscera, making them ready for digestion of the meal; (4) are important in the cessation of eating since they promote satiety; and (5) make possible the pleasure that is anticipated from eating. He recommends that the food industry recognize and measure the usefulness of sensory stimuli and that they preserve desirable flavors during processing and create new and useful flavors in foods by proper processing and handling. Rather than direct measurement of sensory stimuli he recommends measurement of flow of saliva, flow and composition of gastric juice, and motility of the stomach and intestine.

In spite of the voluminous literature on thirst, no theory can explain drinking under all conditions. Among the multiple factors involved are osmotic pressure, solute, taste, timing, other stimuli, and alimentary, nervous, and endocrine factors. It has been suggested (see Wayner and Sporn, 1963) that there is an interaction between thirst and hunger which may be determined centrally as well as peripherally.

A. FOOD HABITS

During World War II a major study was made of our national food habits (Committee on Food Habits, 1943). This study analyzed dietary deficiencies and evolved methods of improving food habits. The approach was generally from the point of view of cultural anthropology, where food habits are viewed as a set of culturally standardized behaviors, although the possibility was taken into account that combinations of foods influence response. Man's individual likings and aversions toward foods are extremely varied. Some are very deeply rooted and capable of producing distressing involuntary reactions. The factors which influence food preference are extremely varied—from the caprices of fashion to the prevalence of dentures.

Some of the food patterns identified (other than those of specific immigrant groups) were: European peasant status concept (white bread, much sugar, daily meat), Puritan tradition of healthful food being disliked (leading to use of delicious food as a reward for eating healthful but disliked food), Southeastern emphasis on personal taste, emphasis on appearance (in contrast to taste), preference for packaged, processed, or highly refined foods with no waste, emphasis on purity and packaging, etc.

The importance of cultural patterns in determining food preferences and tastes must be stressed. Even within the United States there are some differences in patterns of food consumption in different parts of the country as well as significant local patterns among subgroups of nationals. There are also important variations among social classes.

In a survey carried out in Norway by Ogrim and Homb (1960), more meat, vegetables, fruit, eggs, cream, and butter were used by groups with high income and small family. These groups also had a higher consumption of more expensive items within each food group and a wider choice of foods in general. The consumption of sweets and expenditures for vitamin concentrates were also higher in the higher-income groups. The same trends were observed in several occupations. The occupational groups of farmers and forest workers had a higher ratio of meat to fish consumption than the professional men or industrial workers. A large part of the meat consisted of pork. As expected, fishermen had the highest consumption of fish. Some regional divisions were also noted in consumption patterns.

Idiosyncratic variables may also influence food likes and aversions most profoundly. Fischer and Griffin (1959) and Fischer *et al.* (1961) suggested that sensitivity for 6-*n*-propylthiouracil and quinine was related to a number of food dislikes, i.e., bitter-sensitive individuals have the most food dislikes. More information would be desirable on such correlations (see Chapter 2, Section XIII,D).

Gottlieb and Rossi (1961) noted the importance of emotions on food habits. They cited cases of anxiety, early childhood experiences, use of food as a substitute gratification for love, security, or companionship, involvement of oral and gastrointestinal activities, and other psychogenic factors in food acceptance or rejection.

The effect of variations in climate and the general physical status of the individual on food consumption is well known. The specific environment, both social and psychological, may also have a marked influence on food consumption. Further, group situations may lead to rejection or complaints about foods or to acceptance and even preference. Methods of food preparation and serving are also important. Food habits are influenced greatly by food availability, a good example being the preference of Eskimos for fish blubber. The flora and fauna of a region, as well as man's physiological needs, vary with climate and influence food selection. In this country, more ice cream but fewer pancakes are eaten in the summer than in the winter.

Lewin (1943) reported that one answer to what people eat in a family situation is that they eat what is on the table. A change in food acceptability requires a change of the individual's frame of reference. Group decisions were more effective than official requests in changing consumption patterns. The degree to which the individual is identified with a group is also of importance.

Some methods of change which have been studied are: altering the relative or absolute availability of foods, substitute sources (home gardening and canning), substitute foods (glandular foods, sponsored by lower ration-point values during World War II), changing the frame of reference of a food (nutritional emphasis or modifying the idea that it is a "fuss" food), and appeals to "togetherness" or group-eating habits. These can be promulgated by the radio, newspapers, billboards, television, etc. Threats of punishment or democratic "group" decisions could be used.

Gottlieb and Rossi (1961) have reviewed the literature on bases for changing food attitudes. A detailed summary of methods for studying food habits was worked out by the Committee on Food Habits of the National Research Council (Anonymous, 1945). The importance of education in changing food habits cannot be overemphasized. Usually a survey is conducted to determine what the prejudice is, and a campaign is then devised to remove it. Doctors, dentists, and nutrition experts may be approached through professional journals. Salesmen and retailers can be reached by trade journals, conventions, personal contact, etc. Finally, the public itself may be indoctrinated by the multiple and often subtle ministrations of the government and Madison Avenue.

A recent symposium on changing food habits has been edited by Yudkin and McKenzie (1964). They carefully distinguish food preferences (the particular foods an individual likes or dislikes), food choice (the foods selected by an individual at a given time), and food habits (the sum of the food choices of an individual, constituting his total diet). New concepts introduced are economic availability, and doubt as to the effectiveness of some advertising. It seems to be easier to increase the consumption of nutritionally desirable foods than to discourage the use of nutritionally undesirable foods. Nutrition education is recommended as a promising method for changing food habits.

The possibility of changing food habits, particularly in a military situation, has been studied by Peryam (1963). He concluded that prospects are poor of altering food behavior of groups at will. However, some changes may occur through adaptation to alterations in the environment. Specifically, novel foods have each to be studied separately. Even if general food habits cannot be changed, the behavior of a group toward a particular item or group of items can be influenced.

There is, of course, substantial historical evidence that food habits can and do change: acorns are no longer eaten in Europe; TV dinners have become common in America. However, some food prejudices persist for long periods. Racial, "status," religious, and moral prejudices may be tenacious and difficult to alter. The socio-psychological aspects of food acceptance have been noted by Harper (1962). Personal aspirations and identifications apparently play a role which may be stronger than the Veblian factor of "conspicuous waste." We agree with Harper that more information is needed on world food habits, the relation of likes and dislikes to sensory, perceptual, physicochemical, and cultural data, and the possibility of stimulation of interest in unfamiliar foods.

B. DIET SELECTION

In reviewing a large amount of data on food-seeking behavior, Young (1949a) pointed out that "although food selections often are in accord with nutritional needs, the correlation between need and acceptance is far from perfect. Food acceptance is regulated by the characteristics of the food object (palatability), by the environmental surroundings of the food object, by established feeding habits, as well as by intraorganic chemical conditions which themselves may or may not be directly related to metabolic needs."

Does man have an instinct which enables him to select a diet according to his needs? Richter (1942) says "yes" and Remington (1936) says "no." Food habits, obviously, have a physiological basis. Food deprivation leads to hunger. Moreover, work of Davis (1928), Dove (1935, 1939), Richter (1941a,b, 1943), and others did suggest that appetite, if not affected by established food patterns, can lead to a nutritionally adequate diet. However, Scott and Verney (1948, 1949), Scott *et al.* (1948), and others reported little significant relationship between appetite and physiological or nutritional need.

It is, therefore, by no means certain that man eats what he needs. There is no good evidence that man will balance his diet instinctively, and there are instances where he does not. Quantitative and qualitative nutritional deficiencies can and do occur in areas with an adequate food supply. No doubt the stress of modern living interferes with the free selection of available food. In areas of food deficiency the problem is more complicated. Seasonal deficiency is certainly common in many regions and pandemic in others.

Richter (1942) has given a compresensive review of his studies of self-regulatory functions of animals. He credited Bernard and Cannon with the concept that external body needs determine physiological requirements. Richter's experiments showed that the behavior of the organism also contributed to a constant internal environment, i.e., homeostasis. Thus, he says "operative removal of the adrenal glands from animals eliminates their physiological control of sodium metabolism, and as a result large amounts of sodium are excreted as salt in the urine and the internal environment is greatly disturbed. If given access only to a stock diet, such animals die in 8–15 days. However, if given access to salt in a container separate from their food they will take adequate amounts to keep themselves alive and free from symptoms of insufficiency." The effect of adrenalectomy on consumption is clearly demonstrated in Fig. 1.

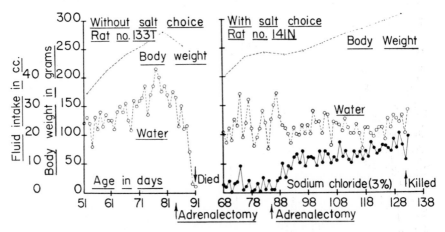

FIG. 1. Salt intake of rats following adrenalectomy. Source: Richter (1942).

Rats have been shown to differentiate between distilled water and dilute alcohol solutions (Richter and Campbell, 1940). Figure 2 shows data from one rat (typical for 13 out of 17). Richter (1942) asked, "Do

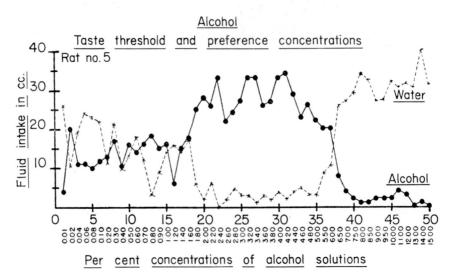

FIG. 2. Influence of concentration on alcohol consumption by the rat. Source: Richter and Campbell (1940).

rats eat certain substances because the ingestion of these substances makes them feel better, and avoid others because their ingestion produces discomfort or pain? Or does the taste of the substance determine the choice? In other words, does appetite serve as a guide to the selection of a beneficial diet? It is not possible to give definite answers to these questions at the present time. Certainly the selections may depend on both factors. The evidence at hand, however, indicates that taste plays a very important part."

But, are the responses due to increased metabolic needs or to other factors? There are many examples of increased intake owing to dietary deficiencies, but this is by no means universal. Richter (1942) observed that children preferred cod-liver oil up to 5 years of age, but thereafter did not. This was true whether they had had cod-liver oil before or not. Nemanova (1941) was able to condition taste discriminations in infants just over a month in age, and established thresholds for sucrose, diluted lemon juice, and sodium chloride.

Richter noted that failure of the self-regulatory mechanism to account for food intake may be due to: (1) the use of purified chemical substances which may confuse choice; (2) the availability of highly refined foods that may not furnish sufficient vitamins, minerals, etc., no matter how adequate the self-regulatory mechanism; and (3) inherited and acquired defects of the sensory mechanism that lead to poor dietary selections. Possibly genetic factors are important in food intake (see Chapter 2, Section XIV). Cultural influences, he concluded, probably account for most failures to make beneficial dietary selections. Finally, there may be breakdowns in the self-regulatory mechanisms themselves with age, disease, accident, etc.

Richter's results may be due to a learning technique. Although adrenalectomized rats eat more salt, Harriman and MacLeod (1953) doubt if this is due to increased receptor sensitivity. With a reward and punishment technique, normal rats showed very low thresholds which were not reduced by adrenalectomy. The actual threshold does not change, i.e., there is no peripheral change in the sensitivity of the taste receptors between adrenalectomized and normal rats. Taste and intragastric factors influence intake. The current opinion is that feeding behavior may be, but is not necessarily, directed toward the physiological well-being of the organism.

Smith and Duffy (1957) showed that initially hungry rats consume more sucrose than satiated rats. With saccharin this difference between hungry and satiated rats did not occur. However, over a 24-hour period hungry rats consumed more sugar and saccharin than satiated rats. Hunger was not the primary factor, but represents some form of learned response. The ingestion of saccharin is apparently more of a reinforcing behavior for hungry rats than for satiated rats. Reduction of need is seemingly not a factor. Le Magnen (1959) reported that odor and taste did not condition satiety as evidenced by food consumption of rats.

The evidence is obviously conflicting. Young and Chaplin (1949) showed that intake of sodium chloride varies with the concentration of the sodium chloride solution. This was true both for normal rats and for adrenalectomized rats, who presumably have a greater need for salt. Intake is thus dependent on need (functioning of the adrenal gland) and on the characteristics of the solution. Do rats therefore take what they need, or do they take what they like?

The influence of caloric need on intake of glucose and saccharin has been studied by Carper and Polliard (1953). They found that under conditions of caloric need rats increased their consumption of glucose and of saccharin. Intake of saccharin is not a matter of fulfilling body needs, since it has no food value. This has also been tested by Sheffield and Roby (1950), who found that hungry rats consumed much more saccharin than satiated rats. The saccharin was given as a reward when a maze problem was solved. For a typical result, see Fig. 3. Richter

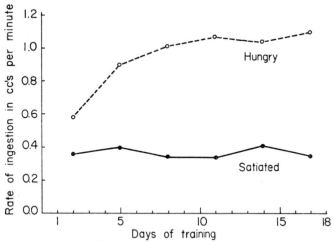

FIG. 3. Acquisition of drinking of saccharin solution (in response to a specific cue-pattern accompanying availability of the solution). Source: Sheffield and Roby (1950).

has been a proponent of the theory that sensitivity increases with need. Meyer (1952) tested this for glucose, sodium chloride, and quinine sulfate during and after deprivation for 34 hours. There was no change in thresholds, which casts doubt on Richter's theory. Irvin and Goetzl

(1952) and Goetzl *et al.* (1950), although using questionable methods, reported significant decreases in thresholds for sodium chloride and sucrose in human subjects as the time after a meal increased. This difference is disturbing and should be resolved—particularly from the point of view of removing another variable in experiments on the sensory properties of foods.

Young (1948) has summarized the evidence that rats can learn to take one path to food when hungry and another to water when thirsty, discriminating on the basis of their organic state. Young's general conclusions are:

> Dietary need is a nutritional concept. When a component of the diet which is required for normal growth, reproduction, activity, or for survival itself, is removed a pattern of deficiency symptoms appears. Deficiency symptoms are not drives. No one has been able to demonstrate that for each specific deficiency there exists a specific form of food-seeking or food-selecting behavior.
>
> There are, however, behavioral manifestations of depletion as well as structural changes. A specific deprivation may change the level of activity, the time and error scores in maze learning, the liability to fits, or the functional capacity of the sense organs.
>
> Habits of seeking particular foods appear to rest directly upon the effects of ingesting these foods. The term *palatability* implies an effective reaction to foodstuffs which stimulate the head receptors. There are also delayed and remote after-effects of food ingestion which, under some circumstances, may be the basis of dietary habits.
>
> An established feeding habit may persist regardless of the bodily needs. On the other hand, new habits tend to form which will meet bodily needs.
>
> The environmental determinants of food acceptance can be classified as palatability factors and non-palatability factors. Palatability factors are characteristics of the food itself such as the kind of food, concentration of solution, temperature of the food, texture, etc. The experimental study of palatability is of great importance in the practical art of feeding men and animals.
>
> Closely related to palatability in the regulation of food acceptance are such determining conditions as size of food object, quantity of food, position of food, degree of contamination, kind of container, laboratory apparatus through which food is obtained, etc. Environmental factors not directly related to palatability but modifying the feeding process are temperature of the surroundings, distractions, emotionally disturbing shocks and noises.
>
> Strength of drive, as measured by the time required to approach and accept a food, is positively correlated with the degree of palatability of the incentive. Animals run faster in approaching a highly palatable food than in approaching one of low palatability.
>
> The rate of habit growth, however, is not dependent upon the degree of palatability of the incentive. Learning depends upon the frequency and distribution of reinforcements.

> There are three main groups of conditions which must be controlled: conditions within the organism (appetitive conditions); conditions within the nutritive environment (palatability and nonpalatability determinants); conditions within the previous behavior of an organism (feeding habits).

Young (1949a,b) applied these results to differentiation between palatability and appetite. He first determined the daily intake for salt and sucrose and found that the level of intake depended on the concentration of the solutions presented. He made the point that intake thus depends on stimulus concentration. This he called "palatability." It includes the temperature and kind of food, texture of food, etc., and involves stimulating receptors in the head. Appetite, in contrast, has to do with intraorganic conditions (need produced by deprivation, satiation produced by continued ingestion, glandular balance, etc.). He demonstrated appetite by showing that rats preferred 50% sucrose solutions over 47% solutions immediately after being deprived of sucrose. But if offered a free choice of several concentrations without prior deprivation, they will select the lower concentration. Palatability and appetite are not motivational units, but rather two interdependent groups of parameters relating to the acceptance and rejection of foods. Appetite itself, however, is a motivational concept. Food habits and addictions are also important (Young and Greene, 1953).

The factors that influence feeding have been shown to be different at the beginning as compared to the end of the feeding period. Appetite and satiety are thus distinct phenomena, according to Brobeck (1955). The internal system which helps the body maintain a steady, or a regularly increasing, body weight is not known. A variety of internal processes apparently control feeding, as reflected in the various indices of "hunger."

The internal factors that influence food acceptance have been stressed by Lepkovsky (1953). He noted that some foods which are normally unacceptable become highly acceptable when a state of stress is developed. He also believed that some foods which are acceptable under normal conditions may become unacceptable under conditions of stress. He suggested that stress factors may act to make foods more or less acceptable by: (1) affecting the flavor of a food, either increasing or decreasing its perception; (2) affecting motor phenomena in the digestive tract and thus increasing or decreasing peristalsis, gastric emptying time, etc.; (3) influencing the flow of gastric juices positively or negatively; and (4) changing the composition of body fluids which bathe the hypothalamus and other tissues which play a role in the basic phenomena of food intake, such as hunger, appetite, and palatability.

Using the brief-exposure technique, Young and Falk (1956) found that nonthirsty rats preferred solutions in the range of 0.75–1.5%. When offered a choice below this range, rats preferred the more concentrated solutions, and above this range they preferred the less concentrated. Thirsty rats preferred water or the weaker of salt pairs and were more variable in their preferences.

Jacobs (1961) noted the difference between long-term (at least 24 hours) and short-term preference studies. In the former, consumption increased to about 10% sucrose and then decreased at higher concentrations. In short-term experiments, consumption increased with concentration in a linear fashion. The difference in the results is generally attributed to postingestion factors, particularly osmotic pressure. Over a brief period, response is determined by taste alone. Once drinking starts, however, a simple feedback system goes into operation. If the animal continues to drink the hypertonic solution to obtain maximum sweetness, it will become dehydrated. Over a period the animal attempts to maximize taste and minimize dehydration. Jacobs believes the results could be explained on the basis of calories.

Pfaffmann (1956) reported that water balance was a factor in feeding studies such as those of Richter. Rats will consume high amounts of salt if permitted large amounts of water. He noted that caloric deficiency increased sugar and saccharin intake, but not sodium chloride intake. When starvation was prolonged, however, sugar was preferred to saccharin. The methodology used in such tests is obviously very important. Bacon *et al.* (1962) obtained higher saccharin and water intake under restricted daily diets and greater preference for saccharin at higher concentrations. For water and salt, Stellar *et al.* (1954) indicated that the three most important regulative factors were taste and other sensory mechanisms located in the mouth, gastric distention, and dehydration of cells.

Mardones (1960) reviewed the genetic factor in rats which produces ethyl alcohol "drinker" and "nondrinker" strains. Deprivation of most of the water-soluble vitamins and of an unidentified factor, N_1, increased alcohol consumption. Thioctic acid or glutamine decreased consumption. When a sugar solution or fat was offered as a third choice, alcohol intake decreased. For effects of other substances, reference should be made to the original paper. The general point is that, for alcohol at least, dietary factors influence intake.

Using adrenalectomized (salt-needy) animals and recording the afferent nerve impulses at the chorda tympani (through which most of the taste fibers pass), Pfaffmann (1957) found a preference for salt over sucrose, quinine, or hydrochloric acid at all concentrations. The electrophysiological threshold for salt remained unchanged. He therefore believes the altered behavior reflects a change in the central neural processes rather than in peripheral afferent neural messages. Similar results were reported by Nachman and Pfaffmann (1963).

Chambers (1956) found that rabbits could learn to perform a task with intravenous injection of glucose as reinforcement. Obvious secondary clues were eliminated. Epstein and Teitelbaum (1962) trained rats to feed themselves by direct intragastric injection so that oropharyngeal and olfactory sensations were eliminated. There still might be regurgitation of food and stimulation of the taste or olfactory receptors but their tests showed that including quinine in the liquid did not change the amount of consumption. The rats were able to regulate their weight and food intake for as long as 44 days. Apparently the taste and smell of the food or water is not necessary. Jacobs (1962) showed that the satiety effect of intragastric glucose loads was independent of gastric distention or potential osmotic effects. Response to glucose and sucrose loads (in the rat) indicated a preabsorptive chemoreceptor system. He considers hunger and thirst as a unitary problem. Classically non-metabolic factors such as bulk and osmotic potential have been identified with thirst, and metabolic factors such as nutrients, flavor, and energy with hunger.

Schutz and Pilgrim (1958) and Siegel and Pilgrim (1958) showed that food monotony, as expressed by lowered consumption, was primarily a function of repetition. A 3-day cycle of self-planned diet and a 6-day cycle of preplanned diet were both found superior to a shorter (3-day cycle) preplanned diet by Kamen and Peryam (1961), but the differences were not large. Using the hedonic-scale method (Chapter 8, Section III), Peryam and Haynes (1957) found that laboratory and field food preferences ratings had satisfactory reliability. Studies such as these can be expected to become more important as food scientists assume more control over the preparation of complete meals. The interrelationships of food preferences are very complex. Preparation of special foods for soldiers, for reducing regimens, or for salt-free or low-sugar or low-cholesterol diets requires special attention to factors such as taste, color, odor, texture, and psychological factors (Harper, 1957).

Preference can account for only 30–50% of the variability in consumption, according to Peryam et al. (1960). Other variables that may influence food acceptance include sensory, physiological, and environmental factors. Preference itself may be a result of all three factors. Pilgrim and Kamen (1963) found that 75% of the variability of food acceptance could be accounted for by four variables: satiety, preferences, percent fat, and percent protein.

Gordon (1957) emphasizes that palatability per se is not to be relied upon in the selection of a balanced diet. Some foods are palatable when consumed with certain foods but are unpalatable alone or in connection with other foods. Palatability differs between the satiated and the ravenous individual. However, palatability decisions do not necessarily have any connection with physiological needs. Gordon concludes: "Is it true to say that 'a little of what you fancy does you good'? The answer seems to be that it may do you good because you fancy it, but it is doubtful whether you fancy it because it does you good."

Dove (1939, 1946) emphasized that food production must be devised to provide proper nutrition. He showed a definite correlation between dental defects and food production. He devised a technique of measuring the food habits of individuals of superior growth ("aggridants") as a measure of dietary needs. Slow-growing individuals had a more variable preference for different foods and tended to lack discrimination. The pattern of food-getting varied with age, but the fast-growing individuals made the wisest selections in terms of growth-promoting substances. In Dove's opinion, food needs should be studied on an individual, not average, basis. This is too often neglected by food producers.

A tentative model (Fig. 4) of the components influencing food ac-

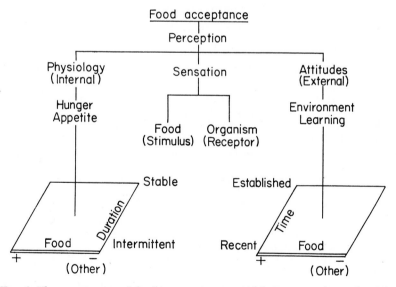

FIG. 4. The components of food acceptance—a model. Source: Pilgrim (1957).

ceptance was given by Pilgrim (1957). Note that this includes physiology, sensation, and attitudes. The relation of these to each other is unknown. The elucidation of these interrelations remains one of the important problems in the sensory examination of foods.

V. Summary

This chapter stresses the antiquity of the importance of sensory stimulants, and describes some modern odor and flavor problems of the food industry.

A general discussion of the senses is presented, emphasizing their number and sensitivity, followed by a general review of texts concerned with the senses and the sensory analysis of foods. The importance of the senses in establishing and maintaining food habits is emphasized. The cultural basis of food habits, as well as psychological, climatic, and other factors, are also noted. The possibility of changing food habits is introduced.

Finally, the concept of the physiological basis of diet selection (appetitive, stress, etc.) is discussed, recognizing the controversy on the self-regulatory mechanisms. Palatability and non-palatability environmental factors as well as feeding habits are noted, with distinction made between palatability and appetite. Genetic factors, satiety, and food monotony are also considered, as well as preferences and individual differences. A model for food acceptance is presented.

REFERENCES

American Physiological Society. 1959. "Handbook of Physiology," Vol. I, Sect. 1, Neurophysiology, 779 pp. (see pp. 356–620). Am. Physiol. Soc., Washington, D. C.

Anonymous. 1945. Manual for the study of food habits. *Bull. Natl. Research Council* (*U. S.*) **111**, 1–142.

Bacon, W. E., H. L. Snyder, and S. H. Hulse. 1962. Saccharine preference in satiated and deprived rats. *J. Comp. and Physiol. Psychol.* **55**, 112–114.

Bedichek, R. 1960. "The Sense of Smell," 264 pp. Doubleday, New York.

Beidler, L. M. 1961. The chemical senses. *Ann. Rev. Psychol.* **12**, 363–388.

Beidler, L. M. 1962. Taste receptor stimulation. *Progr. in Biophys. and Biophys. Chem.* **12**, 106–151.

Beythien, A. 1949. "Die Geschmackstoffe der menschlichen Nahrung," 150 pp. Steinkopff, Dresden.

Bienfang, R. 1946. "The Subtle Sense," 147 pp. Univ. of Oklahoma Press, Norman, Oklahoma.

Boring, E. G. 1942. "Sensation and Perception in the History of Experimental Psychology," 644 pp. Appleton, New York.

Brobeck, J. R. 1955. Neural regulation of food intake. *Ann. N. Y. Acad. Sci.* **63**, 44–55.

Bronshtein, A. I. 1950. "Vkus i Obonianie" (Taste and Smell),306 pp. Akad. Nauk. S. S. S. R., Moscow.

Brožek, J. 1957. Nutrition and behavior. *In* "Symposium on Nutrition and Behavior," Nutrition Symposium Ser. No. 14, 1–124. Natl. Vitamin Foundation, Inc., New York (see also *Am. J. Clin. Nutrition* **5**, 332–343, 1957).

Buddenbrock, W. von. 1953. "Die Welt der Sinne," 147 pp. (see pp. 6–14, 93–109, 109–117). Springer, Berlin.

Buddenbrock, W. von. 1958. "The Senses," 167 pp. (see pp. 9–53, 107–135). Univ. of Michigan Press, Ann Arbor, Michigan.

Carlson, A. J. 1916. "The Control of Hunger in Health and Disease," 172 pp. Univ. of Chicago Press, Chicago, Illinois.

Carper, J. W., and F. Polliard. 1953. A comparison of the intake of glucose and saccharin solutions under conditions of caloric need. *Am. J. Psychol.* **66,** 479–482.

Cartwright, L. C., and P. H. Kelley. 1954. Scheme for odor identification with examples of its use. *Ann. N. Y. Acad. Sci.* **58,** 187–192.

Caul, J. F. 1956. The profile method of flavor analysis. *Advances in Food Research* **7,** 1–40.

Chambers, R. M. 1956. Effects of intravenous glucose injections on learning, general activity and hunger. *J. Comp. and Physiol. Psychol.* **49,** 558–564.

Cloquet, H. 1815. "Dissertation sur les Odeurs, sur le Sens et les Organes de l'Olfaction," 1st ed. (2nd ed. 1821; title varies). Paris.

Cohn, G. 1914. "Die organischen Geschmacksstoffe," 936 pp. Franz Siemenroth, Berlin.

Committee on Food Habits. 1943. The problem of changing food habits. *Bull. Natl. Research Council (U. S.)* **108,** 1–177.

Davis, C. M. 1928. Self-selection of diet by newly weaned infants. *Am. J. Diseases Children* **36,** 651–679.

Dawson, E. H., J. L. Brogdon, and S. McManus. 1963. Sensory testing of differences in taste. I. Methods. II. Selection of panel members. *Food Technol.* **17,** 1125–1129, 1131, 1251–1253, 1255–1256.

Dawson, E. H., and B. L. Harris. 1951. Sensory methods for measuring differences in food quality. *U. S. Dept. Agr. Infor. Bull.* **34,** 1–134.

Dethier, V. G., and L. E. Chadwick. 1948. Chemoreception in insects. *Physiol. Rev.* **28,** 220–254.

Dove, W. F. 1935. A study of individuality in the nutritive instincts and of the causes and effects of variation in the selection of food. *Am. Naturalist* **69,** 469–544.

Dove, W. F. 1939. The relation of man and animals to the environment. *Maine Agr. Expt. Sta. Bull.* **397,** 726–773.

Dove, W. F. 1946. Developing food acceptance research. *Science* **103,** 187–190.

Dove, W. F. 1947. Food acceptability—its determination and evaluation. *Food Technol.* **1,** 39–50.

Epstein, A. N., and P. Teitelbaum. 1962. Regulation of food intake in the absence of taste, smell, and other oropharyngeal sensations. *J. Comp. and Physiol. Psychol.* **35,** 753–759.

Fischer, R., and F. Griffin. 1959. On factors involved in the mechanism of "taste-blindness." *Experientia* **15,** 447–448.

Fischer, R., F. Griffin, S. England, and S. M. Garn. 1961. Taste thresholds and food dislikes. *Nature* **191,** 1328.

Geldard, F. A. 1950. Somestheses and the chemical senses. *Ann. Rev. Psychol.* **1,** 73–86 (see pp. 80–81).

Geldard, F. A. 1953. "The Human Senses," 365 pp. Wiley, New York.

Goetzl, F. R., M. S. Abel, and A. J. Ahokas. 1950. On the occurrence in normal individuals of diurnal variations in olfactory acuity. *J. Appl. Physiol.* **2,** 553–562.

Gordon, J. G. 1957. Palatability in relation to physiological needs. *Advance. of Sci.* **13,** 296–299.

Gottlieb, D., and P. H. Rossi. 1961. A bibliography and bibliographic review of food and food habit research. *Quartermaster Food and Container Inst. Library Bull.* **4**, 1–112. (Also in *Progr. Rept., Contract DA* **19-129-QM-1117**, 1–115. July 1958.)

Haller, A. von. 1763. "Elements Physiologiae," Vol. V, pp. 99–124 and 125–185. Lausanne.

Harper, R. 1957. Psychological aspects of food acceptance. *Advance. of Sci.* **13**, 297–299.

Harper, R. 1962. The psychologist's role in food-acceptance research. *Food Technol.* **16**, 70, 72–73.

Harriman, A. E., and R. B. MacLeod. 1953. Discriminative thresholds of salt for normal and adrenalectomized rats. *Am. J. Psychol.* **66**, 465–471.

Harrison, J. W. E., K. S. Konigsbacher, W. H. Danker, J. W. Hein, G. J. Cox, S. W. Leung, and R. Heggie. 1953. A practical evaluation of chlorophyll in controlling breath odors. *J. Soc. Cosmetic Chemists* **4**, 9–32.

Henning, H. 1916. "Der Geruch," 1st ed., 533 pp. Barth, Leipzig.

Henning, H. 1924. "Der Geruch," 2nd ed., 434 pp. (see pp. 4–23). Barth, Leipzig.

Hollingworth, H. L., and A. T. Poffenberger, Jr. 1917. "The Sense of Taste," 200 pp. Moffat, Yard and Co., New York.

Irvin, D. L., and F. R. Goetzl. 1952. Diurnal variations in acuity of sense of taste for sodium chloride. *Proc. Soc. Exptl. Biol. Med.* **79**, 115–118.

Jacobs, H. L. 1961. The osmotic postingestion factor in the regulation of glucose appetite. *In* "Physiological and Behavioral Aspects of Taste" (M. R. Kare and B. P. Halpern, eds.), pp. 16–17. Univ. of Chicago Press, Chicago, Illinois.

Jacobs, H. L. 1962. Some physical, metabolic and sensory components in the appetite for glucose. *Am. J. Physiol.* **203**, 1043–1054.

Juran, J. M. 1962. Specification of quality. *In* "Quality Control Handbook" (J. M. Juran, ed.), 2nd ed. pp. 3–52 to 3–65. McGraw-Hill, New York.

Kalmus, H., and S. J. Hubbard. 1960. "The Chemical Senses in Health and Disease," 95 pp. Thomas, Springfield, Illinois.

Kamen, J. M., and D. R. Peryam. 1961. Acceptability of repetitive diets. *Food Technol.* **15**, 173–177.

Kare, M. R., and B. P. Halpern. 1961. "Physiological and Behavioral Aspects of Taste," 149 pp. Univ. of Chicago Press, Chicago, Illinois.

Laboratory Practice. 1964. Sensory food analysis. *Laboratory Practice* **13**, 596–641, 700–738.

Le Magnen, J. 1949. "Odeurs et Parfums," 128 pp. Presses Universitaires, Paris.

Le Magnen, J. 1959. Le rôle des stimuli olfacto-gustatifs dans la régulation du comportement alimentaire du mammifère. *J. Psychol. Norm. Pathol.* **56**, 137–160.

Lepkovsky, S. 1953. Nutritional stress factors and food processing. *Advances in Food Research* **4**, 105–132.

Lepkovsky, S. 1963. Challenge to the food industry. *Food Technol.* **17**(4), 10, 14.

Lewin, K. 1943. Forces behind food habits and methods of change. *Bull. Natl. Research Council* (*U. S.*) **108**, 35–65.

McCord, C. P., and W. N. Witheridge. 1949. "Odors—Physiology and Control," 405 pp. McGraw-Hill, New York.

McIndoo, N. E. 1927. Smell and taste and their applications. *Sci. Monthly* **25**, 481–503.

Marchand, L. 1903. "Le Goût," 331 pp. O. Doin, Paris.

Marcuse, R. 1954. "Organoleptisk Laboratorieanalys," 87 pp. Göteborg, Sweden.

Mardones, J. 1960. Experimentally induced changes in the free selection of ethanol. *Intern. Rev. Neurol.* **2**, 41–76.

Masuyama, G., and S. Miura. 1962. "Handbook for Sensory Tests in Industry," 601, 68 pp. JUSE Publishers, Tokyo, Japan. (In Japanese.)

Meyer, D. R. 1952. The stability of human gustatory sensitivity during changes in time of food deprivation. *J. Comp. and Physiol. Psychol.* **45**, 373–376.

Michels, K. M., D. S. Phillips, R. H. Wright, and J. Pustek, Jr. 1961. "Odors and Olfaction," A Bibliography, 1948–1960, 179 pp. Purdue Univ., Lab. of Physiol. Psychol., Lafayette, Indiana. (See also *Perceptual and Motor Skills* **15**, 475–529, 1962.)

Moncrieff, R. W. 1946. "The Chemical Senses," 1st ed., 424 pp. Wiley, New York.

Moncrieff, R. W. 1951. "The Chemical Senses," 2nd ed., 538 pp. Leonard Hill, London.

Moulton, D. G. 1960. Studies in olfactory acuity. 5. The comparative olfactory sensitivity of pigmented and albino rats. *Animal Behavior* **8**, 129–133.

Nachman, M., and C. Pfaffmann. 1963. Gustatory nerve discharge in normal and sodium-deficient rats. *J. Comp. and Physiol. Psychol.* **56**, 1007–1011.

Nemanova, T. P. 1941. Conditioned reflexes to taste stimuli in children in the first months of life. *Fisiol. Zhur. S. S. S. R.* **30**, 478–483.

Ogrim, M. E., and E. Homb. 1960. "Kostvaner og Maeringstilforsel Hos Grupper av Norske Familier," 173 pp. Bergen Universitetsforlaget, Oslo, Norway.

Pangborn, R. M. 1964. Sensory evaluation of foods: A look backward and forward. *Food Technol.* **18**, (9), 63–67.

Parker, G. H. 1922. "Smell, Taste and Allied Senses in the Vertebrates," 192 pp. Lippincott, Philadelphia, Pennsylvania.

Parker, G. H., and W. J. Crozier. 1929. Chemical senses. *In* "The Foundations of Psychology" (C. Murchison, ed.), pp. 350–391. Clark Univ. Press, Wooster, Massachusetts.

Paschal, G. 1952. "Odors and the Sense of Smell, a Bibliography, 320 b.c.–1947," 342 pp. Airkem, New York.

Patton, H. D. 1960. Taste, olfaction and visceral sensation. *In* "Medical Physiology and Biophysics" (T. C. Ruch and J. F. Fulton, eds.), 1232 pp. (see pp. 369–385). Saunders, Philadelphia, Pennsylvania.

Peryam, D. R. 1963. The acceptance of novel foods. *Food Technol.* **17**, 711–715, 717.

Peryam, D. R., and J. G. Haynes. 1957. Prediction of soldiers' food preferences by laboratory methods. *J. Appl. Psychol.* **41**, 2–6.

Peryam, D. R., B. W. Polemis, J. M. Kamen, J. Eindhoven, and F. J. Pilgrim. 1960. "Food Preferences of Men in the U. S. Armed Forces," 160 pp. Dept. of the Army, Quartermaster Research and Engineering Command, Chicago, Illinois.

Pfaffmann, C. 1956. Taste and smell. *Ann. Rev. Psychol.* **7**, 391–408.

Pfaffmann, C. 1957. Taste mechanisms in preference behavior. *Am. J. Clin. Nutrition* **5**, 142–147.

Pfaffmann, C. 1961. Preface. *In* "Physiological and Behavioral Aspects of Taste" (M. R. Kare and B. P. Halpern, eds.), 1149 pp. (see pp. vii–xi). Univ. of Chicago Press, Chicago, Illinois.

Piéron, H. 1952. "The Sensations, Their Functions, Processes and Mechanisms," 469 pp. Yale Univ. Press, New Haven, Connecticut.

Pilgrim, F. J. 1957. The components of food acceptance and their measurement. *Am. J. Clin. Nutrition* **5**, 171–175.

Pilgrim, F. J., and J. M. Kamen. 1963. Predictors of human food consumption. *Science* **139**, 501–502.

Prosser, C. L. 1954. Comparative physiology of nervous systems and sense organs. *Ann. Rev. Physiol.* **16**, 103–124.

Remington, R. E. 1936. The social origins of dietary habits. *Sci. Monthly* **43**, 193–204.

Renou, Y. 1962. Les qualités organoleptiques des viandes. *Ann. nutrition et aliment.* **16**(3), 1–58.

Richter, C. P. 1941a. Behavior and endocrine regulation of the internal environment. *Endocrinology* **28**, 193–195.

Richter, C. P. 1941b. Decreased carbohydrate appetite of adrenalectomized rats. *Proc. Soc. Exptl. Biol. Med.* **48**, 577–579.

Richter, C. P. 1942. Total self regulatory functions in animals and human beings. *Harvey Lectures* **38**, 63–103.

Richter, C. P. 1943. The self selection of diets. *In* "Essays in Biology," pp. 409–506. Univ. of California Press, Berkeley, California.

Richter, C. P., and K. H. Campbell. 1940. Sucrose taste thresholds of rats and humans. *Am. J. Physiol.* **128**, 291–297.

Rosenblith, W. A. 1961. "Sensory Communication," 844 pp. M. I. T. Press, Cambridge, Massachusetts; Wiley, New York.

Schutz, H. G., and F. J. Pilgrim. 1958. A field study of food monotony. *Psychol. Repts.* **4**, 559–565.

Scott, E. M., and E. L. Verney. 1948. Self selection of diet. VIII. Appetite for fats. *J. Nutrition* **36**, 91–98.

Scott, E. M., and E. L. Verney. 1949. Self selection of diet. IX. The appetite for thiamine. *J. Nutrition* **37**, 81–91.

Scott, E. M., S. J. Smith, and E. L. Verney. 1948. Self selection of diet. VII. The effect of age and pregnancy on selection. *J. Nutrition* **35**, 281–286.

Sheffield, F. D., and T. B. Roby. 1950. Reward value of a non-nutritive sweet taste. *J. Comp. and Physiol. Psychol.* **43**, 471–481.

Siegel, P. S., and F. J. Pilgrim. 1958. The effect of monotony on the acceptance of food. *Am. J. Psychol.* **71**, 756–759.

Simoons, F. J. 1961. "Eat Not This Flesh," 241 pp. Univ. of Wisconsin Press, Madison, Wisconsin.

Skramlik, E. von. 1926. *In* "Handbuch der Physiologie der niederen Sinne," Vol. 1: Die Physiologie des Geruchs- und Geschmackssinnes, 532 pp. Thieme, Leipzig.

Smith, M., and M. Duffy. 1957. Consumption of sucrose and saccharine by hungry and satiated rats. *J. Comp. and Physiol. Psychol.* **50**, 65–69.

Stellar, E., R. Hyman, and S. Samet. 1954. Gastric factors controlling water- and salt-solution drinking. *J. Comp. and Physiol. Psychol.* **47**, 220–226.

Sternberg, W. 1906. "Geschmack und Geruch," 149 pp. Springer, Berlin.

Stewart, G. F., M. A. Amerine, and R. H. Vaughn. 1965. "Introduction to Food Science." (In press)

Tepperman, J. 1961. Metabolic and taste interactions. *In* "Physiological and Behavioral Aspects of Taste" (M. R. Kare, and B. P. Halpern, eds.), 149 pp. (see pp. 92–98). Univ. of Chicago Press, Chicago, Illinois.

Tilgner, D. J. 1957. "Analiza Organoleptyczna Zywności," 364 pp. Wydawnictwo Przemysłu Lekkiego i Spożywczego, Warsaw.

Wayner, M. J., Jr., and E. M. Sporn. 1963. Thirst: regulation of body water. *Science* **141**, 741–743.

Weddell, G. 1955. Somesthesis and the chemical senses. *Ann. Rev. Psychol.* **6**, 119–136.

Wenger, M. A., F. N. Jones, and M. H. Jones. 1956. "Physiological Psychology," 472 pp. Holt, New York.

Wenzel, B. M. 1954. The chemical senses. *Ann. Rev. Psychol.* **5**, 111–126.

Young, P. T. 1948. Studies of food preference, appetite, and dietary habit. VIII. Food-seeking drives, palatability, and the law of effect. *J. Comp. and Physiol. Psychol.* **41**, 269–300.

Young, P. T. 1949a. Food-seeking drive, affective process and learning. *Psychol. Rev.* **56**, 98–121.

Young, P. T. 1949b. Studies of food preference, appetite, and dietary habit. IX. Palatability versus appetite as determinants of the critical concentrations of sucrose and sodium chloride. *Comp. Psychol. Monograph* **19**, 1–44.

Young, P. T., and J. P. Chaplin. 1949. Studies of food preference, appetite and dietary habit. X. Preferences of adrenalectomized rats for salt solutions of different concentrations. *Comp. Psychol. Monograph* **19**, 45–74.

Young, P. T., and J. L. Falk. 1956. The relative acceptability of sodium chloride solutions as a function of concentration and water need. *J. Comp. and Physiol. Psychol.* **49**, 569–575.

Young, P. T., and J. T. Greene. 1953. Relative acceptability of saccharine solutions as revealed by different methods. *J. Comp. and Physiol. Psychol.* **46**, 295–298.

Yudkin, J., and J. C. McKenzie. 1964. "Changing Food Habits," 144 pp. Macgibbon & Kee, London.

Zotterman, Y. 1957. Electrophysiological investigations of the functions of gustatory nerve fibres. *Advance. of Sci.* **13**, 292–295.

Zotterman, Y. 1961. Studies in the neural mechanism of taste. *In* "Sensory communication" (W. A. Rosenblith, ed.), 844 pp. (see pp. 205–216). M. I. T. Press, Cambridge, Massachusetts; Wiley, New York.

Zotterman, Y. 1963. "Olfaction and Taste," 396 pp. Macmillan, New York.

Zotterman, Y., and H. Diamant. 1959. Has water a specific taste? *Nature* **183**, 191.

Zwaardemaker, H. 1895. "Die Physiologie des Geruchs," 324 pp. Engelmann, Leipzig.

Zwaardemaker, H. 1925. "L'Odorat," 305 pp. Doin, Paris.

Chapter 2

The Sense of Taste

In French, German, English, and several other languages the word "taste" means not only sensory response to soluble materials in the mouth but also esthetic appreciation. Hollingworth and Poffenberger (1917) noted that the words for the other senses are also employed figuratively: "odorous" for something reprehensible, "vision" for something impersonal and intuitive, "touch" for an expression of sympathy or pity, and "warmth" or "chill" for a depth of emotion. "Taste" is reserved for judgments involving harmony, especial fitness, critical capacity, or quality in general.

It has been noted many times that, among the human senses, taste might be called the "poor relation." Perhaps it is because taste contributes so few important qualities to the sum of human experience when compared to vision or audition. Geldard (1953) noted that topics which are of lesser importance in human affairs do not gain intensive study from scientists. Certainly fewer scientific studies have been made on taste than on vision or hearing. Many intriguing problems remain in connection with taste, and are interestingly discussed by Pfaffmann [1961, 1962, 1964; see also Kalmus (1958a)]. From the viewpoint of the food processor and food scientist, the sense of taste commands interest because of its role in food recognition, selection, and acceptance, in addition to its pleasurable aspects.

Taste, or some aspect of it, is very important for lower animals: If life originated in the ocean, the chemical senses functioned as warning and as feeding mechanisms. Moncrieff (1951) devotes an entire chapter to chemical sensibility in sea animals, insects, birds, reptiles, and non-human mammals. Hasler and Wisby (1951) and Hasler (1954, 1960a,b) noted the importance of a chemical sense for homing in migrating salmon, and Kleerekoper and van Erkel (1960) reported on a similar sense for orientation and feeding in the lamprey. Apparently, as land animals developed, taste became secondary to smell. The importance of taste in rats has been stressed by Harlow (1932), who showed that complete removal of the olfactory bulbs did not result in any dietary deficiencies, whereas, presumably, removal of the taste buds would. Preference must, therefore, have been based on gustatory or tactual clues. For man, both taste and smell contribute to the enjoyment of food.

Although taste was defined as one of the five senses by Aristotle, Haller did not write the chapter "Gustus" in his book on the senses, until 1763, according to Boring (1942). The various forms of papillae are described therein, and since they were the only visible specialized structures on the tongue it seemed logical to consider these the organs of taste. Taste is initiated by contact of an aqueous solution of a chemical with the taste buds on the surface of the tongue and the adjacent regions of the mouth and throat. In this, taste differs from smell, which reacts primarily to chemicals in gases. However, Tucker (1961) reported that "odorants" introduced into a saline solution were effective in stimulating the olfactory receptors of the land tortoise.

Taste and olfactory sensations should be considered separately. This is difficult since we are conditioned to speak of the "taste" of a peach. Actually, a peach has only sweet, slightly acid, and very slightly bitter *tastes*. Likewise, all tactile sensations should be excluded, even though they are important in the sensory examination of foods (see Chapter 4). Experimentally, the taste sense can be demonstrated by plugging the nose and keeping the temperature of the test substance at body temperature. Dilute taste substances affect only the tongue, whereas stronger solutions elicit sensations of pain and sharpness in all parts of the mouth, including the tongue. (We do not exclude the possibility that the central nervous system mediates a quality called "flavor" which is neither taste nor odor.)

The sense of taste has been approached from three directions: behavioral, electrophysiological, and molecular (Beidler, 1952). Behavioral responses constitute the main volume of studies made to date, and have provided useful information on palatability. Increasing numbers of electrophysiological studies have yielded results of great utility in elucidating the nature of the gustatory process. Molecular approaches are still in their infancy.

The salivary glands are important in tasting, particularly in dissolving or diluting tasteful substances and carrying them to the receptors. Saliva also buffers acids and helps control temperature by means of the relatively high specific heat content of the water component (Beidler, 1962). Saliva is secreted by three pairs of glands—the parotid, submaxillary, and sublingual—reinforced by numerous small buccal glands. In man, parotid saliva is watery and has a high digestive power, whereas the secretions from the other glands are more viscous and higher in mucin. The rather high potassium content has been suggested as a sensitizer of taste receptors. Thiocyanate ion, which is present in relatively high concentrations in saliva, has been shown by Ehrenberg and Güttes (1949) to raise the threshold for sweet and decrease that for bitter. Chewing stimulates salivary secretion, as do stimuli brought about by the thought, sight, or odor of food. Chauncey and Shannon (1959) indicated that the rate of salivary secretion was a linear function of the log of the bolus volume of the masticatory stimuli and of the application rate of the taste stimuli. More work is needed on the enzymic functions and the effect of the composition of saliva on taste responses. Human salt thresholds have been found to reflect the state of adaptation to salivary sodium (McBurney and Pfaffmann, 1963). Bartoshuk *et al.* (1964) demonstrated that the tongue could be adapted to various concentrations of sodium chloride. Adapting solutions became tasteless; solutions weaker than the adapting concentration tasted sour or bitter, and stronger solutions were sweet or salty. (See Chapter 2, Section XIV for the effect of saliva on the taste of phenylthiocarbamide.)

The tongue itself probably facilitates tasting by its muscular movements, which bring the taste materials into contact with the taste buds. The movement of the tongue also constantly disturbs concentration gradients near the receptors and thus tends to prevent adaptation to a given stimulus intensity.

I. Anatomy

According to Boring (1942), the raised portions of the tongue, the papillae, were selected as the organs of taste by Haller, in 1763. Various experiments in the nineteenth century clarified their anatomy and dif-

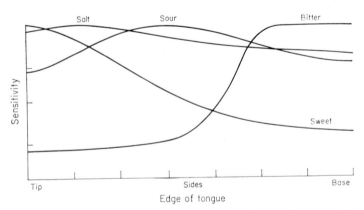

FIG. 5. Sensitivity of areas of taste on the tongue. Source: Hänig (1901).

ferentiation. In 1803 Charles Bell demonstrated that the tongue was insensitive to taste in the regions where there were no papillae; gustatory sensibility was confined mainly to the tip and edges, and was absent in the middle of the tongue. Figure 5 illustrates the sensitivity of different areas.

Four kinds of papillae are found on the human tongue: foliate, circumvallate, fungiform, and filiform (Figs. 6 and 7). Filiform papillae,

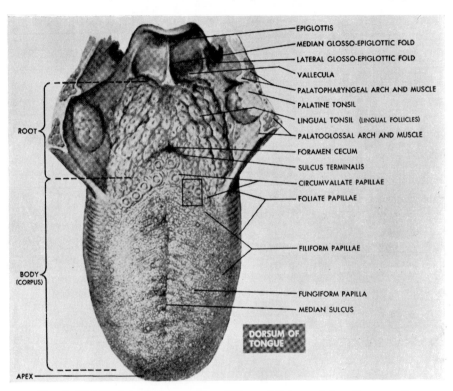

FIG. 6. Distribution of circumvallate, filiform, foliate, and fungiform papillae on the human tongue. Source: Netter (1959).

evenly distributed on the anterior two thirds of the tongue, are the most numerous but have no taste buds. Fungiform papillae, large and round, and mushroomlike in appearance (0.8–1.0 mm in diameter, and 1.0–1.5 mm high), are greater in number at the tip and sides of the tongue. They are scattered over the anterior two thirds of the tongue. It is estimated that they number 150 to 400. The foliate papillae on the posterior third of the tongue (in folds on the sides) are not well developed in man and have little function. The circumvallate papillae form a V-shape

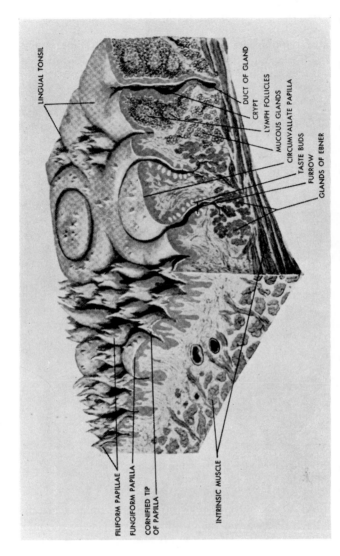

FIG. 7. Schematic stereogram of posterior section of human tongue showing the circumvallate papillae. Source: Netter (1959).

on the back of the tongue. There are usually 6 to 15 of these present. They are large (2 mm high, 1–1.5 mm in diameter, and 1–1.5 mm deep) and easily visible. The name arises from their shape—a small mound surrounded by a ditch. Figure 8 shows the location of papillae near the

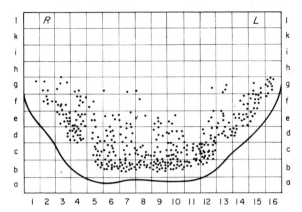

Fig. 8. Distribution of papillae near the end of the tongue. Each square represents 0.25 cm². Source: Skramlik (1926).

tip of the tongue. The location of the fungiform papillae has been studied by Skramlik (1926), who listed the number on the left and right sides of the tongue as follows:

Subject	Left	Right
1	139	99
2	120	119
3	195	178

With age, the number of papillae varies, becoming less in number and more restricted in distribution (Pfaffmann, 1959a).

In adults, the taste buds, containing the receptors, are located mainly in depressions or moats of the papillae, except for the fungiform type, but in children they may also be found in the cheeks. A few are found on the larynx and pharynx. Besides the taste buds in the papillae there are a few in the mucosa of the soft palate, and in children on the sides and even roof of the mouth. Henning (1924) suggested that taste buds occur even in the nose. The taste buds of the fungiform papillae occur on their upper surface, whereas those of the foliate and circumvallate papillae lie in their grooves. According to Beidler (1962), the taste stimulus is apparently "carried down into the grooves by convection forces exerted by the contraction and expansion of the grooves due to the dynamics of

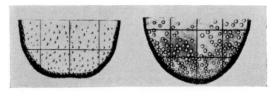

FIG. 9. Distribution of papillae on tongue of children 12 (left) and 5 (right) years old (each square represents 0.25 cm²). Source: Skramlik (1926).

the musculature of the tongue." The distribution of taste buds in children is shown in Fig. 9. According to Heiderich (1906), the number of taste buds per papillae in the human varies from 33 to 508, averaging about 250.

The taste buds, also called "taste-beakers" or "taste onions," were first described over one hundred years ago (see Beidler, 1962). The term "taste-beaker" arose from their resemblance in form to a modern brandy snifter; the "taste-onion" term refers to the spindle-shaped cells bulging out at the root and coming together at the taste-pore, very much like the petals of a bud. Each bud contains a number of taste cells, 5 to 18, together with other cells, which may be immature taste cells. Human taste buds are about 0.07 mm long and 0.05 mm wide at their widest diameter (see Fig. 10 for detail of a taste bud). Within the taste bud are sustentacular cells and gustatory cells (or a mixture of the two in a

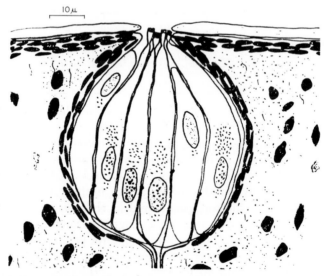

FIG. 10. Drawing of taste bud of the rat. (The nerve fibers enter at the bottom and end on one or two receptor cells about one-third the distance from the base.) Source: Beidler (1952), after Lenhossek.

transitional state from one to the other), arranged to enclose a small chamber, i.e., grouped together into a budlike structure.

Murray and Murray (1960) found only one type of gustatory cell in the taste buds of rhesus and cynomolgus monkeys. Beidler (1960, 1961a) reported that the cells had a relatively brief life. They appear to be produced by mitotic division of epithelium at the edges of the bud and to be in a continuous state of flux and change, with a "turnover" rate of only 6 to 8 days. From each receptor cell a fine hair was formerly believed to project into the chamber and above its inner surface. Since these have not been observed with electron microscopy, Beidler (1961b, 1962) believes they were artifacts, noting, however, that the apical processes of many of the cells of the taste bud bear numerous microvilli, each of which is about 2μ long and 0.12μ wide, and extends into the taste pore. The absence of projecting hairs gives more importance to the region of the taste bud. Murray and Murray (1960) suggested that the cementing substance (or terminal bars) might seal off the chemical activity to this region. The microvilli could facilitate rapid absorption of the taste substance.

The taste bud is innervated by myelinated nerve fibers, arising from the subepithelial plexus, which wind around the taste cells and terminate in knoblike projections on the cell. About two nerves innervate each taste bud of a fungiform papilla (Foley, 1945). For example, the intact tympani of the cat contained 1955 sensory and motor axons, and that of the dog 3347; of these, respectively 1157 and 2205 were sensory axons. The majority of the sensory and motor axons in these cases are myelinated. For further details see the electron photomicrographs of Lorenzo (1958) and Murray and Murray (1960).

For gustation, according to Erickson (1958), there is a chain of three stages of neurons from the periphery to the cortex. The first-order neurons originate in the tongue and terminate in the second-order neurons in the medulla oblongata. The second-order neurons presumably terminate in the thalamus on the third-order neurons which end on the neurons in the cerebral cortex. Krarup (1959), on the basis of clinical findings, indicates that in all cases the taste fibers from the anterior part of the tongue have the following course: lingual nerve, chorda tympani, facial nerve, and intermedius of Wrisberg. The general arrangement is shown in Fig. 11.

Cutting the nerve connections results in degeneration of the whole bud. Guth (1957) found that bilateral glossopharyngeal nerve transection in the rat led to a rapid decrease in the number of taste buds. An unusual property of the end organs of taste is that the nerve fibers regenerate and new taste buds are formed from epithelial tissue. The

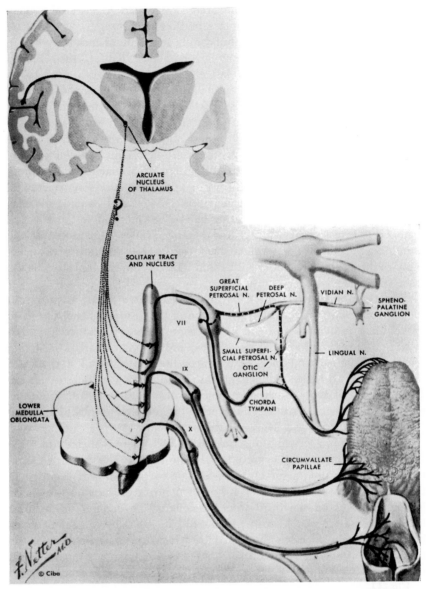

F$_\text{IG}$. 11. Neural pathways of circumvallate papillae. Source: Netter (1959).

mechanism of this transformation is not known, but Beidler (1962) notes that it is possible that the human sensory nerve induces epethelial cells to form taste cells. It does demonstrate the close connection between the taste buds and their nerve supply.

The anterior two thirds of the tongue and the filiform and fungiform papillae are innervated by a portion of the nervus intermedius division of the seventh cranial (facial) nerve. These taste fibers branch away from the lingual nerve to become a part of the chorda tympani nerve, which then passes through the middle ear and enters the brain stem as a part of the seventh cranial nerve. The posterior third of the tongue and the foliate and circumvallate papillae are innervated by the glossopharyngeal (ninth cranial) nerve. Bohm and Strang (1962) reported that, in some individuals, taste sensations may be conveyed almost completely by fibers of the seventh rather than the ninth nerve. Halpern (1959) reported that chemical stimulation of the anterior portion of the tongue yielded the same over-all response functions in both the chorda tympani nerve and medulla oblongata. Posterior tongue stimulation with quinine hydrochloride gave larger bulbar response than did sodium chloride stimulation. The vagus nerve may receive a few taste fibers from the epiglottis and pharynx.

In addition to electrophysiological, neuroanatomical, and behavioral data from lower animals, the nerve pathways for taste have also been determined from intracranial division of isolated cranial nerves in humans (Lewis and Dandy, 1930; Cameron, 1947; Pfaffmann, 1959a). The trigeminal nerve (fifth cranial nerve) is not involved, since its cutting does not affect taste. Cutting of the sensory portion, nervus intermedius, of the facial nerve, so as to control facial tic, results in complete and permanent abolition of taste sensations from the anterior two thirds of the tongue (see, however, Chapter 2, Section XVII).

In the brain, the region of the cortex of the operculum, insula, and supratemporal planes of the temporal lobe are involved in taste but there is no special primary cortical receiving zone with exclusive gustatory functions (Pfaffmann, 1959a). The medulla oblongata and the thalamus are also involved (Halpern, 1959; Frommer, 1961; Ables and Benjamin, 1960). Cameron (1947) noted a report that in 22 cases of head injury involving alterations in smell only 14 also had taste alterations.

Although no anatomical differences have been observed among the taste buds, histochemical studies show localization of esterase, hexosediphosphatase, yeast adenylase, acid phosphatase, lipase, muscle adenylase, and ribonuclease in or near the gustatory regions (Baradi and Bourne, 1953, 1959a,b). However, it must be admitted that, so far, our knowledge of the cellular morphology and biochemistry of the taste buds contributes little to our knowledge of their operation.

Dzendolet (1962) has succeeded in stimulating a single human papilla. In the rat there is only one taste bud per fungiform papilla, so that stimuli experiments have been made with a single taste bud (Kimura and Beidler, 1956 and Tateda and Beidler, 1964). These investigators inserted ultra-microelectrodes into taste buds and found no simple classification of receptors possible, i.e., sucrose did not always give a response, and the effects of quinine and divalent actions were sometimes larger and sometimes smaller than the effect of sodium chloride. Kimura and Beidler (1961) also showed that single receptors responded to all four taste qualities. With other species, the experimental difficulties of determining which bud is stimulated, for how long, by what concentration, and how the stimulus acts upon the receptor are enormous.

The sensitivity of the papillae to different stimuli varies. Using solutions of sucrose, tartaric acid, and quinine (salt solutions were unsuitable), Öhrwall (1891) reported the number of papillae sensitive to different tastes as follows:

Taste	Number of papillae
Sweet, sour, and bitter	60
Sweet and sour	12
Sweet and bitter	4
Sour and bitter	7
Sweet only	3
Sour only	12
Bitter only	0
No taste	27
	125

Öhrwall did not use papillae from the base of the tongue, where bitter-sensitive papillae have been found. This test demonstrates the distinct physiological responses to the three tastes, that many taste buds are involved, and that the taste effect obtained is the result of the stimulation of many papillae.

A further study of the distribution of taste sensitivity along the edge of the tongue was made by Hänig (1901), who used tiny brushes to apply the taste substances. His results (Fig. 5) show that sensitivity is the reciprocal of the threshold value and is plotted so that maximum sensitivity equals 1. Note that salt and sour are not clearly differentiated but that sweet and bitter are antithetical and differentiated not only from each other but from saline and sour. This research proves not that there are only four basic tastes, but that these four, at least, appear to be distinct from each other. In general, sweet and salt are best tasted at the tip of the tongue and some candies are made so that the tip of the tongue is used most. Bitter is best tasted at the back of the tongue;

therefore, many substances do not taste bitter until swallowed. The sour taste is best appreciated along the edges of the tongue. Zaiko (1961) reported the number of functional papillae decreased rapidly after ingestion of food, but the technique needs refining.

II. Classification

Boring (1942) has given the history of the classification of tastes (Wundt is quoted directly) shown in Table 3. Note that odors were

TABLE 3
Various Attempts at Classification of Tastes

Bravo (1592)	Linnaeus (1751)	Haller (1751)	Haller (1763)	Wundt (1910)
Sweet	Sweet	Sweet	Sweet	Sweet
—	—	Spiritous	Spiritous	—
—	—	Aromatic	—	—
Acid	Acid	Acid	Acid	Acid
—	Astringent	—	—	—
Sharp	Sharp	Sharp	Sharp	—
Pungent	—	Pungent	—	—
Harsh	—	Harsh	—	—
—	Viscous	—	—	—
Fatty	Fatty	—	—	—
Bitter	Bitter	Bitter	Bitter	Bitter
Insipid	Insipid	Insipid	—	—
—	Aqueous	—	—	—
Saline	Saline	Saline	Saline	Saline
—	—	Urinous	—	—
—	Nauseous	Putrid	—	—
—	—	—	—	Alkaline?
—	—	—	—	Metallic?

Source: Boring (1942) and Wundt (1910).

confused with taste in the earlier studies. Henning's classical taste prism is given in Fig. 12. Modern physiological psychologists would question such a simple representation of the taste modalities. Pfaffmann (1961) notes that the concept of only four fundamental taste qualities was derived largely from the elementaristic view of life of the introspective psychologists of the nineteenth century. As we shall see, the receptor cells are differentially sensitive to chemicals but are not rigidly specific.

Other tastes have been postulated, particularly alkaline and metallic. Probably these sensations are more tactile than taste, or are at least fusions of taste and touch, and possibly of smell. A mixture of concentrated solutions of salt and sugar will approximate the alkaline taste.

Sour and salt together simulate the metallic taste, but not exactly, probably because of the lack of tactual sensation. Kloehn and Brogden (1948) determined the limens for sodium hydroxide for 8 subjects and found that the tip was more sensitive than the mid-dorsal surface.

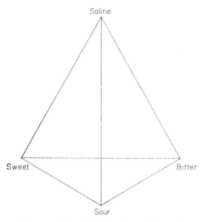

FIG. 12. Taste tetrahedron. The four principal qualities of taste are shown. Intermediate qualities lie on the edges or on the surfaces. Source: Henning (1924).

Kloehn and Brogden believed that pain or the so-called common chemical sense, or both, were factors, along with taste. In any case, alkaline is not considered to be a primary taste. Further tests are needed in this field.

Pfaffmann (1956) reviewed the evidence for a water taste. Weak salt solutions do not taste salty, although they can be distinguished from distilled water. For sodium fluoride, for example, the difference threshold was $0.00013\ M$ (0.000546%), which was far below the recognition threshold. Furthermore, some nerve fibers responded to water but not to saline solutions, and others to saline but not to water. Thus there may be specific nerve endings responding to water. With the rabbit, Pfaffmann found that the chorda tympani nerve gave a greater response to water than to saline solutions. Water reactivity was always associated with the response to other stimuli and was influenced by the previous history of stimulation—being less after saline and more after acid solutions. He concludes: "It would appear that the response to water in mammals does not reflect specific sensitivity to water, but rather excitability differences towards particular ions in which sodium appears to play a particular role." Diamant and Zotterman (1959) and Zotterman (1961), however, reported that cats, dogs, pigs, and monkeys possess nerve fibers in the chorda tympani which respond to application of water to the tongue. Kitchell *et al.* (1959) and Halpern (1962) reported electrophysiological responses to water applied to the tongue of chickens. With rats and human subjects, water did not elicit any positive specific neural sensation. Konishi and Zotterman (1961) found seven groups of taste fibers in the carp, none of which were stimulated by water. From a behavioral standpoint, failure to respond to water may be because the organism is continually adapted to it. Electrophysiological responses may be due to a hypotonic reaction.

III. Four Tastes

The number of distinct tastes is very large but many believe they are only combinations of four basic tastes.

Skramlik (1921) reported that inorganic salt solutions with multiple tastes, i.e., sweet, salty, sour, and bitter, could be duplicated by suitable mixtures of sucrose, sodium chloride, tartaric acid, and quinine. The proportions of the match changed with concentration and varied with the individual. Of 56 equations reported, 33 contained three components, 21 involved two, and 2 contained all four.

Experiments on the effects of narcotics furnish evidence that there are four tastes (Shore, 1892; Kiesow, 1894a). When applied to the tongue, the juice of gymnema leaves markedly reduced sensitivity to sweet and bitter substances without interfering with the sour and saline tastes. Stovaine produces similar effects to a lesser degree. If a 5–10% solution of cocaine is applied to the tongue several times, the tastes disappear in a definite order—first sour, and, after a few minutes, bitter. The sour taste returns before the bitter. Others report the order to be pain, bitter, sweet, saline, sour, and touch, and this is now generally accepted (Wenger *et al.*, 1956). Whether such specificity is a direct result of the action of the drug on the taste cell itself or on the innervating fibers of the cell has not been determined. However, electrophysiological studies show that the nerve fibers responding to bitter compounds are smaller and the action of the drugs appears to be dependent on nerve diameter. Pfaffmann (1959a) reported that when a single fiber is stimulated by sucrose and sodium chloride, gymnemic acid suppressed the response to the former but not to the latter. This is evidence of separate modalities of taste but could also be explained on the basis that different sites on the cell membrane are differentially sensitive.

Allen and Weinberg (1925), often quoted in support of the four tastes, stimulated the human tongue with electrical excitation and reported unique results corresponding to four tastes. The critical frequency of gustation at different frequencies and voltages was believed to fall on four curves when plotted. The curve with the larger number of points represented the sour taste. They then applied gymnemic acid, which removed the sweet and reduced the bitter taste, and found only three curves, the shortest of which they identified as the bitter curve. These data were not substantiated by Ross and Versace (1953), using frequencies of 20 to 2000 cycles per second and up to 3 volts. Above 1 volt, complex sensations of cold, sour, and bitter were observed, and above 3 volts some tactile, kinesthetic, or vibratory sensations. Jones and Jones (1952) also failed to substantiate Allen and Weinberg's results, although some subjects reported a sour taste. Pfaffmann (1959a) believes the effect to be tactile, since it can be demonstrated in regions of the mouth and lips where there are no taste buds. It has been suggested that the wave produced in Allen and Weinberg's apparatus was not actually a square wave, since the inductance and capacitance of the circuit would cause a distortion and the wave probably included high-frequency harmonics. The polarization of the electrodes would also affect the type of wave produced. Since Jones and Jones used different stimulating waves, this may partially explain the difference in the results, but the data of Allen and Weinberg seem anomalous. More recently, Dzendolet (1962) reported results which do not support the hypothesis of direct stimulation of either the receptors or nerves. Anodal pulses much above threshold, and threshold cathodal pulses, evoked sensations which could be classified as either tactile or pain rather than as taste. The threshold appeared to be a function of the rate at which ions were presented to the receptors. For earlier work on the "taste" following electrical stimulation, see Bujas and Chweitzer (1938).

Halpern (1959) noted that "When an adequate stimulus impinges on a receptor, neural activity develops in a number of peripheral nerve fibers. This multi-unit activity leads to trans-synaptic depolarization and discharge in many neurons within the central nervous system. Electrophysiological recording from populations of cells or fibers which comprise the afferent systems may represent a reasonable approximation to the multi-unit afferent barrages which occur in these systems under physiological conditions."

The earlier data could be interpreted in support of the four-modality theory as indicated by Beidler (1952):

> The most striking evidence in support of the four modality theory has been presented by Pfaffmann. Taste nerve strands containing a single active nerve fiber were dissected from the taste nerves innervating the tongue of the cat. The electrical activity was then recorded from the single fiber as various solutions were dropped on the surface of the tongue. Not all the nerve fibers tested responded in the same manner to a given number of solutions. Three different fiber groups were classified by Pfaffmann according

to the solutions to which they responded. The first group consisted of the acid fibers, which responded to potassium chloride, acetic acid, and hydrochloric acid. The second group, the acid-salt fibers, responded to potassium chloride, sodium acetate, calcium chloride, hydrochloric acid, acetic acid, and sodium chloride. The third group, the acid-quinine fibers, responded to acetic acid, hydrochloric acid, and quinine. Of the salts, only sodium chloride, which gave no response, was tested on the third group. Saturated sucrose did not stimulate the fibers tested by Pfaffmann, although it has recently been demonstrated, using different electrophysiological techniques, that taste nerve activity in the cat can be recorded in response to sucrose, the threshold being under 0.25 M. It is concluded that the sour taste is mediated when all three fiber groups are stimulated simultaneously. Stimulation of the acid-salt fiber group alone would mediate a salt response, whereas the acid-quinine group would mediate a bitter response. The single nerve fiber experiments indicate that the four taste modalities are reflected peripherally to the presence of receptors that are somewhat specific to compounds associated with the modalities, but not exclusively sensitive to compounds associated with any one modality.

Later, Pfaffmann (1954, 1955, 1956) reported on the electrical impulses in nerve stimulation of the rat by the four basic tastes. The neural activity followed a sigmoid function of the logarithm of the concentration; the stimulus-concentration response-magnitude function differed with the chemical used. There is no one-to-one correspondence between the four so-called basic taste stimuli and sensory nerve response if individual nerve fibers are employed. Individual fibers may respond to all four. There was nothing in the discharge that was characteristic of the chemical employed. If a single fiber does not discriminate different stimuli by some sort of modulation of its discharge, then the qualitative discrimination must be accomplished by the sense organ as a whole.

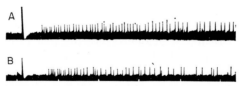

FIG. 13. Oscillographic record of a single nerve fiber preparation responding to acid on the cat's tongue. (A) Stimulus 0.5 N acetic acid; (B) stimulus 0.01 N hydrochloric acid. Each interval mark at base of record B indicates 0.1 second. Source: Pfaffmann (1941).

Different stimuli would set up characteristic patterns of activity among the fibers of the sensory nerve trunk, according to this view (see Pfaffmann, 1941). An example of typical data is given in Fig. 13. Therefore, as Pfaffmann (1959a) noted, "the taste receptors do not always fall into four basic receptor types corresponding to the basic taste qualities. The individual sensory cells are differentially sensitive to chemicals, probably because of differences at sites on the cell membrane. The chemical specificity of the taste cell can best be described as a cluster of sensitivities which varies among different receptor cells. Any one cell is reactive to a varying degree to a number of different chemical stimuli, many of which fall in two or more of the classical basic taste categories."

Even when microelectrodes were thrust directly into taste buds, Kimura and Beidler (1956) were unable to classify the receptors on the basis of the potential changes evoked by the four basic stimuli. It is of interest to note that in Pfaffmann's early work with cat tongue, no fibers that responded to sugar were noted. Pfaffmann (1956) stated: "Thus, although any one fiber responds differentially to the four basic taste stimuli, it may show any one of a wide variety of patterns of sensitivity. Discrimination presumably would depend upon such patterning of the gustatory afferent input. . . . The neuroanatomical data did not support the thesis that particular . . . qualities are determined by particular types of morphological endings. Rather, the primary . . . qualities are convenient descriptive headings rather than actual entities." Pfaffmann (1964) recently described the sensory input for taste as a "neural profile." Some sensory neural units are specific to one class of chemicals, others respond to several of the primary tastes or even a wide range or "spectrum" of tastes. "The neural discharge in any one sensory channel would have a different meaning depending upon the concurrent activity in other parallel sensory channels at the same time. The sensory code appears to be reflected in the ratios of frequencies simultaneously present in a number of taste fibers."

Furthermore, neural responses as measured by electrical currents may not correlate with behavior. Adrian (1953) specifically noted: "The physiology of the sense organs tells us very little about our sensations." Pfaffmann (1956) reviewed evidence showing that rabbits and rats prefer salt concentrations well above those giving an electrophysiological response. In the range where preference begins, the response to salt is a depression of activity (see also Chapter 2, Section XIII,B). Water, on the other hand, gives a marked response that may continue for some time. Here, a reduction in neural response rather than an increase appears to favor salt ingestion (see Chapter 1, Section IV,B).

Wenger *et al.* (1956) gave the following summary of data in favor of four primary taste modalities:

(1) Introspective evidence: the ability of normal individuals when deprived of sense of smell to describe their gustatory sensations in terms of these four qualities.

(2) Differential distribution of taste qualities on the surface of the tongue. This *seems* to indicate different sensory systems.

(3) Differential effect of narcotics.

(4) Fibers sensitive to certain tastes.

(5) Interactions of tastes to change each other's threshold. A subliminal concentration of acid on one side of the tongue becomes intensely acid-tasting when the other side is coated with a subliminal concentration of sucrose.

Applying factorial analysis to responses to the basic tastes at near-threshold concentrations, Yoshida (1963) concluded that four categories best fitted the data. Similarly, on the basis of presenting taste and temperature stimuli to the left and right sides of the tongue to secure additive or separate sensations, Békésy (1964) observed that the four primary taste sensations, and temperature response formed two well-differentiated groups: bitter, sweet, and warm, and sour, salty, and cold.

In summary, on the basis of recent electrophysiological data, there seems to be little physiological ordering of chemoreceptors into four categories, and there are unspecific responses where single peripheral gustatory units respond to a variety of compounds. The afferent neural code apparently depends on some sort of patterning of input, and this provides a basis for taste discrimination. According to Erickson (1958), discrimination would depend on the relative amounts of activity in several parallel afferent fibers. From a behavioral standpoint, however, the four-modality classification still appears useful.

IV. Taste Qualities

The four fundamental taste qualities give variable sensations of pleasantness and unpleasantness, depending on concentration. Engel (1928) noted that the pleasantness of sucrose increased as the concentration increased, and at a rather high concentration it decreased slightly. Solutions of sodium chloride, tartaric acid, and quinine sulfate increased in pleasantness over a small range of increasing concentration, and then gave an unpleasant sensation. Engel reported that 100% of the subjects found 9% sugar ($0.263 M$) pleasant, above 66% found 0.28% ($0.0186 M$) tartaric acid pleasant, about 54% found 2% ($0.342 M$) salt pleasant, and only 24% considered 0.0007% ($0.00000937 M$) quinine sulfate pleasant. In mixtures of tastes, however, pleasantness or unpleasantness is less predictable. (See, for example, the great variability in "gusts" in various foods, Chapter 2, Section V. See, however, the information on desirable bitterness in certain foods Chapter 2, Section XIII,D).

With colors, a neutralization may occur in mixtures of colors or new color tones, with the components of the mixture no longer identifiable.

That is not entirely true with taste, where the components of a mixture may be discerned within limits. If, however, one taste is at or near the threshold and the other very strong, the lesser will not be perceived even by the most sensitive subject. Likewise, in practice, we reduce the strong sensation of one taste with another: salt on melons to reduce the sweet taste, sugar in tea to mollify the bitter taste, sugar in lemonade to ameliorate the sour taste, etc. Therefore, although one taste may modify another it does not neutralize it.

Contrast phenomena are also easy to demonstrate with taste. For example, salt on one side of the tongue will cause distilled water on the other side to taste sweet or insipid. Application of salt to one side of the tongue and only a subliminal concentration of sucrose to the other, causes the latter to be easily recognized as "sweet"—or even "very sweet." A sugar solution on one side will enhance the saltiness reaction on the other. Salt also sensitizes to salt. Bitter has little tendency to contrast with the other tastes. See also Chapter 2, Section XVII.

Recently Bartoshuk *et al.* (1964) showed that subjects adapted to sodium chloride reported weaker sodium chloride solutions tasted sour or bitter and stronger solutions sweet or salty. The taste of water and weak sodium chloride solutions thus depends on prior adaptation. The tongue is normally adapted to saliva, which in man contains relatively low concentrations of salt. Thus it is near the lower limit of the adapting level at which it is possible to get the subadapting taste. This is one reason why water usually tastes flat or nearly tasteless. Bartoshuk *et al.* (1964) attribute the sour-bitter taste of water, after adaptation to sodium chloride, to a gustatory afterimage.

V. Relative Intensity

Lewis (1948) constructed psychological scales of taste intensity. This suggested comparisons of the taste intensity of the different tastes. Beebe-Center and Waddell (1948) used two subjects who could match the relative strength of solutions of quinine sulfate, tartaric acid, or sodium chloride against 1% sucrose. In cross-qualitative matching, there was considerable variability. The concentration that matched 1% sucrose was called a "gust." The gust values of compounds at various concentrations are given in Table 4. The data in Fig. 14 show a match of sodium chloride and sucrose intensity over a range of concentrations.

Beebe-Center (1949) prepared 9 concentrations of the four basic tastes in quarter-log gusts. The subjects then tasted foods and matched them against standards. The "gust" content of various foods was also determined by Beebe-Center (1949), as shown in Table 5. Quinine sulfate alone was predominantly unpleasant at a concentration of 0.0011%,

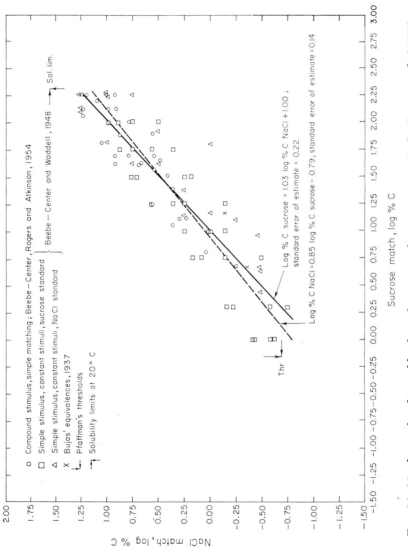

FIG. 14. Matching of sodium chloride and sucrose solutions. Source: Beebe-Center *et al.* (1955).

TABLE 4
Gust Values for Various Concentrations of Four Compounds

Gusts	Sucrose[a]	Quinine sulfate[a]	Tartaric acid[a]	Sodium chloride[a]
1	1.00	0.00020	0.0085	0.30
1.8	1.62	0.00043	0.0142	0.46
3.2	2.76	0.00087	0.0234	0.70
5.6	4.68	0.00174	0.0389	1.15
10	8.32	0.00339	0.0661	2.00
18	15.5	0.00646	0.118	3.80
32	28.8	0.0120	0.209	7.41
56	56.2	0.0224	0.407	15.9
100	115.0	0.0417	0.794	34.7

[a] Concentrations in grams per 100 cc.
Source: Beebe-Center (1949).

which was only 5 gusts, whereas commercial ale had a bitterness of 28.2 gusts. Note that the addition of 5% sucrose raised the sweetness of coffee by only 2.2 gusts but reduced the bitterness by 18.5 gusts. Beebe-Center therefore concluded that sweetness had no advantage over sourness or bitterness in determining acceptability. This conclusion is too

TABLE 5
Gust Values for Various Foods

Food	Sweet	Bitter	Acid	Salty	Total
Consommé	1.4	1.3	4.5	7.9	15.1
Alsacian wine	1.0	7.5	6.7	1.3	16.5
Cola drink	11.2	2.2	5.0	1.3	19.7
Pickles	1.0	1.8	18.0	3.2	24.0
Beer (ale)	2.5	28.2	10.0	1.3	42.0
Grapefruit juice	3.2	2.0	35.5	2.0	42.7
Coffee (no sugar)	1.0	42.3	3.2	1.0	47.5
Coffee (5% sucrose)	3.2	23.8	3.2	1.3	31.5
Honey	56.4	2.4	1.8	1.3	61.9

Source: Beebe-Center (1949).

general, though, and further data should be collected. It is also questionable whether these so-called "gusts" are additive, as indicated in the final column of Table 5.

Gridgeman (1958) was able to get comparisons of relative intensity of sucrose, sodium chloride, citric acid, and quinine hydrochloride. His comparison of 1:14:220:2300 is similar to that of Beebe-Center even though they used different methods.

VI. Reaction Time

The reaction time to taste, i.e., the interval between initial stimulation of the receptors and the report of a reaction, was estimated at 0.02–0.06 sec in electrophysiological studies (Pfaffmann, 1955), compared to oral-response reaction times of 0.307 sec for salt, 0.446 sec for sweet, 0.536 sec for sour, and 1.082 sec for bitter (Kiesow, in: Hollingworth and Poffenberger, 1917). Electrophysiological reaction time, in seconds, to other sensory stimuli include 0.013–0.045 (0.189) for vision, 0.0127–0.0215 (0.146) for hearing, and 0.00024–0.0089 (0.149) for touch. Figures in parentheses are from Hollingworth and Poffenberger (1917) for oral-response reaction times. Note that taste has the slowest reaction time. The faster the reaction the shorter the persistence. The over-all response depends somewhat on concentration and the stimulus: for sodium chloride, 0.370 to 1.007 sec; for citric acid, 0.480 to 1.32 sec; the minimum is about 0.25 sec. However, Beidler (1953), Pfaffmann (1955), and Nejad (1961) reported that the time for adequate chemical stimulation leading to nerve impulses is only 0.020–0.030 sec for sodium chloride, and somewhat longer for sucrose. For electrical stimulation the latency of response is 15 msec or less. Nejad (1961) reported that the response latency to sodium chloride decreased as the concentration increased.

The effect of concentration on reaction time was studied by Bujas (1935a) for citric acid, sodium chloride, and saccharin. When i was the concentration and t the time between stimulation and response, the relation

$$it = at^v$$

held over a short concentration range (a and v are constants). This was simplified to

$$t = c/i^n$$

where c and n are constants. For citric acid and sodium chloride, n equals $\frac{3}{2}$, and for sucrose 2. Bujas (1935b) extended the work to other solutions, but recorded only one observer and four to eight responses. The work should be repeated with more subjects and more observations.

Bujas and Ostojcic (1939) showed that taste intensity increased rapidly after a sapid solution was applied to the tongue, then more slowly, and finally showed no further increase. For salty and bitter, the concentration did not influence the maximum intensity attained. For sweet, the time to reach the maximum increased with concentration. However, the beginning of a sensation is quicker at higher concentrations. The time required to establish a sensation was greatest with bitter and least with salty. In electrophysiological studies with salt and acids the response rises rapidly to a peak and then falls off to some steady resting level. With sugar and quinine the initial peak is absent. Halpern *et al.* (1962) reported that the neural response to sugars resembles responses to amino acids: a relatively slow response build-up with sensitivity to configuration. The responses differ in that sugars adapt more rapidly than do amino acids. According to Beidler (1953) and Pfaffmann (1955), the magnitude of the total nerve response as recorded with an integrator circuit was typically an increasing sigmoid function of the logarithm of the stimulus concentration.

Holway and Hurvich (1938) studied the relationship between reaction time and pressure on area stimulated, and reported considerable variability in the results, possibly because of leakage of solution from the tube. The reaction time was longer at lower pressures on small areas than at greater pressures on larger areas. One of the two observers was more responsive than the other. Bujas and Ostojcic (1941) reported less spatial summation of response for sweet and bitter than for salt and acid. The product of threshold intensity times area stimulated, to a power between 0.37 and 1.62, was reasonably constant. With a single subject, at supraliminal concentrations of salt, the rate of summation was clearly lessened.

The methodology of studying taste reaction time is an important factor in the results obtained. The punctate method, which uses small brushes, has already been mentioned. Integrative stimulation techniques, in which the stimulus is allowed to flow over a large area of the tongue, are employed frequently. In certain experiments, precise control of area, pressure, temperature, and duration may be required, such as glass applicators in which the taste solution flows in and out of the applicator. Hara (1955) found that the threshold concentrations for a variety of compounds were exponential functions of the negative value of the area stimulated. The reaction time to suprathreshold concentrations decreased linearly with the area of the tongue stimulated, and logarithmically with the concentration of the stimulus. The equation $IS^x = K$ approximately described the relation between threshold intensity, I, and surface area, S, with exponents, x, of 0.73 for sodium chloride, 0.6 for citric acid, 0.93 for sucrose, and 1.42 for quinine hydrochloride.

Ichioka and Hara (1955) concluded that, at the threshold, the total number of gustatory nerve responses per second is at a maximum for a definite area, and gustatory reaction time is at a minimum. In general: $T = p - qN^r$, where T is the reaction time, N is the frequency of impulses, and p, q, and r (>1) are constants.

Afterimages in vision are well known, but it is unlikely that any similar mechanism operates for taste. Aftertastes do persist, some of the same quality as the preceding sensation and some quite different. Sweet compounds often have a bitter aftertaste, and vice versa. Washing the mouth with water after tasting potassium chloride solution produced a sweet taste, according to Nagel (1896). If dilute sulfuric acid is tasted, and then distilled water, the latter will taste sweet. These spatial and time effects should be repeated with modern techniques, since the problem of aftertastes needs further elucidation.

VII. Effect of Disease

Disease and accident may result in ageusia, hypogeusia, or parageusia (loss of, decreased, or altered taste sensations). These may be temporary or permanent, and uni- or bilateral. Cameron (1947) summarized some of these data as in Table 6 (the sweet taste was absent in all cases).

TABLE 6

Alterations in Three Taste Sensations as a Result of Disease

Condition	Response to		
	Bitter	Salt	Sour
Multiple gliomata	Delayed (RS)[a]	Absent (LS)[a]	Normal
?	Normal	Lessened	Absent
?	Slight	Absent	Absent
Tic douloureux	Delayed	Absent	Delayed
Tic douloureux	Delayed	Absent	Delayed
Tic douloureux	Absent	Delayed	Delayed
Tic douloureux	Absent	Absent	Sl. delayed
Tic douloureux	Absent	Delayed	Sl. delayed

[a] RS, right side; LS, left side.
Source: Cameron (1947).

The relation of disease to tasting ability has been discussed by Kalmus and Farnsworth (1959) and Kalmus and Hubbard (1960). They noted that irradiating the side of the tongue of a patient with cobalt source or X-rays reduced taste sensitivity to all tastes except sour. Recovery took about 2 months. In electrophysiological studies, Pfaffmann (1961) found X-rays did not grossly affect the response in the chorda tympani nerve until after the sixth day. Response to sodium chloride decreased slowly, but response to sucrose remained constant or even increased. On the sixth to seventh day, response to both dropped off rapidly.

In many individuals the lesions of the fifth cranial nerve reduce or cause a temporary loss of taste sensitivity from the front of the tongue.

Taste sensitivity returns after a short or longer period. Apparently dual functioning of the fifth cranial nerve and the chorda tympani and petrosal nerves is responsible for gustatory sensations from the front of the tongue. As previously indicated the fifth cranial nerve may also serve the posterior part of the tongue instead of the glossopharyngeal nerve.

In cases of diabetes, Hollingworth and Poffenberger (1917) reported that a sweet taste may be experienced in the absence of stimuli on the tongue. A bitter taste was reported in the case of jaundice. Bartley (1958) found a tingle and metallic taste at the tip of the tongue within a few seconds of intravenous injection of nicotinic acid. Henkin and Solomon (1962) and Henkin et al. (1962) have shown that patients with adrenal insufficiency exhibit increased sensitivity to salt, sweet, bitter, and sour tastes. Treatment with carbohydrate-active steroids (prednisolone) resulted in a return to the normal thresholds within 18–48 hours. Henkin and Powell (1962) also reported greater sensitivity in patients with cystic fibrosis. Confusing data on the effect of diabetes on taste were reviewed by Joergensen and Buch (1961), who concluded that the sense of taste was not altered, even in pregnant diabetics. They interpreted the craving of pregnant diabetics for certain foods to be related to perversion of the sense of smell (see Chapter 3, Section VIII).

The effect of adrenalectomy does not appear to be due to a decreased taste receptor threshold (Pfaffmann and Bare, 1950) or a lowered psychological threshold (Carr, 1952; Harriman and MacLeod, 1953). Some central mechanism apparently mediates such spontaneous taste preference behavior. Herxheimer and Woodbury (1960) reported that the salt preference threshold of rats decreased following treatment with deoxycorticosterone. Whether the effect is due to the change in intracellular electrolyte distribution in the brain or to a direct effect on the taste receptors is not known, but the former seems more likely (see also Chapter 1, Section IV,B). Pfaffmann (1964) has suggested that changes in salivary sodium level may affect the threshold for solutions of sodium chloride.

After prolonged vitamin A depletion, rats showed a decrease in degree of rejection of quinine sulfate solutions (Bernard et al., 1961). The rejection of sodium chloride increased toward the end of the depletion period. Following vitamin A injection, the depleted rats regained their normal sodium chloride but not their quinine sulfate preference. The possibility was suggested that vitamin A has a direct effect on the functioning of the taste cells.

Weiss Valbranca and Pascucci (1946) reviewed literature on the influence of defects on taste, and reported that sugar in the blood (diabetic or added) reduced sensitivity to sweetness. In addition, they demonstrated that sensitivity to citric acid increased with increased ascorbic acid deprivation. In pregnant women, citric acid thresholds were also low, prompting the investigators to conclude that their findings contributed to Richter's theory that sensitivity depended on need (Chapter 1, Section IV,B). Noferi and Guidizi (1946) reported a lowered threshold for acids and a reduced sensitivity to lemon odor during gestation.

VIII. Taste Thresholds

Measurement of thresholds is the most common procedure for studying the psychophysics of taste. The absolute threshold, S_o or, better, the absolute limen, t_o, is the minimum detectable concentration. The limen is not a sharply defined stimulus increment; since subjects vary in sensitivity and attention from measurement to measurement, the limen can only be defined as a statistical measure. The absolute or sensitivity limen is usually set as the stimulus magnitude at which the subject can identify a difference in taste in half of his attempts in a paired test. Difference limens can be defined at 25% (or greater) success.

The "recognition" threshold is the concentration at which the specific taste can first be recognized and is higher than the "sensitivity" threshold concentration. These thresholds have not always been distinguished, particularly in tests where the observers knew the identity of the taste substance. In these cases, there is a strong tendency to identify the taste at the "sensitivity" threshold level. Gridgeman (1959) defines another threshold, higher than the above two, where the taste sensation is sufficiently strong for the subject to assign an intensity. Gregson (1962) presented evidence that there may be many psychologically defined thresholds, the limit being the number of statement forms one is able to conceptualize. For example, he used the following rating scale: "same as water," "doubtful if pure water," "a very faint taste, can't say what," "a very faint sour (or sweet) taste," "a faint sour taste," "a weak sour taste," and "a clear sour taste." Assigning integers from 1 to 7, respectively, he considered the recognition threshold to be the concentration with a score equal to or greater than 4. One problem with this procedure is not knowing whether the steps on the rating scale are psychologically equidistant on the stimulus scale.

Skramlik and Schwarz (1959) reported that the absolute threshold and the recognition threshold were much closer together for bitter-tasting than for sweet- or sour-tasting compounds (see also Chapter 5, Section IV). Since most substances produce a mixed sensation, one is never certain that the response is really the threshold for a particular type of taste receptor. For example, Skramlik (1926) found that potassium chloride gives a response before sodium chloride although the latter is more salty (Table 7).

Thousands of taste thresholds are reported in the literature. The data are not always comparable, because of differences in technique employed, impurities in the chemicals, inadequate numbers of tests or insufficient statistical analyses of their validity, and the effect of undetermined factors such as order of presentation, temperature, extraneous

TABLE 7

Response to Taste of Sodium Chloride and Potassium Chloride

Concentration (M)	NaCl (%)	KCl (%)	Taste	
			Sodium chloride	Potassium chloride
0.009	0.0526	0.0671	No taste	Sweet
0.010	0.0584	0.0745	Slight sweet	Sweeter
0.015	0.0877	0.1118	Sweeter	Still sweeter
0.020	0.1169	0.1491	Sweet	Sweet, bitter
0.030	0.1754	0.2236	Strong sweet	Bitter
0.040	0.2338	0.2982	Salty sweet	Bitter
0.050	0.2922	0.3727	Salty	Bitter, salty
0.070	0.4091	0.5218	Saltier	Bitter, salty
0.100	0.5845	0.7455	Still saltier	Bitter, salty
0.200	1.1690	1.5910	Pure salty	Bitter, salty, sour
0.500	2.9225	3.7275	Pure salty	Bitter, salty, sour

Source: Skramlik (1926).

noise, time of day, experience, physical condition, age, sex, and area stimulated. Even from day to day, using the same subject and method, there are variations in the taste threshold to a given compound. Thresholds have been given in this text as percent and in moles. Dove (1953) proposed a logarithmic scale, but this does not appear practical to us (see Chapter 8, Section VII,B).

The data of Richter and MacLean (1939) for sodium chloride are indicative of the effect of the method of measurement (Table 8). In the "drop" method, three drops were placed on the protruded tongue; in the "swallow" procedure, 10 cc were swallowed; in "comparison No. 1," 10 cc of the salt solution were compared with 10 cc of distilled water; and in "comparison No. 2" as much salt solution and distilled water as desired were available.

Note that the "sensitivity" threshold is much lower than the "recognition" threshold by all methods, but particularly so when unlimited quantities of salt solution and water are available for comparison. The

TABLE 8

Influence of Method of Measurement on Sensitivity and Recognition Thresholds for Sodium Chloride

Method	No. of subjects	Sensitivity threshold		Recognition threshold	
		Range	Av.	Range	Av.
Drop	17	0.045–0.225% 0.0077–0.0385 M	0.135% 0.0231 M	0.120–0.350% 0.0205–0.0599 M	0.192% 0.0328 M
Swallow	24	0.015–0.150% 0.0026–0.0256 M	0.047% 0.0080 M	0.040–0.400% 0.0068–0.0684 M	0.167% 0.0286 M
Comparison 1	28	0.007–0.080% 0.0012–0.0137 M	0.037% 0.0063 M	0.030–0.300% 0.0051–0.0513 M	0.080% 0.0137 M
Comparison 2	53	0.007–0.060% 0.0012–0.0103 M	0.016% 0.0027 M	0.020–0.250% 0.0034–0.048 M	0.087% 0.0149 M

Source: Richter and MacLean (1939).

large range in thresholds is also noteworthy. Linker *et al.* (1964) showed in simple taste threshold experiments that nonsensory events effected the responses. Therefore, a more complex model is needed for establishing psychophysical thresholds.

Using the magnitude of the electrical activity of the chorda tympani in response to the activation of a group of receptors on the tongue, the data in Fig. 15 were obtained. Note the saturation level where no further

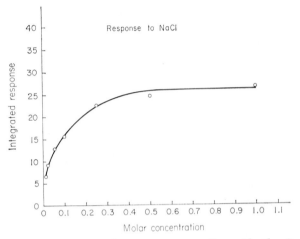

FIG. 15. Integrated response of taste nerve to sodium chloride. Curve showing the electrical activity of the taste nerve (integrated response) as various concentrations of sodium chloride solutions are flowed over the tongue of the rat. Source: Beidler (1953).

response is elicited. Each salt appears to have a unique saturation level, which indicates that the properties of the receptors are important, not merely the total number of available molecules. However, as Bernard (1962) has shown, strong behavioral responses in the calf may exist where electrical response of the appropriate nerve is slight or nil, and vice versa. One cannot, therefore, predict behavior on the basis of neural response.

Some ranges and average values will be given in discussion of the individual tastes, but the limitations indicated above should be kept in mind. The wide differences in sensitivity of individuals to the four basic tastes should also be noted (Schutz and Pilgrim, 1957).

Skouby and Zilstorff-Pedersen (1955) showed that acetylcholine in amounts of 1 to 100 μg per milliliter decreased the taste threshold by 20 to 63%. Menthol in amounts of 0.4 to 400 μg per milliliter had a similar effect. Actual taste substances were not used. The amount of anodal current required to produce an acid sensation was the test used. Strychnine (0.1–10 mg per milliliter) and higher concentrations of acetylcholine and menthol increased the threshold as measured by this procedure. With the latter two substances a direct effect on the receptors is believed responsible. The data would be more convincing if actual taste materials had been used.

The thresholds for rats obtained by Koh and Teitelbaum (1961) were: sucrose, 0.0099 M; sodium chloride, 0.00074 M; hydrochloric acid, 0.00046 M; and quinine hydrochloride, 0.000012 M. For sucrose the values compare well with those of Richter and Campbell (1940a), who used a preference threshold measurement, and those of Hagstrom and Pfaffmann (1959), who used an electrophysiological technique.

A. Effect of Sleep and Hunger

Lack of sleep, up to 72 hours, did not affect the thresholds to salt and sweet in the experiment of Furchtgott and Willingham (1956). Lack of sleep for 48 and 72 hours raised the sour threshold significantly.

In studies on hunger by Yensen (1959), sensitivity to the four basic taste qualities was greatest at 11:30 A.M. There was a significant decrease in sensitivity for about 1 hour after a meal, followed by an increase in 3 or 4 hours. The degree of decrease appeared to be related to the caloric value of the meal. Depletion of body salt content increased the sensitivity to salt but did not affect the other taste thresholds. Loss of body water caused a decrease in sensitivity to salt but did not affect the sour threshold. Gusev (1940) seemed to find an increase in sensitivity 1½ and 8 hours after fasting began, but Pick (1961) doubts if the results are statistically significant. The same objection may be made to the results of Goetzl *et al.* (1950) and Zaiko (1956). Meyer (1952) found no change in sensitivity to taste up to 34 hours of fasting.

Pangborn (1959) has reviewed this literature, and has made extensive consumer tests with peaches, and laboratory tests with apricot nectar and pure solutions. Hunger had little, if any, influence on preferences of 11,456 consumers for peaches varying in sugar and acid content. Detection of differences in sweetness of apricot nectar by trained judges was likewise not influenced by hunger. Fasting from breakfast until 4:30 P.M. did not influence absolute thresholds or difference thresholds of a trained panel for the four primary tastes in 7 out of 8 subjects. In data reported by Furchtgott and Friedman (1960), withholding lunch resulted in slightly lowered thresholds for sucrose, hydrochloric acid, and sodium chloride (see also Chapter 3, Section X,C). The development of better methodologies might lead to better results. Complete control of the diet would seem desirable.

B. AGE

Beidler (1961b) noted conflicting results on the effect of age on thresholds. The newborn apparently have little taste differentiation until about 35–40 days. However, response to saltiness has been demonstrated in 2-day-old children (Jensen, 1932). Richter and Campbell (1940a) found a much higher sweet threshold in a 52- to 85-year group than in a 15- to 19-year group. Cooper *et al.* (1959), using subjects 15 to 87 years old, found that curves for development and decline of sensitivity for the four basic tastes were the same. This decline started in the late 50's, and affected sour less than the other tastes (Table 9). Degenerative changes in the taste receptors are believed to be responsible. Aubek (1959), using only 100 subjects (25 from 15 to 29 years of age, 16 from 30 to 44, 23 from 45 to 59, 27 from 60 to 74, and 9 from 75 to 89), reported no significant impairment of taste sensitivity prior to 60 years of age. Above this there were significant decreases in sensitivity to salty, sour, sweet, and bitter. No sex differences were observed, but the population was small.

In contrast, Tilgner and Barylko-Pikielna (1959) found women to have a higher sensitivity than men for sweet and salty but less for sour and no difference between the sexes for bitterness. Decreases in sensitivity with age were reported for sweet and sour, and no change for salty and bitter.

A decrease in taste sensitivity after 60 years of age was reported by Lumía (1959). However, the differential sensitivity was less in children 7–11 years old than in people 20–30 or 70–90 years old.

According to Moore (1962), the number of taste buds per papilla drops from an average of 245 in young adults to 88 in subjects 70–85 years old. Cohen and Gitman (1959) reported more complaints among the aged (65–94 years) regarding ability to recognize basic tastes, but did not actually find any gross impairment in the pattern of taste perception with aging. Similar results were reported by Byrd and Gertman (1959), who stated that when older persons complain of loss of appetite one should investigate problems of environment, the patients' attitude toward self, and the possibility of hypogeusia.

C. SMOKING

Bronte-Stewart (1956) hypothesized that smoking could affect taste preferences via the taste mechanism. Krut *et al.* (1961) found no differences between smokers and nonsmokers in their thresholds for sweet, sour, or salty, but the mean threshold for bitter was significantly ($p <$ 0.001) higher for smokers. However, for PTC (phenylthiocarbamide) the

TABLE 9

Threshold Values in Percentage Concentrations for the Four Taste Qualities

Age group:	15–29		30–44		45–59		60–74		75–89		F ratio
N:	25		16		23		27		9		
Taste thresholds											
Sucrose	0.540	(0.016)[a]	0.522	(0.015)	0.604	(0.018)	0.979	(0.029)	0.914	(0.027)	6.142***
Sodium chloride	0.071	(0.012)	0.091	(0.016)	0.110	(0.019)	0.270	(0.046)	0.310	(0.053)	6.827***
Hydrochloric acid	0.0022	(0.0005)	0.0017	(0.0005)	0.0021	(0.0006)	0.0030	(0.0008)	0.0024	(0.0007)	1.618
Quinine sulfate	0.000321	(0.0000043)	0.000267	(0.0000036)	0.000389	(0.0000052)	0.000872	(0.0000116)	0.000930	(0.0000125)	7.540***
Difference thresholds											
Sucrose	0.275	(0.008)	0.268	(0.008)	0.281	(0.008)	0.430	(0.013)	0.396	(0.012)	
Sodium chloride	0.032	(0.005)	0.036	(0.006)	0.047	(0.008)	0.123	(0.021)	0.101	(0.017)	
Hydrochloric acid	0.0012	(0.0003)	0.0009	(0.0002)	0.0009	(0.0002)	0.0026	(0.0007)	0.0012	(0.0003)	
Quinine sulfate	0.000176	(0.0000024)	0.000094	(0.0000013)	0.000111	(0.00000015)	0.000623	(0.0000083)	0.000196	(0.0000026)	

[a] ( ) M values.

*** Significant at 0.001 level.

Source: Cooper et al. (1959).

distribution and average threshold of the PTC tasters was about the same for both groups. This contradicts the conclusion of Thomas and Cohen (1960), who reported more PTC tasters among the heavy cigarette smokers (65.9%) than among the nonsmokers (42.7%). This was not true of Negro smokers or nonsmokers. Age did not affect the percentages. The immediate effect of smoking did not seem to influence taste thresholds in work by Krut *et al.* (1961). The decrease in sensitivity was progressive with age and thus appears to be the result of prolonged addiction. They made the suggestion that the nicotine and other alkaloids in cigarette smoke fatigue the mechanisms for perception of bitter.

Freire-Maia (1960) noted no effects of smoking or of smokers versus nonsmokers on PTC sensitivity: "Concluding, we can say that in the large amount of data now available, obtained by different authors in different populations and here analyzed, there is no evidence of any smoking effect on taste sensitivity to PTC." Any effect in distribution of tasters and nontasters between smokers and nonsmokers appeared to be an age effect. Hopkins (1946), Tilgner and Barylko-Pikielna (1959), Aubek (1959), and Cooper *et al.* (1959) also reported that smoking had no significant effect on the taste receptors.

In studies by Sinnot and Rauth (1937), sugar and salt thresholds were higher among smokers than among nonsmokers, but the levels were the same if the smokers abstained for several hours. Laird (1939) found that female smokers 50 to 68 years old generally preferred tart juice. No differences were observed in taste preferences between male smokers and non-smokers of any age, of females up to 40, and in nonsmoking females from 50 to 68.

Using only six female college students as subjects (three smokers and three nonsmokers), Arfmann and Chapanis (1962) attempted to determine ability to evaluate vanilla taste intensity in the mouth after vanilla was sprayed into the nostrils. Just what the subjects "tasted" is not clear (possibly alcohol?), and the experiment should be repeated with some material which has a true taste and odor. They interpreted their results as showing reduced "taste" sensitivity among smokers.

D. OTHER FACTORS

Henning (1921) reported that taste sensitivity to sucrose was not affected by chronic alcoholism, excessive smoking, badly infected gums, marked tooth decay, mild head colds, hay fever, or allergy.

Water, unless specially purified, has a taste, according to Anderson (1959). Very sensitive subjects frequently note a "taste" or "flavor" in distilled water. These impurities could influence the results of threshold tests.

TABLE 10

Taste Thresholds for Selected Compounds

Investigator	Sucrose	Caffeine	Glutamic acid	Tartaric acid	Citric acid	Sodium chloride
Knowles and Johnson (1941)	0.0192 M (0.657%)	0.0008 (0.0155%)	0.0010 (0.0147%)	0.00026 (0.0039%)	— —	0.0199 (0.116)%
Hopkins (1946)	0.0195 M (0.667%)	0.0018 (0.0350%)	0.0008 (0.0118%)	0.00020 (0.0030%)	— —	0.0192 (0.112%)
Pfaffmann (1951)	0.02 M (0.685%)	— —	— —	— —	— —	0.035 (0.205)%
Pangborn (1959)	0.022 M^a (0.753%) 0.008 M^b (0.274%)	0.0014 (0.0272%) 0.0004 (0.0078%)	— —	— —	0.00116 (0.0223%) 0.00005 (0.00096%)	0.021 (0.123%) 0.008 (0.047%)

[a] First determination.
[b] Sixth determination.

Related to thresholds is the ability to distinguish intermediate concentrations. Lewis (1948) asked subjects to find the half-concentration of a standard from a series of comparison solutions. At the lower concentrations the solution chosen as the half-strength was actually greater than half in concentration (expressed as grams per 100 ml); at higher values the solution selected was less than half. Quinine sulfate was an exception, the half solution being nearly half. From these and other data Lewis showed that discriminable increments in gustatory intensity increase in size with increase in stimulus concentration. This is related to the Weber ratio (see Chapter 5, Section IV,A).

In all thresholds determinations, practice is a factor; one probably learns to fix one's attention on the proper taste so that taste cues are recognized at lower concentrations with increased familiarity with the stimuli (Pangborn, 1959).

E. TYPICAL VALUES

Hopkins' (1946) threshold values agreed fairly well with those obtained by Knowles and Johnson (1941), Pfaffmann (1951), and Pangborn (1959), as shown in Table 10. Pfaffmann's threshold for hydrochloric acid was $0.002 M$ (0.0073%), and for sodium saccharate was $0.00002 M$ (0.00045%). By statistical analyses, Hopkins showed that the threshold values for his data and those of Knowles and Johnson were normally distributed, and that the median thresholds at or below which 50% reacted agreed for the two groups except for bitter, where the observed difference exceeded by three times its standard error. In view of the close agreement for the others he believes some difference in the caffeine solutions employed might have been involved. For Knowles and Johnson's and Hopkins' data the association of sensitivities to the primary tastes, using χ^2 for 2×2 contingency tables, was:

Test substance	Glutamic acid	Sodium chloride	Sucrose
Caffeine	2.16*	0.01	0.17
Glutamic acid	—	3.31**	3.23**
Sodium chloride	—	—	2.20*

* Significant at 5% level.   ** Significant at 1% level.

Thus, there was a significant degree of correlation for the same individual for sour, salt, and sweet substances, but sensitivity to bitterness was associated only feebly with sourness, and not at all with saltiness or sweetness. In these tests, females were more sensitive to sourness than males.

It is of interest to note that Hopkins (1946) was unable to find any correlation between taste acuity and palatability judgments. He attributed this to the fact that olfactory and tactile sensations are involved in palatability—plus the purely subjective reactions based on training, prejudice, and other factors.

Because of these differences one would expect great variations between individual thresholds. Warren (1963) recently demonstrated the typical preference-aversion curve with mice for sucrose octaacetate. One mouse actually had a preference at saturation, whereas others rejected low concentrations. Similar variation in animal behavior was reported by Kare (1961). It is of interest that sucrose octaacetate is not a nutritive and has a negligible effect on osmotic pressure.

IX. Effect of Temperature

The influence of temperature on taste is not uniform (Cameron, 1947; Pfaffmann, 1959a). Optimums have been reported of 35°–50°C for sucrose and hydrochloric acid, 18°–35°C for saltiness, and 10°C for quinine. Sodium chloride tasted bitter at 10°C, presumably at or near its threshold concentration. Increasing temperature appears to increase the response to sweet and decrease it to salty and bitter. Hahn and Günther (1932) and Hahn (1936a) noted that study of the effect of temperature requires control of the area stimulated and the rate with which the liquid passes over the tongue. Although there were some exceptions, Hahn found that the threshold for sweetness of glycerol decreased from 2.3% $(0.25\,M)$ at 17°C to 0.25% $(0.27\,M)$ at 37°C, above which it increased. The dulcin threshold was 0.00085% $(0.000047\,M)$ at 17°C, 0.00015 $(0.0000083\,M)$ at 34.5°–37°C, and 0.00029 $(0.000016\,M)$ at 42°C. The hydrochloric acid threshold $(0.003\,M)$ and that of glycine were not affected by differences in temperature between 17° and 42°C. The thresholds for salty and bitter tastes increased throughout the temperature range. Sodium chloride had a threshold of 0.002% $(0.00034\,M)$ at 17°C and rose fairly steadily to 0.005 $(0.00085\,M)$ at 42°C. The threshold of quinine sulfate increased more rapidly at the higher temperatures— 0.00015% $(0.0000020\,M)$ at 17°–22°C, 0.0002% $(0.0000027\,M)$ at 32°C, and 0.0005% $(0.0000067\,M)$ at 42°C. Maurizi and Cimino (1961), in contrast, found the thresholds for bitter, acid, and salt to be lower at 35°–40°C than at 15°–20°C.

The effect of temperature on electrophysiological response was studied by Nejad (1961). He found it necessary to use a three-dimensional model to represent the temperature effect.

Adaptation is also a function of temperature. Warming a 10% sucrose solution from 17° to 32°C reduced the absolute threshold before adaptation, and shifted the adaptation curve downward. Five seconds of continuous stimulation by the warmer solution elevated the threshold half as much as the cooler one, but, in either case, adaptation was complete in 15 seconds. This temperature effect indicates a peripheral rather than a central locus of adaptation. Typical data on the effect of temperature on taste are given in Fig. 16. Extremes of temperature apparently de-

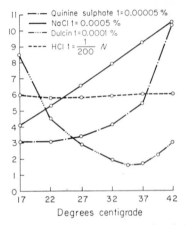

FIG. 16. The effect of temperature on taste thresholds for sodium chloride, quinine sulfate, dulcin, and hydrochloric acid. The ordinate gives the thresholds in arbitrary units. The value of one unit on the ordinate differs for each of the four substances, as shown by the key in the figure. For example, one unit for sodium chloride equals 0.0005%. Source: Hahn (1936b).

sensitize the receptors for certain sensations momentarily, so that a temperature effect may not be noted.

Pfaffmann (1959a) observed that some data obtained by electrophysiological methods show that sensitivity to sodium chloride decreased with increasing temperature, particularly above 22°C, whereas in other cases there was little change. Pfaffmann noted that with extreme cooling or excessive heating there may be irreversible changes, and stated that "temperature increase does not increase all taste sensitivity. There is no simple temperature coefficient in the usual sense." Nejad (1961) showed that change of temperature caused little or no change of ΔF in electrophysiological studies of the chorda tympani of the rat. Nejad postulated that the small effect of temperature (within the physiological range) that he observed might have been due to a secondary taste mechanism such as physiological processes in the cell and/or of the taste cell membrane. According to Sato (1962), the chorda tympani and lingual nerves of frog's tongue gave the same response to water at 10°, 20°, 30°, 40°, and 50°C, a maximum response to Ringer's solution at 10°C, and a decreasing response to sodium chloride as concentration increased above 1 *M*.

In view of the lack of adequately controlled experimentation with a sufficient number of subjects and compounds, it is difficult to generalize on the effect of the temperature of the stimuli on the resultant taste response in the human. It appears difficult to separate taste, temperature, and pain effects. In addition, the temperature of the receptor may be of more critical importance than the temperature of the sapid substance.

X. Effect of Taste Medium

In only a few isolated cases has the interrelationship of the tactile and gustatory properties of oral stimuli been investigated. Several theories, without benefit of substantiating data, appear in the early literature. One of the earliest is the statement by Skramlik (1926) that the intensity of taste was greater in aqueous media than in paraffin oil, a condition which may be related to the combined effects of viscosity, solubility of the compounds in oil and of the oil in saliva. Crocker (1945) speculated that the physical state of a food influenced taste by partially controlling the quantity of sapid matter reaching the taste receptors in a given time. He further theorized that the viscosity of a fluid thickened with algin, gum tragacanth, flaxseed, or other source of mucilaginous material, interferes with diffusion of soluble substances to the receptors. According to Tritton (1939) pectin depresses free hydrogen ions, thereby reducing apparent sourness in food products. Although the presence of pectin may reduce apparent sourness, Tritton has given no evidence of reduction of free hydrogen ions; it is probable that the physical characteristics of the pectin in solution may reduce diffusion of protons or hinder their adsorption on the receptors.

In experiments conducted by Mackey and Valassi (1956), taste thresholds for sucrose, sodium chloride, caffeine and tartaric acid were lower in water solutions than in tomato juice and custard, each prepared as liquids, gels, and foams. The added taste substances were easiest to detect in the liquid state, most difficult in the gel, and intermediate in the foam. Unfortunately it was not indicated whether the volume concentration of a component was the same in each medium. Moreover, if the composition of each medium was identical, as stated in the report, the temperature of the gelatin-containing media would have had to vary from the sol to the gel state.

Later, Mackey (1958) observed that the tastes of caffeine, quinine, and saccharin were more easily detected in water than in mineral oil, and theorized that the lipid inhibited the solubility of the taste compounds in the saliva. When methylcellulose was added to water to give the same viscosity as that of the oil (115 cps at 25°C) ease of detection of the three compounds was intermediate between water and oil. Although only a limited number and type of taste stimuli were tested and only eight evaluations per sample were collected, the results clearly indicated that the methylcellulose interfered with taste perception.

Wick (1963) reported that judges' accuracy in ranking sweetness intensity in aqueous solutions, sucrose-starch powder mixtures, 7% gelatin gels and whipped 7% gelatin gels averaged, respectively, 75, 47, 43, and 33%. Citric acid and naringin were more easily detected and identified in aqueous solutions than in a 7% gel or a fondant, but responses to sodium chloride were unaffected by the physical nature of the medium.

Unpublished data of Simone (1962) indicated that, at threshold concentrations, sensitivity to sodium chloride was lower in agar solutions than in pure water. Conversely, at a level of 0.5% sodium chloride, ability to detect differences in saltiness was greater in the agar than in water solutions. In a food medium, white sauce, there was no evidence that increased viscosity influenced sensitivity to differences in saltiness. Pangborn (1963) observed that, on a weight basis, fructose was sweeter than sucrose in water, but the reverse was true when both sugars were compared in pear nectars at various levels of citric acid, a result which may have been related to viscosity.

XI. Taste and Chemical Configuration

As with most biological phenomena, taste responses are related to chemical specificity. For example, there are taste differences between o-, m-, and p-tolylurea (Fig. 17). The compound p-anisonitrile

$$CH_3O-\langle\bigcirc\rangle-CN$$

is sweet, whereas p-ethoxybenzonitrile

$$C_2H_5O-\langle\bigcirc\rangle-CN$$

is bitter. The stereoisomers sorbitol and dulcitol are not equally sweet. With amino acids, Kaneko (1938) found that D-tyrosine compounds were sweet and the L-compounds bitter or disagreeable. The taste was related not to the optical rotation but to the stereo structure. In 1937 Neri and Grimaldi showed how the introduction of various groups into the molecule affects their sweet and bitter tastes (see also Cohn, 1915).

Ferguson and Lawrence (1958) and Lawrence and Ferguson (1959) observed that the D-configurations of leucine, isoleucine, valine, histidine, tryptophan, and asparagine were sweet, whereas the L-forms were not. Galvin (1948) and Berg (1953) summarized findings on the tastes of various amino acids. For the rat, Halpern *et al.* (1962) reported that the "natural" L-form of several amino acids gave lower electrophysiological responses than did the D-forms. They noted that the neural responses to sugars resemble those to amino acids; rats, however, begin to select

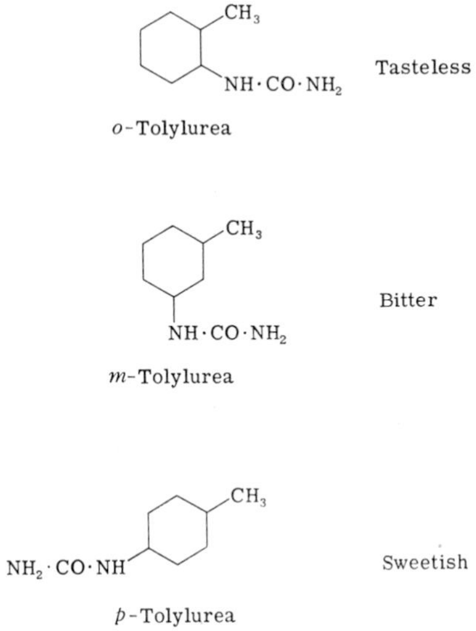

o-Tolylurea — Tasteless

m-Tolylurea — Bitter

p-Tolylurea — Sweetish

FIG. 17. Effect of chemical structure on taste. Source: Berlinerblau (in Moncrieff, 1951).

amino acids at concentrations far below those to which human beings respond. The response magnitude, at concentrations close to the solubility limits, was DL-methionine < DL-tryptophan < DL-valine < DL-alanine < glycine < 0.1 M sodium chloride. Stimulation by several amino acids reduced the response to sodium chloride for as long as 20 hours. It appeared that glycine and alanine affected different receptors more than did sodium chloride, but all three may affect some common receptor type.

Ferguson and Lawrence (1958) found that isomaltose (6-α-D-glucopyranosyl-D-glucose) was sweet whereas its anomer, gentiobiose (6-β-D-glucopyranosyl-D-glucose), was bitter. They studied several physical properties which could have been controlling factors of the taste sensation, but were unable to identify any consistent pattern. Application of enzyme inhibitors, sodium azide, potassium fluoride, sodium iodoacetate, and sodium cyanide modified the sweet taste, but none obliterated it completely. α-Galactose is reported to be sweeter than β-galactose, but β-fructose is sweeter than α-fructose. Boyd and Matsubara (1962) reported that 5 of 8 observers found L-mannose less sweet than D-mannose, and L-glucose not sweet but slightly salty. These were presumably tasted in crystalline form, but no information is given on the methods used.

In an intensive study of the effectiveness of various carbohydrates in stimulating labellar and tarsal hairs of the blowfly, *Phormia regina,* Dethier (1955) found that α-nitroglucose and α-methylglucoside were respectively more effective than β-nitroglucose and β-methylglucoside. Compound sugars with an α-D-glucopyranoside link were the most effective carbohydrate stimuli. Once again, enzyme inhibitors such as azide, iodoacetate, phlorizin, and fluoride did not prevent stimulation.

Cameron (1947) reported that a 10% solution of α-D-glucose had a sweetness equal to or more than that of a 10.5% equilibrium solution. Those results were verified by Pangborn and Gee (1961), who also noted that the α-configuration of galactose was significantly sweeter than the β-forms, whereas the reverse was true for fructose and lactose.*

Recently, Steinhardt *et al.* (1962) observed that the α-anomer of D-mannose was sweet whereas the β-anomer was bitter. From Tsuzuki's rule that the sweeter isomer has *cis*-hydroxyl groups on the carbonyl and adjacent carbon atom (in the less sweet isomer the hydroxyls are *trans*), it was predicted that the α-form would be less sweet than the β-form. This was confirmed by Tsuzuki and Mori (1954).

Shallenberger (1963) proposed that the sweetness of sugars is influenced by hydrogen bonding. When hydroxyl groups, which elicit sweet taste, are hydrogen bonded, the ability of the compound to cause a sweet taste appears restricted. As Shallenberger noted, this does not rule out the possibility that other parameters, such as resonance energy, vibratory hydrogen, solubility, and rate of diffusion into taste-bud receptor sites, may not also be related to the sweet taste. These various studies emphasize the high degree of physicochemical stereospecificity of the taste receptors.

On the basis of studies of the taste of 80 saccharin derivatives, Hamor (1961) suggested that a "lock and key" relationship at the receptor site is perhaps necessary for taste. Among the many interesting taste alterations resulting from addition or substitution on the saccharin structure was the observation that doubling the molecule produced a tasteless compound (see also Mee, 1934; Neri and Grimaldi, 1937).

XII. Taste Theories

Beidler (1952) suggested that any theory of taste must account for the following: (1) the taste receptors respond rapidly to a chemical

* In that paper the first compound in Table 1 should read β-D-fructose and the values under "Alpha sweeter" should be under "Beta sweeter."

stimulus; (2) all substances tasted must be in a liquid (soluble) form; (3) a variety of substances stimulate the taste receptors; (4) the threshold concentrations for stimulation are not large; (5) many taste substances are nonphysiological, i.e., they do not result in any rapid deterioration of the receptor cells; this is true of 0.1 M sodium chloride, 10 mM strychnine, and acids with a pH down to about 2.5; (6) the taste receptor rapidly elicits a steady level of response with a magnitude that is a function of the concentration of the applied substance; (7) the response to many substances remains constant over a long period of adaptation; (8) receptor stimulation must be followed by electrical depolarization of the nerve membrane, and possibly preceded by depolarization of the end organ itself; (9) a water rinse rapidly reduces the taste response; (10) the receptors are the site of the chemical specificity; and (11) there are genetic variations in taste ability. To these he added (1962): (1) the taste receptor response of the rat to sodium chloride is almost independent of temperature between 20° and 30°C, and of pH between 3 to 11; (2) the presence of saliva is not necessary; and (3) different species reveal different cationic series of taste-receptor excitability.

Warfield (1954), like many others, searched for a common molecular factor related to taste. He proposed a "taste couple"—a proton and a neighboring unshared electron pair. Details of his scheme, which he admits to be tentative, are not available, but with inorganic salts, sweetness, and bitterness a pattern of quantitative differences did emerge. He suggested that a "direct-reading" chemical sense may be involved—the stimulus being a trigger process with very specific absorption and little energy. The receptors might be sensitive to fine details of molecular structure which are not readily perceived by physical methods. This theory obviously needs a fuller elucidation.

Lasareff (1922) considered that each receptor was responsive to a single taste and that the applied stimulus caused decomposition of a material in the cell. This decomposition produced ions which stimulated the nerve endings. Equations were derived and experiments gave good agreement with these equations. According to Beidler (1962), however, those experiments were based on a change in adaptation which is not seen at the receptor level.

A. ENZYME THEORY

The location of 6 main sites of enzyme activity in the papilla foliata of the rabbit prompted Baradi and Bourne (1953) to hypothesize that enzyme activity in the vicinity of nerve fibers produces ionic changes which induce the formation of nerve impulses. The taste substance

would inhibit enzymes in some sites, leaving enzymes in other sites unaffected, thereby producing a change in the pattern of impulses reaching
the brain. Different tastes could thus be distinguished. One advantage of
this theory is that it provides an explanation of why substances of widely
differing chemical composition can have similar tastes. However, the
enzyme theory would seem to deny the association of gustatory nerve
fibers with specific taste sensations. The observed functioning of nerve
fibers would not easily fit the enzyme theory relative to sensations being
caused by inhibition of spontaneous discharges of some nerve fibers
and increases in the rate of discharge of others. The main criticism is
that the magnitude of taste response is fairly independent of temperature whereas enzyme reactions are very dependent on temperature.
Although enzymes may not be involved in the initial reaction of the
stimulus with the receptor, enzymatic processes are most certainly involved in over-all maintenance of the integrity of the receptor.

Hagstrom (1958), using the hamster and recording action potentials
of the chorda tympani following taste stimulation of the anterior part
of the tongue, found no evidence that the mechanism of sugar stimulation is an enzymatic process. Rather, it appears to be related to some
physical property of the cell surface and probably involves sites of
action different from those for salt stimulation. Dethier (1956, 1962)
noted how little the sugar threshold of various insects could be changed
by changes in temperature. This, together with the lack of inhibition of
phlorizin, fluoride, azide, iodoacetate, and cyanide by stimulation with
sugars, appears to rule out many enzymatic reactions as the limiting
reaction. He thus favors the hypothesis for stimulation by sugars, at least
in insects, that there is a combination of the sugar molecule with a specific receptor substance or site by weak forces, such as van der Waals'
forces, resulting in a complex which depolarizes the membrane, after
which the sugar is removed passively by a shift in concentration gradient.
Thus, multiple sites seem required. For monovalent salts, on the other
hand, there seems to be a single site on the receptive surface.

B. BEIDLER'S THEORY

Beidler (1954) believes that taste sensation is dependent on: (1)
the particular types of chemoreceptors that are activated; (2) the magnitude of their response; and (3) the pattern of the nerve discharge over
each taste nerve fiber. With salt receptors the reactions involved are in a
time-independent state and stimulation is probably in thermodynamic
equilibrium; the reaction is very rapid and reversible; both cations and
anions enter the reaction (although the magnitude of response is determined chiefly by the cations); a saturation level is reached which is

different for different compounds; and the receptors respond to diverse substances.

The different peripheral innervations of the fungiform, foliate, and circumvallate papillae suggest that there may be different spatial representations of the taste of chemical compounds on this basis alone (Halpern, 1959).

Halpern also found that mixtures of sucrose and acetic acid and of sodium chloride and potassium chloride did not show algebraic summations of their separate electrophysiological responses in the medulla oblongata but did with the chorda tympani. With greater depth the sucrose function recorded in the anterior tongue region showed an increase in response relative to sodium chloride. Large sucrose responses were found only within a narrow bulbar region. Such differences in sucrose response, Halpern suggests, are indicative of spatial representation for stimulus quality within the bulbar taste region. Erickson (1958) believed that first- and second-order neurons did not differ significantly in patterns of sensitivity to chemical stimulation. The distinction between tastes might be due to the number of impulses resulting from discharge, the fibers stimulated, and the pattern in time of the discharge.

Another possible theory is that taste substances participate in an adsorption process, possibly with proteins, at the surface of the receptor. This results in a rapid depolarization of the receptor surface which spreads to the attached nerve fiber and excites it.

In investigations on the application of sodium salts to rat tongues, Beidler (1954) assumed that the gustatory reaction follows the mass-action law. He assumed further that, if the mass-action law applies, the interaction of a stimulus with a given substance of the receptor is expressed by the equation

$$Kc = \frac{n}{S - n} \tag{1}$$

where $n =$ the total number of ions or molecules that react with the receptors at concentration c of applied stimulus, S, the maximum number of ions or molecules that can react, and K, the equilibrium constant. If the magnitude of the response, R, is proportional to the number of ions or molecules that have reacted, then $R = an$, where a is a constant. For maximum response, $R_m = aS$. Substituting in Eq. (1),

$$Kc = \frac{R}{R_m - R} \quad \text{or} \quad \frac{c}{R} = \frac{c}{R_m} + \frac{1}{KR_m} \tag{2}$$

This equation relates magnitude of response to the concentration of the applied stimulus.

Note that $c = 1/K$ when $R = R_m/2$.

If c/R is plotted against c, a straight line should result with slope equal to $1/R_m$ and a y intercept equal to $1/KR_m$. This equation is similar to the adsorption isotherm of Langmuir, and similar equations have been used to express the binding of ions by proteins.

Using Eq. (2), Beidler plotted c/R versus c for the electrochemical response of chemoreceptors of rats' tongues to sodium salts. Straight-line plots resulted, as postulated. Agreement between a mathematical equation and a set of data does not prove a theory to be correct, but it is at least a point in its favor. Beidler believes that weak physical forces of about 1.0 to 2.0 kcal bind the sodium salts to a polyelectrolyte-like structure, possibly a nucleoprotein, at the receptor surface. Beidler's data do not favor the theory that an enzymatic reaction is involved. The K value is not the same as for enzyme reactions, and receptor response varies little between 20° and 25°C. The low ΔF values, also, do not favor an enzyme theory (see also Nejad, 1961). The cation was more important than the anion. The reaction was pH-independent from pH 3.0 to 11.0; therefore, Beidler believes that the reacting anionic groups of the receptors are strong acidic radicals. The weak carboxyl radical of a protein could not be a reacting group. The phosphate and sulfate radicals of nucleic acids and even polysaccharides can bind cations in this manner.

Nejad (1961) showed that change in temperature caused little or no change in ΔF as calculated in the Beidler equation. This he takes as support of the adsorption theory as the primary taste mechanism. The slight effect of temperature on the taste response of the rat (within the physiological range), he believes, is due to some secondary taste mechanism, such as physiological processes in the cell and in the taste-cell membrane.

Using primary taste-receptor cells in the blowfly rather than secondary neurons in the chorda tympani, Evans and Mellon (1962) were able to show that the magnitude of the response to stimulus intensity followed Beidler's equation. The free-energy change of the reaction between salt and receptor site was in the range of 0 to -1 kcal per mole. Again, the salt-combining sites of the receptor appear to be anionic and strongly acidic, and they concluded that the cation of the salt largely dominates stimulation. They used activity rather than molarity in their calculations. About 10^7 molecules appeared to be necessary for a response. This recalls Lasareff's (1922) and Hahn's (1936b) earlier idea that taste represents a first-order reaction between the taste material and some unknown substrate on the surface of the tongue or in the receptors.

Beidler considers that the presence of nucleic acids in cellular membranes is additional evidence for his theory. It has been shown that deoxypentose nucleic acid from calf thymus binds cations much more than anions, and that the extent of the binding does not change with depolymerization. Beidler (1961a) feels that this adsorption results in a slight change in the spatial configuration of the receptor molecule. A leakage follows of some ionic species, probably potassium, from the interior, decreasing the normal potential across the receptor membrane. The spread of this local polarization over the rest of the cell surface may stimulate the innervating nerve, either by chemical or electrical means, such that the frequency of nerve impulses generated is proportional to the magnitude of receptor depolarization. Quality discrimination, Beidler believes, is due to the complex pattern of a number of single taste-nerve fibers.

If the concentration of the stimulus is reduced, the value of c/R_m approaches zero, and the taste equation reduces to

$$R_t = c_t K R_m$$

where R_t and c_t are at the threshold. Thus, the threshold concentration, c_t, depends not only on the strength with which the stimulus is attached to the receptor site but also on the number of sites available to the particular stimulus. For this reason, the effectiveness of the response may vary at low and high concentrations.

Iur'eva (1957) reported that cadmium chloride decreased sensitivity to taste substances. Since cadmium chloride blocks the sulfhydryl groups of protein complexes, this was considered evidence that proteins participate in gustatory reception. He (1961) later showed that guanidine nitrate sensitized taste receptors of frogs' tongues to gustatory substances (increase in intensity and duration of pulses). This effect was eliminated by blocking the sulfhydryl groups with cadmium chloride. Nejad (1961) found that chloride solutions of copper, iron, cadmium, and nickel had only a slight effect on the neural response to sodium chloride. However, sodium cyanide inhibited response to sodium chloride but the inhibition was reversible and recovery occurred in about 20 minutes. Five percent iodoacetic acid inhibited activity of the taste receptors unless the tongue was previously soaked with cysteine, in which case no inhibition occurred. On the other hand, when a 0.2% solution of phlorizin was employed it had no noticeable effect on taste activity.

Generally, these theories are too broad to permit any direct proof or disproof. Furthermore, there is little reason to assume that there is only one type of stimulating mechanism for all types of taste substances. This is emphasized by the fact that sour and salty tastes are primarily elicited by electrolytes, whereas bitter and sweet tastes may be elicited by either.

C. OTHER THEORIES

Frings (1951, 1954) believes that the so-called primary tastes are merely points of familiarity on a taste "spectrum." The determining factor in taste quality is thought to depend on: (1) the stimulative effectiveness of the substance; and (2) the penetration or adsorption of the compound by the receptors. The population of receptors is variably sensitive to stimulation, with sweet least stimulating, then salt, bitter, and sour. The receptors are differently susceptible to penetration or adsorption. Frings' taste-spectrum concept does not exclude regional localization of end organs of quantitatively different susceptibility. As suggested by Frings, there are two series of stimulatory substances: polar and nonpolar. By this theory, a substance which is both sweet and sour would be difficult to explain. Wenger *et al.* (1956) simply noted that chemical groupings permit very little taste prediction. The decrease in sensitivity to salt and bitter above 30°C makes a simple chemical theory of taste untenable. Those investigators suggested that promising lines of research would be measurement of the size of the molecules which can pass through a cell membrane, and measurement of the effect resulting from the adsorption of sapid molecules on the cell membrane.

Beidler (1961a) favors a biophysical rather than a biochemical explanation of the taste mechanism. For sweetness, no physicochemical factors appear to be correlated with intensity. Beidler (1962) showed that the number of potential sites on the microvillus of the taste cell is adequate to account for the various types of taste. He has also given a stimulating discussion of unsolved problems and research needs in this field.

Pfaffmann (1959b) now believes in a one-to-one relation between nerve fiber and sensory quality: "In the two-fiber example . . . low concentrations of salt will discharge only A, higher concentrations will discharge both A and B, but activity in A will be greater than that in B. Low concentrations of sugar will activate only B, higher concentrations will activate both B and A, but B will be greater than A." Sensory quality is thus determined by a pattern of fibers excited rather than by one specific type of fiber. The units of the pattern are fibers and their receptors. The differential sensitivity of the receptor can be described only in terms of the physical dimensions that correspond to the sensory qualities sweet, sour, bitter, or salty. For a more complete statement of the pattern of discrimination, see Pfaffmann (1962).

XIII. The Basic Tastes

A. SOUR

Along with saltiness, sour is considered to be a primitive taste and is a true taste since we can taste concentrations lower than those which affect the common chemical sense. Not all acids are sour: amino acids are often sweet, and picric acid is very bitter. The apparently sour taste of carbon dioxide may be an artifact representing nongustatory sensations.

Mosel and Kantrowitz (1952) reported a threshold for tartaric acid of 0.0075 M (0.1125%) for 4 tasters. Knowles and Johnson (1941) reported tartaric acid thresholds of 0.00012 M (0.00180%) to 0.003 M, (0.0450%), with a medium of 0.00045 M, (0.00675%) whereas Crocker and Henderson (1932) gave 0.00125 M (0.01876%).

Berg *et al.* (1955a) reported the following acid thresholds for $p = 0.001$ and for $p_c = 0.50$ (in parentheses) as g/100 ml: sulfurous, 0.001 (0.0011); sulfuric, 0.0015 (0.0013); tartaric, 0.0025 (0.0027); citric, 0.0025 (0.0023); potassium acid tartrate, 0.0075 (0.0090); lactic, 0.004 (0.0038); malic, 0.0030 (0.0026); and succinic, 0.0035 (0.0034) (p and p_c refer to probabilities; see Chapter 10, Section I). Fabian and Blum (1943) gave lower values for tartaric, citric, malic, and acetic acids. Schutz and Pilgrim (1957) reported a threshold for citric acid of 0.004% (0.000208 M). Tilgner and Barylko-Pikielna (1959) reported average thresholds for tartaric acid from 0.008 to 0.017% (0.000533–0.001132 M). For some original data with four tasters, see Skramlik and Schwarz (1959). Table 11 shows the most reliable data as summarized by Pfaffmann (1959a).

Berg *et al.* (1955a) determined the minimum detectable difference in suprathreshold concentrations of acid: For D-tartaric acid of 0.25 g/100 ml, a difference of 0.05 g/100 ml was necessary; for 0.30 g/100 ml of potassium acid tartrate, a difference of 0.10 g was needed; for 0.21 g/100 ml of citric acid, 0.07 g; for 0.23 g/100 ml of malic, 0.05 g; and for 0.002 g/100 ml of sulfurous acid, 0.004 g.

The reaction time to acid was given as 0.536 sec by Kiesow (1903) and as 0.3315 sec by Vintschgau and Hönigschmied (1877a). Such differences are to be expected with variations in the volumes and concentrations used, the specific portion of the tongue exposed, the temperature of the solution, and individual variability. The order of intensity of common organic acids is usually given as: tartaric, citric, malic, hydrochloric, lactic, and acetic but this is subject to various variables.

Ever since the concept of hydrogen ion activity was introduced, the acid (or sour) taste has been attributed to it (Paul, 1916). Thus, Richards (1898) pointed out that weak acids have a lower hydrogen ion concentration and taste less sour. He showed that addition of sodium acetate to hydrochloric acid reduced the acid taste yet the thresholds are not equal to the pH if various acids are tested. Acetic acid is more sour than hydrochloric at the same pH, but at the same molar concentration the stimulus is the reverse. Near-threshold equinormal solutions of organic and inorganic acids taste equally sour, according to Baráth and Vándorfy (1926). The threshold for weak organic acids is about pH 3.7 to 3.9, whereas for strong organic acids it is about 3.4–3.5. Clendenning (1940a,b,c) claimed that it is possible to raise the pH with sodium salts and not change the acid taste. This should be verified.

TABLE 11

Taste Threshold for Selected Acids

	Range		Median	
Acid	N	%	N	%
Hydrochloric	0.00005–0.01	0.00018–0.036	0.0009	0.0033
Nitric	0.001–0.0063	0.0063–0.040	0.0011	0.0069
Sulfuric	0.00005–0.002	0.000245–0.0098	0.001	0.0049
Formic	0.0007–0.0035	0.0032–0.0161	0.0018	0.0083
Acetic	0.0001–0.0058	0.0006–0.0348	0.0018	0.0108
Butyric	0.0005–0.0035	0.0044–0.0308	0.0020	0.0176
Oxalic	0.0020–0.0032	0.0090–0.0144	0.0026	0.0117
Succinic	0.0016–0.0094	0.0094–0.0555	0.0032	0.0189
Lactic	0.00052–0.0028	0.0047–0.0252	0.0016	0.0144
Malic	0.0013–0.0023	0.00871–0.0154	0.0016	0.0107
Tartaric	0.000025–0.0072	0.000188–0.0543	0.0012	0.00905
Citric	0.0013–0.0057	0.00858–0.0376	0.0023	0.0152

Source: Pfaffmann (1959a).

According to Richard's theory, reaction of hydrogen ions at the receptor surface causes the sour taste, and, as hydrogen ions are used up, more appear from the dissociation of the acids. This would indicate that repeated tasting of subthreshold concentrations of an acid should produce a sour taste (see Kahlenberg, 1900). Harvey's (1920) work indicated that total acidity as well as pH is a factor and this appears reasonable to us. Others believe that titratable acidity is the main factor.

Using citric acid as the standard, Pangborn (1963) collected data on the relative sourness of suprathreshold levels of four organic acids (Table 12). At the threshold level, Hahn and Ulbrich (1948) found the sourness of different acids to be additive.

Taylor *et al.* (1930) believed that for equi-sour concentrations of different acids the cell pH is the same, even though the external pH

TABLE 12
Relative Sourness of Organic Acids

Concen-	Citric			Acetic			Tartaric			Lactic		
tration[a]	pH	%	M	pH	%	M	pH	%	M	pH	%	M
I	3.64	0.005	0.00026	3.62	0.004	0.00067	3.97	0.004	0.00027	3.69	0.004	0.00044
II	3.40	0.010	0.00052	3.36	0.008	0.00133	3.81	0.009	0.00060	3.54	0.008	0.00089
III	3.21	0.020	0.00104	3.16	0.017	0.00283	3.66	0.016	0.00107	3.26	0.018	0.00200
IV	3.00	0.040	0.00208	2.98	0.031	0.00516	3.50	0.031	0.00207	3.08	0.035	0.00388

[a] Values represent levels of equal sourness within each concentration, unbuffered solutions.
Source: Pangborn (1963).

may be different. Beatty and Cragg (1935) tried to correlate the intensity of sourness with buffer action. They titrated 0.0001–0.005 M solutions of acids to a pH of 4.45 in 10 ml of a phosphate buffer (3.24 g $NaH_2PO_4 \cdot H_2O$, 0.48 g $Na_2HPO_4 \cdot 12H_2O$, and 20 ml of approximately normal sodium hydroxide made to one liter—final pH 7.05). For acetic acid, the concentrations were 0.0005–0.006 M (0.0030–0.0360%). The amount of acid required to bring the pH from 7.05 to 4.45 was plotted against the pH. Figure 18 gives some typical results. Note that a line

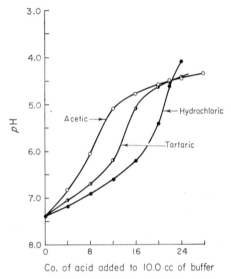

Fig. 18. Acid required to change pH of buffer. Source: Beatty and Cragg (1935).

drawn from any point on the vertical axis parallel to the horizontal axis bisects the buffer titration curves at equi-sour molar concentrations. This method was also used by Fabian and Blum (1943). Their data are shown in Table 13.

The values agree very well except for tartaric acid, where concentration by taste is about 30% higher than that by titration. The relation does not apply to salty or sweet solutions.

At 0.01 N, hydrochloric is stronger than acetic acid. In more dilute solutions, however, acetic may taste more acid, according to Baráth and Vándorfy (1926). In electrophysiological studies the response to 0.001 M (0.0060%) acetic acid is at least as large as that to 0.001 M (0.00365%) hydrochloric acid (Halpern, 1959). With rat neurons, Erickson (1958) found that the total concentration of acids (molarity) was more equivalent to stimulating efficiency than to concentrations of hydrogen ion. Other factors, e.g., chain length, may modify this.

Sugar may enhance or depress sourness (see Chapter 2, Section XVII), but it would not be expected to change the buffer titration value as demonstrated by Fabian and Blum (1943). Therefore, in the presence of other substances the phosphate buffer titration values do not correlate well with sourness. Berg *et al.* (1955a) noted that the pH of the threshold concentrations for a variety of acids varied from 3.55 to 4.15, suggesting that the anion and undissociated acid may have an effect.

TABLE 13

Equi-sour Concentrations of Various Acids as Determined by Taste and by Titration

Acid	Equi-sour by taste		Equi-sour by titration	
	M	%	M	%
Hydrochloric	0.00078	0.00284	0.00078	0.00284
Lactic	0.00085	0.00766	0.00078	0.00703
Malic	0.00075	0.01006	0.00065	0.00872
Tartaric	0.00070	0.01051	0.00048	0.00720
Acetic	0.00210	0.01261	0.00230	0.01381
Citric	0.00070	0.01345	0.00062	0.01191

Source: Fabian and Blum (1943).

Cragg (1937a,b) demonstrated that differences in the sourness of an acid could be correlated with variations in the pH of the saliva. Tasters with a more alkaline saliva required more concentrated hydrochloric acid solutions to match standard acetic acid solutions. The sour taste of buffers, or of solutions of monobasic salts of organic acids, can be detected at pH values below those of inorganic solutions. Buffer solutions also retain their acid taste in the mouth longer than pure acid solutions. If a solution of acetic acid is held in the mouth it will change pH less than a solution of hydrochloric acid. Both Cragg (1937a) and Pfaffmann (1959a) pointed out that response to different acids is not associated with the buffering effect of saliva.

Langwill (1948, 1949) tested the pH of the saliva of 499 people and considered that it did not influence the ability of the individual to differentiate the four tastes; most of the pH values were in the range 6.8–7.1, and so were most of the correct and incorrect taste identifications. Actually, inspection of her data shows a slight tendency for correct identification to increase with saliva pH up to about 7.4. This study should be expanded and repeated under more closely controlled experimental conditions.

Beidler (1952) summarized the pH-taste relation as follows:

> If, however, a weak organic acid such as acetic acid is placed on the tongue, the buffering effect of the saliva is not as great, since the acetic acid tends to dissociate to produce more hydrogen ions if those already present react with the buffer. Thus the buffer effect of the saliva present on the tongue allows the solutions containing weakly dissociated organic acids to be more effective in stimulating the acid receptors than solutions of the same pH containing strong acids. Liljestrand found that buffer mixtures of acetic acid and sodium acetate could be prepared so that a sour threshold would be found at pH 5.6, whereas the threshold for acetic acid alone was pH 3.9. He concluded that the sour taste is due to the titratable acidity of the solution. It should be remembered, however, that Pfaffmann found a large number of single taste fibers that responded to both acid and salt stimulation of the tongue of the cat. It is therefore possible that the salt of the buffer mixture itself contributes to the threshold measured by Liljestrand.
>
> The second interpretation assumes that the acids must enter the receptor cell and, therefore, pass through a lipid phase. Taylor has studied the taste thresholds of various acids and concludes that those weak acids that are more lipid-soluble are also the acids which elicit a sour sensation at a hydrogen ion concentration lower than the strong acids that are not appreciably lipid-soluble. One difficulty with this explanation is that acids usually enter cells rather slowly, whereas the sour receptors of the rat can respond to an acid solution well within 50 msec after the solution is applied to the tongue.

Beidler (1958) studied neural responses in saliva-free preparations in the rat. With nineteen organic and inorganic acids, equal-response concentrations varied from 2.2 to 180 mM at various pH's from 2.6 to 6.0. The greater response of organic acids can be accounted for by the facilitative action of the undissociated acid which is adsorbed to the receptor sites.

Nybom (1963) found a better correlation between the acid taste of apples and their titratable acidity than between acid taste and pH. This he attributes to the buffering effect of the saliva. The best correlation was given by the following equation: acid taste $= 1.75 + 0.4$ (titratable acidity) $- 0.3$ (soluble solids $-$ titratable acidity). He reported that the tasters' sensitivity and preference were influenced by the composition of the apples.

On the tongue, the sourness of an acid appears to depend on the buffering action of the saliva and the characteristics of the acid. The acidity of the solution around the cell depends on: (1) the nature of the acid; (2) the rate at which the acid is released from the bulk of the food during mastication; and (3) the amount of saliva. In behavioral studies, removing the saliva causes the thresholds for acids to be equinormal, according to Hahn *et al.* (1938). This should be investigated further.

Crozier (1916, 1918, 1934) and Taylor (1928a) believed that the intensity of the sour taste of an acid was due to the speed at which the acid penetrated the cells. However, Rosenbaum (1925) was not able to correlate penetration with acidity. Taylor did find some correlation between the order of speed of penetration of acids into tissue and the acid taste (Table 14). The amount of acid adsorbed on charcoal was

TABLE 14

Relative Concentration Gradients of Undissociated Acids Across Living Tissues Compared to Those of Formic Acid

Acid	Taste		Penetration (Crozier)
	(Taylor)	(Paul)	
Formic	1.00	1.00	1.00
Acetic	0.17	0.43	0.60
Propionic		0.53	0.36
Butyric	0.17	0.068	0.24
Isovaleric	0.21		0.10
Caprylic			
Caproic			
Bromoacetic		6.1	
Chloroacetic		7.5	5.95
Dichloroacetic			
Lactic	0.54	2.9	1.12
Benzoic			0.52
Salicylic			3.76
Succinic	0.34	0.48	0.93
Malic		1.9	4.26
Tartaric	1.60	1.1	8.00
Oxalic	6.3		6.5
Malonic			8.8
Glutaric	0.38		
Carbonic		0.019	

Source: Taylor (1928a).

also related to sourness. This order of penetration is nearly the same as that for relative sourness reported by Fabian and Blum (1943). Of course, these adsorption data could be taken to support Richard's hypothesis. In general, sour stimulation is associated with increasing lipoid solubility, with increased chain length, and with certain functional groups which reduce water solubility. Introduction of polar groups to organic acids reduces their penetrating power, and apparently their sourness.

Acid taste is much more complicated in complex biological fluids than in simple pure solutions. Moir (1936) reported differentiation between 0.2, 0.3, 0.4, and 0.5% citric in 15% sucrose; between 0.25 and 0.50% citric in 20% sucrose; and between 0.8, 0.9, 1.0, and 1.1% citric in 30% sucrose. Crisci (1930) noted that sugars, alcohols, glycerin, salts, tannin, etc., influence the sour taste of wines, in addition to pH and titratable acidity. For example, if wine is diluted with water the pH changes very little but the acid taste is much less, and addition of organic acids may not modify the pH but will make the wine more sour.

In interpreting these data one should remember that the percent dissociation decreases as the concentration increases, whereas the pH increases arithmetically with an exponential rise in hydrogen ion concentration. The relative strengths of acids depend primarily on the percent dissociation, but they are certainly modified by a number of factors.

The report of Skramlik and Schwarz (1959) that sour-tasting compounds elicited a pain sensation (which bitter or sweet compounds did not) should be investigated further. Possibly some of the anomalies of sour response to acids may be due to the interference of pain sensations.

B. SALTY

The saline taste is typified by sodium chloride. The chlorides, bromides, iodides, nitrates, and sulfates of potassium and lithium are also salty, but usually give a mixed taste. Potassium chloride is salty *and* bitter (see Chapter 2, Section VIII). The particular taste depends not only on the salt employed but on its concentration. It can also be shown that it is the ions that give the taste. Salty compounds are all soluble salts of positive and negative ions. The anion series for sodium salts is $SO_4 > Cl > Br > I > HCO_3 > NO_3$. Pfaffmann (1959a) noted that the anion has a smaller effect in the rat, in which the following series was observed in the chorda tympani: $Cl = Br > NO_3 >$ citrate $> SO_4 > CO_3$. Species differences have been attributed to differences in the detailed configurations of the reacting molecular sites on the receptor surfaces. If electrical nerve response of the chorda tympani nerve of the rat is measured, it can be shown that the cation has the predominant effect on the ability of a salt to stimulate salt receptors (Beidler, 1952). The effect of the anion on stimulative behavior is nevertheless important. Sodium chloride at $0.04\,M$ is salty whereas sodium acetate of the same molarity is not. The sodium is present in the ionic form in both, indicating a predominant effect of the chloride ion. As the molecular weight of salts increases there appears to be more bitter receptor stimulation.

Hahn *et al.* (1938) concluded that human thresholds for a just-perceptible salty taste are about equimolar for all sodium salts. Beidler

(1953) reported a much more uniform electrophysiological response to a series of sodium salt of equimolar concentration than for a cation series. From these results he suggested that salts may act in an undissociated form in a medium of low dielectric constant.

Deutsch-Renner (1937) reported a threshold range for sodium chloride of 0.0058 to 0.049 g/100 ml of solution. Bailey and Nichols, in 1888, reported 0.045% (0.0077 M). An early value of 0.001% for difference (by Venable, 1887) is the lowest value noted. Mosel and Kantrowitz (1952) obtained 0.0075 M (0.0438%) as a recognition threshold for four tasters. Knowles and Johnson (1941) reported sodium chloride thresholds of 0.001–0.08 M (0.0058–0.468%), median 0.0217 M (0.127%). Previously they reported ranges of 0.0214–0.0854 M (0.125–0.494%) and 0.0218–0.0256 M (0.127–0.150%), with respective medians of 0.04 and 0.03 M (0.234 and 0.175%). Fabian and Blum (1943) determined the sensitivity and recognition thresholds for sodium and calcium chlorides as shown in the following tabulation:

	Sensitivity	Recognition
Sodium chloride	0.011 M (0.064%)	0.039 M (0.228%)
Calcium chloride	0.0076 M (0.084%)	0.0126 M (0.140%)

These values were based on the geometric mean of 15 judges, each tasting twice. The concentrations of the solutions employed is not given, nor the range of sensitivities. In this study, calcium chloride appeared less strong than sodium chloride for sensitivity, but the taste threshold was less for the former. Fabian and Blum concluded that both cation and anion play a part in the saline taste. Schutz and Pilgrim (1957) reported an absolute threshold of 0.089% (0.0152 M) for sodium chloride. Tilgner and Barylko-Pikielna (1959) found average thresholds between 0.1 and 0.18% (0.017 and 0.0308 M). Skramlik and Schwarz (1959) give thresholds for a number of salts, but for only four subjects.

Skramlik (1926) obtained taste matches for taste intensity for various salts against mixtures of sodium chloride, quinine hydrochloride, tartaric acid, and glucose (Table 15). See also Chapter 2, Section III.

The saltiness of different salts was found to be additive (Hahn and Ulbrich, 1948). Gley and Richet (1885b) studied the saline taste of mixtures of various chlorides, and reported a synergistic action. Mixtures of chlorides, bromides, and iodides also indicated a synergistic effect. They found some evidence that the degree of saline taste was proportional to molecular weight. Skramlik and Klosa (1957) found the diammonium salt of adipic acid, $COOH(CH_2)_4COOH$, had about the same saltiness as sodium chloride. From 1 to 8 CH_2 groups can be present.

TABLE 15
Matching Taste Intensities

Subject	Salt	Matching solution (M)			
		Quinine hydrochloride	Sodium chloride	Tartaric acid	Glucose
1	KCl, 0.268 M (2.00)[a]	0.000019 (0.00070)[a]	0.273 (1.59)[a]	0.0012 (0.0150)[a]	—
2		—	0.410 (2.39)	0.000475 (0.00716)	—
3		0.000063 (0.00233)	0.410 (2.39)	0.00095 (0.01435)	—
1	KBr, 0.336 M (4.00)	0.000107 (0.00395)	0.342 (2.00)	0.00238 (0.0359)	—
2		0.000252 (0.00930)	0.496 (2.90)	0.00238 (0.0359)	—
3		0.000095 (0.00351)	0.342 (2.00)	0.00179 (0.0270)	—
1	NaI, 0.215 M (3.21)	0.000006 (0.00021)	0.103 (0.602)	0.000595 (0.00898)	0.078 (1.405)[a]
2		0.000403 (0.0149)	0.274 (1.59)	—	0.09 (1.620)
3		0.0005 (0.0185)	0.119 (0.695)	—	—

[a] ( ) % values.
Source: Skramlik (1925).

TABLE 16
Threshold Values for Selected Salts

Substance	Range M	Range %	Median M	Median %
Lithium chloride	0.009–0.04	0.038–0.170	0.025	0.106
Ammonium chloride	0.001–0.009	0.0053–0.048	0.004	0.021
Sodium chloride[a]	0.001–0.08	0.0058–0.468	0.01	0.058
Sodium chloride[b]	0.003–0.085	0.175–0.497	0.03	0.175
Potassium chloride	0.001–0.07	0.0075–0.522	0.017	0.127
Magnesium chloride	0.003–0.04	0.0286–0.381	0.015	0.143
Calcium chloride	0.002–0.03	0.0222–0.333	0.01	0.111
Sodium fluoride	0.001–0.04	0.0042–0.168	0.005	0.021
Sodium bromide	0.008–0.04	0.0823–0.412	0.024	0.247
Sodium iodide	0.004–0.1	0.0600–1.499	0.028	0.420

[a] Sensitivity threshold.
[b] Recognition threshold.
Source: Pfaffmann (1959a).

Pfaffmann (1959a) summarized the threshold values for salts as shown in Table 16.

The cation strength for chlorides has been variously reported. The generally accepted order is $NH_4 > K > Ca > Na > Li > Mg$. In electrophysiological studies the order of response for carnivores is $NH_4 > Ca > Sr > K > Mg > Na > Li$, and for rats it is $Li > Na > NH_4 > Ca > K > Sr > Mg$. Note that sodium is much more effective for rodents

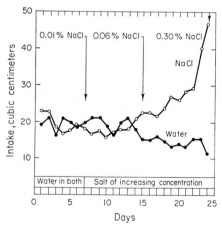

FIG. 19. Salt preference thresholds of 12 rats. At 0.06% the animals begin to show a definite preference for salt solution, which becomes greater as the concentration increases. Source: Bare, quoted in Pfaffmann (1948).

than for carnivores whereas potassium is relatively ineffective for *both*. Beidler *et al.* (1955) reported that the sodium:potassium ratios in the red blood cells were 0.12 for rodents, compared to 16.1 for carnivores, indicating a possible species difference in membrane specificity. Beidler (1962) later failed to find any correlation of the sodium:potassium ratio with taste response in sheep.

With rats the preference threshold for sodium chloride begins at 0.01–0.06%, but peak preference is 0.5–1.0%. Above this, salt intake diminishes, and little salt is taken above 3.0% (see Fig 19). For adaptation to salt, see Chapter 5, Section V and Abrahams *et al.* (1937). The data of Irvin and Goetzl (1952) seemed to show a diurnal fluctuation in sensitivity to salt.

C. Sweet

The sweet taste is produced by a variety of nonionized aliphatic hydroxy compounds, particularly alcohols, glycols, sugars, and sugar derivatives. Electrolytes such as beryllium and some lead salts are sweet, and many α-amino acids are also sweet, although the β- and, particularly, the γ-forms are usually not. β-Glucose derivatives are more bitter than α-glucose derivatives, but both are sweet.

Saccharin is the best known synthetic sweetening agent, being 200–700 times as sweet as sucrose. Its sweetness is presumably due to the anion

Other sweet substances are dulcin, cyclamate, and the 4-alkoxy-3-amino-nitrobenzenes. Dulcin (or *p*-ethoxyphenylurea) is over 300 times as sweet as sucrose at low concentration. Kamen (1959) showed that mixtures of sucrose and calcium cyclamate were significantly sweeter at *moderate concentrations* than would be predicted from simple additiveness. He noted that this might be explained if the sweet receptors were differentially sensitive to the two compounds. Mixtures of the two would then excite a larger number of receptors and appear more intense in sweetness. Or, if the cyclamate has a bitter note that tends to suppress the sweet taste, this bitter note would be more dilute in mixtures and the solution would appear sweeter. For the sweetness of cyclamate and saccharin, see Vincent *et al.* (1955).

Many glycols are sweet; erythritol is more than twice as sweet as sucrose. The lower homologs of halogenated hydrocarbons are usually sweet, and increasing the number of halogen atoms in the molecule tends to increase the sweetness. Most amides are bitter, but the introduction of groups such as halogen, phenyl, or hydroxyl tends to give a sweet taste. A few aldehydes and ketones are sweet. Many esters are sweet, but some are bitter or produce burning sensations. Esters of low-molecular-weight alcohols and inorganic acids are usually sweet, and increasing the molecular weight tends to increase the sweetness. Furane derivatives and nitriles are often sweet, as are hydrazides and substituted benzenes. The *n*-propyl derivative of 4-alkoxy-3-aminonitrobenzene is about 5000 times as sweet as sucrose, and is also toxic. See Petersen and Müller (1948) for other sweet compounds of this type. Some substituted naphthoisotriazines are sweet. The sweetness of some synthetic compounds approaches the intensity of bitterness of some bitter compounds. For further data on sweetness see Cohn's (1914) and Lawrence and Ferguson's (1959) compilations.

Not all mammals show gustatory neural responses to sugars. Electrical records from taste fibers, however, generally show a response, as the data in Table 17 indicate. According to Carpenter (1956),

TABLE 17

Relative Magnitude of Neural Response

Stimulus	M	%	Rat	Ham-ster	Guinea Pig	Dog	Cat	Rabbit
Ammonium chloride	0.5	2.1	—	—	—	1.0	1.0	1.0
Sodium chloride	0.1	0.58	1.0	1.0	1.0	—	—	—
Hydrochloric acid	0.01	0.037	0.61	0.85	0.44	0.16	0.36	0.56
Sucrose	0.5	17.1	0.21	0.75	0.62	0.27	0–0.20	0.52
Quinine-HCl	0.02	0.072	0.20	0.33	0.24	0.09	0.31	0.48

Source: Beidler *et al.* (1955).

cats can be conditioned to taste sugar (although they do not show a preference for it), probably, as Prosser (1954) suggests, by nerves other than those used to make the electrical recordings mentioned above.

Recordings from the chorda tympani of the dog showed the following order of decreasing stimulating ability: D-fructose > sucrose > L-sorbose > D-mannose > D-glucose > maltose > D-galactose > lactose (Andersen *et al.*, 1962), which agrees quite well with psychophysiological investigations.

Determining individual sugar thresholds, a complicated problem, has been attacked by a variety of techniques—with an equal diversity of results. Pfaffmann (1948) reported encountering two subjects who disliked 9% sugar solutions. It would be valuable to determine whether thresholds are influenced by individual preferences. The main procedures have been: (1) the absolute threshold; and (2) the method of successive approximations or comparisons. The threshold procedure allows for rapid determination, but thresholds vary with individuals and are difficult to determine accurately. Furthermore, threshold sugar concentrations give no information of supraliminal sweetness. Richter and Campbell (1940a) reported that the following tastes were noted by subjects in below-threshold concentrations of sucrose solutions: 12 bitter, 8 sour, 7 salty, 6 acid, 6 "chemical," 5 "medicine," 4 "lemon," 3 "peppermint," etc. The purity of the sugars used, and possibly the appetite of the tasters, may have been a factor. Two children did not recognize the sweetness of a 10% (0.292 M) sucrose solution! Young adults (45) had taste thresholds of 0.41% (0.0119 M); 58 children, 0.68% (0.0198 M); 52 elderly patients, 1.23% (0.0356 M). Richter and Campbell (1940b) showed that rats could distinguish between water and solutions of various sugars at the following concentrations: maltose, 0.06% (0.0016 M); glucose, 0.20% (0.0111 M); sucrose, 0.57% (0.0167 M); and galactose, 1.60% (0.0888 M). Schutz and Pilgrim (1957) reported a threshold for sucrose of 0.35% (0.0102 M). Tilgner and Barylko-Pikielna (1959) reported average values of between 0.1 and 0.4% (0.0029–0.0116 M). Pfaffmann (1959a) has summarized some of the threshold data as shown in Table 18.

TABLE 18
Thresholds for Selected Sweet Compounds

	Range		Median	
Substance	M	%	M	%
Sucrose[a]	0.005–0.016	0.171–0.548	0.01	0.342
Sucrose[b]	0.012–0.037	0.411–1.267	0.017	0.582
Glucose	0.04–0.09	0.721–1.621	0.08	1.442
Saccharin (Na)	0.00002–0.00004	0.00041–0.00082	0.000023	0.00047
Beryllium chloride	—	—	0.0003	0.0024
Sodium hydroxide	0.002–0.012	0.0080–0.0480	0.008	0.0320

[a] Detection threshold.
[b] Recognition threshold.
Source: Pfaffmann (1959a).

The sweetness of a sugar is related, in part, to its solubility. Attempts to relate sweetness to a "contraction coefficient" (sum of atomic volumes/molecular volume) have not been very successful. Bronshtein (1950) reported that an oxygen deficiency decreased sensitivity to sugar. Oxygen deficiency first increased, but later reduced, sensitivity to the other taste qualities.

At suprathreshold concentrations, care must be exercised in determining sweetness. It was first observed in the confectionary trade that the relative sweetness of sucrose and glucose varied with concentration. Lichtenstein (1948) showed that the sweetness of 10% sucrose was equivalent to that of 15.5% glucose, and that 40% sucrose was equivalent to 48.1% glucose. Thus, at 10% sucrose, glucose was 65% as sweet; at 25%, 71% as sweet; and 40%, 83% as sweet. A mixture of two-thirds sucrose and one-third glucose gave a sweetness equivalent to that calculated from the above. At high percentages glucose was bitter and burned the throat, which suggests that sweetness may not have been the only factor involved. Much data of this type have been collected and summarized by Cameron (1947), who employed the method of "right and wrong answers" to determine equisweetness. For a sucrose solution equisweet to 15% galactose he obtained the results given in Table 19. Based on these calculations, Cameron concluded that 15%

TABLE 19

Determination of Amount of Sucrose Equivalent in
Sweetness to 15% Galactose

Sucrose %	Tasters %	Reporting sucrose sweeter %
7.5	100	0
8.5	100	3
9.5	100	37
10.5	100	70
11.5	100	90
12.5	100	100
Difference 5	Sum 600	Sum 300

Calculation: $300 \times 5/600 = 2.5$; $12.5 - 2.5 = 10.0$.
Source: Cameron (1947).

galactose was equivalent in sweetness to 10.0% sucrose. The data were based on 15 trained judges, all of whom participated in each test. Judges were allowed to indicate that the paired samples were equal in sweetness and their judgments were then divided between the sucrose and the galactose. The method gives only an approximation of equivalent sweetness, since it is based on the assumption that, if the number of tasters is sufficiently large, there will be an even distribution of results about the calculated mean value.

Cameron's curves for equisweetness to sucrose are shown in Fig. 20. For equisweetness to glucose, see Fig. 21. Differences from earlier data

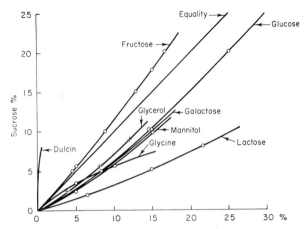

FIG. 20. Curves showing the sweetness of various compounds compared with sucrose. Data for fructose include Dahlberg and Penczek's (1941) values. The dulcin curve only approximates to the values found. Source: Cameron (1947).

may have arisen from using too few tasters and failing to take the mutarotation of glucose and other sugars into account (Cameron, 1947; Pangborn and Gee, 1961).

The concept of changing sweetness with concentration is well established, but the relative sweetness of glycerol, glucose, galactose, and lactose remains relatively stable, as the logarithmic curves show (Fig.

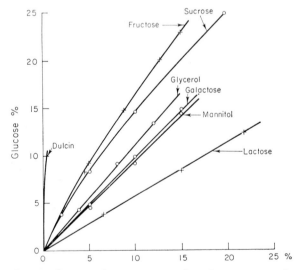

FIG. 21. Curves showing the sweetness of various compounds compared to sucrose. Source: Cameron (1947).

22). Cameron (1947) noted that very sensitive tasters may be misled by additional taste sensations such as bitterness, in comparing relative sweetness.

Mixtures of sucrose and glucose are sweeter than anticipated if calculated in terms of sucrose, but not if calculated in terms of glucose. Cameron calculated the sweetness of mixtures in terms of sucrose. With

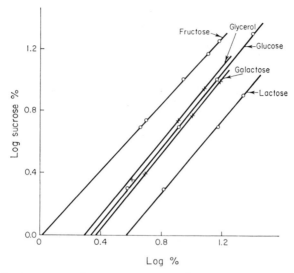

Fig. 22. Equisweetness of various sugars on a logarithmic scale. Source: Cameron (1947).

amino acids, the sweetness of the mixtures was less than calculated, and no compound formation was noted. Pfaffmann (1959a) noted that when such mixtures are computed in terms of equisweet glucose concentrations the sweetness of the mixture is the sum of the components. If the magnitude of nerve impulse discharge determines the magnitude of the sweet taste directly, the sensory effect of glucose is linearly proportional to concentration but that of sucrose is curvilinear, i.e., negatively accelerated. Figure 23 gives a graphical solution of the results of addition of 0.2 M sucrose. The total sensory effect of the mixture should be the sum of the two functions at point B, which is equal to 62 units, a magnitude of response that could be produced by either 0.34 sucrose or 0.94 glucose, individually. The empirical match in the original mixture can be stated as:

$$0.2G + 0.2S = 0.34S \qquad (3)$$

In sucrose-equisweet solutions, where $0.2G = 0.04S$, Eq. (3) becomes:

$$0.04S + 0.2S = (\text{sucrose match})$$

Since the arithmetic sum of 0.04S + 0.2S is 0.24 and not 0.34 (a difference of 0.10), there is supplemental action; that is, the empirical match shows a stronger sucrose concentration than could be predicted by the simple addition of equisweet sucrose solutions. Expressing Eq. (3) in terms of glucose, where $0.2S = 0.74G$, $0.2G + 0.74G = 0.94G$ (and $0.94G = 0.34S$).

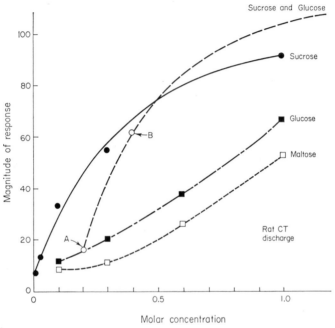

FIG. 23. Response of rat chorda tympani nerve to different concentrations of various sugars. The dashed sucrose and glucose line is the summated response to be expected when sucrose solutions are added to 0.2 M glucose. Source: Hagstrom in Pfaffmann (1959a).

According to Pfaffmann, "The arithmetic sum of $0.2G + 0.74G$ equals exactly 0.94G which is the same as the equivalent glucose value to match 0.34 sucrose. There is no supplemental action by this computation. The apparent supplemental action with one set of transformations but not the other is due to the attempt to add arithmetically one linear to another nonlinear function. . . . The additive analysis is theoretical except that the response curves for the individual sugars are based upon experimental points."

A similar situation occurs for glucose and galactose, where the sweetness is additive if expressed relative to either of these sugars but is not when expressed relative to sucrose. For invert sugar below 10%, sucrose

TABLE 20
Sweetness of Various Glucose Concentrations

Concentration (%)	Sweetness (relative to sucrose)
1	45.5
2	50
5	58
10	66
15	72.5
20	78
25	82
30	86
35	90
40	93.5
45	97
50	100

Source: Nieman (1960).

inversion slightly reduces sweetness, but above 10% increases it. Finally, Cameron calculated that $S = KC^m$ or $\log S = \log K + m \log C$, where S is sweetness, C is concentration, and K and m are constants. Figure 22 shows a plot of log sweetness versus log concentration which gives additional support to Weber's law (Chapter 5, Section IV,A).

Nieman (1958) criticized earlier summaries of the relative sweetness of sugars because they included data which had been obtained by uncritical methods. Concentrations of about 5–15% glucose are about

TABLE 21
Relative Sweetness of Various Concentrations of Glucose Syrups
of Two Dextrose-Equivalent (DE) Ratings

Concentration (%)	Relative Sweetness	
	DE = 42%	DE = 64%
5	30.5	42
10	33	49
15	36	53
20	39	63.5
25	41.5	69.5
30	44	75.5
35	47	81
40	50.5	85
45	54	89
50	58	91

Source: Nieman (1960).

60–79% as sweet as a 10% sucrose solution. There are wide divergencies in the data, however. The reasons for these differences are methodological, chemical, and subjective.

Schutz and Pilgrim (1957) found that glucose had a minimum sweetness at about 8%, corresponding to a 4% sucrose solution. Nieman (1960) summarized his values in Table 20. For glucose syrups with "dextrose" equivalents (DE) of 42 and 64%, the relative sweetness values were as shown in Table 21.

For fructose, Nieman (1958) gave the following values:

Concentration (%)	Relative sweetness
5.0	111.5
10.0	115
15.0	118.5

The relative sweetness of dulcin and saccharin at different concentrations was summarized by Nieman (1958) as shown in Table 22. He

TABLE 22
Relative Sweetness of Sucrose, Dulcin, and Saccharin[a]

Sucrose (%)	Dulcin		Saccharin	
	1[b]	2[b]	1	3[b]
1.7	—	—	—	67,500
2.0	38,500	—	55,600	—
2.7	—	—	—	55,300
3.0	26,300	—	49,200	—
3.4	—	26,800	—	—
3.9	—	—	—	39,900
4.0	15,400	—	41,700	—
4.1	—	16,400	—	—
4.6	—	9,200	—	—
5.0	10,900	—	35,200	—
6.0	9,100	—	29,400	—
6.2	—	—	—	31,700
7.0	8,100	—	25,600	—
8.0	7,600	—	22,300	—
9.0	7,100	—	20,300	—
10.0	6,900	—	18,900	—
10.2	—	—	—	26,100
15.0	—	—	—	19,200

[a] Relative to 100 for sucrose.

[b] 1, Täufel and Klemm (1925); 2, Cameron (1947); 3, Magidson and Gorbachow (1923).

also summarized similar data for lactose, maltose, fructose, galactose, mannitol, and glycerol.

When glucose is used as the comparison solution, the results are somewhat different. The curves for fructose, sucrose, glycerol, and galactose are close to that for glucose (Fig. 20). In other words, the different sugars appear more nearly equally sweet when compared to glucose. It is unlikely that glucose will become the reference sugar, so common is the use of sucrose for the standard.

Nieman (1958, 1960) has summarized the best data in the relative sweetness of different sugars compared to 10% sucrose (see Table 23).

TABLE 23
Relative Sweetness of Sugars

Sugar	Relative sweetness	Sugar	Relative sweetness
Raffinose	22	α,β-D-Glucose	69
Rhamnose	33	Glycerol	79
Lactose	39	Invert sugar	65
Dulcitol	41	D-Fructose	114
Maltose	46	Glycyrrhizin	15,000
D-Sorbitol	51	Steviosid	30,000
D-Mannose	59	Calcium cyclamate	3,380
Galactose	63	Dulcin	9,000
D-Xylose	67	Saccharin	30,000
D-Mannitol	69	(Kristallose)	70,000

Source: Nieman (1958).

The special problem of the relative sweetness of invert sugar should be considered. After hydrolysis, 10% sucrose would be 10.53% invert sugar, corresponding to 5.26% glucose and 5.26% fructose. If Nieman's

TABLE 24
Additive Sweetness in Mixtures

Sucrose (%)	Dulcin (%)	Saccharin (%)	Total relative sweetness
4.6	0.0030	0.0063	43,000
5.0	0.0041	0.0081	41,000
6.0	0.0052	0.0102	39,000
7.0	0.0065	0.0131	36,000
8.0	0.0079	0.0170	32,000
9.0	0.0090	0.0220	29,000
10.0	0.0099	0.0289	26,000

Source: Nieman (1958).

TABLE 25
Comparative Sweetness of Sucrose and Sucrose-Glucose Mixtures

Sucrose (%)	Mixture of equal sweetness		Relative sweetness of glucose[a]
	Sucrose (%)	Glucose (%)	
15.0	10.0	5.3	94
15.0	10.0	5.5	91
15.0	5.0	11.8	85
20.0	10.0	10.15	98
20.0	15.0	7.00	70
20.0	10.0	13.3	75
25.0	16.7	8.3	100
40.0	26.7	13.0	102

[a] Assumes sucrose at 100.

Source: Niemann (1958).

(1958) values of 56 and 112 for the relative sweetness are used, the invert sugar solution should have a relative sweetness of 1.053 × 84, or 88. In practice, the relative sweetness is higher, about 95.

This additive effect of mixtures was demonstrated by Paul (1922). The equivalent-sweetness data in Table 24 illustrate the effect. Since a 0.146% dulcin solution or a 0.053% saccharin solution is equisweet to sucrose, it is obvious that mixtures of the two are much sweeter (0.0099 and 0.0289 being equisweet). Niemann (1958) summarized results from Roederer (1952) and other workers for sucrose and glucose (see Table 25).

The influence of increasing temperature of the solution on increasing apparent sweetness is especially important. Tsuzuki and Yamazaki (1953) and also Yamazaki *et al.* (1947) gave the following values for D-fructose at suprathreshold concentrations:

Temperature (°C)	Relative sweetness
5	143.7
18	128.5
40	100.0
60	79.0

Parker (1922) and Crocker and Henderson (1932) gave a threshold value of 0.02 M (0.685%) for sucrose. Bailey and Nichols (1888) reported 0.5% (0.0146 M), which was probably a sensitivity value, not a recognition value. Henning's (1921) summary gave values of 0.009–0.5% (0.00026–0.0146 M). Mosel and Kantrowitz (1952) reported 0.0175 M

(0.5985%) for four tasters. King (1937) reported 0.0128 *M* (0.438%). Knowles and Johnson (1941) reported thresholds for sucrose of 0.003 *M* (0.103–0.171%), median 0.0224 *M* (0.767%). Fabian and Blum (1943) reported the relatively high thresholds shown in Table 26.

TABLE 26
Thresholds of Sugars

Sugar	Sensitivity		Identification	
	M	%	*M*	%
Sucrose	0.016	0.56	0.037	1.30
Glucose	0.045	0.80	0.090	1.63
Fructose	0.020	0.35	0.052	0.94
Maltose	0.038	1.36	0.080	2.89
Lactose	0.072	2.60	0.116	4.19

Source: Fabian and Blum (1943).

Deutsch-Renner (1937) reported relative sweetness (not threshold) values of 1.005 for fructose, 0.53 for glucose, 0.48 for glycerol, and 0.27 for lactose when sucrose was given an arbitrary value of 1.00. He reported thresholds for glucose to vary from 0.072 to 0.144 g/100 g of solution. Different values in the literature may be due to the difficulty of purifying the sugars.

Berg *et al.* (1955a) reported the following thresholds (as grams per 100 ml):

	$p = 0.001$	$p_c = 0.50$
Fructose	0.15	0.13
Glucose	0.40	0.44
Sucrose	0.30	0.31
Glycerol	0.38	0.44

In this case, p_c is the concentration where the difference could be detected 50% of the time, based on the psychologically justified assumption that the percent of correct judgments is a measure of intensity of sensation or a measure of the difference in intensity between two samples. Pangborn (1963), using a similar technique, obtained the data shown in Table 27.

Wykes (1952) reported that honeybees preferred sucrose and glucose to fructose. An equal mixture of the three was preferred to any one, any two, or unequal mixtures of the three. For uptake, the order was sucrose, glucose, maltose (not present in nectar), and fructose. The

TABLE 27
Sweetness of Fructose, Glucose, and Lactose as Compared to Sucrose

	Threshold concentrations (%)			
	Sucrose	Fructose	Glucose	Lactose
Absolute threshold[a]	0.017	0.016	0.132	0.160
$p = 0.001$	0.064	0.059	0.242	0.220

	Suprathreshold concentrations (%)[b]			
	Sucrose	Fructose	Glucose	Lactose
	0.5	0.42	0.89	1.90
	1.0	0.76	1.84	3.46
	2.0	1.66	3.57	6.54
	5.0	4.19	8.28	15.74
	10.0	8.62	13.86	25.92
	15.0	12.97	20.00	34.60

[a] Concentration at which 50% of the responses correctly distinguished the solution containing sugar from a distilled-water blank (paired comparison).
[b] Values represent levels of equal sweetness within each concentration.
Source: Pangborn (1963).

equal mixture was again preferred. Evans (1961) showed that fructose in the media during rearing of the larvae of the blowfly greatly depressed the sensitivity of the resulting adults to fructose and also to sucrose.

An internal scale for sweetness has been constructed by MacLeod (1952), who found log I glucose = 0.681 log I sucrose + 0.439. Such a scale needs to be tested by application to practical problems. If substantiated, it would be very useful.

Of interest besides relative sweetness levels are the differences that tasters can detect. Berg et al. (1955a) reported the following data for glucose:

Concentration (g/100 ml)	Difference for $p = 0.001$	Difference for $p_e = 0.50$
1.0	0.4	0.7
5.0	0.6	0.8
10.0	0.8	0.8
15.0	1.0	1.1

Those investigators (1955b) also studied the influence of tartaric acid and ethyl alcohol on the sweet taste. Table 28 summarizes some of their

TABLE 28

Effect of Ethyl Alcohol and Acid on Minimum Detectable Concentration Differences for Sucrose

Sucrose (g/100 ml)	In water	% alcohol: % acid[a]							
		10:0	20:0	0:0.3	0:0.6	10:0.3	10:0.6	20:0.3	20:0.6
0[b]	0.3	0.4	0.5	0.6	0.6	0.8	0.7	0.8	0.8
1[c]	0.4	0.6	0.7	0.5	0.5	0.7	0.7	0.9	0.9
5[c]	0.5	1.0	1.0	0.6	0.6	0.8	1.0	1.5	1.5
10[c]	0.6	1.8	2.4	1.0	0.9	1.4	1.5	2.6	2.6
15[c]	0.9	2.7	—	1.4	—	—	—	—	—

[a] Mixture of lactic, succinic, malic, and tartaric acids.
[b] Absolute threshold.
[c] Difference threshold.
Source: Berg *et al.* (1955b).

data. It can be seen that the difference threshold increased with concentration, as expected from Weber's ratio (Chapter 5, Section IV,A). Acidity raised the difference threshold slightly, and the absolute threshold to a greater extent. Alcohol did not change the absolute threshold as much as the difference thresholds. A solution of 10% alcohol and 8% sucrose was as sweet as a 10% aqueous sucrose solution; 20% alcohol and 7% sucrose was equivalent in sweetness to 10% sucrose. Olfactory stimulation by the alcohol may have influenced these results. Berg *et al.* (1955b) showed that sugar tended to raise the alcohol difference threshold in water but not in red wines.

Sucrose (g/100 ml)	Alcohol difference threshold		
	10% Alcohol	10% Alcohol: 0.3% acid	Red table wine
0	2.0	2.5	4.0
5	3.0	2.5	4.0
10	4.0	3.5	4.0

Some significant interactions in taste, with and without tannin, were found at different levels of sugar. For the effect of acids on sugar difference thresholds in foods, see Pangborn *et al.* (1959, 1960).

Moir (1936) says tasters should be able to distinguish between 18 and 22% sucrose. Dahlberg and Penczek (1941), however, found experienced tasters who could detect differences between 2.00 and 2.07, 10.00 and 10.25, 20.0 and 20.5, 30.0 and 31.0, 40.0 and 41.5, and 50.0

and 52.0% sucrose. Sale and Skinner (1922) reported four tasters who could distinguish between 2.0 and 2.1% sucrose solutions accurately and consistently, whereas Biester *et al.* (1925), with untrained tasters, required greater differences. In the latter study, only 59.6% of the tasters could distinguish between 0.75 and 4.00% sucrose, 46.9% differentiated between 5.25 and 10.00% sucrose, and 58.4% between 0.75 and 9.75% sucrose. Since those individuals' thresholds were also high (0.6 for sucrose, 0.58 for fructose, and 1.25 for glucose), there were, perhaps, problems in methodology or insensitive tasters. The data of Cameron (1947) do not substantiate those of Berg *et al.* (1955a) or of Dahlberg and Penczek (1941). Using triangular testing, Cameron found that only 49% of 179 students could distinguish between 8 and 10% sucrose in two successive trails. However, in this case triangular testing may have given less sensitive discrimination than paired testing. Also, trained subjects are more sensitive than untrained.

In an experiment with jams where 25% of the sucrose was replaced by glucose (on a weight basis), a panel was unable to distinguish the all-sucrose from the sucrose-glucose jams (Gridgeman, 1956). Furthermore, with the particular panel, there did not seem to be any correlation between sweetness and preference, although some subjects did associate the two.

The reaction time for sucrose is 0.446 sec, according to Kiesow (1903). An earlier value (0.384 sec) by Vintschgau and Hönigschmied (1877b) is not very different.

It has already been noted that the amount of sugar consumed appears to be related to the blood sugar level. Mayer-Gross and Walker (1946) have also shown that tasters with blood sugar at a normal level found 30% sucrose sickeningly sweet whereas tasters with blood sugar at one half the normal level found that the same concentration tasted very good. They pointed out that stress may influence acceptability by changing palatability, the flow of digestive juices, motor phenomena in the digestive tract, or the composition of body fluids. The method used affects the results in animal studies, according to Pfaffmann (1956). For example, when saccharin solutions were presented in six concentrations, 0.25% was favored unless the rats were thirsty; then the 0.075% solution was preferred. Some animal experiments show that sucrose is preferred over glucose in approximately the ratio of its relative sweetness. Electrophysiological data also show greater apparent nerve discharge to sucrose than to equimolar solutions of glucose. Recording the unit activity of single neurons of hypothalamic centers of dogs, obtained electroencephalographically through implanted electrodes, Anand *et al.* (1962) indicated that increases in blood glucose increase the activity of the satiety-center neurons and decrease the activity of feeding-center neurons.

Ever since saccharin was prepared by Fahlberg and Remsen in 1879, its remarkable sweet taste has been known, but a bitter off taste was noted by Stutzer (1886), and later by Helgren *et al.* (1955) and Hamor (1961) and by the general public. The off taste has been ascribed to thermal decomposition, trace impurities of synthesis inter-mediates, age of the solution, and other factors, but variations in tech-nique probably account for the lack of concordant results. A careful study by Helgren *et al.* (1955) did not substantiate that any of the above factors were responsible for the "off taste," but rather that, for sensitive tasters, it is intrinsic in the saccharin molecule. They found six of 51 tasters (about 12%) to be insensitive to the off taste. For the remaining tasters the relation of off taste and concentration was as listed in Table 29.

TABLE 29

Off Taste of Saccharin as Related to Concentration

Sodium saccharin concentration (%)	People finding off taste	
	No.	%
0.01	0	0
0.02	7	13.7
0.04	18	35.3
0.08	27	52.9
0.16	37	72.5
0.32	45	88.2

Source: Helgren *et al.* (1955).

They also found no difference in off taste when they used calcium saccharin or sodium saccharin prepared by a new synthesis. A 0.026% saccharin solution is roughly equivalent to a 10% sucrose solution. At this concentration, about 25% of the population can be expected to find the off taste. In an effort to reduce this percentage, mixtures of saccharin and sodium cyclamate (Sucaryl) have been studied. A 1:10 mixture was best. It is of interest that the relative sweetness of sodium cyclamate is 350 times that of sucrose when near the absolute threshold but that the relative strength decreases as the concentration increases. Täufel and Klemm (1925) showed that the sweetness of sodium saccharate and of dulcin relative to sucrose increased in 20, 29, and 40% alcohol. Beidler (1962) reported that the equilibrium constant for the reaction of sac-charin in taste cells was about 1700, compared to constants of only 0.5 to 15.0 for most other stimulus-receptor reactions. He therefore postulated that saccharin does not necessarily combine with the same sites as sucrose. A variety of evidence shows that rats and human beings do not react the same to sweet substances. Solutions of sodium cyclamate that humans preferred to saccharin were rejected by rats.

Although sweetness recognition thresholds are of interest, they are of only limited application in food products, where concentrations are usually much higher than the threshold. Chappell (1953), for example, tested 25% solutions on two occasions with 20 tasters. The results are shown in Table 30 (the tasters marked only one, but some chose none).

TABLE 30
Acceptability of Selected Sugars

	Test 1			Test 2		
Sugar	Sweetest	Least sweet	Most acceptable	Sweetest	Least sweet	Most acceptable
Maltose	0	1	1	0	1	2
Lactose	0	9	1	0	19	2
Glucose	0	4	1	0	0	1
Sucrose	8	0	12	4	0	8
Fructose	12	0	0	16	0	4

Source: Chappell (1953).

There were 17 complaints about the flavor of maltose. Sucrose was the most acceptable sugar, and maltose the least. Fructose was about 25% sweeter than sucrose, and lactose 40% less sweet. The most popular concentrations were 15% for fructose and 20 or 25% for sucrose. If small amounts of lemon or orange oil (0.05 ml/100 ml) were added, a wider range of sucrose solutions was acceptable and the 25% solution was the most popular. It is of interest to note that at higher concentrations of sugar the panels indicated that the lemon and orange flavors were more intense even though the concentrations were the same. This is probably a factor which operates in the flavor of liqueurs.

Young and Greene (1953a,b) reported that preference was influenced by the type of test. When a single sample was presented, 9% sucrose was preferred to 36%. When both solutions were presented simultaneously, however, 36% was preferred to 9%. Single-stimulus presentation measures relative acceptability, not preference, since the latter implies choice.

Fatigue may be a factor in testing sugars. Using two triangular tests in succession with maple syrup, Elder (1955) reported significantly less success with the second triangle than with the first. This observation differs from that of Dawson *et al.* (1963), who found that acuity of perception of solutions of sucrose, caffeine, sodium chloride, and tartaric acid was greater in the second three than in the first three sets of triangle tests presented at one tasting session. In a second study, the number of correct identifications was greater in a second five than in a first five sets of paired presentations. In this latter study, however, the intensities were considerably lower than those in maple syrup.

Hahn *et al.* (1940) showed that the time required for adaptation increases with concentration. Dethier (1952), using an insect, found time required for adaptation to sucrose increased as the logarithm of concentration.

Pfaffmann (1959a) reported that an observed reduction in sweetness and bitterness from the action of gymnema leaf extract was substantiated by a lesser electrical activity in the chorda tympani. Since individual afferent receptor neural units respond to both salt and sucrose, and since gymnema blocks only the sweet and bitter sensations, this difference strongly suggests that there are sites on the receptor cell which the gymnema does and does not block. Pfaffmann also noted that the response to sugar was resistant to enzyme poisons and pH change but not to surface-active competitive inhibitors. Warren and Pfaffmann (1959) suggested that in the events leading to sweet and bitter sensation there is a common step which can be blocked by gymnemate. This field should certainly be explored more widely.

It is of interest to note that gustatory desensitization reduces sugar preference and quinine aversion. Pfaffmann (1964) notes that the sweet taste certainly instigates ingestion and also serves as a reward or reinforcement for learning. The vigor of response to sugar solutions as reflected in the rate of response appears to be determined by the strength of the taste stimulus reinforcing that response.

Pangborn (1960a) found sweetness discrimination not to be influenced by red, green, or yellow coloring of aqueous solutions. With pear nectar, however, sweetness was associated less with green color than with uncolored, or red, yellow, or blue samples. There was a tendency for apricot- and cherry-flavored aqueous solutions to be marked somewhat sweeter than they really were, especially when the sugar concentrations were small. Red illumination interfered with discrimination more with trained judges than with untrained judges. Using wines colored to simulate five wine types, Pangborn *et al.* (1963) observed that experienced wine tasters ascribed greater sweetness to pink wines, whereas naive subjects had no color-sweetness association.

D. Bitter

The typical bitter stimuli are alkaloids such as quinine, caffeine, and strychnine. The bitter taste is often associated with compounds harmful to man, but no single class of chemical compounds is characteristically bitter. Several electrolytes (magnesium and ammonium salts, for example) are bitter. Some low-molecular-weight salts are sweet, whereas higher-molecular-weight substances are bitter. Salts of cesium or rubidium are bitter, as are iodide salts. Nitro compounds, such as picric acid, are often bitter and the bitterness increases as the number of nitro groups increases. According to Kaneko (1939) and Berg (1953), the L-isomers of the α-amino acids are generally bitter to man. The rat, however, selected L- and DL-alanine but rejected the D-forms (Halpern *et al.*, 1962). In man, the amino group may obliterate the taste of a bitter substance. If there are enough amino groups to make the compound distinctly alkaline, the taste is bitter. Most amides are bitter. Glucosides, benzamide, and the substituted benzamides are usually bitter, as are some aldehydes and ketones, esters, nitriles, isocyanides, urethans, N,N'-hydrazinedicarboxylic acids, and substituted benzenes and naphthoisotriazines.

The bitter and sweet tastes are frequently associated; both sensations are inhibited by the action of gymnemic acid, and there is a change in taste from sweet to bitter in the homologous series of hydroxy aliphatic alcohols. Ethylene glycol and trimethylene glycol are sweet, propylene glycol is slightly sweet, tetramethylene glycol is barely sweet, and hexamethylene glycol is bitter. Some compounds are first bitter and then sweet, e.g., o-benzoylbenzoic acid, p-aminoazobenzene sulfonic acid, L-leucyl-D-tryptophan, and phenolphthalein. Tetrachloroethyl ether and 2,3-dichlorohexane are bitter *and* slightly sweet. Hexenylglycerin is slightly bitter and sweet. Sodium ethyl sulfonate is bitterish and later slightly sweet. Phenylurea, $C_6H_5NHCONH_2$, is bitter, but p-tolylurea, $p\text{-}CH_3C_6H_4NHCONH_2$, is sweet. Glycol, CH_2OHCH_2OH, is sweet, but phenylglycol, $C_6H_5CHOHCH_2OH$, is bitter. The close interrelationship between bitter and sweet sensations raises the question of whether these "basic" tastes are qualitatively or only quantitatively different.

Using 6 subjects, Engel (1928) indicated almost 100% "unpleasant" response to 0.001% quinine sulfate solutions. However, as Harper (1962) noted, the panel was very small, and nonalcoholic beverages containing considerable quinine are quite popular. Responses are not necessarily the same to blended stimuli as to aqueous solutions (see also Pangborn, 1963).

Moncrieff (1951) suggested that the introduction of a phenyl group produces a bitter taste because of the increase in molecular weight. Addition of methoxy groups has a tendency to convert tasteless substances into bitter ones, with some exceptions. The group —CO—NH—N:C= is bitter in aqueous solutions. Urea is bitter, but α-dimethylurea is sweet and the diethyl compound is also sweet. Thus the influence of structure on bitterness is complicated. Intensive, systematic investigations are needed before theories can be formulated.

Urea   α -Dimethylurea

It is generally considered that bitterness is a taste sensation which can be evoked by the lowest concentrations. The idea that all poisonous substances are bitter is not correct, as shown by Richter's (1950) data (Table 31). Note the lack of taste of poisonous substances and the absence of a relation between solubility and taste.

TABLE 31
Detection of Bitterness by Rats and Humans

| Substance | Solubility[a] | Percent able to taste | | LD$_{50}$[b] |
		Rats	Humans	
Strychnine sulfate	3200	100	100	5
Mercuric chloride	6900	100	93	40
Phenyl thiourea	260	100	100	9
Barium carbonate	Ins.	0	0	1480
Zinc phosphide	Ins.	0	61-(odor?)	40
Thallium sulfate	4870	0	0	16

[a] Milligrams per 100 ml.
[b] Lethal dose for 50% of wild Norway rats, mg per kg.
Source: Richter (1950).

Using 38 subjects, Harris and Kalmus (1949–1950b) employed solutions of quinine sulfate and reported thresholds (as quinine) from 2.4×10^{-4} to $5.7 \times 10^{-6} M$ (7.79×10^{-1} to $1.85 \times 10^{-4}\%$). Moncrieff (1951) reported quinine thresholds of 4×10^{-5} to $1.5 \times 10^{-6} M$ (1.30×10^{-3} to $4.87 \times 10^{-5}\%$). Lugg (1955) gave a value of $1.3 \times 10^{-6} M$ ($4.22 \times 10^{-5}\%$), and this appears to be the lowest recorded threshold for quinine. However, Deutsch-Renner (1937) observed a threshold for quinine hydrochloride of $2 \times 10^{-7} M$ ($7.22 \times 10^{-6}\%$). An earlier value for quinine hydrochloride was $0.0004 M$ ($1.44 \times 10^{-2}\%$), given by Parker (1922). Quinine itself was reported by Bailey and Nichols (1888) to have a threshold of 0.00025% ($7.71 \times 10^{-6} M$). Henning (1921) summarized the quinine sulfate threshold values to that date as 0.00005–0.0005% (6.69×10^{-7} to $6.69 \times 10^{-6} M$). Mosel and Kantrowitz (1952) reported thresholds of $1.5 \times 10^{-5} M$ ($5.41 \times 10^{-4}\%$) for two tasters for quinine hydrochloride, and $4.6 \times 10^{-5} M$ ($1.66 \times 10^{-3}\%$) for two others. These were markedly reduced by exposure to monosodium glutamate (Chapter 2, Section XVI).

On a weight basis, brucine has been found to be twelve times as bitter as quinine and four times as effective as strychnine. Using the value of twelve times as effective, the threshold for brucine should be about $1 \times 10^{-7} M$ ($3.94 \times 10^{-6}\%$). Caffeine was reported by Deutsch-Renner (1937) to have a threshold of $1.5 \times 10^{-4} M$ ($2.91 \times 10^{-3}\%$). Knowles and Johnson (1941) reported caffeine thresholds of $2 \times 10^{-4} M$ to $5 \times 10^{-3} M$ (3.88×10^{-3} to $9.71 \times 10^{-2}\%$), median $1.5 \times 10^{-3} M$ ($2.91 \times 10^{-2}\%$). Crocker and Henderson (1932) reported a threshold of $2 \times 10^{-4} M$ ($3.88 \times 10^{-3}\%$) for caffeine, but King (1937) observed a higher threshold, of $3 \times 10^{-3} M$ ($5.83 \times 10^{-2}\%$). Tilgner and Barylko-Pikielna (1959) gave averages of $1.86 \times 10^{-4} M$ to $1.96 \times 10^{-4} M$ (3.61×10^{-3} to $3.81 \times 10^{-3}\%$), whereas Pangborn (1959) found $8 \times 10^{-5} M$ to $2 \times 10^{-4} M$ (1.55×10^{-3} to $3.88 \times 10^{-3}\%$) for trained judges. Values from Schutz and Pilgrim (1957) were $1 \times 10^{-4} M$ ($1.94 \times 10^{-3}\%$).

The thresholds for a variety of alkaloid substances given by Gley and Richet (1885a) were (as percent or grams per liter): strychnine monochloride, 0.0006; strychnine, 0.0008; nicotine, 0.003; quinine, 0.004; colchicine, 0.0045; atropine, 0.03; and cocaine, 0.15. They noted little relationship between toxicity and bitterness. Quinine is less toxic than atropine but it is more bitter.

Tannins occur frequently in foods, imparting bitterness and astringency. Bokuchava and Novozhilov (1946) studied tea tannins and noted that different fractions had differing degrees of bitterness. Bitterness is sometimes a positive quality factor, as in tea, red wines, beer, certain cocktails, vermouth, and quinine waters. But it can, in certain products, be a negative quality factor, as in white wines and orange juice (Coote, 1956). Using grape seed tannin in water, Berg et al. (1955a) reported a threshold of 0.020 g/100 ml, which is considerably higher than for other bitter substances, but the tannin used may have been more or less modified in processing. Pfaffmann (1959a) summarized the best data for the threshold for bitter compounds as given in Table 32.

The reaction time for quinine was found to be 1.082 sec (Kiesow, 1903). Earlier, Vintschgau and Hönigschmied (1877b) gave 0.4129 sec. The reaction time, of course, varies with temperature and the part of the tongue tested, and possibly with the composition of the subject's saliva. Neilson (1958) reported that the aftereffects of dilute quinine solutions were dissipated in about 50 seconds.

The mechanism of human sensitivity to the bitter taste is not as well understood as that to the other tastes. In fact, tasters often find consider-

TABLE 32

Taste Thresholds for Bitter Compounds

Substance	Range		Median	
	M	$\%$	M	$\%$
Quinine sulfate	0.0000004–0.000011	2.99×10^{-5}–8.22×10^{-4}	0.000008	5.98×10^{-4}
Quinine hydrochloride	0.000002–0.0004	7.22×10^{-5}–1.44×10^{-2}	0.00003	1.08×10^{-3}
Strychnine monohydrochloride	—	—	0.0000016	6.51×10^{-5}
Nicotine	—	—	0.000019	3.08×10^{-4}
Caffeine	0.0003–0.001	5.83×10^{-3}–1.94×10^{-2}	0.0007	1.36×10^{-2}
Urea	0.116–0.13	6.97×10^{-1}–7.81×10^{-1}	0.12	7.21×10^{-1}
Magnesium sulfate	0.0042–0.005	5.06×10^{-2}–6.02×10^{-2}	0.0046	5.54×10^{-2}

Source: Pfaffmann (1959a).

able difficulty in identifying dilute bitter solutions, confusing them with other tastes, particularly sour solutions.

XIV. The Special Case of Phenylthiocarbamide (PTC)

In 1926, Williams and Laselle reported that creatine, a constituent of muscle, was tasteless to some people and bitter to others. They noted that lean meat may contain 2 g of creatine per pound, enough to taste bitter to creatine-sensitive individuals. Since soups made from lean meats may be high in creatine content, bitterness may be detectable in them. This aspect of the problem does not seem to have been studied further. The related compound *sym*-diphenylguanidine does not taste bitter to about 25% of the population, according to Snyder and Davidson (1937), but sensitivities to this compound and to PTC are not related.

In 1931, while Fox was preparing PTC, some of the chemical blew into the air with a gust of wind. His colleague, Noller, complained of a very bitter taste, yet Fox found the crystals tasteless. Fox (1931) tested many people and reported that about 40% of the Caucasian American population was "taste blind" to PTC. From this discovery there developed a voluminous literature. Figure 24 shows the distribution of taste threshold for PTC and a variety of other substances. Note that only PTC has a bimodal distribution.

PTC has the formula

Paraethoxyphenylcarbamide, of similar structure,

is bitter except to persons insensitive to PTC. It is of interest that replacing the sulfur atom in the latter compound with oxygen gives dulcin, which is over 300 times as sweet as sucrose. Fox (1932) and Hopkins (1942) investigated a large series of compounds and reported that the bitter taste was determined by the C:S linkage, or, more specifically, the $=N-C(=S)-$ group. Harris and Kalmus (1949–1950b) and Harris and Kalmus (1949) found that PTC, phenylthiourea, *sym*-diphenylurea, thiourea, thioglyoxaline, thiouracil, and other compounds gave similar responses but that the sensitivity to these compounds was unrelated to urea, phenylurea, or uracil. Barnicot *et al.* (1951) showed that the taste

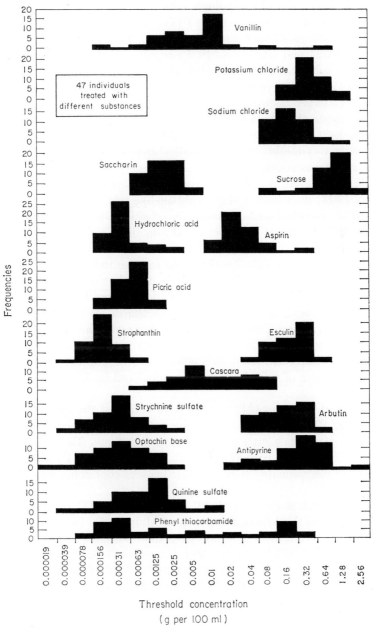

FIG. 24. Distribution of thresholds for 47 individuals. Source: Blakeslee and Salmon (1935).

sensitivity of a variety of compounds with the $=N-C(=S)-$ group was highly correlated with sensitivity to PTC.

Not all individuals find the taste of PTC bitter or neutral. Blakeslee and Fox (1932) and Blakeslee (1935) reported that some people found PTC sweet whereas others found it salty, sour, camphory, or sulfury. Skude (1959, 1960a) reported that about 7–9% of a population tested found PTC sweet tasting, and he considered this to be an autosomal dominant mode of inheritance. When the subjects were tested repeatedly, however, he (1960b) found considerable individual variation and admitted that this might affect his earlier analysis of the data and that further study was required.

At first, Blakeslee and Fox believed that these odd reactions were due to odors (PTC does have a slight cabbagelike odor). Blakeslee and Salmon (1935) reported wide variation in sensitivity to PTC for the same individual. Ten subjects were examined four times a day for 4 to 9 days. The thresholds for one individual varied more than 10,000%. Even at 15- and 5-minute intervals the threshold for one individual varied. One person was insensitive to PTC crystals in 1933 but could taste a 0.005% solution in 1934. The thresholds for PTC do not correlate with those for quinine, picric acid, hydrochloric acid, saccharin, or salt, according to Blakeslee (1932) and Cook (1933). Blakeslee and Salmon (1935) found that 47 PTC-sensitive individuals were more sensitive to 17 other substances, but there were many exceptions and the population was small. Data on the taste of PTC have been summarized by Cohen and Ogdon (1949a).

Harris and Kalmus (1949–1950a) have reviewed the methodology of determining PTC thresholds, preferring a Fisher tea experimental setup to the use of crystals or a serial dilution technique. They took as the threshold the lowest concentration at which all four PTC-containing samples are discriminated from the four beakers containing only distilled water.

In sorting trials between distilled water and PTC solutions, three male Negritos in the Kintak Bong area of Malay, ages 15, 17, and 18, respectively, derived a taste sensation from solutions containing 0.00003965, 0.00000991, and 0.00001982 g per liter (Lugg, 1955, 1957). At these concentrations all subjects called the taste sour instead of bitter. The lowest threshold was 9.91 μg per liter ($6.5 \times 10^{-8}\ M$). Two females of the same ethnic group could not taste 2.6 g per liter—emphasizing a wide range in acuity for PTC even in relatively primitive areas.

Ainu and Japanese subjects manifested even lower thresholds in the tests by Lugg (1962). He pointed out that, if Moncrieff's estimate that 0.05 ml of solution is sufficient for a taste test, then 6×10^{10} to 2×10^{12}

molecules were sufficient to give a reaction with his subjects. Figure 25 summarizes the data of Setterfield *et al.* (1936) on numbers of tasters at different concentrations.

Thieme (1952) studied 3229 Puerto Ricans of 10 ethnic groups in 15 geographic regions, and found 12% nontasters, with no significant variations between the regions or groups. Temperature does not have much effect, although PTC is sparingly soluble and there may be a delayed action in cold solutions. Blakeslee (1932) reported that some nontasters

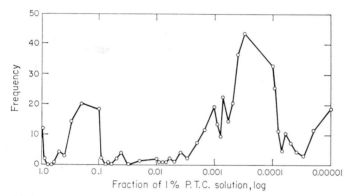

Fig. 25. Variation in sensitivity to phenylthiocarbamide (PTC). Source: Setterfield *et al.* (1936).

could taste when the temperature was raised and the concentration was high enough. The interaction of concentration and taste has not been studied systematically. Cameron (1947) tested 48 students with PTC crystals on the tongue, and found that 31% were nontasters.

Saliva did not seem to be a factor in the ability to taste PTC in a test in which saliva was transferred from a nontaster to a taster. However, Cohen and Ogdon (1949b) found that tasters could not perceive PTC in the absence of their own saliva, and if no saliva was used there was no taste.

Taylor (1961) studied the "taste patterns" (areas of the tongue responding to PTC) of 105 male and 105 female university students, and reported the following distribution:

	Area of tongue stimulated				
	Entire	Central	Root	Tip	Tip + root
Males	27	17	15	8	5
Females	35	17	11	11	3
	62	34	26	19	8

Taylor speculated that there might exist a relation between reported differences in response to the basic tastes and the areas of the tongue responding to PTC.

Generally, women are more sensitive to PTC than are men (Soltan and Bracken, 1958). In Wales, the highest ratio of female to male tasters was 1.66. The hereditary sensitivity to PTC is apparently not sex-linked. Age, likewise, does not appear to be a factor. One 82-year-old had a good acuity. However, Harris and Kalmus (1949–1950a) administered to 441 men and boys an increasing-concentration test in which four samples of water and four containing PTC were to be distinguished. Mean thresholds were 2.54 mg per liter for the 10-to-19-year group, 2.54–5.08 mg for the 20- to 49-year group, and 10–16 mg for the over-50 group. Hall and Blakeslee (1945) reported that smoking reduced acuity to PTC, and that the recovery time after smoking varied; 58% returned to normal acuity within one hour of smoking.

Based on studies of families and twins, "taste blindness" was first reported to be a simple recessive character. Harris and Kalmus (1951), however, presented evidence from brother-sister studies that this was too simple an explanation. Most identical twins have the same PTC sensitivity. Brandtzaeg (1958) found that taste dimorphism and sensitivity to PTC depend on a pair of genes in which the recessive one in homozygous condition causes inability to taste. The sensitivity to bitterness is reported to be greater for the homozygous tasters than for the heterozygous tasters.

Recent data by Das (1958) suggest that a simple, unifactorial recessive inheritance of taste deficiency is not possible. Kalmus (1958b) suggested that the PTC threshold be corrected by measuring the threshold for an unrelated bitter compound and also by correcting for sex, age, and loss of taste. He believes that homozygous (TT) tasters can be distinguished from heterozygous (TE). Even chimpanzees have been found to be sensitive or insensitive to PTC, in approximately the same percentages as humans (Fisher *et al.*, 1939).

Kalmus and Trotter (1962) tested the PTC sensitivity of 110 subjects 10 to 15 years after the initial test. There were 61 increases in threshold, 22 decreases, and 27 with no change. The correlation between the original and retest values was high. But the rate of change could not be correlated with age, thyroid condition, or taster status. In women deterioration was more rapid than in men. The mean annual increase in threshold was about 3%.

Anthropologists have been interested in possible ethnological factors in PTC sensitivity (see Table 33). The variation, 60–82% tasters for Caucasian Americans, for example, is probably due to differences in technique. Cardullo and Holt (1951) even suggest applying the test to infants in cases of doubtful paternity.

Boyd (1950) found in turnips, cabbage, and other plants a natural substance, 1,5-vinyl-2-thiooxazolidone, having a taste characteristic paralleling that of PTC. With 21 individuals, seven were nontasters, 13 were

TABLE 33
Distribution of Tasters of PTC

Group	Number	Percent tasters
Caucasians (American)	?	60
Arabs (Syria)	400	63
Armenians (Syria)	294	68
Northern Jews (Palestine)	245	68
Semenites (Palestine)	59	68
Caucasians (American)	283	68
Caucasians (American)	439	69
Caucasians (American)	440	69
Caucasians (American)	3,643	70
Southern Jews (Palestine)	175	72
Caucasians (American)	1,025	73
Egyptians	208	76
Negroes (Alabama)	533	77
Caucasians (American)	232	80
Caucasians (American)	477	82
Caucasians (Jews)	82	85
Formosans (Chinese origin)	5,933	89
U. S. Indians (mixed blood)	110	90
Negroes (American)	3,156	90
Negroes (Kenya)	110	91
Japanese	921	91
Negroes (American)	107	92
Japanese	8,824	93
Chinese	167	94
U. S. Indians (full blood)	183	94
Formosans (Aborigines)	1,756	95
Egyptian Sudan natives	805	96
Koreans	55	97

Source: Cohen and Ogdon (1949a).

tasters, and 1 had a delayed reaction to both. This finding, since it relates to an actual food product, should be investigated further. A wide variety of other compounds have been investigated for their bitterness properties.

Fischer and Griffin (1959) consider that the amount and composition of the soluble enzyme system tyrosine iodinase in saliva is related to taste-blindness. PTC and related compounds containing the $=N-C$ $(=S)-$ group are apparently specific inhibitors of this system. The nature of the mechanism is not known, but they reported (1960) a differential reactivity of saliva from tasters and nontasters and that if thyroxine precursors were added to 6-n-propylthiouracil there was an increase in acuity to this compound except with extreme nontasters. Fischer and Griffin (1963) found 3 levels of sensitivity to quinine in each of which there were tasters and nontasters of PTC or of 6-n-propylthiouracil. This appears to be a useful classification, especially if related to food preferences.

Fraser (1961) found an unusually high percentage of nontasters in children with athyrestic cretinism. Some deep-seated variation in the metabolism and disposal of antithyroid substances may cause nontasting. Presumably it would also lead to euthyroid goiter or to a destruction of the thyroid gland and consequent athyrestic cretinism.

Taylor's (1928b) theory of sweet and bitter taste may be pertinent here. He noted that the cell membrane is composed of fatty materials. Bitter materials, e.g., morphine, codeine, quinine, and cocaine, are soluble in organic liquids and readily pass through fatty membranes, but at lower concentrations these same anesthetic compounds are stimulating. Taylor concluded that the sweet taste corresponds to a condition of facilitation and the bitter taste to one of inhibition. Hence, bitter substances should be sweet at low concentrations. Rhamnose, methylphloroglucinol, m-nitrobenzoic acid, etc., taste sweet but have bitter aftertastes. Nearly insoluble substances such as the α-anti-aldoxime of perillaldehyde are very sweet.

XV. Sodium Benzoate

Fox (1954) reported that sodium benzoate is variously sweet, sour, salty, bitter, or tasteless and that when response to this compound was combined with that for PTC it was correlated to the individual's food preferences. However, Hoover (1956) found that the response to sodium benzoate of an individual varied as tasting was repeated.

Peryam (1960) made a detailed study to determine whether the response to sodium benzoate was variable and, if so, whether this was a function of differences among people or a function of differences in stimulus strength. He found that, except at low concentrations, the overall flavor intensity was linearly related to concentration. Figure 26 plots the taste intensity of the four primary tastes in sodium benzoate solutions against sodium benzoate concentration. Salt and sweet intensities increased with concentration, bitterness decreased and then increased, and sour showed little change. Analysis of variance following orthogonal comparisons showed significant subject-quality and concentration-quality interactions. The individual data indicated that these tasters varied widely in the number and level of tastes which they found in sodium benzoate solutions. Peryam concluded that "taste" was much more variable for sodium benzoate than for other common substances. Since people vary in response, the sodium benzoate-PTC method is not a reliable way of classifying a population.

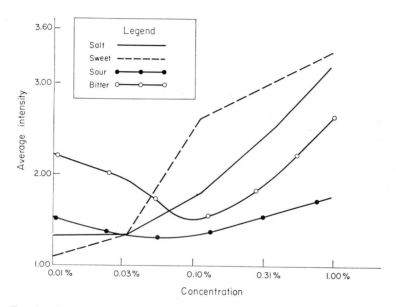

Fig. 26. Average intensity of four taste qualities of sodium benzoate solution in relation to concentration. Source: Peryam (1960).

The neural response of rat taste receptors to potassium benzoate is somewhat anomalous, according to Beidler (1962). Neural activity decreased following initial application of potassium benzoate; rinsing the rat's mouth with water increased neural activity over that at a resting level. At higher concentrations of potassium benzoate, neural response did decline with repeated applications.

XVI. The Taste of Monosodium Glutamate (MSG)

In 1908, Ikeda (1912), of Tokyo University, discovered glutamic acid in the edible seaweed used in Japanese cookery. Its flavor-enhancing properties were recognized at once, and there was substantial production of MSG in Japan within 10 years. The Oriental soya sauce was found to contain ammonium glutamate. Marshall (1948) gives an interesting history of the manufacture of glutamate in this country, Japan, and China.

Crocker (1948) reported that pure glutamates are odorless. Glutamates therefore do not increase the "meatiness" of meats, since meatiness is almost entirely odor. Fellers (1948) reported, however, that monosodium glutamate (MSG) is commonly used in fish products, such as chowder, to improve their flavor. The meaty aroma of the early lots of glutamate produced in this country was apparently due to impurities resulting from protein hydrolysis. Some food technologists held the opinion that MSG had no flavor of its own, as would a condiment or seasoning, but acts to increase the acuity of the taste receptors or promotes and prolongs sensory acuity for the natural flavor [see, however, Mosel (1954)]. Others asserted that MSG suppressed acuity to undesirable flavors: the sharpness in onion flavor, rawness in vegetables, fishy taste in lima beans, bitter taste in freshly opened canned vegetables, etc. Sjöström and Crocker (1948), Cairncross (1948), and Melnick (1950) favored the hypothesis that MSG is a general sensitizer for taste acuity, but they did not present convincing supporting data.

Pure MSG has a distinct taste—a pleasant, mild flavor with a persistent sweet and salty taste and some tactile sensation. The oral sensation has been described as "mouth satisfaction." In the amounts commonly added to foods, MSG is itself not detectable, but the enhanced flavor occurs even with subthreshold concentrations. Galvin (1948) reported that glutamate was slightly sweet and salty at concentrations of 0.05 to 1.0%, but that if salt was already present there was an enhanced flavor with a maximum effect at pH 6 to 8. Other amino acids do not replace glutamate and may have flavor effects of their own. Even if a synthetic MSG taste is made up from compounds having the four primary tastes, it does not enhance food flavor. Crocker, however, prepared a synthetic glutamate taste from compounds having 0.6 times the threshold of sweet, 0.7 of saltiness, 0.3 of sourness, and 0.9 of bitterness. These reasons are not sufficient to rule out the possibility that MSG has a flavor of its own, particularly since adequate experimental proof is lacking. Furthermore, some evidence indicated that threshold concentrations of salt were increased in saltiness but that subthreshold concentrations were not. In many of these reports there is confusion between palatability, an indefinite term, and acuity. However, Mosel and Kantrowitz (1952) did show that MSG increased the sensitivity to sour by a factor of about 1.7 and to bitterness by a factor of 1.8 (for the least sensitive pair of subjects) to 30 (for the most sensitive pair). These data contradict those of Lockhart and Gainer (1950), who determined thresholds for sucrose, sodium chloride, and monosodium glutamate for eight tasters in a triangular test. Addition of MSG to the sugar and salt solutions did not lower thresholds. Van Cott *et al.* (1954) employed concentrations of MSG at 0.75 times the threshold, and found a reduction in thresholds for sweet and salt but not for bitter and sour. Mosel and Kantrowitz (1952) reported no change in threshold for salt and sweet following a 7-second exposure to 15 ml of a 0.004 M solution of MSG. The recognition threshold of MSG was 0.00085 M. The thresholds for sour, and especially for bitter, were reduced. Table 34 summarizes Mosel and Kantrowitz' threshold results for four tasters.

TABLE 34

Taste Thresholds before and after Administration of Glutamate

Substance	Pre-glutamate		Post-glutamate	
	M	%	M	%
Sodium chloride	0.0075	0.0438	0.0075	0.0438
Sucrose	0.0175	0.5985	0.0175	0.5985
Tartaric acid	0.00075	0.01125	0.00045	0.00675
Quinine hydrochloride				
Tasters A and B	0.00015	0.000539	0.000005	0.000036
Tasters C and D	0.000046	0.001643	0.0000260	0.000935

Source: Mosel and Kantrowitz (1952).

Wenzel (1954) criticized the lack of controls and the insufficiency of the statistical analyses.

Pilgrim *et al.* (1955) studied the influence of MSG on absolute threshold, then on differential threshold, and finally on subjective intensity. For subjective intensity, using paired samples, their results were:

No. of tests	Taste and substance	% with MSG judged stronger	p^{50}
35	Sweet (sucrose, 2%)	34	0.09
48	Sour (HCl, 0.021%)	62	0.11
30	Salty (NaCl, 0.2%)	80	0.002
48	Bitter (caffeine, 0.00015%)	81	0.001

where p^{50} equals the probability that the difference from expected distribution of 50:50 occurred by chance. Salt and bitter seem to be intensified (i.e., their thresholds were lowered), but sour and sweet were not affected significantly. For determining thresholds, Pilgrim *et al.* used the method of constant stimuli with seven concentrations in the range of the taster's threshold. In this case, 0.068% MSG was used as a rinse before tasting. The thresholds, with and without the rinse, were as follows:

Taste	Threshold (%) without rinse	Threshold (%) with rinse	p
Sweet[a]	0.27	0.32	0.05
Sweet[b]	0.34	0.43	0.01
Sour[b]	0.00128	0.00171	0.001

[a] Method of limits.
[b] Method of constant stimuli.

Here, acuity for sweet and sour seem to be decreased.

For differential thresholds, 0.8, 0.9, 1.0, and 1.1% (0.137, 0.154, 0.171, and 0.188 M) sodium chloride were used with an MSG (0.01 M) (0.169%) rinse. For bitter, the method of constant-stimulus differences was employed, with 0.020 M (0.388%) caffeine as the standard to be compared with solutions of 0.0014, 0.0016, 0.0018, 0.0022, 0.0024, and 0.0026 M (0.0237, 0.0271, 0.0304, 0.0372, 0.0406, and 0.0440%) MSG. No significant differences were found. These results do not support the idea that MSG acts as an intensifier. Since MSG did increase preference, the investigators concluded that it acts as a seasoning, adding its flavor to that of the food.

The threshold for glutamic acid was reported by Knowles and Johnson (1941) to vary from 0.0001 M to 0.003 M (0.00169–0.0507%), median 0.0015 M (0.0254%). Sanders (1948) reported an MSG threshold of 0.0632% (0.00373 M) with a purified salt, and was unable to duplicate Crocker's synthetic MSG. Sanders reported that another laboratory obtained a threshold of 0.0588% (0.00347 M). Mosel and Kantrowitz (1952) reported a recognition threshold of monosodium glutamate of 0.00075 M (0.0127%) for 380 subjects in two trials, and of 0.00095 M (0.0161%) for four tasters in ten trials. The distinction (from water) thresholds were slightly lower.

Fagerson (1954) showed that foods that have the greatest flavor effect from MSG have pH's from 5.0 to 6.5. He showed that there is an equilibrium between four ionic species of glutamate depending on pH; the desirable species is not formed in solution below pH 4.

Heintze and Braun (1958) also demonstrated a quantitative relation between amount of glutamate taste and the pH. Coating peas and beans with a dilute calcium hydroxide solution improved taste through the formation of calcium glutamate. Not all varieties of beans were improved, however. Van Duyne et al. (1957) found no effect of MSG (in Ac'cent) on the palatability of fresh or cooked frozen broccoli, corn, peas, snap beans, or spinach. They believe that the level of free glutamic acid in the vegetables used may account for the differences in the results of various investigators, and they agree with Pilgrim *et al.* (1955) that MSG acts as a seasoning, i.e., does not change sensory acuity. The favorable results of Norton *et al.* (1952) and others may have been due to their use of low-glutamate vegetables. The occurrence of free glutamic acid in foods has been demonstrated by Hac *et al.* (1949). With canned or frozen meats or poultry, samples with 0.15–0.25% added MSG were generally preferred. Norton *et al.* (1952), Giradot and Peryam (1954), Kemp (1955), and Rogers *et al.* (1956) also reported a preference for samples containing MSG. Sather *et al.* (1958) observed that untrained tasters had no consistent preferences for canned and frozen green beans or wax beans processed with and without 0.125 or 0.200% MSG.

Hanson *et al.* (1960a) found glutamate ion to have a specific flavor effect. Their trained panel could detect glutamate added to chicken broth at levels ranging from 0.015 to 0.04%. They, too, reported that detection of added glutamate was more difficult in foods that normally contain low levels of glutamate. Detection was also more difficult when a single sample was presented than when paired comparisons were made.

Hanson *et al.* (1960b) reported that 0.15 and 0.35% monosodium glutamate did not prevent or delay off flavor development at 10°F in a variety of meats and meat products, nor did its presence mask flavor changes. Glutamate is not destroyed in normal canning operations, and hence may be added before processing.

A specific synergistic action between MSG and several nucleoside-5'-monophosphates has been reported by Sakaguchi (1961). Even a small amount of these latter materials added to MSG increased its flavor-enhancing properties as much as thirty times. He suggested their use in foods and beverages that contain natural glutamate.

The disodium salt of inosinic acid (hypoxanthine riboside-5-phosphoric acid) has been recommended as a flavor enhancer by Wagner *et al.* (1962), who based their opinion on previous work by several Japanese investigators, including Kuninaka (1960, 1961). In water, the compound imparted a brief, mouth-filling sensation followed by an astringent, drying sensation. It did not stimulate salivation. Disodium inosinate added to soup resulted in a fuller flavor and an *impression* of increased viscosity. Sulfidelike flavors were suppressed by the compound in some foods; sourness was modified in many products (Wagner *et al.*, 1962). The primary effect thus seems to be tactile.

A summary of the present status of the flavor of the 5'-ribonucleotides was recently published by Kuninaka *et al.* (1964). The threshold level appears to vary from 0.0035 to 0.025%, depending on the particular compound. They are being used commercially in Japan—usually in conjunction with MSG. Shimazono (1964) emphasized that appreciable quantities of some of the 5'-ribonucleotides are normally present in food, e.g., inosinic acid in meats, and guanylic acid in shiitake extract. The compounds, as sodium salts, are stable and do not decompose under the usual cooking or storage conditions.

XVII. Interaction of Tastes

Although threshold tests for individual tastes are of interest we seldom encounter this problem in practice. Foods contain two or three or probably all the basic tastes. Heymans (1899), in a systematic study of the effect of the four basic tastes on each other, showed that the presence of increasing amounts of another taste raised its threshold. For example, the threshold for hydrochloric acid in the presence of increasing amounts of sodium chloride was as follows:

NaCl	Threshold (%) for HCl
0.0	0.0034
0.625	0.0031
1.25	0.0041
2.5	0.0051
5.0	0.0065
7.5	0.0083
10.0	0.0118
12.5	0.0128

Kiesow (1894b) used a brush technique on the surface of the tongue and reported that all the tastes enhanced each other. Hahn and Ulbrich (1948) observed a reduction in saccharin thresholds by adding to the test solution subliminal concentrations of quinine sulfate, sodium chloride, and hydrochloric acid. On the other hand, Hambloch and Püschel (1928) showed that the effect of one taste on another depended on their relative concentrations. If one component is present in a very much higher concentration than the other its taste tends to predominate. In the intermediate range one may still predominate but its tone will be modified or both may be tasted. In some cases one component is tasted first and then the other.

The effect on a threshold of previous exposure to another taste substance was determined by Mayer (1927). Threshold increased with time of previous exposure up to 1 to 2 minutes; the effect on the threshold increased with increasing concentration. The ratio of adapted threshold to the normal threshold was 11.4 for sucrose, 3.6 for quinine hydrochloride, 1.6 for sodium chloride, and 1.2 for hydrochloric acid.

Bujas (1934) applied flowing solutions of salt on one side of the tongue, and sugar on the other (all exposures 7 sec). At low sugar levels, the salt sensitivity is increased; high sugar levels had a reverse effect (Fig. 27).

Bujas (1939) used two areas on the tongue for stream flow of sodium chloride solutions of various concentrations. In the first experiment, only one stream was used until adaptation was achieved. Then the threshold was tested, and was found to be higher than normal. In the second test, both areas were stimulated to adaptation and then washed with water

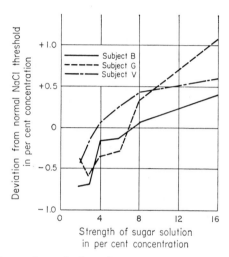

FIG. 27. Taste interactions of salt and sugar. Source: Bujas (1934).

for 50 seconds, and the threshold redetermined. A slightly lower threshold was obtained, i.e., a contrast effect. In the third experiment one area was continuously supplied with the adapting sodium chloride solution and the threshold was determined on the other. The threshold was much lower, i.e., a large contrast effect. Thus, adaptation to salt is due to decreased sensitivity of the receptors. The cerebral effect tended to increase sensitivity and offset the adaptation effect.

In Hahn's (1936b) experiment, a stream of a supraliminal solution of sodium chloride, acetic acid, glycerol, or glycine was placed on the tongue for 2 to 50 seconds. The tongue was then washed with water, and dilute solutions of the same substances were applied to test for the effect on the threshold for all substances, with time of previous exposure up to about 40 seconds. Washing with water for 30 seconds brought the salt threshold back nearly to normal.

Hahn *et al.* (1938) studied the effect of exposure to salts with three subjects on the threshold for each of the salts. Previous exposure to a specific salt raised the threshold for that salt but not for the others. They suggested that adaptation was not a necessary concomitant of stimulation. Adaptation to a salt apparently is a process distinct from stimulation. They therefore suggested that adaptation to a salt may involve a selective decrease in the permeability of the receptor cell to this substance. With sweet and bitter compounds, exposure to any single compound raised the thresholds for all compounds possessing the same taste quality. The threshold of a substance increased with increasing concentration of the adapting solution up to the "absolute adaptation limit" of the substance. Some substances (dulcin, for example) showed no "absolute adaptation limit" within the range of concentrations employed. Reversing the solutions, i.e., the adapting solution and the adapting threshold solution, produced curves which were not necessarily the same in form. See also Chapter 5, Section V.

Dallenbach and Dallenbach (1943) reported that adaptation to quinine hydrochloride reduced sensitivity to sucrose, sodium chloride, and acids. The concentration of the bitter solution did not appear to influence the effect. Hahn and Ulbrich (1948) reported little effect of adaptation for many compounds although there were a few instances of reduced sensitivity and some of increased sensitivity. There was also some variation in response among their three subjects. Hahn *et al.* (1940) also studied the adaptation effects of six acids with only three subjects. Previous exposure to any of the acids raised the threshold for the acid and for all other acids.

Fabian and Blum (1943) studied the competitive and compensatory actions that subthreshold levels of one taste had on suprathreshold levels of another when the two were mixed together. "Compensatory" action was the term used when a second substance added to a taste substance prevented matching this with another solution of the same concentration. The term "competitive action" was used when the second substance did not influence the basic taste. (These terms seem inappropriate.) The experimental technique was to mix a below-threshold concentration of substance *A* with an above-threshold concentration of substance *B*. This solution was then compared to a series of solutions of substance *B* alone until a supposed match was obtained. If the actual concentrations of *B* differed, however, then substance *A* was reducing or increasing the taste effect of substance *B*. The number of replications was limited, with results as follows:

(1) Subthreshold levels of sodium chloride reduced the sourness of acetic, hydrochloric, and citric acids moderately, and of lactic, malic, and tartaric acids markedly.

(2) Sodium chloride increased the sweetness of sugars in the order

maltose, lactose, fructose, glucose, and sucrose (on a weight basis). (This effect had been noted earlier by Kremer, 1917.)

(3) Hydrochloric acid did not influence the taste of sodium chloride. This is unexpected if chloride is responsible for the salty taste. If sodium is responsible, then it should reduce the salty taste, owing to the common ion effect. All other acids increased the salty taste.

(4) Acids did not influence the sweetness of glucose except hydrochloric and acetic, which reduced its sweetness. The sweetness of sucrose was increased by lactic, malic, citric, and tartaric acids, but remained unchanged with hydrochloric and acetic acids. Inversion was not a factor in these results. The sweetness of fructose was reduced by all the acids except hydrochloric and citric, where no change was noted.

(5) Sugars reduced the salty and sour tastes. The sour taste of malic and tartaric acids was reduced more by sucrose than by other sugars. The different sugars reduced the sourness about the same for the other acids.

The above results are summarized in Fig. 28.

Quinine hydrochloride was shown by Kremer (1917) and others to reduce sweetness. Subjects were first adapted to the taste, and thresholds were then determined. Thus, adaptation to sweetness reduced thresholds for salt, to a lesser extent for sourness, and even less for bitterness.

The effects of sodium chloride and sugars on sourness might be due to some effect on the phosphate buffer titration value (Chapter 2, Section XIII,A). Fabian and Blum (1943), however, found no correlation between the phosphate buffer titration values or pH and sourness. Parker (1922) and Öhrwall (1891) believed that true compensation never occurs, but that these enhanced or modified effects are due to sensitization or desensitization of the receptors. Fabian and Blum believed that their data showed true compensatory action of one taste on another.

Using a sipping procedure with two subjects, Anderson (1950) obtained increases in sodium chloride thresholds in the presence of sucrose, hydrochloric acid, and quinine hydrochloride. Less definite, but usually inhibitory, relations were derived from pairings of stimuli, more for sugar and quinine than for acid or salt. In the supraliminal range, more distinct effects were reported. Acids appeared to increase the saltiness of salt and the sweetness of sugar, but to reduce the sourness of acids. Since, however, there were only two subjects and they sometimes reacted in opposite directions, generalizations are difficult.

Hopkins (1953) found no effect of quinine sulfate on the salty taste although high salt concentration (1.5%) seemed to decrease bitterness at low quinine values and increase it at high. The effects were small, however. A subliminal concentration of sodium chloride lowered the sucrose

Competitive or Compensatory Action of Substances Tasted

Substance tasted	Contrasting substances in sub-taste-threshold concentration											
	Sodium chloride	Hydrochloric acid	Citric acid	Acetic acid	Lactic acid	Malic acid	Tartaric acid	Sucrose	Glucose	Fructose	Lactose	Maltose
Sodium chloride.........	−[1]	±[1]	+	+	+	+	+	−[1]	−	−	−	−
Hydrochloric acid	−	−	−	−	−	−	−	−	−	−	−	−
Citric acid	−	−	−	−	−	−	−	−	−	−	−	−
Acetic acid...........	−	−	−	−	−	−	−	−	−	−	−	−
Lactic acid...........	−	−	−	−	−	−	−	−	−	−	−	−
Malic acid	−	−	−	−	−	−	−	−	−	−	−	−
Tartaric acid	−	−	−	−	−	−	−	−	−	−	−	−
Sucrose	+	±	+	±	+	+	+	−	−	−	−	−
Glucose	+	−	±	−	±	±	±	−	−	−	−	−
Fructose.............	+	±	±	−	−	−	−	−	−	−	−	−
Maltose	+	−	−	−	−	−	−	−	−	−	−	−
Lactose	+	−	−	−	−	−	−	−	−	−	−	−

[1] ± Competitive action; + or − compensatory action, ▬ No test made.

FIG. 28. Competitive and compensatory action of taste substances. Source: Fabian and Blum (1943).

threshold, according to Anderson (1955). A subliminal concentration of calcium chloride increased the sucrose threshold, as did a mixture of calcium and sodium chlorides. Cameron (1947) noted that even a slight addition of a bitter substance will reduce sweetness. Hinreiner *et al.* (1955) showed that sugar tended to minimize the effect of tannin (see also Chapter 2, Section XIII,C). In Chappell's (1953) experiments with strong sugar solutions, the presence of 0.2 g salt per 100 ml along with 0.35 ml of orange oil increased the apparent sweetness, flavor, and acceptability of the solutions.

Beebe-Center *et al.* (1959) found some enhancement of sweetness by small additions of sodium chloride. The principal effect was one of masking of saltiness by sucrose, and vice-versa. Pangborn (1960b) reviewed previous contradictory results and made an extensive study of the taste interrelationships of subthreshold, threshold, and suprathreshold concentrations of the four primary tastes, using Fabian and Blum's technique with ten highly trained tasters. In general, each compound depressed the intensity of each of the others, although in some comparisons there was little interference of one taste with another. In one case, an untrained panel found an enhancing effect of sodium chloride on sweetness whereas a trained panel did not. In particular, citric acid reduced the sweetness of sucrose, and vice versa. With apricot and pear nectars, increased sugar or acid content decreased the ability of tasters to match a standard sample. In a more detailed study with a highly trained panel, using paired stimuli and single-stimulus methods, Pangborn (1961) again found that citric acid in the range of 0.007–0.073% depressed the perceived sweetness of 0.5–20.0% solutions of sucrose. The effect was greater at *lower* concentrations than at higher. Pangborn (1962) has also shown, again with highly trained panels, that the apparent saltiness of 0.36–3.24% sodium chloride was reduced by 1.5–13.5% sucrose. With 0.75, 2.25, and 6.75% sucrose, 0.2–0.4% sodium chloride enhanced sweetness. Above 0.4% sodium chloride, sweetness was reduced. All levels of salt depressed the sweetness of 20.25% sucrose. Note that in this case the depressing effect of saltiness was greater at the *higher* concentrations.

Kamen *et al.* (1961) also reviewed the problem in considerable detail. Caffeine had no significant effect on saltiness or sweetness but enhanced sourness significantly. Sodium chloride had no effect on the bitterness of caffeine although there were significant interactions between the components. Those researchers suggested that, in view of the large error term between judges, the experiment should be repeated. Sodium chloride appeared to mask sweetness, but the interpretation was complicated by significant interactions and the effect was least—or even opposite—at low sucrose concentrations; more study at just-above-threshold concentration was recommended. Sodium chloride affected the sourness of citric acid in a complicated fashion. The highest and lowest salt concentrations had less effect than the middle concentration, but significant interactions were found. Salt tended to enhance the sourness of lower concentrations of citric acid but reduced the sourness of higher concentrations. The higher the acid concentration the later these two stages appeared (in terms of increasing salt concentration). Sucrose appeared to reduce the intensity of bitterness, especially at higher concentrations, but two specific solutions (0.45% sucrose and 0.76% caffeine, and 1.9% sucrose and 0.50% caffeine) deviated from the general trend. Sucrose had no general enhancing or masking effects on saltiness, but it reduced the sourness of citric acid. Citric acid markedly enhanced bitterness, saltiness, and sweetness.

Kamen *et al.* (1961) summarized their results as follows: (1) caffeine did not affect saltiness, and vice versa; (2) caffeine did not affect sweetness, but sucrose depressed bitterness; (3) caffeine enhanced the effect of salt, and vice versa; (4) salt decreased sweetness but the opposite effect was not found; (5) salt did not have a monotonic effect on sourness, but citric acid increased saltiness; and (6) sucrose decreased sourness but citric acid enhanced sweetness. Kamen *et al.* noted that their experimental design, using 72 tasters (most of whom tasted only once), did not permit complete replication of all comparisons. This led to rather large error terms in some cases. On the other hand, Pangborn's design permitted replication of all comparisons, and the trained judges tasted many times. Pangborn noted lack of reproducibility in untrained subjects and therefore prefers highly trained panels. Kamen *et al.* reported variable difficulties in rating—saltiness being least ambiguous, sweetness next, and bitterness and sourness most difficult for their panel to evaluate. Obviously, more experimentation is indicated, particularly with more complicated mixtures. The probable causes for discrepancies, Pangborn (1962) suggested, are differences in methods and in the sensitivity of the tasters.

Reviewing the data of Kamen *et al.* (1961) and Pangborn (1960b, 1962), Gregson and McCowen (1963) concluded that individual judge variation could account for lack of agreement among laboratories. Their results showed that some tasters found citric acid increased sweetness whereas other tasters indicated decreased sweetness. Two distinct groups of tasters seemed to be involved, and Gregson and McCowen object to treating all the tasters as equivalent. Perceptual processes play as great a part, in their opinion, in determining responses to very weak tastes as do the stimuli themselves. Therefore, controls and measures of the taster's prior relevant behavior are necessary. Individual differences might indeed influence responses, as subsequently reported by Pangborn and Trabue (1964) and Pangborn and Chrisp (1964).

Using information theory analysis, Beebe-Center *et al.* (1959) concluded that when sugar and salt were tasted together the judgments were still entirely independent. However, the total information transmission for two-dimensional judgments was substantially larger than for either dimension alone, even though it appears that the information transmission from each dimension is less. Garner (1962) noted that the greater information transmission occurs even if the stimulus dimensions are correlated.

Carpenter (1956) found that behavioral responses and electrophysiological data did not correspond very well. The discrepancies may have been due to the fact that the neural data of the chorda tympani represent only the anterior two thirds of the tongue whereas behavioral studies reflect the action of receptors from all parts of the tongue. Additionally, the method used for collecting the data may contribute to the results. Finally, responses that disturb fluid balance may be influenced by processes of the central nervous system. Carpenter suggested that the intake of fluids may depend on taste at very low concentrations but may result from the interaction of taste and osmotic effects at approximately isotonic levels. The taste preference-avoidance behavior of the rabbit, hamster, and cat was similar for potassium chloride and quinine hydrochloride but differed for sodium chloride, sucrose, and saccharin.

XVIII. Summary

Taste should be clearly differentiated from odor as being exclusively the sensation perceived by the receptors on the tongue. The fact that the posterior third of the tongue is innervated by one nerve and the anterior two thirds by another should be kept in mind in studies on taste sensitivity or quality. One must also consider the differential sensitivity to taste materials of receptors in different regions of the tongue.

There is strong behavioral evidence for the existence of four basic taste modalities: sweet, sour, salty, and bitter. The actual receptors, however, are less easily categorized. Individual nerve fibers may respond to all four, and there does not appear to be anything in the nature of the discharge that is characteristic of the taste material applied.

Cross matching of taste intensity appears possible and might be useful in studies with foods if subjects could be trained. Ageusia (absence of sense of taste) is not common, but taste acuity and acceptability may be affected by disease. A variety of kinds of thresholds can be defined and measured. Various factors (age, for example) influence taste acuity, but hunger and smoking do not appear to be important. Increase in temperature does appear to improve sensitivity to sugar and to decrease sensitivity to salt and bitter. Sour is not affected much. Water seems to be the best medium for sensitivity tests. Taste responses to many organic compounds are highly specific; the anomers of some sweet-tasting sugars are bitter. Stereoisomers may have very different tastes. The best explanation of a taste mechanism seems to be that the taste substance is adsorbed, possibly on a protein at the surface of the receptor. This results in a rapid depolarization of the receptor surface which spreads to the nerve fiber and excites it.

Data on the four basic tastes have been summarized. There is still no clear-cut evidence as to the nature of the stimulus. For the sour sensation, hydrogen ion concentration, percent dissociation, buffer effect, and the anion all have an influence. Saltiness is clearly associated with salts, and sweetness and bitterness with organic compounds. The variety of organic compounds with a sweet or bitter taste is very wide. The non-additivity of sweetness for sugar solutions is one of their characteristics that is of interest to the food industry. Also important are changes in relative sweetness with concentration and the effects of various compounds and environmental conditions on absolute and difference sugar thresholds. Much more attention should be given to these matters with more complex mixtures, particularly simulated foods.

The bitter taste is likewise associated mainly with organic compounds and is the taste modality to which we are most sensitive. The bitter taste of PTC may be of some importance in classifying tasters, especially if the classification could be shown to be related to taste preference. The same is true of sodium benzoate.

As indicated above, the interaction of tastes is a subject of great potential interest to the food industry. At or near the threshold the effect of one taste on another is a slight reduction in intensity if trained panels are used. At higher concentrations the effects are more marked, probably owing to psychological factors. Nevertheless, reports have been made of enhanced sweetness in the presence of certain acids. We feel that the training of the subjects and differences in methodology may possibly be involved, but we nevertheless should point out that consumers are seldom trained and presumably might behave like an untrained laboratory panel.

REFERENCES

Ables, M. F., and R. M. Benjamin. 1960. Thalamic relay nucleus for taste in the albino rat. *J. Neurophysiol.* **23**, 376–382.

Abrahams, H., D. Krakauer, and K. M. Dallenbach. 1937. Gustatory adaptation to salt. *Am. J. Psychol.* **49**, 462–469.

Adrian, E. D. 1953. Flavour assessment. *Chem. & Ind.* (*London*) **48**, 1274–1276.

Allen, F., and M. Weinberg. 1925. The gustatory sensory effect. *Quart. J. Exptl. Physiol.* **15**, 385–420.

Anand, B. K., G. S. Chhina, and B. Singh. 1962. Effect of glucose on the activity of hypothalamic "feeding centers." *Science* **138**, 597–598.

Andersen, H. T., M. Funakoshi, and Y. Zotterman. 1962. Electrophysiological investigation of the gustatory effect of various biological sugars. *Acta Physiol. Scand.* **56**, 362–375.

Anderson, C. D. 1955. The effect of subliminal salt solutions on taste thresholds. *J. Comp. and Physiol. Psychol.* **48**, 164–166.

Anderson, R. J. 1950. Taste thresholds in stimulus mixtures. *Microfilm Abstr.* **10**(4), 287–288.

Anderson, R. J. 1959. The taste of water. *Am. J. Psychol.* **72**, 462–463.

Arfmann, B. L., and N. P. Chapanis. 1962. The relative sensitivities of taste and smell in smokers and non-smokers. *J. Gen. Psychol.* **66**, 315–320.

Aubek, J. P. 1959. Intellectual and sensory processes in the aged: a terminal report. *Med. Serv. J. Can.* **15**, 731–733.

Bailey, E. H. S., and E. L. Nichols. 1888. On the sense of taste. *Science* 11, 145–146.

Baradi, A. F., and G. H. Bourne. 1953. Gustatory and olfactory epithelia. *Intern. Rev. Cytol.* 2, 289–330.

Baradi, A. F., and G. H. Bourne. 1959a. New observations on the alkaline glycerophosphatase reaction in the papilla foliata. *J. Biophys. Biochem. Cytol.* 5, 173–174.

Baradi, A. F., and G. H. Bourne. 1959b. Histochemical localization of cholinesterase in gustatory and olfactory epithelia. *J. Histochem. and Cytochem.* 7, 2–7.

Baráth, E., and J. Vándorfy. 1926. Experimentelle Untersuchungen über die physikalisch-chemischen Grundlagen der Geschmacksempfindung nach Säurelösungen. *Biochem. Z.* 176, 473–477.

Barnicot, N. A., H. Harris, and H. Kalmus. 1951. Taste thresholds of further eighteen compounds and their correlation with PTC thresholds. *Ann. Eugenics* 16, 119–128.

Bartley, S. H. 1958. "Principles of Perception," 482 pp. (see pp. 337–348). Harper, New York.

Bartoshuk, L. M., D. H. McBurney, and C. Pfaffmann. 1964. Taste of sodium chloride solutions after adaptation to sodium chloride: Implications for the "water taste." *Science* 143, 967–968.

Beatty, R. M., and L. H. Cragg. 1935. The sourness of acids. *J. Am. Chem. Soc.* 57, 2347–2351.

Beebe-Center, J. G. 1949. Standards for the use of the gust scale. *J. Psychol.* 28, 411–419.

Beebe-Center, J. G., and D. Waddell. 1948. A general psychological scale of taste. *J. Psychol.* 26, 517–524.

Beebe-Center, J. G., M. S. Rogers, and W. H. Atkinson. 1955. Intensive equivalences for sucrose and NaCl solutions. *J. Psychol.* 39, 371–372. (The 1954 data of these authors are cited here.)

Beebe-Center, J. G., M. S. Rogers, W. H. Atkinson, and D. N. O'Connell. 1959. Sweetness and saltiness of compound solutions of sucrose and NaCl as a function of the concentration of solutes. *J. Exptl. Psychol.* 57, 231–234.

Beidler, L. M. 1952. Our taste receptors. *Sci. Monthly* 75, 343–349.

Beidler, L. M. 1953. Properties of chemoreceptors of tongue of rat. *J. Neurophysiol.* 16, 595–607.

Beidler, L. M. 1954. A theory of taste stimulation. *J. Gen. Physiol.* 38, 133–139.

Beidler, L. M. 1958. Acid stimulation of taste receptors. *Physiologist* 1(4), 4.

Beidler, L. M. 1960. Physiology of olfaction and gustation. *Ann. Otol. Rhinol. & Laryngol.* 69, 398–409.

Beidler, L. M. 1961a. Biophysical approaches to taste. *Am. Scientist* 49, 421–431.

Beidler, L. M. 1961b. The chemical senses. *Ann. Rev. Psychol.* 12, 363–389.

Beidler, L. M. 1962. Taste receptor stimulation. *Progr. in Biophys. and Biophys. Chem.* 12, 109–151.

Beidler, L. M., I. Y. Fishman, and C. W. Hardiman. 1955. Species differences in taste responses. *Am. J. Physiol.* 181, 235–239.

Békésy, G. v. 1964. Duplexity theory of taste. *Science* 145, 834–835.

Berg, C. P. 1953. Physiology of the D-amino acids. *Physiol. Rev.* 33, 145–189.

Berg, H. W., F. Filipello, E. Hinreiner, and A. D. Webb. 1955a. Evaluation of thresholds and minimum difference concentrations for various constituents of wines. I. Water solutions of pure substances. *Food Technol.* 9, 23–26.

Berg, H. W., F. Filipello, E. Hinreiner, and A. D. Webb. 1955b. Evaluation of thresholds and minimum difference concentrations for various constituents of wines. II. Sweetness: the effect of ethyl alcohol, organic acids and tannin. *Food Technol.* **9,** 138–140.

Bernard, R. A. 1962. An electrophysiological study of taste reception in the calf. 74 pp. Thesis. Cornell Univ., Ithaca, New York.

Bernard, R. A., B. P. Halpern, and M. R. Kare. 1961. Effect of vitamin A deficiency on taste. *Proc. Soc. Exptl. Biol. Med.* **108,** 784–786.

Biester, A., M. W. Wood, and C. S. Wahlin, 1925. Carbohydrate studies. I. The relative sweetness of pure sugars. *Am. J. Physiol.* **73,** 387–396.

Blakeslee, A. F. 1932. Genetics of sensory thresholds: taste for phenylthiocarbamide. *Proc. Natl. Acad. Sci. (U. S.)* **18,** 120–130.

Blakeslee, A. F. 1935. A dinner demonstration of threshold differences in taste and smell. *Science* **81,** 504–507.

Blakeslee, A. F., and A. L. Fox. 1932. Our different taste worlds. *J. Heredity* **23,** 97–110.

Blakeslee, A. F., and T. N. Salmon. 1935. Genetics of sensory thresholds: individual taste reactions for different substances. *Proc. Natl. Acad. Sci. (U. S.)* **21,** 84–90.

Bohm, E., and R. R. Strang. 1962. Glossopharyngeal neuralgia. *Brain* **85,** 371–388.

Bokuchava, M. A., and N. P. Novozhilov. 1946. Taste qualities of various fractions of tea tannin and their significance in tea quality (transl.). *Biokhim. Chainogo Proizvodstva, Akad. Nauk S. S. S. R., Inst. Biokhim. im. A. N. Bakha, Sbornik* **5,** 190–196. (*Chem. Abstr.* **46,** 2712.)

Boring, E. G. 1942. "Sensation and Perception in the History of Experimental Psychology," 644 pp. (see especially pp. 449–458, 460–462). Appleton, New York.

Boyd, W. C. 1950. Taste reactions to antithyroid substances. *Science* **112,** 153.

Boyd, W. C., and S. Matsubara. 1962. Different tastes of enanthiomorphic hexoses. *Science* **137,** 669.

Brandtzaeg, M. B. 1958. Taste sensitivity of P.T.C. in 60 Norwegian families with 176 children: confirmation of the hypothesis of single gene inheritance. *Acta Genet. et Statist. Med.* **8,** 115–128.

Bronshtein, A. I. 1950. "Vkus i obonianie" (Taste and smell). 306 pp. Akad. Nauk S. S. S. R., Moscow.

Bronte-Stewart, B. 1956. Smoking and the cardiovascular system. *Brit. Med. J.* **4968,** 659.

Bujas, Z. 1934. Quelques remarques sur le contraste et l'inhibition à la suite d'excitations gustatives simultanées. *Compt. rend. soc. biol.* **116,** 1304–1306 (see also pp. 1307–1309).

Bujas, Z. 1935a. Le rapport entre les quantités liminaires et le temps d'action pour les excitations gustatives. *Compt. rend. soc. biol.* **119,** 835–837.

Bujas, Z. 1935b. Le temps de réaction aux excitations gustatives d'intensité différente. *Compt. rend. soc. biol.* **119,** 1360–1362.

Bujas, Z. 1939. Kontrast- und Hemmungserscheinungen bei disparaten simultanen Geschmacksreizen. *Ind. Psychotech.* **16,** 81–89.

Bujas, Z., and A. Chweitzer. 1938. Les modifications électrotoniques d'excitabilité pour le goût électrique. *Compt. rend. soc. biol.* **127,** 1071–1072.

Bujas, Z., and A. Ostojcic. 1939. L'évolution de la sensation gustative en fonction du temps d'excitation. *Acta Inst. Psychol. Univ. Zagreb.* **3**(1), 1–24.

Bujas, Z., and A. Ostojcic. 1941. La sensibilité gustative en fonction de la surface excitée. *Acta Inst. Psychol. Univ. Zagreb.* **5**(13), 1–19.

Byrd, E., and S. Gertman. 1959. Taste sensitivity in aging persons. *Geriatrics* **14**, 381–384.

Cairncross, S. E. 1948. The effect of monosodium glutamate on food flavor. *In* "Flavor and Acceptability of Monosodium Glutamate," Symposium on Monosodium Glutamate, 92 pp. (see pp. 32–38). Food and Container Inst., Chicago, Illinois.

Cameron, A. T. 1947. The taste sense and the relative sweetness of sugars and other sweet substances. Sugar Research Foundation Rept. No. 9, 1–72. New York.

Cardullo, H. M., and L. E. Holt, Jr. 1951. Ability of infants to taste P.T.C.: its application in cases of doubtful paternity. *Proc. Soc. Exptl. Biol. Med.* **76**, 589–592.

Carpenter, J. A. 1956. Species differences in taste preferences. *J. Comp. and Physiol. Psychol.* **49**, 139–144.

Carr, W. J. 1952. The effect of adrenalectomy upon the NaCl taste threshold in rat. *J. Comp. and Physiol. Psychol.* **45**, 377–380.

Chappell, G. M. 1953. Flavour assessment of sugar solutions. *J. Sci. Food Agr.* **4**, 346–350.

Chauncey, H. H., and I. L. Shannon. 1959. Parotid gland secretion rate as a method for measuring response to gustatory and masticatory stimuli in humans. School of Aviation Med., USAF, Randolph AFB, Texas Bull. No. **59–66**, 1–7.

Clendenning, T. 1940a. Flavor in confections. I. The physiological aspects. *Mfg. Confectioner* **20**(1), 17–19.

Clendenning, T. 1940b. Flavor in confections. II. Methods of evaluation. *Mfg. Confectioner* **20**(2), 23–25.

Clendenning, T. 1940c. Flavor in confections. III. Taste-provoking agents. *Mfg. Confectioner* **20**(3), 21–22.

Cohen, J., and L. Gitman. 1959. Oral complaints and taste perception in the aged. *J. Gerontol.* **14**, 294–298.

Cohen, J., and D. P. Ogdon. 1949a. Taste blindness to phenyl-thio-carbamide and related compounds. *Psychol. Bull.* **46**, 490–498.

Cohen, J., and D. P. Ogdon. 1949b. Taste blindness to phenyl-thio-carbamide as a function of saliva. *Science* **110**, 532–533.

Cohn, G. 1914. "Die organischen Geschmacksstoffe," 936 pp.. Franz Siemenroth, Berlin.

Cohn, G. 1915. "Geschmack und Konstitution bei organischen Verbindungen," 100 pp. Enke, Stuttgart.

Cook, R. C. 1933. Inherited variations in the sense of taste. *Am. Mercury* **28**, 67–69.

Cooper, R. M., I. Bilash, and J. P. Zubek. 1959. The effect of age on taste sensitivity. *J. Gerontol.* **14**, 56–58.

Coote, G. G. 1956. Analysis of scores for bitterness of orange juice. *Food Research* **21**, 1–10.

Cragg, L. H. 1937a. Relation between sourness and pH of the saliva. *Proc. Trans. Roy. Soc. Canada* **31**, 1–7.

Cragg, L. H. 1937b. Sour taste. *Proc. Trans. Roy. Soc. Canada* **31**, 131–140.

Crisci, P. 1930. Intorno alla pretesa proporzionalità fra il pH e il sapore acido delle soluzioni acquose con speciale riguardo ai vini. *Ann. chim. appl.* **20**, 566–583.

Crocker, E. C. 1945. "Flavor," 172 pp. McGraw-Hill, New York.

Crocker, E. C. 1948. Meat flavor and observations on the taste of glutamate and other amino acids. *In* "Flavor and Acceptability of Monosodium Glutamate,"

Symposium on Monosodium Glutamate, 92 pp. (see pp. 25–31). Food and Container Inst., Chicago, Illinois.

Crocker, E. C., and L. F. Henderson. 1932. The glutamate taste. *Am. Perfumer Essent. Oil Rev.* **27**, 156–158.

Crozier, W. J. 1916. The taste of acids. *J. Comp. Neurol.* **26**, 453–462.

Crozier, W. J. 1918. Sensory activation by acids. *Am. J. Physiol.* **45**, 323–341.

Crozier, W. J. 1934. Chemoreception. *In* "Handbook of General Experimental Psychology" (C. Murchison, ed.), 1125 pp. (see pp. 987–1036). Clark Univ. Press, Worcester, Massachusetts.

Dahlberg, A. C., and E. S. Penczek. 1941. The relative sweetness of sugars as affected by concentration. *N. Y. State Agr. Expt. Sta. Tech. Bull.* **258**, 1–12.

Dallenbach, J. W., and K. M. Dallenbach. 1943. The effects of bitter-adaptation on sensitivity to other taste-qualities. *Am. J. Psychol.* **56**, 21–31.

Das, S. R. 1958. Inheritance of the P.T.C. taste character in man: an analysis of 126 Rárhi Bráhmin families of West Bengal. *Ann. Human Genet.* **22**, 200–212.

Dawson, E. H., J. L. Brogdon, and S. McManus. 1963. Sensory testing of differences in taste. I. Methods. *Food Technol.* **17**(9), 45–51.

Dethier, V. G. 1952. Adaptation to chemical stimulation of the tarsal receptors of the blowfly. *Biol. Bull.* **103**, 178–189.

Dethier, V. G. 1955. The physiology and histology of the contact chemoreceptors of the blowfly. *Quart. Rev. Biol.* **30**, 348–371.

Dethier, V. G. 1956. Chemoreceptor mechanisms. *In* "Molecular Structure and Functional Activity of Nerve Cells" (R. G. Grenell and J. L. Mullins, eds.), IX, 169 pp. (see pp. 1–33). Am. Inst. Biol. Sci., Washington, D. C.

Dethier, V. G. 1962. Chemoreceptor mechanisms in insects. *Symposia Soc. Exptl. Biol.* **16**, 180–195.

Deutsch-Renner, H. 1937. Die Sinneswahrnehmungen an Nahrungs- und Genussmitteln. *Das Weinland* **9**, 36–38, 76–77, 114–116, 142–143.

Diamant, H., and Zotterman, Y. 1959. Has water a specific taste? *Nature* **183**, 191–192.

Dove, W. F. 1953. A universal gustometric scale in D-units. *Food Research* **18**, 427–453.

Dzendolet, E. 1962. Electrical stimulation of single human taste papillae. *Perceptual and Motor Skills* **14**, 303–317.

Ehrenberg, R., and H. J. Güttes. 1949. Über die Wirkung von Rhodaniden und Sulfaten auf die Schwellenwerte des Geschmacks. *Arch. ges. Physiol.* **251**, 644–671.

Elder, L. W. 1955. Flavor perception by consumers. *Virginia J. Sci.* **6**, 33–38.

Engel, R. 1928. Experimentelle Untersuchungen über die Abhängigkeit der Lust und Unlust von der Reizstärke beim Geschmackssinn. *Arch. ges. Psychol.* **64**, 1–36.

Erickson, R. P. 1958. Responsiveness of single second order neurons in the rat to tongue stimulation. 98 pp. Ph.D. Thesis. Brown Univ., Providence, Rhode Island. [See also *Dissertation Abstr.* **19**, 1835 (1959).]

Evans, D. R. 1961. Depression of taste sensitivity to specific sugars by their presence during development. *Science* **133**, 327–328.

Evans, D. R., and D. Mellon, Jr. 1962. Stimulation of a primary taste receptor by salts. *J. Gen. Physiol.* **45**, 651–661.

Fabian, F. W., and H. B. Blum. 1943. Relative taste potency of some basic food constituents and their competitive and compensatory action. *Food Research* **8**, 179–193.

Fagerson, I. S. 1954. Possible relationship between the ionic species of glutamate and flavor. *J. Agr. Food Chem.* **2**, 474–476.

Fahlberg, C., and I. Remsen. 1879. Ueber die Oxydation des Orthotoluolsulfamids. *Chem. Ber.* **12**, 469–473.

Fellers, C. R. 1948. The use of monosodium glutamate in sea food products. *In* "Flavor and Acceptability of Monosodium Glutamate," Symposium on Monosodium Glutamate, 92 pp. (see pp. 44–88). Food and Container Inst., Chicago, Illinois.

Ferguson, L. N., and A. R. Lawrence. 1958. Physicochemical aspects of the sense of taste. *J. Chem. Educ.* **35**, 436–444.

Fischer, R., and F. Griffin. 1959. On factors involved in the mechanism of "taste-blindness." *Experientia* **15**, 447–448.

Fischer, R., and F. Griffin. 1960. Differential reactivity of saliva from "tasters" and "non-tasters" of 6-*n*-propylthiouracil. *Nature* **187**, 417–419.

Fischer, R., and F. Griffin. 1963. Quinine dimorphism: a cardinal determinant of taste sensitivity. *Nature* **200**, 343–347.

Fisher, R. A., E. B. Ford, and J. Huxley. 1939. Taste-testing the anthropoid apes. *Nature* **144**, 750.

Foley, J. O. 1945. The sensory and motor axons of the chorda tympani. *Proc. Soc. Exptl. Biol. Med.* **60**, 262–267.

Fox, A. L. 1931. Six in ten "tasteblind" to bitter chemical. *Sci. News Letter* **19**, 249.

Fox, A. L. 1932. The relation between chemical constitution and taste. *Proc. Natl. Acad. Sci.* (*U. S.*) **18**, 115–120.

Fox, A. L. 1954. A new approach to explaining food preferences. *Abstr. Papers Am. Chem. Soc. 126th Meeting, Div. Agr. and Food Chem. New York, N. Y., 1954* p. 14A.

Fraser, G. R. 1961. Cretinism and taste sensitivity to phenylthiocarbamide. *Lancet* **1**, 964–965.

Freire-Maia, A. F. 1960. Smoking and P.T.C. sensitivity. *Ann. Human Genet.* **24**, 333–341.

Frings, H. W. 1951. Sweet taste in the cat and the taste-spectrum. *Experientia* **7**, 424–426.

Frings, H. W. 1954. Gustatory stimulation by ions and the taste spectrum. *Abstr. Papers Am. Chem. Soc. 126th Meeting, Div. Agr. and Food Chem., New York, N. Y., 1954* p. 14A.

Frommer, G. P. 1961. Electrophysiological analysis of gustatory, tongue temperature, and tactile representation in thalamus of albino rat. Ph.D. Thesis. Brown Univ., Providence, Rhode Island. Quoted *In:* "The Physiological and Behavioral Aspects of Taste" (M. R. Kare and B. P. Halpern, eds.), 149 pp. (see pp. 50–65). Univ. of Chicago Press, Chicago, Illinois.

Furchtgott, E., and M. P. Friedman. 1960. The effects of hunger on taste and odor RLs. *J. Comp. and Physiol. Psychol.* **53**, 576–581.

Furchtgott, E., and W. W. Willingham. 1956. The effect of sleep-deprivation upon thresholds of taste. *Am. J. Psychol.* **69**, 111–112.

Galvin, S. L. 1948. The taste of monosodium glutamate and other amino acid salts in dilute solutions. *In* "Flavor and Acceptability of Monosodium Glutamate," Symposium on Monosodium Glutamate, 92 pp. (see pp. 39–44). Food and Container Inst., Chicago, Illinois.

Garner, W. R. 1962. "Uncertainty and Structure as Psychological Concepts," ix, 369 pp. (see pp. 137). Wiley, New York.

Geldard, F. A. 1953. "The Human Senses," 365 pp. (see pp. 295–323). Wiley, New York.

Girardot, N. F., and D. R. Peryam. 1954. MSG's power to perk up foods. *Food Eng.* **26**, 71–72, 182, 185.

Gley, E., and C. Richet. 1885a. De la sensibilité gustative pour les alcaloides. *Compt. rend. soc. biol.* **37**, 237–239.

Gley, E., and C. Richet. 1885b. Action chimique et sensibilité gustative. *Compt. rend. soc. biol.* **37**, 742–746.

Goetzl, F. R., A. J. Ahokas, and J. G. Payne. 1950. Occurrence in normal individuals of diurnal variations in acuity of sense of taste for sucrose. *J. Appl. Physiol.* **2**, 619–626.

Gregson, R. A. M. 1962. A rating-scale method for determining absolute taste thresholds. *J. Food Sci.* **27**, 376–380.

Gregson, R. A. M., and P. J. McCowen. 1963. The relative perception of weak sucrose-citric acid mixtures. *J. Food Sci.* **28**, 371–378.

Gridgeman, N. T. 1956. A tasting experiment. *Appl. Stat.* **5**, 106–112.

Gridgeman, N. T. 1958. Application of quantal-response theory to the cross-comparison of taste-stimuli intensities. *Biometrics* **14**, 548–557.

Gridgeman, N. T. 1959. Sensory item sorting. *Biometrics* **15**, 298–306.

Gusev, N. K. 1940. Change in taste sensitivity in connection with a dynamic demand for food (transl.). *Leningrad, Trudy Inst. V. M. Bekhterova Izuchen. Mozga* **13**, 156–168.

Guth, L. 1957. The effects of glossopharyngeal nerve transection on the circumvallate papilla of the rat. *Anat. Record* **128**, 715–731.

Hac, L. R., M. L. Long, and M. J. Blish. 1949. The occurrence of free *l*-glutamic acid in various foods. *Food Technol.* **3**, 351–354.

Hänig, D. P. 1901. Zur Psychophysik des Geschmackssinnes. *Phil. Studien (Wundt)* **17**, 576–623.

Hagstrom, E. C. 1958. Nature of taste stimulation by sugar. *Dissertation Abstr.* **18**, 676.

Hagstrom, E. C., and C. Pfaffmann. 1959. The relative taste effectiveness of different sugars for the rat. *J. Comp. and Physiol. Psychol.* **52**, 259–262.

Hahn, H. 1936a. Die unmittelbare Ursache der Temperaturempfindung. *Klin. Wochschr.* **15**, 931–933.

Hahn, H. 1936b. Über die Ursache der Geschmacks-Empfindung. *Klin. Wochschr.* **15**, 933–935.

Hahn, H., and H. Günther. 1932. Über die Reize und die Reizbedingungen des Geschmackssinnes. *Arch. ges. Physiol.* **231**, 48–67.

Hahn, H., and L. Ulbrich. 1948. Eine systematische Untersuchung der Geschmacksschwellen. *Arch ges. Physiol.* **250**, 357–384.

Hahn, H., G. Kuckulies, and H. Taeger. 1938. Eine systematische Untersuchung der Geschmacksschwellen. *Z. Sinnesphysiol.* **67**, 259–306.

Hahn, H., G. Kuckulies, and A. Bissar. 1940. Eine systematische Untersuchung der Geschmacksschwellen. *Z. Sinnesphysiol.* **68**, 185–260.

Hall, A. R., and A. F. Blakeslee. 1945. Effect of smoking on taste thresholds for phenyl-thio-carbamide (PTC). *Proc. Natl. Acad. Sci.* (*U. S.*) **31**, 390–396.

Halpern, B. P. 1959. Gustatory responses in the medulla oblongata of the rat. 77 pp. Ph. D. Thesis, Brown Univ., Providence, Rhode Island. (See also *Dissertation Abstr.* **20**, 2397, 1961.)

Halpern, B. P. 1962. Gustatory nerve responses in the chicken. *Am. J. Physiol.* **203**, 541–544.

Halpern, B. P., R. A. Bernard, and M. R. Kare. 1962. Amino acids as gustatory stimuli in the rat. *J. Gen. Physiol.* **45**, 681–701.

Hambloch, H., and J. Püschel. 1928. Ueber die sinnlichen Erfolge bei Darbietung von Geschmacksmischungen. *Z. Psychol. Physiol. Sinnesorg.* (Abt. 2) **50**, 136–150.

Hamor, G. H. 1961. Correlation of chemical structure and taste in the saccharin series. *Science* **134**, 1416.

Hanson, H. L., M. Bushway, and H. Lineweaver. 1960a. Monosodium glutamate studies. I. Factors affecting detection of and preference for added glutamate in foods. *Food Technol.* **14**, 320–327.

Hanson, H. L., M. Bushway, and H. Lineweaver. 1960b. Monosodium glutamate studies. II. Evaluation of a possible flavor stabilizing effect of glutamate in frozen foods and of the stability of glutamate to commercial canning process. *Food Technol.* **14**, 328–332.

Hara, S. 1955. Interrelationship among stimulus intensity, stimulated area and reaction time in the human gustatory sensation. *Bull. Tokyo Med. Dental Univ.* **9**, 147–158.

Harlow, H. F. 1932. Food preferences of the albino rat. *J. Genet. Psychol.* **41**, 430–438.

Harper, R. 1962. The psychologist's role in food-acceptance research. *Food Technol.* **16**, 70, 72–73.

Harriman, A. E., and R. B. MacLeod. 1953. Discriminative thresholds of salt for normal and adrenalectomized rats. *Am. J. Psychol.* **66**, 465–471.

Harris, H., and H. Kalmus. 1949. Genetic differences in taste sensitivity to phenylthiourea and to anti-thyroid substances. *Nature* **163**, 878–879.

Harris, H., and H. Kalmus. 1949–1950a. The measurement of taste sensitivity to phenylthiourea. *Ann. Eugenics* **15**, 24–31.

Harris, H., and H. Kalmus. 1949–1950b. Chemical specificity in genetical differences in taste sensitivity. *Ann. Eugenics* **15**, 32–45.

Harris, H., and H. Kalmus. 1951. The distribution of taste thresholds for phenylthiourea of 384 sib pairs. *Ann. Eugenics* **16**, 226–230.

Harvey, R. B. 1920. The relation between the total acidity, the concentration of hydrogen ion, and the taste of acid solutions. *J. Am. Chem. Soc.* **42**, 712–714.

Hasler, A. D. 1954. Odour perception and orientation in fishes. *J. Fisheries Research Board, Canada* **11**, 107–129.

Hasler, A. D. 1960a. Homing orientation in migrating fishes. *Ergeb. Biol.* **23**, 94–115.

Hasler, A. D. 1960b. Guideposts of migrating fishes. *Science* **132**, 785–792.

Hasler, A. D., and W. J. Wisby. 1951. Discrimination of stream odors by fishes and its relation to parent stream behavior. *Am. Naturalist* **85**, 223–238.

Heiderich, F. 1906. Die Zahl und die Dimension der Geschmacksknospen der Papilla vallata des Menschen in den verschiedenen Lebensaltern. *Nachr. Ges. Wiss. Göttingen Math.-physik Kl.* (Heft 1) **1906**, 54–64.

Heintze, K., and F. Braun. 1958. Beziehungen zwischen der geschmacklichen Wahrnehmung von Glutamat und dem pH-Wert. *Deut. Lebensm.-Rundschau* **54**, 25–28.

Helgren, F. J., M. J. Lynch, and F. J. Kirchmeyer. 1955. A taste panel study of the saccharin "off-taste." *J. Am. Pharm. Assoc.* **44**, 353–355; also 442–446.

Henkin, R. I., and G. F. Powell. 1962. Increased sensitivity of taste and smell in cystic fibrosis. *Science* **138**, 1107–1108.

Henkin, R. I., and D. H. Solomon. 1962. Salt-taste threshold in adrenal insufficiency in man. *J. Clin. Endocrinol. and Metabolism* **22**, 856–858.

Henkin, R. I., J. R. Gill, Jr., F. C. Bartter, and D. H. Solomon. 1962. On the presence and character of the increased ability of the Addisonian patient to taste salt. *J. Clin. Invest.* **41**, 1364–1365.

Henning, H. 1921. Physiologie und Psychologie des Geschmacks. *Ergeb. Physiol.* **19**, 1–78.

Henning, H. 1924. "Der Geruch," 2nd ed., 434 pp. Barth, Leipzig.

Herxheimer, A., and D. M. Woodbury. 1960. The effect of deoxycorticosterone on salt and sucrose taste thresholds and drinking behavior in rats. *J. Physiol. (London)* **151**, 253–260.

Heymans, G. 1899. Untersuchungen über psychische Hemmung. *Z. Psychol. Physiol. Sinnesorg.* **21**, 321–359.

Hinreiner, E. H., F. Filipello, A. D. Webb, and H. W. Berg. 1955. Evaluation of thresholds and a minimum difference concentration for various constituents of wines. III. Ethyl alcohol, glycerol and acidity in aqueous solution. *Food Technol.* **9**, 351–353.

Hollingworth, H. L., and A. T. Poffenberger, Jr. 1917. "The Sense of Taste," 200 pp. (see pp. xiii–xvii, 1–195). Moffat, Yard and Co., New York.

Holway, A. H., and L. M. Hurvich. 1938. On psychophysics of taste: pressure and area as variants. *J. Exptl. Psychol.* **23**, 191–198.

Hoover, E. F. 1956. Reliability of phenylthiocarbamide-sodium benzoate method of determining taste classification. *J. Agr. Food Chem.* **4**, 345–348.

Hopkins, C. Y. 1942. Taste differences in compounds having the NCS linkage. *Can. J. Research* **20B**, 268–273.

Hopkins, J. W. 1946. Precision of assessment of palatability of foodstuffs by laboratory panels. *Can. J. Research* **24F**, 203–214.

Hopkins, J. W. 1953. Laboratory flavor scoring: two experiments in incomplete blocks. *Biometrics* **9**, 1–21.

Ichioka, M., and S. Hara. 1955. On the reaction time of the human gustatory sensation. *Bull. Tokyo Med. Dental Univ.* **2**, 159–165.

Ikeda, K. 1912. The taste of the salt of glutamic acid. *Orig. Comm. 8th Intern. Congr. Appl. Chem.* **18**, 147.

Irvin, D. L., and F. R. Goetzl. 1952. Diurnal variations in acuity of sense of taste for sodium chloride. *Proc. Soc. Exptl. Biol. Med.* **79**, 115–118.

Iur'eva, G. Iu. 1957. Oroli reaktionykh grupp belkovykh kompleksov v vozbozhdenii vkusovogo retseptora (On the role of reactive groups of protein complexes in the excitation of the taste receptor). *Biofizika* **2**, 665–669.

Iur'eva, G. Iu. 1961. New data on the role of sulfhydryl groups in taste sensitivity. *Biophysics* **6**(2), 29–31.

Jensen, K. 1932. Differential reactions to taste and temperature stimuli in newborn infants. *Genet. Psychol. Monograph* **12**, 361–479.

Jones, M. H., and F. N. Jones. 1952. The critical frequency of taste. *Science* **115**, 355–356.

Joergensen, M. B., and N. H. Buch. 1961. Sense of smell and taste in pregnant diabetics. *Pract. Oto-Rhino-Laryngol.* **23**, 390–396.

Kahlenberg, L. 1900. The relation of the taste of acid salts to their degree of dissociation. *J. Phys. Chem.* **4**, 33–37.

Kalmus, H. 1958a. The chemical senses. *Sci. American* **198**(4), 97–102, 104–106.

Kalmus, H. 1958b. Improvement in the classification of the taster genotypes. *Ann. Human Genet.* **22**, 222–230.

Kalmus, H., and D. Farnsworth. 1959. Impairment and recovery of taste following irradiation of the oropharynx. *J. Laryngol. and Otol.* **73**, 180–182.

Kalmus, H., and S. J. Hubbard. 1960. "The Chemical Senses in Health and Disease," 95 pp. Thomas, Springfield, Illinois.

Kalmus, H., and W. R. Trotter. 1962. Direct assessment of the effect of age on P.T.C. sensitivity. *Ann. Human Genet.* **26**, 145–149.

Kamen, J. M. 1959. Interaction of sucrose and calcium cyclamate on perceived intensity of sweetness. *Food Research* **24**, 279–282.

Kamen, J. M., F. J. Pilgrim, N. J. Gutman, and B. J. Kroll. 1961. Interactions of suprathreshold taste stimuli. *J. Exptl. Psychol.* **62**, 348–356.

Kaneko, T. 1938. Taste and constitution of amino acids. *J. Chem. Soc. Japan* **59**, 433–439.

Kaneko, T. 1939. Taste and constitution of α-amino acids. II. Stereochemistry of α-amino acids. *J. Chem. Soc. Japan* **60**, 531–538.

Kare, M. R. 1961. Comparative aspects of the sense of taste. *In* "Physiological and Behavioral Aspects of Taste" (M. R. Kare and B. P. Halpern, eds.), 149 pp. (see pp. 6–15). Univ. of Chicago Press, Chicago, Illinois.

Kemp, J. D. 1955. The use of monosodium glutamate in frozen pork sausage. *Food Technol.* **9**, 340–341.

Kiesow, F. 1894a. Ueber die Wirkung des Cocain und der Gymnemasäure auf die Schleimhaut der Zunge und des Mundraums. *Phil. Studien (Wundt)* **9**, 510–527.

Kiesow, F. 1894b. Beiträge zur physiologischen Psychologie des Geschmackssinnes. *Phil. Studien (Wundt)* **10**, 523–561.

Kiesow, F. 1903. Ein Beitrag zur Frage nach den Reaktionszeiten der Geschmacksempfindungen. *Z. Psychol. Physiol. Sinnesorg.* **33**, 453–461.

Kimura, K., and L. M. Beidler. 1956. Microelectrode study of taste bud of the rat. *Am. J. Physiol.* **187**, 610–611.

Kimura, K., and L. M. Beidler. 1961. Microelectrode study of taste receptors of rat and hamster. *J. Cellular Comp. Physiol.* **57**, 131–139.

King, F. B. 1937. Obtaining a panel for judging flavor in foods. *Food Research* **2**, 207–219.

Kitchell, R. L., L. Ström, and Y. Zotterman. 1959. Electrophysiological studies of thermal and taste reception in chickens and pigeons. *Acta Physiol. Scand.* **46**, 133–151.

Kleerekoper, H., and G. A. van Erkel. 1960. The olfactory apparatus of *Petromyzon marinus. Can. J. Zool.* **38**, 209–223.

Kloehn, N. W., and W. J. Brogden. 1948. The alkaline taste: a comparison of absolute thresholds for sodium hydroxide on the tip and mid-dorsal surfaces of the tongue. *Am. J. Psychol.* **61**, 90–93.

Knowles, D., and P. E. Johnson. 1941. A study of the sensitiveness of prospective food judges to the primary tastes. *Food Research* **6**, 207–216.

Koh, S. D., and P. Teitelbaum. 1961. Absolute behavioral taste thresholds in the rat. *J. Comp. and Physiol. Psychol.* **54**, 223–229.

Konishi, J., and Y. Zotterman. 1961. Taste functions in the carp. *Acta Physiol. Scand.* **52**, 150–161.

Krarup, B. 1959. Electrogustometric examination in cerebellopontine tumors and taste pathways. *Neurology* **9**, 53–61.

Kremer, J. H. 1917. Influence de sensations du goût sur d'autres spécifiquement différentes. *Arch. néerl. physiol.* **1**, 625–634. (See also *Ned. Tijdschr. Geneesk.* **2**, 1284–1286, 1917.)

Krut, L. H., M. J. Perrin, and B. Bronte-Stewart. 1961. Taste perception in smokers and non-smokers. *Brit. Med. J.* No. **5223**, 384–387.

Kuninaka, A. 1960. Studies on the taste of ribonucleic acid derivatives. *J. Agr. Chem. Soc. Japan* **34**, 489–492.

Kuninaka, A. 1961. Tasting effects and production methods of 5'-nucleotides. Biochemical considerations. *Tampakushitsu Kakusan Koso* (*Protein, Nucleic Acid, Enzyme*) **6**, 403.

Kuninaka, A., M. Kibi, and K. Sakaguchi. 1964. History and development of flavor nucleotides. *Food Technol.* **18**, 287–293.

Laird, D. A. 1939. Effect of smoking on taste preferences. *Med. Record N. Y.* **149**, 404.

Langwill, K. E. 1948. Taste perception and taste preferences of the consumer. *Canner* **105**(25), 26, 30, 32.

Langwill, K. E. 1949. Taste perception and taste preferences of the consumer. *Food Technol.* **3**, 136–139.

Lasareff, P. 1922. Untersuchungen über die Ionentheorie der Reizung. III. Ionentheorie der Geschmacksreizung. *Arch. ges. Physiol.* **194**, 293–297; also **197**, 468–470, 1923.

Lawrence, A. R., and L. N. Ferguson. 1959. Exploratory physicochemical studies on the sense of taste. *Nature* **183**, 1469–1471.

Lewis, D., and W. E. Dandy. 1930. The course of the nerve fibers transmitting sensations of taste. *Arch. Surgery* **21**, 249–288.

Lewis, D. R. 1948. Psychological scales of taste. *J. Psychol.* **26**, 437–446.

Lichtenstein, P. E. 1948. The relative sweetness of sugars: sucrose and dextrose. *J. Exptl. Psychol.* **38**, 578–586.

Linker, E., M. E. Moore, and E. Galanter. 1964. Taste thresholds, detection models and disparate results. *J. Exptl. Psychol.* **67**, 59–66.

Lockhart, E. E., and J. M. Gainer. 1950. Effect of monosodium glutamate on taste of pure sucrose and sodium chloride. *Food Research* **15**, 459–464.

Lorenzo, A. J. de. 1958. Electron microscopic observations on the taste buds of the rabbit. *J. Biophys. Biochem. Cytol.* **4**, 143–150.

Lugg, J. W. H. 1955. Some notably high acuities of taste for phenylthiocarbamide. *Nature* **176**, 313–314.

Lugg, J. W. H. 1957. Taste thresholds for phenylthiocarbamide of some population groups. II. The thresholds of two uncivilized ethnic groups living in Malaya. *Ann. Human Genet.* **21**, 244–253.

Lugg, J. W. H. 1962. Some extremely high acuities of taste for phenylthiocarbamide. *Nature* **194**, 980.

Lumía, V. 1959. Sulla sensibilità gustativa dell'uomo in età senile. *Arch. fisiol.* **59**, 69–84, 279–287.

McBurney, D. H., and C. Pfaffmann. 1963. Gustatory adaptation to saliva and sodium chloride. *J. Exptl. Psychol.* **65**, 523–529.

Mackey, A. O. 1958. Discernment of taste substances as affected by solvent medium. *Food Research* **23**, 580–583.

Mackey, A. O., and K. Valassi. 1956. The discernment of primary tastes in the presence of different food textures. *Food Technol.* **10**, 238–240.

MacLeod, S. 1952. A construction and attempted validation of sensory sweetness scales. *J. Exptl. Psychol.* **44**, 316–323.

Magidson, O. J., and S. W. Gorbachow. 1923. Zur Frage der Süssigkeit des Saccharins. Das o-Benzoylsulfimid und seine elektrolytische Dissoziation. *Chem. Ber.* **56B**, 1810–1817.

Marshall, A. E. 1948. The history of glutamate production. *In* "Flavor and Acceptability of Monosodium Glutamate," Symposium on Monosodium Glutamate, 92 pp. (see pp. 4–14). Food and Container Inst., Chicago, Illinois.

Maurizi, M., and A. Cimino. 1961. L'influenza delle variazioni termiche sulla sensibilità gustativa. *Boll. mal. orecchio, gola, naso* **79**, 626–634.

Mayer, B. 1927. Messende Untersuchungen über die Umstimmung des Geschmackswerkzeugs. *Z. Psychol. Physiol. Sinnesorg.* (Abt. 2) **58**, 133–152.

Mayer-Gross, W., and J. W. Walker. 1946. Taste and selection of food in hypoglycaemia. *Brit. J. Exptl. Pathol.* **27**, 297–305.

Mee, A. J. 1934. Taste and chemical constitution. *Sci. Progr.* **29**, 228–235.

Melnick, D. 1950. Monosodium glutamate: improver of natural food flavors. *Sci. Monthly* **70**, 199–204.

Meyer, D. R. 1952. The stability of human gustatory sensitivity during changes in time of food deprivation. *J. Comp. and Physiol. Psychol.* **45**, 373–376.

Moir, H. C. 1936. Some observations on the appreciation of flavour in foodstuffs. *Chem. & Ind.* (*London*) **55**, 145–148.

Moncrieff, R. W. 1951. "The Chemical Senses," 2nd ed., 538 pp. Leonard Hill, London.

Moore, R. A. 1962. Quoted by N. W. Shock. The physiology of aging. *Sci. American* **206**(1), 100–110.

Mosel, J. N. 1954. Absolute sensitivity to the glutamic taste. *J. Gen. Psychol.* **51**, 11–18.

Mosel, J. N., and G. Kantrowitz. 1952. The effect of monosodium glutamate on acuity to the primary tastes. *Am. J. Psychol.* **65**, 573–579.

Murray, R. G., and A. Murray. 1960. The fine structure of the taste buds of rhesus and cynomolgus monkeys. *Anat. Record* **138**, 211–219.

Nagel, W. A. 1896. Über die Wirkung des chlorsauren Kali auf den Geschmackssinn. *Z. Psychol. Physiol. Sinnesorg.* **10**, 235–239.

Neilson, A. J. 1958. Time-intensity studies. *In* "Flavor Research and Food Acceptance." A. D. Little, Inc., ed., 391 pp. (see pp. 88–93). Reinhold, New York.

Nejad, M. S. 1961. Factors involved in the mechanism of stimulation of gustatory receptors and bare nerve endings of the tongue of the rat. 188 pp. Ph.D. Thesis. Florida State Univ., Tallahassee, Florida. [See also *Dissertation Abstr.* **22**, 2855–2856 (1962).]

Neri, A., and G. Grimaldi. 1937. Contributo allo studio del rapporto tra sapore e constituzione chimica. Richerche nel gruppo delle naftoisotrizine. *Gazz. chim. ital.* **67**, 273–282, also 448–453.

Netter, F. H. 1959. "The CIBA Collection of Medical Illustrations," Vol. 3: Digestive System; Part I: Upper Digestive Tract, 206 pp. CIBA, New York.

Nieman, C. 1958. Relative Süsskraft von Zuckerarten. *Zucker- u. Süsswarenwirtsch.* **11**(9), 420–422, 465–467, 505–507, 632–633, 670–671, 752–753, 791–792, 840–841, 878–879, 933–934, 974, 1051, 1088–1089.

Nieman, C. 1960. Sweetness of glucose, dextrose and sucrose. *Assoc. Intern. Fabricants Confiserie, Assemblée Gén., Münich, June 15–17, 1960* pp. 3–22. [See also *Zucker- u. Süsswarenwirtsch.* **13**(14), 620, 629–630, 674–678, 706–707, 756–760.]

Noferi, G., and S. Guidizi, 1946. Le variazioni della sensibilità gustativa in particolari situazioni fisiologiche ed in alcuni stati morbosi; le variazioni della soglia gustativa per l'acido e della soglia olfattiva per l'odore limone durante la gravidanza. *Riv. clin. med.* (*Suppl. 1, Margin. otolaryngol.*) **5,** 89–100.

Norton, K. B., D. K. Tressler, and L. D. Farkas. 1952. The use of monosodium glutamate in frozen foods. *Food Technol.* **6,** 405–411.

Nybom, N. 1963. Hur surt är ett äpple? *Inst. Växtförädling Frukt Och Bär Balsgård* (*Sweden*), *Meddelande* No. **62,** 117–134.

Öhrwall, H. 1891. Untersuchungen über den Geschmackssinn. *Skand. Arch. Physiol.* **2,** 1–69.

Pangborn, R. M. 1959. Influence of hunger on sweetness preferences and taste thresholds. *Am. J. Clin. Nutrition* **7,** 280–287.

Pangborn, R. M. 1960a. Influence of color in the discrimination of sweetness. *Am. J. Psychol.* **73,** 229–238.

Pangborn, R. M. 1960b. Taste interrelationships. *Food Research* **25,** 245–256.

Pangborn, R. M. 1961. Taste interrelationships. II. Suprathreshold solutions of sucrose and citric acid. *J. Food Sci.* **26,** 648–655.

Pangborn, R. M. 1962. Taste interrelationships. III. Suprathreshold solutions of sucrose and sodium chloride. *J. Food Sci.* **27,** 495–500.

Pangborn, R. M. 1963. Relative taste intensities of selected sugars and organic acids. *J. Food Sci.* **28,** 726–733.

Pangborn, R. M., and R. B. Chrisp. 1964. Taste interrelationships. VI. Sucrose, sodium chloride, and citric acid in canned tomato juice. *J. Food Sci.* **29,** 490–498.

Pangborn, R. M., and S. C. Gee. 1961. Relative sweetness of α- and β-forms of selected sugars. *Nature* **191,** 810–811.

Pangborn, R. M., and I. M. Trabue. 1964. Taste interrelationships. V. Sucrose, sodium chloride, and citric acid in lima bean purée. *J. Food Sci.* **29,** 233–240.

Pangborn, R. M., S. Leonard, M. Simone, and B. S. Luh. 1959. Freestone peaches. I. Effect of sucrose, citric acid and corn syrup on consumer acceptance. *Food Technol.* **13,** 444–447.

Pangborn, R. M., G. L. Marsh, W. R. Channell, and H. Campbell. 1960. Consumer opinion of sweeteners in frozen concentrated lemonade and orange juice drink. *Food Technol.* **14,** 515–520.

Pangborn, R. M., H. W. Berg, and B. Hansen. 1963. The influence of color on discrimination of sweetness in dry table-wine. *Am. J. Psychol.* **76,** 492–495.

Parker, G. H. 1922. "Smell, Taste, and Allied Senses in the Vertebrates," 192 pp. (see pp. 110–166, 175–185). Lippincott, Philadelphia.

Paul, T. 1916. Beziehung zwischen saurem Geschmack und Wasserstoffionen-Konzentration. *Chem. Ber.* **49,** 2124–2137.

Paul, T. 1922. Physikalische Chemie der Lebensmittel. VI. Physikalisch-chemische Untersuchungen über die sauere Geschmacksempfindung. *Z. Elektrochem.* **28,** 435–446.

Peryam, D. R. 1960. The variable taste perception of sodium benzoate. *Food Technol.* **14,** 383–386.

Petersen, S., and E. Müller. 1948. Über eine neue Gruppe von Süsstoffen. *Chem. Ber.* **81,** 31–38.

Pfaffmann, C. 1941. Gustatory afferent impulses. *J. Cellular Comp. Physiol.* **17,** 243–258.

Pfaffmann, C. 1948. Studying the senses of taste and smell. *In* "Methods of Psychology" (T. G. Andrews, ed.), 716 pp. (see pp. 269–279). Wiley, New York.

Pfaffmann, C. 1951. Taste and smell. *In* "Handbook of Experimental Psychology" (S. S. Stevens, ed.), 1436 pp. (see pp. 1143–1171). Wiley, New York.

Pfaffmann, C. 1954. Sensory mechanisms in taste discrimination. *Abstr. Papers Am. Chem. Soc., 126th Meeting, Div. Agr. and Food Chem., New York, N. Y., 1954* p. 17A.

Pfaffmann, C. 1955. Gustatory nerve impulses in rat, cat and rabbit. *J. Neurophysiol.* **18**, 429–440.

Pfaffmann, C. 1956. Taste and smell. *Ann. Rev. Psychol.* **7**, 391–408.

Pfaffmann, C. 1959a. The sense of taste. *In* "Handbook of Physiology," Vol. 1, 779 pp. (see pp. 507–534). Am. Physiol. Soc., Washington, D. C.

Pfaffmann, C. 1959b. The afferent code for sensory quality. *Am. Psychol.* **14**, 225–232.

Pfaffmann, C. 1961. Preface. *In* "Physiological and Behavioral Aspects of Taste" (M. R. Kare and B. P. Halpern, eds.), 149 pp. (see pp. vii–xi). Univ. of Chicago Press, Chicago, Illinois.

Pfaffmann, C. 1962. Sensory processes and their relation to behavior. Studies on the sense of taste as a model S-R system. *In* "Psychology—a Study of a Science" (S. Koch, ed.), Vol. 4: "Biologically Oriented Fields; Their Place in Psychology and in Biological Science," 731 pp. (see pp. 380–416). McGraw-Hill, New York.

Pfaffmann, C. 1964. Taste, its sensory and motivating properties. *Am. Scientist* **52**, 187–206.

Pfaffmann, C., and J. K. Bare. 1950. Gustatory nerve discharges in normal and adrenalectomized rats. *J. Comp. and Physiol. Psychol.* **43**, 320–324.

Pick, H. L., Jr. 1961. Research on taste in the Soviet Union. *In* "Physiological and Behavior Aspects of Taste" (M. R. Kare and B. P. Halpern, eds.), 149 pp. (see pp. 117–126). Univ. of Chicago Press, Chicago, Illinois.

Pilgrim, F. J., H. G. Schutz, and D. R. Peryam. 1955. Influence of monosodium glutamate on taste perception. *Food Research* **20**, 310–314.

Prosser, C. L. 1954. Comparative physiology of nervous systems and sense organs. *Ann. Rev. Physiol.* **16**, 103–124.

Richards, T. W. 1898. The relation of the taste of acids to their degree of dissociation. *J. Am. Chem. Soc.* **20**, 121–126.

Richter, C. P. 1950. Taste and solubility of toxic compounds in poisoning of rats and man. *J. Comp. and Physiol. Psychol.* **43**, 358–374.

Richter, C. P., and K. H. Campbell. 1940a. Sucrose taste thresholds of rats and humans. *Am. J. Physiol.* **128**, 291–297.

Richter, C. P., and K. H. Campbell. 1940b. Taste thresholds and taste preferences of rats for five common sugars. *J. Nutrition* **20**, 31–46.

Richter, C. P., and A. MacLean. 1939. Salt taste threshold of humans. *Am. J. Physiol.* **126**, 1–6.

Roederer, H. 1952. Verdickungsvermögen und Süsskraft von Stärkesirup. *Stärke* **4**, 19–22; **5**, 7–10, 1953.

Rogers, C. J., P. A. Mills, and G. F. Stewart. 1956. Incorporation and distribution of monosodium glutamate in frozen foods. *Food Technol.* **10**, 299–302.

Rosenbaum, H. 1925. Über den Schwellenwert des sauren Geschmacks. *Arch. ges. Physiol.* **208**, 730–731.

Ross, S., and J. Versace. 1953. The critical frequency of taste. *Am. J. Psychol.* **66**, 496–497.

Sakaguchi, K. 1961. "Outline and Characteristics of Japanese Fermentation Industries," 12 pp. Rikaguku Kenkyusho, Tokyo.

Sale, J. W., and W. W. Skinner. 1922. Relative sweetness of invert sugar. *Ind. Eng. Chem.* **14**, 522–525.

Sanders, R. 1948. The significance of thresholds of taste acuity in seasoning with glutamate. *In* "Flavor and Acceptability of Monosodium Glutamate," Symposium on Monosodium Glutamate, 92 pp. (see pp. 70–72). Food and Container Inst., Chicago, Illinois.

Sather, L. A., L. A. Pettit, and R. W. Hirzel. 1958. The influence of added monosodium glutamate on the flavor of processed green beans. *Food Technol.* **7**, 372–374.

Sato, M. 1962. The effect of temperature change on taste receptor activity. *In* "Olfaction and Taste" (Y. Zotterman, ed.), 396 pp. (see pp. 151–164). Macmillan, New York.

Schutz, H. G., and F. J. Pilgrim. 1957. Differential sensitivity in gustation. *J. Exptl. Psychol.* **54**, 41–48.

Setterfield, W., R. G. Schott, and L. H. Snyder. 1936. Studies in human inheritance. XV. The bimodality of the threshold curve for the taste of phenyl-thio-carbamide. *Ohio J. Sci.* **36**, 231–235.

Shallenberger, R. S. 1963. Hydrogen bonding and the varying sweetness of the sugars. *J. Food Sci.* **28**, 584–589.

Shimazono, H. 1964. Distribution of 5′-ribonucleotides in foods and their application to foods. *Food Technol.* **18**, 294, 299–301, 303.

Shore, L. E. 1892. A contribution to our knowledge of taste sensations. *J. Physiol. (London)* **13**, 191–217.

Simone, M. 1962. Private communication.

Sinnot, J. J., and J. E. Rauth. 1937. Effect of smoking on taste thresholds. *J. Gen. Psychol.* **17**, 151–153.

Sjöström, L. B., and E. C. Crocker. 1948. The role of monosodium glutamate in the seasoning of certain vegetables. *Food Technol.* **2**, 317–321.

Skouby, A. P., and K. Zilstorff-Pedersen. 1955. The influence of acetylcholine, menthol and strychnine on taste receptors in man. *Acta Physiol. Scand.* **34**, 250–256.

Skramlik, E. von. 1921. Mischungsgleichungen in Gebiete des Geschmackssinns. *Z. Sinnesphysiol.* **53B**, 36–78, 219.

Skramlik, E. von. 1926. *In* "Handbuch der Physiologie der niederen Sinne," Vol. I: Die Physiologie des Geruchs- und Geschmackssinnes, 532 pp. (see pp. 1–345). Thieme, Leipzig.

Skramlik, E. von, and J. Klosa. 1957. Ein Kochsalzersatz auf organischer Grundlage. *Naturwissenschaften* **44**, 268. (See also *Pharmazie* **12**, 580–582, 1957.)

Skramlik, E. von, and G. Schwarz. 1959. Über die sinnlichen Wirkungen von Geschmackslösungen in der Mundhöhle. *Z. Biol.* **111**, 99–127.

Skude, G. 1959. Sweet taste perception for phenylthiourea (P.T.C.) *Hereditas* **45**, 597–622.

Skude, G. 1960a. On sweet taste perception for P.T.C. *Acta Genet. Med. Gemellolog.* **9**, 99–102.

Skude, G. 1960b. Consistency of sweet taste perception for phenylthiourea (P.T.C.). *Acta Genet. Med. Gemellolog.* **9**, 325–333.

Snyder, L. H., and D. F. Davidson. 1937. Studies in human inheritance. XIII. The inheritance of taste deficiency to di-phenyl-guanidine. *Eugenical News* **22**, 1–2.

Soltan, H., and S. E. Bracken. 1958. The relation of sex to taste reactions for P.T.C., sodium benzoate and four "standards." *J. Heredity* **49**, 280–284.

Steinhardt, R. G., A. D. Calvin, and E. A. Dodd. 1962. Taste-structure correlation with α-D-mannose and β-D-mannose. *Science* **135**, 367–368.

Stutzer, A. 1886. Ueber Saccharin. *Biedermanns Zentr.* **15**, 64–65.

Täufel, K., and B. Klemm. 1925. Untersuchungen über natürliche und künstliche Süsstoffe. I. Studien über den Süssungsgrad von Saccharin und Dulcin. *Z. Untersuch. Nahr. Genussm.* **50**, 264–273.

Tateda, H., and L. M. Beidler. 1964. The receptor potential of the taste cell of the rat. *J. Gen. Physiol.* **47**, 479–486.

Taylor, C. W. 1961. A note on differential taste responses to P.T.C. (phenyl-thiocarbamide). *Human Biol.* **33**, 220–222.

Taylor, N. W. 1928a. Acid penetration into living tissues. *J. Gen. Physiol.* **11**, 207–219.

Taylor, N. W. 1928b. A physico-chemical theory of sweet and bitter taste excitation based on the properties of the plasma membrane. *Protoplasma* **4**, 1–17.

Taylor, N. W., F. R. Farthing, and R. Berman. 1930. Quantitative measurements on the acid taste and their bearing on the nature of the nerve receptor. *Protoplasma* **10**, 84–97.

Thieme, F. P. 1952. The geographical and racial distribution of ABO and Rh blood types and tasters of PTC in Puerto Rico. *Am. J. Human Genet.* **4**, 94–112.

Thomas, C. B., and B. H. Cohen. 1960. Comparisons of smokers and non-smokers. I. A preliminary report on the ability to taste phenylthiourea (P.T.C.). *Bull. Johns Hopkins Hosp.* **106**, 205–214.

Tilgner, D. J., and N. Barylko-Pikielna. 1959. Threshold and minimum sensitivity of the taste sense (transl.). *Acta Physiol. Polon.* **10**, 741–754.

Tritton, S. M. 1939. Pectin in flavoured products. *Flavours* **2**, 9–13, 15.

Tsuzuki, Y., and N. Mori. 1954. Sweetness and configuration in rhamnose. *Nature* **174**, 458–459.

Tsuzuki, Y., and J. Yamazaki. 1953. The sweetness of fructose and some other sugars. *J. Chem. Soc. Japan, Pure Chem. Sect.* **74**, 596–601.

Tucker, D. 1961. Physical variables in the olfactory stimulation process. *Dissertation Abstr.* **22**, 2858.

Van Cott, H., C. E. Hamilton, and A. Littell. 1954. The effects of subthreshold concentrations of monosodium glutamate on absolute taste thresholds. Eastern Psychol. Assoc. 75th Ann. Meeting, New York. Quoted by Pilgrim *et al.* (1955).

Van Duyne, F. O., U. R. Charles, M. C. Titus, and E. H. Wheeler. 1957. Effect of addition of monosodium glutamate on palatability of frozen vegetables. *Food Technol.* **11**, 250–252.

Venable, F. P. 1887. Sensitiveness of taste. *Chem. News* **56**, 221.

Vincent, H. C., M. J. Lynch, F. M. Pohley, F. J. Helgren, and F. J. Kirchmeyer. 1955. A taste panel study of cyclamate-saccharin mixture and its components. *J. Am. Pharm. Assoc.* **44**, 442–446.

Vintschgau, M. von, and J. Hönigschmied. 1877a. Nervus glossopharyngeus und Schmeckbecher. *Arch. ges. Physiol.* **14**, 443–448.

Vintschgau, M. von, and J. Hönigschmied. 1877b. Versuche über die Reaktionszeit einer Geschmacksempfindung. *Arch. ges. Physiol.* **14**, 529–592.

Wagner, J. R., D. S. Titus, and J. E. Schade. 1962. New opportunities for flavor modification. *Food Technol.* **17**(6), 52–55, 57.

Warfield, R. B. 1954. Taste and molecular structure. *Abstr. Papers Am. Chem. Soc.,* *126th Meeting, Div. Agr. and Food Chem., New York, N. Y. 1954* p. 15A.

Warren, R. M., and C. Pfaffmann. 1959. Suppression of sweet sensitivity by potassium gymnemate. *J. Appl. Physiol.* 14, 40–42.

Warren, R. P. 1963. Preference aversion in mice to bitter substance. *Science* 140, 808–809.

Weiss Valbranca, G., and F. Pascucci. 1946. Le variabioni della sensibilità gustativa in particolari situazioni fisiologiche ed in alcuni stati morbosi. I. II. III. *Riv. Clin. Med.* (Suppl. 1, *Marg. Otolaryngol.*) 5, 46–88.

Wenger, M. A., F. N. Jones, and M. H. Jones. 1956. "Physiological Psychology," 472 pp. (see pp. 133–142). Holt, New York.

Wenzel, B. M. 1954. The chemical senses. *Ann. Rev. Psychol.* 5, 111–126.

Wick, E. L. 1963. Sweetness in fondant. Paper presented at the 17th Ann. Prod. Conf., Penn. Mfg. Confectioner's Assoc., Lancaster, Penn., April 25, 1963, 25 pp.

Williams, R. J., and P. A. Laselle. 1926. Identification of creatine. *J. Am. Chem. Soc.* 48, 536–537. (See also *Science* 74, 597–598, 1931.)

Wundt, W. 1910. "Grundzüge der physiologischen Psychologie," Vol. 2, 782 pp. (see p. 59). Engelmann, Leipzig.

Wykes, G. R. 1952. The preferences of honeybees for solutions of various sugars which occur in nectar. *J. Exptl. Biol.* 29, 511–519.

Yamazaki, J., Y. Tsuzuki, and K. Kagami. 1947. Sweetness of fructose. *Science* (*Japan*) 17, 175–176.

Yensen, R. 1959. Some factors affecting taste sensitivity in man. I. Food intake and time of day. II. Depletion of body salt. III. Water deprivation. *Quart. J. Exptl. Psychol.* 11, 221–229, 230–238, 239–248. (See also *Nature* 182, 677–679, 1958.)

Yoshida, M. 1963. Similarity among different kinds of taste near the threshold concentration. *Jap. J. Psychol.* 34, 25–35.

Young, P. T., and J. T. Greene. 1953a. Quantity of food ingested as a measure of relative acceptability. *J. Comp. and Physiol. Psychol.* 46, 288–294.

Young, P. T., and J. T. Greene. 1953b. Relative acceptability of saccharin solutions as revealed by different methods. *J. Comp. and Physiol. Psychol.* 46, 295–298.

Zaiko, N. S. 1956. Regularity in appearance of the functional mobility of the human gustatory apparatus. *Bull. Exptl. Biol. Med.* 41(1), 21–23.

Zaiko, N. S. 1961. K voprosu o fiziologicheskom deĭstvin pishchi raznogo kochestva i kolichestva na vkusovuiu chuvstvitel'nost'. *Voprosy pitania* 20, 9–14.

Zotterman, Y. 1961. Studies in the neural mechanism of taste. *In* "Sensory Communication" (W. A. Rosenblith, ed.), 844 pp. (see pp. 205–216). Wiley, New York.

Chapter 3

Olfaction

Smell is a primitive sense—more primitive than vision and more complex than taste. Man's interpretation of his environment is influenced largely by a complex pattern of sight and sound, with only occasional impressions of odor. This pattern of behavior may differ from that of prehistoric man, whose judgments apparently were based largely upon olfactory, gustatory, and tactile stimuli (Proetz, 1953). As man developed an erect posture, sight and sound became of primary importance, and olfaction became secondary. That the sense of smell is more highly developed than the sense of taste is demonstrated by Parker and Stabler's (1913) observation that the olfactory organ can detect dilutions of alcohol 24,000 times greater than those required to stimulate the organ of taste.

Animals can be classified as macrosmatic or microsmatic, with man belonging to the latter group. According to Proetz (1953), the extent and distribution of the olfactory nerve endings in the nose are related directly to the animal's position on the evolutionary scale; man's receptor area is restricted to a small portion of the olfactory mucosa, whereas dogs, for example, possess highly convoluted turbinals which greatly increase the olfactory area. Bhargava's (1959) studies on the relation between degree of palato-epiglottic overlap and the extent of olfactory development in 23 animals, showed that man, with no overlap, has the least olfactory development.

In most animals, olfaction functions to regulate the nutritive processes in that odors, to some extent, influence food intake (Le Magnen, 1953). The customary odor of the culturally selected food, however, may have a greater effect on intake than alterations in the animal's internal metabolism. Ottoson (1963) has summarized the evidence on the role of odor in the search for food by mammals. Le Magnen (1956) showed that rats ate more when four differently flavored meals were alternately presented than when only one was given. Wright (1964) has summarized the impressive evidence of olfaction as a factor in the "homing" of fish.

145

The effects of odorous materials on endocrine function have been termed "exocrinology" by Parkes and Bruce (1961). They summarized the literature on the role of olfactory stimuli in mammalian reproduction and pointed out that odorous substances emanating from the male mouse excited neurohumoral mechanisms affecting estrus, pregnancy, and pseudopregnancy in the female. Le Magnen (1948, 1952a,b) earlier reviewed the literature on odor and sex in man and in the white rat. The general importance of odors to animals and humans has been summarized by Bienfang (1946), McCord and Witheridge (1949), Buddenbrock (1958), and the naturalist Bedichek (1960).

Newborn infants possess the ability to distinguish between as well as to perceive odors, as demonstrated by Stirniman (1936a,b), who observed the infant's vasomotor and motor reflexes (see also Ciurlo, 1934). Relative to the pleasant and unpleasant aspects of odor stimuli, Stein *et al.* (1958) noted that children 3 to 4 years old rated many odors as pleasant which they later considered unpleasant. It is believed that the odor preferences of the adult are developed after the age of 5.

Relatively little is understood of the mechanism of olfaction. In his Alexander Pedler lecture on olfaction at the Royal Institution, Adrian (1948) stated, "We know so little about the sense of smell that I must excuse myself for choosing such an unusual subject for a lecture." As stated by Mullins (1955a), "Few physiological processes remain today as elusive of analysis and as obscure in mechanism as those involved in olfaction." Ottoson (1963) recently noted, "In spite of all attempts at evaluation of the processes by which smell is perceived, the basic mechanisms of olfaction are still unknown."

Because the perceptive mechanism of olfaction is not understood, descriptive terms for odors are very subjective, a situation which complicates communication. Although everyone knows what odor is, no one has successfully defined it. Furthermore, many odorous materials which are easily perceived by the human are difficult, if not impossible, to measure by conventional chemical or physical methods. We are awed by a mechanism which can differentiate between substances with similar molecular configuration and which can perceive concentrations as dilute as 10^{-13} M. According to Davies and Taylor (1957), about 107 molecules per milliliter of some odorous compounds can be discerned (see also Chapter 3, Section X,E). If one assumes that an odorous material diffuses equally over man's postulated twenty million receptors, only a few hundred molecules are necessary to trigger the olfactory reaction. The molecules per unit time, rather than the total number of molecules, appear to determine the character of the odor (Le Magnen, 1953). With training, odors can be recognized at very low concentrations, and several thousand different odors can be distinguished. Perfumers and tasters of tea, coffee, and wine appear to utilize a highly developed odor memory rather than depending on hypersensitivity.

I. Importance of Odor

The food industry is particularly cognizant of the importance of odors in the acceptance of various food products since odors can attract or repel consumers. Dorn (1954) analyzed the odor problems of food plants processing fish, meat, sugar, grain products, and other foods. Vapor collection and the use of counter-odors, ozone, adsorption agents, and chemical neutralizers have been studied. Odor problems of the paper industry have been described by Reed (1954), of the hotel industry by Kenney (1954), of the cigarette industry by Darkis *et al.* (1954), and of office buildings by Reynolds (1954). Odors as a nuisance in cities were discussed by Gruber (1954), and the importance of odor research in the aviation industry was covered by Spealman (1954). State legislation and typical court cases involving control of off-odors emanating from the by-products and waste disposal of wineries, canneries, slaughterhouses, etc., have been surveyed by McCord and Witheridge (1949).

Hassler (1947), Lawson (1954), and Turk (1954) have reviewed methods of modifying odors with mechanical, physical, or chemical procedures. "Mask" is a technical term for use of an odorous substance to alter an undesirable odor character—the mask being added to the odorous mixture. A perfume is a "mask" which imparts or alters odor. Deodorants may counteract malodors by reacting with them, reducing the original intensity, and leaving a slight residual odor which is reminiscent of neither the deodorant nor the malodor. If the reaction is complete, no odor may remain. Other masking agents may simply cover the offensive odor by a more powerful odor. Zwaardemaker (1895) and Kiesow (1922) showed that certain mixtures of odors tend to cancel each other or to change the original odors markedly. Whether the effect occurs at the sensory receptor or within the chemical mixture is not known. However, the ability of subjects to "analyze" complex odors is well known. Foster and Scofield (1950) reported that mixtures of odors had distinct odor qualities not found in their component parts. Some odor pairs fuse more readily than others. The psychophysical anomaly of apparent increase in odor intensity with dilution was noted (see Chapter 3, Section X,D).

Using a titration technique, Sjöström *et al.* (1957) studied 300 pairs of odorous materials for their effects on each other, and observed the following five categories of classification: (1) mixtures in which some of the major odor characteristics were suppressed or submerged; (2) neutralization, in which the major characteristics of both constituents were nullifying recognizable properties; (3) mixtures in which some of the odor characteristics of one compound were suppressed while the identity of the other survived; (4) a complete blend, in which the identity of both compounds was so altered as to produce an entirely new odor; and (5) a partial blend, in which both compounds retained some identity and a new odor was also produced. Although the results appear reasonable, larger panels and statistical analysis of the results would be desirable.

According to Bartley (1958), when two olfactory stimuli are presented at the same time, any one of six results may ensue: (1) There may be a blending, and a single odor blending the characteristics of each (possibly revealing some new odor note) may be perceived. (2) When two dissimilar odors are presented, both odors may be noted, first one and then the other being the center of attention. (3) If one odor is presented to one nostril and one to the other, the two odors may be smelled in alternation. (4) The odors may be experienced simultaneously but separately. (5) One odor may mask the other. (6) One odor may neutralize the other, although Bartley indicated that some doubt exists as to the reality of neutralization. See Woodworth and Schlosberg (1954) for a history of the controversy over the last point. The problem is important in food preparation and deserves more study (see Guadagni et al., 1963).

New chemicals to modify tastes (Chapter 2, Section XVI) have also been used to alter food odors. Wagner et al. (1963) showed how both monosodium glutamate and the 5'-nucleotides change the odor profiles of foods. Specifically, disodium inosinate seemed to repress the sulfidelike odor note.

Comprehensive bibliographies on odor and olfaction have been prepared by Paschal (1952) for the period 320 B.C. to 1947 A.D., and by Michels et al. (1961) for the years 1948 to 1960. For treatises on odor, see American Society for Testing Materials (1954), Miner (1954), Mullins (1955a), Rosenblith (1961), Ottoson (1963), Zotterman (1963), New York Academy of Sciences (1964), and Wright (1964).

II. Definition of Odor

Sagarin (1954) has struggled with the problem of defining odor. If odor is defined as "that which can be smelled," this needs qualification. Smelled by whom—man or animal? Some animals can smell odors that escape us. Sagarin complained that Moncrieff (1951) and other texts avoid a definition.

Should odor be defined in physical or phenomenological terms?

Sound, for example, can be defined in terms of waves of a given length or frequency, intensity, or energy—a physical definition. At present, this is impossible for odor. Sagarin therefore proposed a phenomenological definition:

"Odor is the property of a substance or substances that is perceived, in the human and higher vertebrates, by inhalation in the nasal or oral cavity; that makes an impression upon the olfactory area of the body; and that, during and as a result of such inhalation, is distinct from seeing, hearing, tasting or feeling, and does not cause or result in choking, irritation, cooling, warmth, drying, wetting or other functions foreign to the olfactory area." *Odorless* would be the verdict when such a sensory stimulus was not received.

A phenomenological definition places the responsibility on the individual. But surely one could not say that onions were odorless just because the observer had a cold and the nasal passages were blocked. Sagarin further defines impure odors as those in which other senses in addition to the olfactory are excited.

One problem is that odors cannot be measured quantitatively by the nose. Subjective terminology such as camphorlike, flowery, etc. are commonly used to describe olfactory sensations. Furthermore, even if two odors appear similar the mechanism of action of two different chemical compounds may, in fact, be different as far as the olfactory region is concerned. Experiments with partial anosmia (absence of sense of smell) indicate that differences in response to odorous compounds occur which are not noted by normal individuals. We therefore favor a physiological definition: sensations perceived from responses of the olfactory nerve or first cranial nerve.

The three elements of odor appear to be intensity, type, and variety. Intensity and type are self-explanatory, whereas variety is the deviation from the main type. Sfiras and Demeilliers (1957) stressed the importance of careful measurement of intensity. Much of the earlier work is suspect because of doubts as to the purity of the compounds used (Beets, 1957).

III. History of Odor Research

Boring (1942) made an extensive survey of the history of research on the sense of smell, from the text of Bravo in 1592 to Haller's "Elementa Physiologiae" (1763), which had 61 pages on *olfactus*. In 1815 Cloquet wrote 758 pages. In 1895, in his "Die Physiologie des Geruchs," Zwaardemaker covered the subject in 324 pages, and Henning, in 1916, wrote 533 pages. In 1926 Skramlik wrote the standard modern text (345 pages). A general review of the sense of smell from the medical point of view was given by Portmann (1951), Proetz (1953), and Fortunato and Nic-colini (1958).

According to Boring (1942) the olfactory region was not discovered until 1862 by Max Schultze. The olfactory cells and their supporting cells were described by von Brunn in 1892. Paulsen (1892) cut cadavers' heads in half to show air passage over the olfactory region.

One of the earliest olfactory thresholds measured was that for mercaptan (presumably ethyl) by Fischer and Penzoldt (1886) in 1884. Their value of 2.5×10^{-10} mg in 50 ml is still quoted. In 1889, Zwaardemaker (1895) reported olfactory compensation. By mutual cancellation, pairs of odors resulted in perception of only one or no odor, even when one odor was released into one nostril and another into the other. Some claim the result was only chemical. Recently, more attention has been brought to this problem through work on adaptation by Cheesman and Mayne (1953) and Cheesman and Townsend (1956). These workers found that homogeneous substances had similar "communities of odour property," while heterogeneous pairs of odors (i.e., dioxan and isopropanol) had varying slopes for their measure of stimulus intensity. For

TABLE 35
Classification of Odors

Linnaeus (1752)	Haller (1763)	Zwaardemaker (1895)		Henning (1916)	
		Type	Example	Type	Example
1. Aromatic		Aromatic	Camphor Citral	Spicy	Clove Anisaldehyde
2. Fragrant		Fragrant (balsamic)	Vanillin	Flowers Fragrant	Heliotrope Coumarin
3. Ambrosiac	Sweet or ambrosiac	Ambrosial	Musk	Resinous	Pinene Turpentine
4. Alliaceous		Alliaceous	Onion Mercaptan		
5. Hircine		Hircine (caprylic)	Strong cheese Caprylic acid		
6. Foul	Stencher	Foul (repulsive)	Some nightshades Bedbug	Putrid (foul)	Hydrogen sulfide Mercaptan
7. Nauseous		Nauseous (fetid)	Feces Skatol		
8.	Intermediate	Ethereal	Fruit Acetic acid Amyl ether	Fruit Ethereal	Fruit Citral
9.		Empyreumatic (burned)	Phenol Pyridine		

Source: Boring (1942).

reviews of recent research see Pfaffmann (1951, 1956), Wendt (1952), Wenzel (1954), Beidler (1961a,b), and Ottoson (1963).

IV. Odor Classification

The classification of odors forms an important chapter in the history of olfaction, as shown in the outline from Boring (1942) in Table 35. Henning's smell prism is shown in Fig. 29. Henning believed that all odors would find a place on the surface of the prism, and Boring (1942)

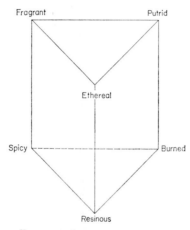

Fig. 29. Henning's smell prism. The six principal qualitative classes of odors are shown. Intermediate qualities lie on the edges or on the surfaces. Source: Henning (1916).

believed that it conformed roughly with the facts but missed many details. Bartley (1958) has summarized the evidence against this concept—mainly the inability of observers to place mixtures of odors properly. Furthermore, dimensions other than odor quality could not be accommodated on the prism. Foster's system (Fig. 30) seems more inclusive.

Crocker and Henderson (1927) proposed a four-modular classification, with eight degrees or intensities for each and a definite chemical compound for each intensity. The compounds with the highest intensity for each of the four classes (each example containing all classes) were:

Basic type	Example
Fragrant	Methyl salicylate (8453)
Acid	20% Acetic acid (3803)
Burnt	Guaiacol (7584)
Caprylic	2,7-Dimethyl octane (3518)

The underlined figures indicate intensities of the basic odor types, in respective order for fragrant, acid, burnt, and caprylic. Boring (1928) obtained good reproducibility with Crocker and Henderson's system. He suggested that the average individual can differentiate 2000 to 4000 different odors. For the aliphatic alcohol series C_3 to C_{12}, Kruger *et al.* (1955b) noted that the intensity of odor and the Crocker-Henderson

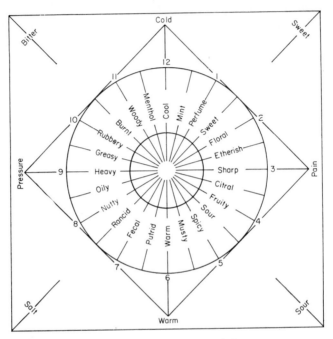

FIG. 30. Foster's odor classification system, including taste, temperature, and tactile sensations. Source: Pilgrim and Schutz (1957).

numbers fell in essentially the same direction, even including the increase in intensity for C_{11}. Nevertheless, the Crocker-Henderson system seems to be inadequate. We believe that independent verification of such systems (or modification when necessary) by other investigators is needed, especially with a wide variety of new compounds or with mixtures of compounds.

Schutz (1964) rejected the Crocker-Henderson system because its reliability and validity have not been established, and also the four odor categories are not the result of either reported physiological or intensive psychological experimentation. He used factor analysis and identified nine odor factors: fragrant (methyl salicylate), burnt (guaiacol), goaty or sulfurous (ethyl disulfide), etherish (1-propanol), sweet (vanillin), rancid (butyric acid), oily (heptanol), metallic (hexanol), and spicy (benzaldehyde). Only the first three correspond to the Crocker-Henderson classification. The words in parentheses indicate the standard chemical used to represent the odor quality. They were undiluted except butyric acid at 3.8% and ethyl disulfide at 0.03%. These standards were used in describing the odor of irradiated beef.

Crocker (1945) classified odors into 14 groups, with vapor pressures of 1.0–3.1 mm Hg at 68°F (20°C) for group A, and less than 0.0010 mm for group N. Substances of low vapor pressure evaporate slowly. Hence, in perfumes, materials of low vapor pressure remain after substances of higher vapor pressure have evaporated.

Wenger *et al.* (1956) concluded that there is no adequate classification of odors. We do not know how many separate odors can be perceived, how many classes, or even whether there are classes or several broad bands. Wenzel (1954) has made the useful suggestion that psychologists should devise a new "nonsensical" vocabulary for odors. This would avoid the semantic problems of describing odors in terms of each other. Johnston (1960) has also indicated the need for an understandable odor language.

Woskow (1964) arranged 25 odors in an "odor space." Whether the judgments were made by taking category means or from the method of successive intervals, they led to essentially the same configuration for the odor space. Factor analysis was used to calculate the interstimulus distances among the 25 odors. The first three factors removed about 86% of the variance from the scalar product matrix, hence a three-dimensional odor space model was constructed. The first dimension seemed to represent pleasantness, the second "coolness" or "woodsiness," and the third defied interpretation. Woskow concluded, "Eventually, one would hope to specify the position of any odor in the space by relating it to a few standards. This was the dream of all odor classifiers. Maybe their lack of success was due to a neglect of the pleasantness of the odors."

Wright (1963) had 84 subjects rate 9 standards of each of 50 chemicals. A 50 × 50 matrix was generated. The matrix was factor analyzed to indicate the possible number and type of olfactory receptors. Although he found no obvious relation between Raman spectra and the original odor data there were significant relationships between the spectral data and the factors obtained by the factor analysis (see Chapter 3, Section XIII,C).

V. Chemical Specificity

Odor is frequently found in compounds containing hydrogen, carbon, nitrogen, oxygen, and sulfur. Some compounds of the halogens and of phosphorus, arsenic, selenium, boron, antimony, and silicon are also odorous. A chemical entity which confers odor on an otherwise odorless compound is called an osmophoric group. Among the strong osmophores are phosphorus, arsenic, sulfur, selenium, chlorine, and bromine. Also good osmophores are carbonyls, esters, amines, imines, and lactones. Double-bond and ring structures are associated with odor, as is the hydroxyl group. However, as molecular weight increases, the influence of the hydroxyl group decreases. Stoll (1957) noted that these rules are valid only in molecules containing one osmophore group. For other theories on the relation of structure and odor, see Ruzicka (1920), Moncrieff (1951), Gerebtzoff (1953), Jones and Jones (1953), and Beets (1957, 1961). Passy (1892a,b) and Cohn (1915) were especially interested in relating odor to chemical structure. Cohn's compilation lists not only organic compounds but also the plant materials in which they are found. The aliphatic alcohol series, methyl (molecular weight 32), ethyl (46), propyl (60), butyl (74), and amyl (88), had relative odor insensities of 1, 4, 100, 1000, and 10,000, respectively. Odor is limited to molecules having neither too low nor too high a molecular weight. The structures of carbon bisulfide and carbon dioxide are similar, but only the compound of higher molecular weight has an odor. (However, the nose may be adapted to such common substances as water and carbon dioxide and thus be insensitive to them.) According to Stoll (1957), compounds with a molecular weight greater than 300 have generally been found to be odorless. This is particularly due to the low volatility of such compounds and partially to differences in structure. The influence of structure on odor is of particular interest since it could provide a clue as to how the odor combines with the receptor to trigger the olfactory sensation (Chapter 3, Sections III–VII).

Henning (1924) believed that spicy odors had the osmophoric group in the *para* position, flowery odors in the *meta* position, resinous odors in a position within the ring, burnt odors with a smooth ring, foul odors with a fragmentary ring, and fruity odors with a forked ring, thus:

For an odor intermediate between spicy and flowery he postulated:

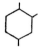

This classification appears to be far too simple. Molecules are often not rigid structures. Furthermore the meaning of words such as spicy, flowery, fruity, resinous, burnt, or foul is far too indefinite for precise classification. We also note that molecules of quite dissimilar structures may have similar odor properties.

In general, the characteristic odor of a chemical compound, which is specific for that compound, decreases with molecular weight in a homologous series. This should not be confused with odor intensity, which increases with increasing molecular weight. The nature of the odor also changes with molecular weight, suggesting that the form and size of the molecule are related to the intensity and character of the odor. Mullins (1955b) showed that rigid molecules of certain shapes are very much more effective olfactory stimuli than flexible molecules. He believes that the odor is specified by the internal attractive forces of the compound and by the size and shape of the molecule (see also Chapter 3, Section XIII,B).

The polarity and form of the molecules also seem to influence odor. When the nonvolatile, odorless heteropolar compounds are removed, heteropolarity favors odor. Aliphatic compounds, with less rigid structures, are less odorous than their corresponding cyclic or polycyclic compounds, with more rigid structures. When isomerism is created by a double bond, the odor of the *cis-* and *trans-*isomers is very distinct but their intensities are about the same. Mullins (1955a) showed that differences in odor between the *cis-* and *trans-*isomers in the butane series were pronounced at low molecular weights, and barely distinguishable with 10 carbon atoms. In such tests, Mullins (1955b) emphasized the importance of using reagent chemicals of the highest purity. He cited the example that the supposed petroleum smell in the normal paraffin series is due to impurities, not to any inherent odor. When the stereoisomerism is the result of a ring, the kinds of odor and their intensity vary. Optical isomers generally have very similar odors. Posvic (1953) found one case where a reputed difference in odor between a pair of optical antipodes was due to an impurity in one of them. Many stereoisomers and even optical stereoisomers have different odors, for example, iso-α-irone-*trans*-2,6-methyl-6-α-ionone versus neo-irone-*cis*-2,6-methyl-6-α-

ionone (Moncrieff, 1954b). It is obvious that the problem of odor differences associated with isomers is still unsolved. Since there is doubt as to the differences reported, further experimentation is clearly desirable.

The quality and intensity of odor are influenced by the position of the double bond in the molecule, the distribution of electrons, resonance or induction of the molecule (particularly in 5- or 6-membered rings), and the kind of group adjacent to the osmophore. In general, molecules with greater adsorption capacity are more odorous.

Some compounds of very different chemical structure have similar, though distinct, odors; the usual example is musk and amber. When more than one osmophore is present, the effect of added groups may vary markedly—increasing the odor in some cases and decreasing it in others. These differences are also affected by molecular weight. Moncrieff (1951, 1954b) summarized a variety of such observations. The 1:3:4 arrangement of substitution in the benzene ring usually results in pleasant odors, although n-methoxyacetophenone has a floral odor. With macrocyclic ketones, 13 atoms in the ring caused a cedarlike odor, 14, 15, or 16 atoms in the ring gave musk odors predominantly, and 17 or 18 atoms gave a civetlike odor. A sulfur atom in the molecule usually leads to a strong or unpleasant odor (as in oil of garlic), but if it is within the ring (as in 2-tolyl benzothiazole) it may lead to pleasant odors. The position of substitution is often very great in effect, e.g., the methyl ester of o-hydroxybenzoic acid has a characteristic wintergreen odor absent in the methyl ester of p-hydroxybenzoic acid. Structure-odor relationships have been discussed extensively by Beets (1957).

Amoore (1952) stipulated that the odorous properties of any compound depend on its volatility and on the size, shape, and electronic status of its molecule. Then he postulated that the corresponding olfactory receptor site possessed complementary properties. Empirically, Amoore named the seven olfactory sites: "A" ethereal; "B" camphoraceous; "C" musky; "D" floral; "E" pepperminty; "F" pungent; and "G" repulsive.

Recently, Amoore (1962a,b, 1963) and Amoore et al. (1964) expanded his theory. The molecular structures of 616 odorous compounds were evaluated on the basis of whether the structure was: (1) invariant (bond-defined); (2) determinate (force-defined); or (3) articulate (ill-defined). Amoore classified the 616 compounds as follows: camphoraceous (20, 33, 53); pungent (32, 19, 44); ethereal (27, 12, 14); floral (3, 33, 35), pepperminty (8, 22, 47); musky (0, 30, 39); putrid (21, 4, 24); almond (4, 19, 7); aromatic (4, 7, 16); aniseed (3, 8, 1); lemon (0, 6, 1); cedar (0, 5, 2); garlic (0, 1, 6); and rancid (0, 1, 5). The values in parentheses refer to the number of invariant, determinate, and articulate compounds, respectively. Amoore made the following assumptions: (1) the olfactory mechanism is the same in all humans; (2) the receptor sites have fixed properties; (3) there are only a small number of primary odors; (4) the sites for any one odor are all the same; and (5) the sites for different primary odors are distinct. The invariant and determinate molecules together were said to be rigid in structure. Considerations of molecular similarity also seemed to divide the compounds. Certain definite molecular properties characterized the first seven odors; the others were considered complex, i.e., with molecules which could satisfy the site requirements of two or more of the primary odors. Amoore (1962b) prepared two-dimensional models of the molecules, each atom being represented by a disk whose radius was proportional to the single-bond covalent radius of the atom portrayed. The over-all size of the molecule and its general shape were the most important factors, but in certain cases the electronic status of the molecule played an essential part in deciding the odor of the compound. For example the camphoraceous molecules were approximately spherical and about 7 Å in diameter. Amoore suggested that the corresponding receptor site must resemble an oval basin in shape. The smallest basin that could fit all the camphorous rigid molecules would be about 9 Å long, 7½ Å wide, and 4 Å deep. The requirement that the molecule fill at least two thirds of the receptor site was not met by a few examples with camphoraceous odor. Association in bimolecular form or hydrogen binding is suggested as a means by which the molecule might fill the site. Amoore noted that odorless molecules which would fit some of the receptor sites are known. Apparently there are requirements in addition to volatility, molecular size, shape, and electronic status which must be met if a molecule is to possess an odor. Rubin *et al.* (1962) prepared a series of cyclohexane compounds and analyzed their structures in terms of the receptor sites proposed by Amoore. Deductions of Amoore as to their probable odor were largely confirmed. Johnston and Sandoval (1962) used trained judges and found that the odors of aromatic musks, tetrolin (1,1,4,4-tetramethyl-6-ethyl-7-acetyl-1,2,3,4-tetrahydronaphthalene), and cyclopentadecanone were confused. This, they believed, supported the postulate that "muskiness" is a primary odor, sensorywise and semantically. Wright (1964) criticized Johnston and Sandoval's results on the basis their judges were "too" normal. He believed that if some people with partial anosmia had been included that different results might have been obtained. This remains to be proven.

Saunders (1962) failed to find a primary odor that contradicted the theory. Nevertheless the Amoore stereochemical theory of olfaction needs much more chemical study. The nature of the receptor-odor trig-

ger is not specified. The matching of structure with the nature of an
odor still does not ensure that a causal relationship exists. Finally, as
Saunders notes, not all the compounds listed as floral are really the
same. In addition to nature of fit, size of molecule, or electronic status,
some other parameters of olfaction will have to be found.

As an example of the complexity of the problem, following are
some thresholds of isomers as determined by Stuiver (1958) (as molecules per cubic centimeter): o-xylene 1.2 × 10^{13}; m-xylene, 2.2 × 10^{12};
p-xylene, 3.2 × 10^{11}; o-toluidine, 6.4 × 10^{11}; m-toluidine, 1.1 × 10^{13};
p-toluidine, 6.6 × 10^{11}; 1,3-xylen-2-ol, 8.0 × 10^{8}; 1,4-xylen-2-ol, 2.6
× 10^{9}; 1,2-xylen-3-ol, 2.6 × 10^{9}. Stuiver noted that, starting with benzene,
addition of a methyl or hydroxyl group generally caused little change in
olfactory threshold but a nitro or amine group decreased the threshold
by a factor of 400 and 10, respectively. Two methyl groups decreased it
by a factor of 10, while two hydroxyl groups markedly increased the
threshold and a methyl and hydroxyl group decreased it by a factor of
10^{4}. The differences in thresholds of ortho-, meta-, and para-isomers, investigated by Stuiver, could not be correlated with their known physical
and chemical characteristics.

Elsberg et al. (1935a) found that the odor coefficients as determined
by the Elsberg apparatus varied directly as the boiling points of the
compounds tested. The boiling point alone is not an indicator of volatility, but vapor pressure is. The technique, however, is open to question
(Chapter 3, Section IX,B).

It is possible to calculate the vapor pressure of a compound from the
Clausius-Clapeyron equation, knowing the heat of vaporization at two
different temperatures. If the heat of vaporization and the vapor pressure
at one temperature are known, the vapor pressure at any other temperature may be calculated. However, as pointed out by Daniels and
Alberty (1955), there are two assumptions: that the heat of vaporization
is constant and the vapor pressure follows the ideal gas law. Those
authors discussed this problem and listed several equations for the calculations. The "Handbook of Chemistry and Physics" (1959–1960) also
contains a listing of compounds and the necessary constants to determine
the vapor pressure of an inorganic or organic material within a specified temperature range. The equation follows:

$$\log_{10} p = - \frac{0.05223a}{T} + b$$

where T is the absolute temperature ($t°C + 273.2$) and a and b are
constants. Jones (1955b) pointed out that a perfect relationship between vapor pressure and threshold cannot be expected in all cases,

because of steric hindrance and of specific structural properties of compounds which may influence adsorption. He suggested that water solubility did not appear to be important, because the concentration of odorous material in the mucus at the threshold was very small and adsorption on the receptor would remove molecules from solution and keep the concentration low [see also Calingaert and Davis (1925) and Davis (1925)].

The relative saturation of the vapor in the vapor phase represents its thermodynamic activity. The biological action exerted should be proportional to the thermodynamic activity. As applied to human olfactory acuity, Gavaudan *et al.* (1948) and Moulton and Eayrs (1960) found that, based on thermodynamic activities, the odor intensity of aliphatic alcohols increased from C_1 to C_4 and then decreased or was essentially constant from C_5 to C_{11}. Ottoson (1963) thus indicates that within a certain range of chain length the odorant potency of homologous compounds closely follows thermodynamic activity. However, discrepancies in some series indicate that other factors influence the action of a substance on the olfactory receptors.

As Beets (1957) wrote, "when one surveys all that has been published concerning the relationship between chemical structure and odour, one is struck by the vastness of the material and by the large number of attempts made to throw light on this difficult problem. . . ." Ehrensvärd (1942) has summarized much of this data.

VI. Anatomy of Olfactory Region

In man, the two nasal cavities are separated by a smooth median septum. The lateral walls of the cavities have a series of folds, approximately horizontal, varying from two to six. The lower fold extends over most of the length of the nasal cavity. The two above this, called conchae, are smaller and protrude into the cavities to provide three channels, the inferior, median, and superior meatus (see Fig. 31). Each meatus is confluent with a large common meatus, which communicates with the olfactory cleft above the superior concha and the septum. These spaces are all connected by very narrow passages with the posterior naris (choana) and with the pharynx. The upper and lower nasal passages are mere slits, nowhere wider than 1–2 mm. Proetz (1953) believes that the slitlike nature of the nasal passages has not been noted because they are widened when examined by a nasal speculum or a pharyngoscope. Using models, Stuiver (1958) estimated that in normal inspiration the fraction of inspired air passing the olfactory slit is at least 5% and at most 10%. For small rates of flow, the number of molecules striking the olfactory region is small because so many are being absorbed by the mucous membranes. For larger rates of flow the fraction striking the sense organ is also small because only a small part of the molecules in the olfactory slit can diffuse to the walls. Stuiver therefore calculated that about 2% of the total odorous molecules reach the olfactory epithelium in normal breathing. When injection or blast techniques are

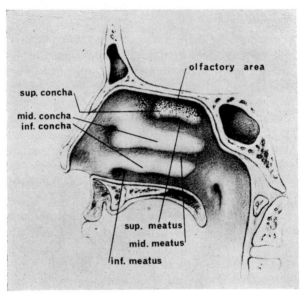

FIG. 31. Cross section of the nose.

used, the amount may reach 4%. Stone (1963) reported that temperature had little effect on olfactory sensitivity to acetic acid presented in air streams maintained at 12.5°–35°C. He correctly attributed this to rapid warming of the odor-laden air to body temperature before it reached the olfactory receptors.

The deeper part of the nasal cavity contains a pseudo-stratified columnar epithelium containing ciliated cells whose cilia beat toward the choana. The cavity also contains many alveolo-tubular glands with mucous cells. The conchae are very vascular and their edges are erectile and capable of enlargement through reflex excitation. Air entering the nasal cavity is warmed and humidified by passage over these surfaces. Proetz (1953) reported that the general pattern of the normal air currents in the nose is determined by three structural elements: the direction of the anterior naris, the essential configuration of the nasal chamber, and the relative sizes of the anterior and posterior nares. During normal breathing, air does not reach the olfactory cleft, and, upon expiration, air normally passes along the lower routes. Once olfaction is begun, sniffing reflexively draws air up into the olfactory cleft. In normal sniffing there is a dilation of the lower orifice by a spreading of the lateral alar cartilage of the nose and a narrowing of the upper orifice by traction of the lateral alar cartilage. As a consequence a greater quantity of air enters at a faster rate, according to Portmann (1951). The odorous materials thus reach the olfactory fissure by diffusion, by direct projection of odoriferous molecules, and by the eddies of air created in the nose at the beginning of inhalation.

Schneider and Wolf (1960) reported that olfactory acuity was impaired when there was a high degree of nasal obstruction or when the mucosa was relatively pale, dry, and shrunken. Thus, smelling is performed best when the mucosa is red, swollen, and wet but not to such a degree as to block air passage substantially. They suggested that the greater acuity for medium values of redness and swelling is due to increased temperature within the nasal cavity so that the volatility and dispersion of odor molecules is increased. Kuehner (1954) noted: "At the onset of a head cold, an operator's (olfactory) sensitivity increases strikingly before it is destroyed by mucous accumulation." Odor may also reach the olfaction region from the mouth and pharynx during expiration of air, during swallowing, or, in the case of very odorous materials, by diffusion. This is one reason for the confusion between taste and odor.

The effect of the shape of the nose on the path of air was noted by Fortunato and Niccolini (1958). They observed considerable variation in the pressure of the inspired air. There was also some variation in the rate at which the air was warmed on entering the nose, depending on volume and humidity of the inspired air, pressure, configuration of the nose, and other factors. Those investigators stressed that the character and strength of an odor depend, to a certain extent, on the observer's anatomy, physiology, and psychology. For summaries of the structure of the olfactory region or its functioning, see Allison (1953), Fortunato and Catalano (1958), Niccolini (1958), Fortunato (1958a,b), and Bartalena (1958a,b). In the Semon lecture of 1955, Adrian (1956) remarked on the bulk of the olfactory region in most mammals, and stressed that a given quantity of odorous material is more effective if it passes through the nose in one second than if it takes twenty seconds. Thus the depth and course of inspiration can control the intensity of the stimulus over a wide range. The differential sensitivity to different odors in areas of the olfactory region may be important (see also Chapter 3, Section VII).

The olfactory region, or olfactory epithelium, is yellow or yellow-brown, in contrast to the reddish hue of the other parts of the nasal cavity. The source and nature of the lipid- or lipid-soluble pigment has been studied by Heusghem and Gerebtzoff (1953), Gerebtzoff and Philippot (1957), and Jackson (1960). Ottoson (1963) considers it highly improbable that the pigments or their autoxidation products are related to the olfactory perception mechanism.

Only the inner face of the superior concha and the adjacent outward face of the septum are innervated by the olfactory nerve—about 2.5 cm² or 500–625 mm² in man (some say as much as 750 mm²). The olfactory region contains basal cells, sustentacular (supporting) cells, and sensory (olfactory) cells. It is estimated that man has 10 to 20 million such receptors; Ottoson (1963) indicates 100 million for the rabbit. The olfactory epithelium as well as the rest of the nasal surface is also innervated by bare nerve fibers from the trigeminal nerve.*

The sensory cells are bipolar neurons with oval-shaped cell bodies. The olfactory rod or dendrite extends from the peripheral part of the cell body, ending in a rounded enlargement, the olfactory vesicle. Very thin hairlike projections protrude from the vesicle into the mucus. The number of these filaments has been variously reported—as 9–16 by Le Gros Clark (1956), and 1000 by Bloom and Engström (1952)—but Ottoson (1963) indicates that it is likely that ciliary processes of cells other than receptor cells may have been confused with olfactory hairs in some studies. They appear to be 1–2 μ long and 0.1 μ wide, but a fine process may extend to 100 μ, according to Gasser (1956), and this increases their total surface enormously. Ottoson (1956) presented evidence that the potential probably originates in the olfactory hairs. As Mateson (1954) indicated, there is no positive evidence that these filaments protrude through the liquid epithelial covering into the gaseous environment of the nasal cavity.

Beidler (1961b) noted that the nuclei of the receptors are situated at different depths in the olfactory mucosa, with olfactory rods, 20–90 μ long, extending to the surface. He and others have suggested that these differences in receptor morphology may be related to differential sensi-

---

* Parker (1922) and others consider that, from the histological point of view, the neurons of the olfactory epithelium (and of the vomeronasal organ) represent "primary" sense cells. Their similarity to the receptor element of primitive forms (in that its nerve cell body is located in the receptive epithelium) is another reason for considering this sense as morphologically "primitive." The receptors of the common chemical sense are "free" nerve terminations in the epithelium of moist surfaces of apertures of the body without specialized end organs. The taste buds are specialized epithelial cells, and their specialization is induced from nerve fibers. The receptive cells of taste buds, then, represent "secondary" sense cells forming groups of elements associated with neuron terminals. The cell bodies of taste buds are, as with the apparent neurons of the common chemical sense, deeply situated in association with the central nervous system. Parker calls this "sensory appropriation."

tivity to odors and might be a basis for odor quality discrimination. The whole region is covered with secretion from numerous branched alveolo-tubular glands which contain both mucous and serous cells. The proximal part of the body of the sensory cell tapers down to a fine process which continues as the olfactory nerve fiber, and finally terminates in the olfactory bulb.

The over-all physiological design for odor perception is schematically outlined in Fig. 32. This chart emphasizes several important aspects of

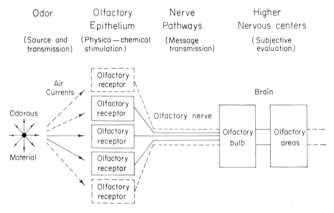

FIG. 32. Diagrammatic scheme of olfactory perception.

odor perception: (1) the prospective odorous material must be volatile; (2) the odor-laden air must reach the olfactory receptors; (3) differences in diffusion rates may be a factor in stimulation; and (4) the odor must dissolve in an aqueous mucus and then diffuse through it. There is, of course, a critical concentration below which there will be no identifiable sensation. The exact definition of a threshold appears to be more difficult in this case than with the other senses. Some believe that the actual threshold is not measured, but only some effect of various external and internal influences. This, of course, increases the day-to-day variability in results. See Chapter 5, Section IV.

VII. Neural Mechanisms

Recent work on the neural mechanisms involved in olfaction has been reviewed by Wenger *et al.* (1956), Pfaffmann (1956), Adey (1959), Beidler (1961a,b), and Ottoson (1963). Those investigators emphasized the constant morphology of the olfactory system throughout the vertebrates. Areas other than the olfactory have been shown to play some role in olfaction. Ogasawara (1954) found no discontinuity between the sensory endings in the mucosa and the cell bodies in the bulb. This is at variance with most results, although it is recognized that the connections are very intimate. The fine, unmyelinated proximate ends of the olfactory cells are the axons which enter the olfactory bulb. Here the sensory cell is both the receiver and conductor, i.e., a primary neuron. These nerve fibers end in a series of intricate basketlike terminations called glomeruli. There they synapse with the large mitral and the tufted cells. Axons from both types form the olfactory tract which then passes along the base of the frontal lobe. The arrangement in the olfactory bulb of cells and axons provides a convergence of pathways and a return route back to the glomerulus by way of collaterals. Hence there is a sort of closed reverberating system, or "feedback," and this may partially account for the great sensitivity of the sense of smell (see Fig. 32). As Ottoson (1963) says: "The structural arrangement of the synaptic connections between primary and secondary neurons in separate units represented by the glomeruli may serve an important function in olfactory discrimination. It was suggested that there is a concentration of fibers from functionally similar receptors onto particular glomeruli." However, much more evidence is needed on the nature of the "feedback" system. From only ten different receptors with a simple two-way response, it has been estimated that 2^{10} odors could be differentiated.

The olfactory membrane develops a slow, negative, purely monophasic potential when stimulated by odorous material (Fig. 33). A wavelike oscillation of 25–30 cycles per second (cps) is a particularly striking feature of the olfactory bulb. Olfactory stimulation initiates long or short bursts of activity. The activity seems to arise peripherally rather than within the neuronal network inside the bulb. Adrian (1955) recorded sine-wavelike oscillatory waves from the olfactory mucosa directly during odor stimulation. The frequency was 30–60 cps, with an amplitude of 0.05–0.1 mv. Adrian noted that the rate-limiting step appeared to be in the neural components of the olfactory bulb and not in the receptors. Thresholds varied with the substance and the region of the olfactory bulb tested (Adrian, 1956). Near-threshold concentrations of amyl acetate, for example, gave an abrupt discharge near the anterior pole. Hydrocarbons resulted in a more gradual discharge, deep in the posterior part. Thus, spatial distribution may be a factor in olfactory stimulation. Fibers which responded to lipoid-soluble substances rarely responded to water-soluble materials, and vice versa. Adrian concluded that he demonstrated two extreme types of electrical responses unevenly distributed over the epithelium of the olfactory region [axon spikes of uniform size and large potential (0.1–0.2 mv) compared to smaller spikes of varying size]. At first Adrian (1955) believed these waves came from the sensory cell and not from the axons. He later

(1957) reported that they appeared to be generated by the dendritic potentials in the glomerular region. Ottoson (1956) demonstrated that the effect elicited in the olfactory receptors increases approximately logarithmically with increasing odor intensity.

Ueki and Domino (1961) reported evidence that bursts of electrical activity in the olfactory structures were synchronous with inspiration in the monkey and with inspiration and expiration in dogs. Odor-free oxygen, nitrogen, or carbon dioxide elicited the discharges. When the

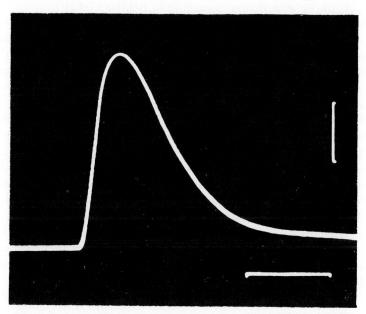

Fig. 33. An electro-olfactogram. Response from nasal mucosa with butanol. Vertical line is 1 mv; time bar is 2 sec. Source: Ottoson (1956).

rate of flow of the odoriferous air was kept constant, an increase in rate of flow of oxygen caused greater electrical response. Obviously the concentration per unit volume of gas decreased. It is not clear whether the effect is one of pressure or flow, and this seems to conflict with the data reported by Beidler (1961b).

Because of the inaccessibility and short length of the olfactory nerve fibers, electrical activity from them is difficult to record. The conduction velocity of the olfactory nerve fibers appears, however, to belong among the slowest-conducting afferent systems in the body, according to Ottoson (1963). It is possible to study the activity of single units of the olfactory nerve, and these show that different units react to odors in different ways.

Walsh (1956) has characterized the single-cell spike discharges in the olfactory bulb of the rabbit as indicating three classes of neurons. Those of classes I and II are not modified by olfactory stimulation (those of class II discharged intermittently in synchrony with passage of air through the nose). It thus appears that only class III cells respond to odors. Some cells of class III respond to some odors and not to others; hence, odor specifically appears to be a fundamental characteristic of the olfactory system. However, the olfactory response may be increased by sympathetic stimulation, according to Beidler (1961b).

Shibuya and Shibuya (1963) recorded single-unit spike discharges in the olfactory epithelium in response to odors such as amyl acetate. The decrement in height, number per minute, and average frequency increased with increasing odor strength. The authors believe these positive spike discharges were from the olfactory cell body rather than from its axonal extension. Different odors did not produce specific patterns of discharge. Shibuya (1964) believes that the negative slow potential is not the generator potential as indicated by Ottoson (1963).

The region of the brain stimulated by odorous substances has also been investigated by electrical measurements. The largest and most stable responses are in the prepiriform and piriform cortex, in the anterior commissure and its branches, the ventral part of the head of the caudate nucleus, the olfactory tubercle, and the anterior limbs of the internal capsule. These are believed to be the direct olfactory system. Potentials with longer latency can also be detected in the claustrum, putamen, globus pallidus and in the lateral control, and basal amygdaloid nuclei. The slowest responses are in the septum and the dorsal part of the caudate nucleus. The foregoing emphasizes the complexity of olfactory central connections.

When wire needles were inserted into the bulb of the rabbit and odorous substances applied, water-soluble odors gave a response in the anterior portion, and fat-soluble stimuli tended to activate the posterior region, again suggesting that different types of odors influence different parts of the olfactory region. There is also some evidence that low-frequency stimulation of nonolfactory regions of the brain may nevertheless result in activity in the olfactory bulb. Mozell (1958) emphasized, however, that the number of spatial and temporal differentiations which can be demonstrated fall far short of the vast number of discriminable odors.

Tucker (1961) noted that nerves other than the olfactory receptors respond to odorants. The olfactory receptors of the land tortoise were responsive to various compounds, and, with the techniques employed, no particular site was more sensitive to any odorant in particular. The odor species, concentration of odor in the air entering the nares, and the nasal flow rate were more important in determining electrophysiological response than temperature, humidity, or the nature of the inert gas carrier. The dependence on flow rate is due to losses in odorous molecules before arrival at the receptors being monitored. With the land tortoise the response of the olfactory receptors appeared to be insensitive to variations in ionic strength, pH, and osmotic pressure.

With olfaction, in contrast to most other sensory systems, there is evidence that amplitude rather than frequency-modulation is important. The number of, and differences between, the odor receptors are not known. Adrian (1951) found that the mitral cells of the cat's olfactory epithelium could be arranged into 10 classes according to response to different chemical stimuli. Beidler (1954) believes that the olfactory receptors do not all respond to odorous stimuli in the same manner. Adrian (1956, 1957) demonstrated a differential odor sensitivity at the mitral cell level which may account for odor quality discrimination. He also suggested that the brain may receive olfactory information via the gray matter as well as through discharges in the large mitral fibers in the olfactory tract. He believes the latter might provide fine discrimination while the former is concerned with arousing olfactory attention. (See Chapter 3, Section V for Amoore's work on olfactory receptor specificity.) The current status of this research is summarized by Beidler (1961a,b), Ottoson (1963), and Zotterman (1963).

Many different smells must be detected with a finite number of receptors. Sumner's (1954) idea (Chapter 3, Section XIII,G) that a limited number of receptors are more or less responsive to a given stimulus is worth considering. Beidler (1954) suggested that such theoretical studies do not provide the information desired regarding the response of individual receptors. Recent work by Gesteland (1961) demonstrated six different types of receptors. One type responded to camphor but was unaffected by the other odors. Each of four receptors responded to a single odor but was inhibited by another odor.

VIII. Olfactory Abnormalities

Among the medical terms employed for olfactory anomalies (which may be uni- or bilateral) are cryptosmia (obstruction in nasal passages), anosmia (temporary or permanent loss of smelling capacity), hemianosmia or hyperosmia (excessive response), merosmia (loss of only certain odors), heterosmia or parosmia (false odors perceived), autosmia (odor sensation in the absence of odor stimuli), and cacosmia (persistent perception of unpleasant odors). Anosmia may be due to mechanical or central injury, or it may be functional. Portmann (1951) reported that some individuals subject to migraine headaches had hyperosmia and that individuals with anosmia usually have defective taste sensitivity. Merosmia is reported to occur after certain operations and may be unilateral. For the effect of accidents on olfactory acuity, see Graf (1961). Borsanyi and Blanchard (1962) and Borsanyi *et al.* (1962) used psychogalvanic skin response to determine whether a person was anosmic. This is based on the fact that the electrical resistance of the skin is affected by the autonomic nervous system through changes in the formation of sweat beneath the electrodes. Since the autonomic nervous system may be affected by emotional stimuli, sound, and pain as well as by smell, it is obvious that the results must be interpreted carefully. Whether the method could be perfected to detect odor thresholds is not known.

Guillot (1958) reported 11 types of anosmia, indicating, he believed, at least 11 specific sensory types of cells. To account for several chemical substances with different structures having the same odor he considered that there are several types of sensory cells specific for each compound but all influencing the same central olfactory region. To explain why a single compound smells different as the physiological state of the observer differs, he theorized that a single sensory cell influences several regions in the central cortex. There may, of course, be two methods of transmission: one where a complex odor stimulates several sensory cells, and one in which simple but specific stimuli operate. He suggested that molecules might have a specific action or, in the case of stereoisomers, qualitative identity but with quantitative differences in intensity.

Patterson and Lauder (1948) tested 4030 high school and college students and found that seventeen were anosmic to butyl mercaptan. Sensitivity to other odors was measured, and their families were investigated. Four types of deficiencies were found: (1) seven cases due to accident or disease; (2) four cases showing inheritance of smell blindness as a recessive character; (3) four anosmic through inheritance as a dominant character; and (4) two "partial" anosmics that exhibited a faint reaction to a very strong solution. Le Magnen (1953) cited other examples of partial anosmia. He also reported that, following anesthesia, there was a different rate of return of sensitivity for various odors, and that the quality of the odor was modified. This type of research should be extended.

Castello (1958) compared odor responses of normal individuals with those of abnormal individuals, particularly the anomalies observed in alcoholics, dope addicts, etc. Ghirlanda (1958) described modifications in olfactory function in individuals with endocrine disorders. Bartalena

(1958b) summarized various types of partial and complete anosmia—both congenital and inherited. Semeria (1958) described olfactory aberrations following accident, disease, or hypnosis.

Le Magnen and Rapaport (1951) found that rats with severe vitamin A deficiency were unable to make odor discriminations. The yellow color of the olfactory region suggests a possible connection between vitamin A and olfaction. Duncan and Briggs (1962) have improved odor sensitivity in some cases of anosmia by treatment with vitamin A. Schneider *et al.* (1958) reported increased sensitivity to citral with two hypogonadal subjects receiving estrogens, and decreased sensitivity in a patient receiving androgens. Local changes in the nasal membranes were suggested as contributing to these differences. Joergensen and Buch (1961, 1962) showed that hyposmia occurred in about 60% of 58 diabetics studied. Whether the cause is peripheral or central has not been established.

According to Henkin *et al.* (1962), patients with adrenal insufficiency exhibited lower odor thresholds than normal subjects. Henkin and Powell (1962) reported that six of eleven patients with cystic fibrosis consistently demonstrated taste thresholds for sodium chloride, potassium chloride, sucrose, hydrochloric acid, and urea that were extremely low in comparison with those of 28 normal controls. It is of interest that nine of the eleven patients had extremely low odor thresholds for these compounds whereas the controls were unable to smell them at any concentration tested. The "odor" thresholds of the afflicted patients for sodium chloride, sucrose, hydrochloric acid, and urea were 0.01, 0.01, 0.006, and 0.08 mole per liter, respectively. Since some of these compounds are generally considered to be nonodorous, it is possible that impurities in the compound or extraneous odors in the containers contributed to these threshold values.

Changes in olfactory sensitivity during pregnancy have been reviewed by Noferi and Guidizi (1946), Salis (1959), and Luvarà and Maurizi (1961). The last researchers found hyperosmia during the first 3 months, whereas hyposmia was observed in the second 3 months and especially in the last 3 months. Immediately after delivery, hyperosmia was again found for a short period. However, the number of patients was limited, the patients were not the same in all trials, and the suspect Elsberg technique was employed. Further experiments would be welcome in view of Salis' (1959) negative results. Ottoson (1963) considers that the changes in olfactory sensitivity which occur during pregnancy can be explained by hormonal effects upon the olfactory mucosa.

There are reports that various substances increase olfactory acuity (caffeine, for example) and that others decrease olfactory acuity or produce anosmia (tyrothricin, acetylcholine). In some cases intravenous injection leads to olfactory sensation, probably, Ottoson (1963) suggests, by being carried to the mucosa by the blood and giving rise to excitation of the olfactory nerve by direct excitation of the end organs.

Hoeven-Leonard (1908) postulated a connection between low color sensitivity and high olfactory acuity, but no definite studies seem to have been made. This reminds us of Fauvelle's (1888) suggestion that forms of life with a prominent naso-labial organ often have limited vision. He believed that this might apply to individuals and races.

Amici and Raschella (1958) noted the close central connection of the olfactory and gustatory senses. The psychic effects of the olfactory sense on the condition of the organism suggested to them further experimentation on the relation of the senses. However, if the gustatory sense is considered to be projected in the somesthetic region of the parental lobes and is thus a specialized skin sense, it is clearly very different from olfaction.

IX. Odor Testing Techniques

A number of techniques and a variety of equipment have been developed for the determination of odor intensity and olfactory sensitivity in animal and in human subjects. The design and construction of such equipment have been reported by Zwaardemaker (1895, 1921a,b, 1925), Woodrow and Karpman (1917), Elsberg and Levy (1935), Gundlach and Kenway (1939), Pfaffmann (1948), Wenzel (1948a,b), Castello (1958), Fortunato and Niccolini (1958), Moncrieff (1951), Portmann (1951), Barail (1952), Neuhaus (1953), Deininger and McKinley (1954), Jones (1954, 1955a), Sfiras and Demeilliers (1957), Nader (1958), Pfaffmann *et al.* (1958), Stuiver (1958), Prince and Ince (1958), Bozza *et al.* (1960), Johnston and Sandoval (1960, 1962), and Ough and Stone (1961). Stone *et al.* (1965) have prepared a critical review of olfactometry, with specific emphasis on food odors.

The failure of many of these approaches to produce a satisfactory theory of olfaction is attributable to the lack of: (1) an understanding of the dimensions of the stimulus or the sensation, which is due partially to the inaccessibility of the olfactory region; (2) satisfactory methods for the control of pain (trigeminal responses at high odor concentrations); (3) control of temperature and humidity during testing; (4) precise control of air-flow pressure and velocity; (5) a supply of odor-free air and highly purified and stable test materials; (6) quantitative control of odor concentration; (7) the use of odorless and easily cleaned construction materials; and (8) a means of expressing the intensity of the stimulus in some common scientific unit. The foregoing conditions, discussed by several investigators, require careful consideration in the construction and use of apparatus for odor testing (Gundlach and Kenway, 1939; Wenzel, 1948a).

Although the physical, chemical, and mechanical problems of olfactometry can be defined and investigated, the subjective response of the observer introduces psychological problems which are not easily defined (see Chapter 5). Stuiver (1958) pointed out that since only a few observations can be made before adaptation occurs, tests must be conducted over a period of time in order to get meaningful information on human olfactory sensitivity. The equipment may be of different design; however, the theory is the same: delivery of an odorous material to a subject and the measurement of his response to intensities, differences, or affective qualities. Individual variation was also emphasized by Jones (1957) and Moulton *et al.* (1960).

A. History

The first investigations, reported by Valentin in 1850 (Wenzel, 1948b), consisted of a measured amount of odorous material sealed in a small thin-walled glass tube placed inside a larger container. The small tube was broken, and the subject opened the container and sniffed the contents. If the subject could detect the odor, the test was repeated with the same quantity of material in larger containers until the odor was no longer recognizable. Major errors associated with this technique include adsorption of the test material on the glass (important at threshold concentrations), dilution when the container was opened, and difficulty in weighing the volatile material (Wenzel, 1948a,b). From this crude but simple serial-dilution method there have developed a large number of similar techniques employing various solvents or diluents, such as air, compressed gas, mineral oil, or glycerol.

Several years later, Zwaardemaker (1895, 1921b) introduced an olfactometer consisting of two tubes, one fitting inside the other, with the inner tube graduated, perforated on the sides, open at both ends, and shaped to fit the subject's nostril. The odorous material was transported through the outer tube, and the subject withdrew the inner rod until the odor was just detected. This length of exposed rod was considered one "olfactie" (unit of odor stimulus), and withdrawing the tube further gave so many more olfacties. In general, an olfactie is defined as the odor stimulus of exactly one threshold odor concentration of any odorant. The ratio of the true concentration divided by the threshold concentration is the number of olfacties of the sample. Both single and double olfactometers were used by Zwaardemaker. In these studies, temperature and humidity were not controlled. Further, it was assumed that a progressive increase in exposure caused a proportional increase in the saturation of the air current. Air becomes saturated with vapor when the partial pressure of the vapor in the air equals the vapor pressure of its liquid at that temperature. If the air is saturated, no increase in concentration of the vapor could occur if the area exposed is increased. In spite of these objections and the lack of a quantitative measure of the odor, the data are believed to indicate the relative intensities of different odor compounds. A modification of the Zwaardemaker instrument by Reuter, using solid odoriferous substances, was described by Portmann (1951).

During this same time, other investigators constructed and experimented with more elaborate testing techniques. Woodrow and Karpman (1917) used air bubbled through test samples at different temperatures and delivered to the subject's nose. Their experiments were concerned with adaptation and were limited to liquids. Recently, Mullins (1955a) noted that sensitivity in olfactory testing was maximum when the odor concentration was raised as rapidly as possible to the desired level. He further noted that, at low flow rates, considerable adsorption could occur on the mucous membranes. Therefore, the supposed relation of duration of odor sensation and odor concentration as reported by Woodrow and Karpman (1917) was due to: (1) low flow velocities; and (2) a continuous increase in concentration with time at the olfactory epithelium.

Another method, described by Allison and Katz (1919), is quite complicated but introduced one of the better olfactometers. The flowmeters used were Venturi tubes so arranged that a measured volume of air could pass at a uniform rate through or over the chemical and could be mixed with a measured volume of pure air, also flowing at a uniform rate. The chemical concentration was determined by measuring the loss in weight after a measured volume of air passed over it. The subject sniffed once and reported "no odor, detectable, faint, noticeable, strong, or very strong."

Hofmann and Kohlrausch (1925) developed a blast-type olfactometer. Saturated vapor was stored over mercury, mixed with air by mercury columns, and then delivered through nosepieces to the subject's nostrils. With pressure, volume, and specific gravity known, the concentration (gram fraction) for 1 cc was calculated. Morimura (1934) modified this apparatus in his experiments on the effects of temperature and various states of anosmia on odor thresholds. His reasons for the modifications were incomplete mixing of air and odor material (with the mercury) and subject variation over long periods. In spite of improvements, the apparatus was subject to several disadvantages: adsorption of the vapor on the tubing, the use of rubber tubing, the use of a large number of containers, and the slow rate of testing.

An apparatus described by Gundlach and Kenway (1939) used manometers to regulate dilution of odorous material obtained by sparging a test liquid. The design was such, however, that changing the concentration required several hours. The technique was slow, saturation of the air was not certain, and the period of sniffing was uncontrolled. Subjects were asked to inhale briefly from each of two nosepieces (one pure air, and the other a test material) while a continuous supply of both was emitted.

B. ELSBERG TECHNIQUE

In 1935, Elsberg and his associates introduced their injection technique. It is interesting to note that Elsberg was concerned primarily with locating brain tumors via partial or complete anosmia of one or both nostrils. The technique involved placing an odorous material under varying amounts of pressure and releasing this directly into the nose while the subject held his breath. Both pressure and volume varied. The smallest identifiable volume was called the MIO (minimum identifiable odor). Elsberg *et al.* (1935b) recommended inhalation tests with ammonia, benzene, menthol, xylol, benzaldehyde, citral, coffee, or oil of turpentine. For blast-injection tests (high rates of steady flow), the last four compounds were recommended. Experimentation over the past several years, however, has indicated that the technique is unreliable and not suitable for further odor investigations (Jones, 1955a; Wenzel, 1948b). Wenzel (1948a), Jones (1953a, 1954), and others modified this technique in an attempt to overcome some of its drawbacks. Wenzel designed an apparatus (Fig. 34) with controlled temperature, pressure, and volume of stimulus which permitted calculation of molecular concentrations delivered to the subjects, and used test materials with known vapor pressures. She was unable to demonstrate a significant difference between odor and pressure judgments, and cautioned against using the technique in differential measurements.

In 1950, Castello (see Fortunato and Niccolini, 1958) constructed an electronic olfactometer based on the blast injection method, with elaborate controls for pressure, temperature, and humidity. Nitrogen was used as the diluent, part of each test sample was bypassed through an ionization chamber, and deflections on a microammeter were noted. The obvious disadvantage of these measurements is that they lack quantitative significance. Results are reported on a time basis and would be of some value for studying olfactory fatigue, but only with this instrument and technique. Fortunato and Niccolini (1958) also employed the Elsberg technique in their studies of olfactory fatigue. Instead of the single bottle, several containers were placed on a revolving plate and different materials could be sampled by revolving the plate. The center of the plate had a vertical column to keep the bottles in place and served as a mounting for the syringe with inlet and outlet valves.

Jones (1953a) theorized that if the Elsberg test measured thresholds of molecular concentrations the MIO should increase with decreasing concentration. Experimental results indicated that concentration did

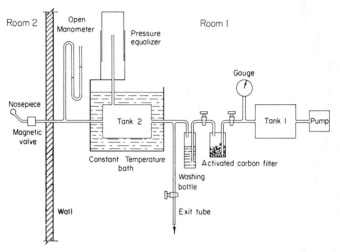

FIG. 34. Wenzel's olfactometer. Source: Wenzel (1948a).

not have a uniform effect, and the data could not be transformed to molecular terms. To avoid pressure differences and obtain molar concentrations, Jones (1954) devised a motor-driven syringe filled with air and test material. Concentrations were varied by changing proportions of each. For two different concentrations of benzene there was a good agreement between subjects, but with methyl salicylate there were wide differences between individuals. Jones emphasized that the Elsberg injection thresholds could not be converted to molar concentrations. It was further concluded that thresholds obtained by the blast-injection method might in some way be related to the aerodynamics of the individual nose. Wenzel (1955) also concluded that the Elsberg injection technique was unreliable for odor testing, for several important reasons: (1) the inability of subjects to perform reliably over long periods despite training; (2) lack of control over the position of internal mouth and throat parts; and (3) the extreme artificiality of the situation (holding the breath).

C. OTHER OLFACTOMETERS

As a replacement, Wenzel suggested the use of an odor-free environment similar to Zwaardemaker's (1895) "camera inodorata," which utilized normal breathing. Controlled amounts of odor are added to the container, and the subject responds at will. Odor concentration is attained by saturation of a stream of pure air with odor by sparging the

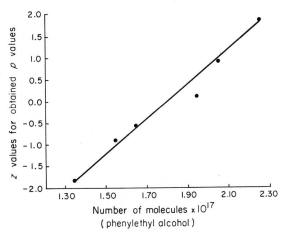

FIG. 35. Relative discrimination to phenylethyl alcohol. The method of plotting transforms the original ogive into a straight line by converting the percentages of "strong" judgments (obtained p values) to normal curve z scores. Source: Wenzel (1948a).

air through the odorous liquid. The test vapor is then released to the subject by electronic timers and valves. The subject breaths normally, no special training is required, and the environment around the subject's head is controlled. Difference thresholds were obtained for phenylethyl alcohol, as shown in Fig. 35.

Similar olfactometers based on this same principle have been used by Stuiver (1958, 1960), Cheesman and Kirkby (1959), Bozza *et al.* (1960), Johnston and Sandoval (1960), Ough and Stone (1961), and Stone *et al.* (1962). In the Cheesman and Kirkby apparatus several points could be supplied independently with controlled concentrations of odorous materials. In the others, manometers were used to supply a wide range of concentrations of the odorous materials but only the last olfactometer (Fig. 36) had the odor-free environment (in the form of a Plexiglas hood around the subject's head). By careful measurement of the air flow rates and the concentrations of odorous material, Ough and Stone (1961) could determine actual concentrations delivered to the

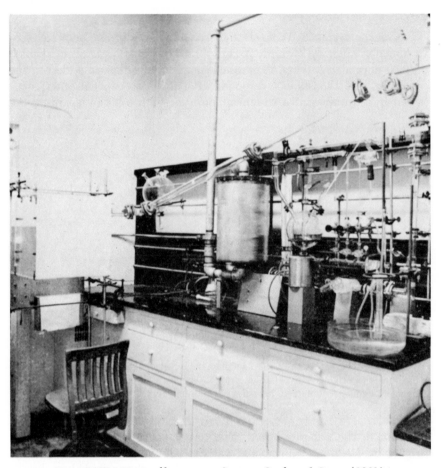

FIG. 36. The Davis olfactometer. Source: Ough and Stone (1961).

subject at any specific setting of the manometer. In the original Wenzel apparatus, the number of molecules could be altered only by changing the rate of flow, but this obviously introduced a second variable. Stuiver (1958, 1960) found that charcoal and silica gel, used as deodorants, actually introduced odors themselves. This should be checked further. In Stuiver's apparatus a nitrogen stream was therefore used to introduce odors at 32% humidity at 17°C. Materials with low thresholds had to be cooled, and very small capillaries used. Some compounds (1,4-xylen-2-ol, for example) adsorbed strongly, and short distances and a preconditioned apparatus had to be employed. In general, Stuiver's apparatus was similar to those of Gundlach and Kenway (1939) and Neuhaus (1953).

The Milan olfactometer (Bozza et al., 1960; Battiston, 1962) is quite similar to the apparatus of Ough and Stone (1961). One unique and desirable feature of their design is the use of solid substances for odorizing the air. The interval between the moment the stimulus is taken away and the disappearance of the sensation is defined as the delay, or persistence, time. This time depends on the concentration, and the threshold is determined by extrapolating the delay concentration curve. The subjective nature of the time interval seems to us a valid objection to this procedure. Its adaptability for mono- and birhinal, as well as homo- and hetero-olfactometry, is an advantage.

The next step beyond this type of olfactometer was the introduction of a glass olfactorium (Foster and Dallenbach, 1948; Foster *et al.*,

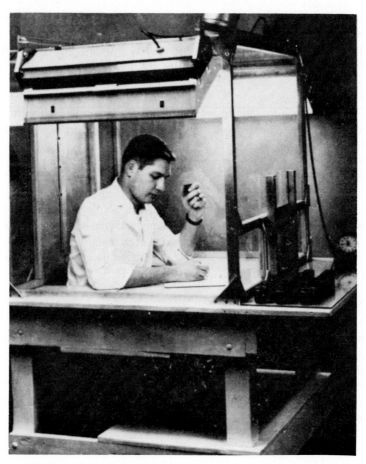

Fig. 37. Olfactorium for presentation of samples for sniffing. Source: Pilgrim and Schutz (1957).

1950). Not only atmospheric odors were controlled; odors emanating from the subjects themselves were minimized by covering the subjects with a plastic envelope. Samples were then introduced by atomizing samples into the entering air stream.

Deininger and McKinley (1954) have also described an olfactorium of sufficient size to permit several subjects to be tested simultaneously. This olfactorium, which they used in conjunction with the flavor profile procedure (Chapter 8, Section V), was protected by an antechamber with 5 oscillating fans to ensure homogeneity in the atmosphere. Samples were introduced by means of an ultramicroburet, with a fan for distribution. To facilitate odor delivery, a meteorological balloon was employed as a gas holder. Schneider and Wolf (1955) described a similar olfactorium, and used citral as the test material. Subsequent studies by Berg *et al.* (1963) indicated that citral lacked stability over a few day's testing. Rennes (1945) released camphor into a room, apparently mainly to detect anosmia. A small "olfactorium" (Fig. 37) was used by Pilgrim and Schutz (1957), but subjects employed a sniffing technique from bottles. The technique of The American Society for Testing Materials (1961) is similar, but is designed for thresholds of industrial odors. The procedure calls for no tobacco, gum chewing, or eating for at least 30 minutes prior to the test.

There are many disadvantages to the olfactorium technique. Since the panel is in the room for some time, olfactory adaptation may very easily occur. Distracting body odors and perfumes could be brought in by the subjects, and are often very difficult to eliminate. In addition, the technique does not lend itself to testing varying concentrations over short intervals. Finally, cleaning the room after each test would be difficult, time consuming, and costly. The results do not seem to justify the construction of such rooms.

D. SNIFFING

The simplest technique, and probably the most popular, for odor determination is sniffing. Baten (1946) showed that there were variations between subjects but that selected subjects were reliable. Jones (1955a,c) concluded that sniffing was an adequate technique for threshold studies. Other workers have also been successful with this technique (Cheesman and Mayne, 1953; Cheesman and Townsend, 1958; Engen and Pfaffmann, 1959). Bags made of odorless plastic and filled with odor have been used for sniffing in odor intensity studies by Reese and Stevens (1960). One difficulty associated with these methods is the preparation of a test series in some stable, inodorous, nonreactive solvent of low viscosity. Calculation of odor concentrations in the vapor may present problems unless an ideal solution is assumed. At low concentrations it is assumed that Henry's Law is obeyed, and knowledge of the vapor pressure and mole fraction of solute permits calculation of the concentration of the odorous material in the vapor above the solute. In spite of the above disadvantages, the technique is popular, inexpensive, and easy to carry out with large numbers of subjects.

Jones (1955a) experimentally compared sniffing with the Elsberg injection procedure and concluded that the two were not directly comparable. In sniffing tests the question of whether the partial vapor pressure is proportional to the amount of substance dissolved is of critical importance. Tables of partial vapor pressures and the amount of substance dissolved in a liquid are available for some chemicals, but these should be determined for each case. The molecules adhering to the walls of the flask could be an interfering variable.

A special type of odor threshold problem is that of the odor of industrial water supplies. One common method is that of the American Society for Testing Materials (1960). This uses a triad-system sniffing technique in which the observer must distinguish the flask containing the water being tested from two flasks containing odor-free water.

Guadagni *et al.* (1963) used a questionable system for determining thresholds. Polyethylene bottles were partially filled with an aqueous solution of the odorous material. A plastic tube connected to the bottle was placed in the nostril. Manual squeezing of the bottle forced odorous air into the nasal passages. They found much lower thresholds with this procedure than with sniffing. Unfortunately, it was difficult to free the polyethylene bottles of all odor and control of pressure is not possible. Teflon bottles are now recommended.

E. Control

In olfactory tests, too little attention has been paid to ensuring that the subjects can breath normally. Coumétou (1959) suggested several simple tests. The Rosenthal procedure demands 15 normal inspirations with both nostrils open, 15 with the left closed, and 15 with the right closed—all with the mouth closed. If, at the end of the 45 inspirations, breathing is without discomfort, the nasal passages can be considered free of obstruction. Breathing onto a polished metal should produce two nearly equal spots of condensation.

Moncrieff (1961) measured the temperature rise when odorized air was passed through an adsorbent. The rise in temperature varied from one compound to another for the same adsorbent, or between adsorbents for the same compound. Moncrieff believes that his instrument gives a simulation of the olfactory act. No tests appear to have been made with nonodorous materials (except water). Water gave a response when a protein film was used as the adsorbent. The instrument might be used in certain plant situations where detection of an odor is necessary, but we do not consider it very useful as a simulant of the olfactory process.

Fatiguing the olfactory sense for one odor reduces the sensitivity to related odors and may cause striking differences in the nature of the odor of the second substance. Where no change in sensitivity occurs, one assumes that the two substances have no primary odor in common (Anonymous, 1950).

X. Thresholds

The apparent olfactory thresholds for the most powerful odors are about 10,000 times lower than the lowest taste thresholds. Differential sensitivity to taste, appears to be finer than it is to odor. Fatigue is also more rapid and permanent with smell than with taste, sight, or hearing.

A. Purity of Compounds

Johnston (1960) emphasized how necessary purity is in threshold tests. He noted that gas chromatography may be used to ensure the purity of compounds. Guadagni et al. (1963) purified compounds for olfactory tests by gas-liquid chromatographic separation and verified the purity by refractive index and gas-liquid chromatography. The purified compounds were used less than 2 hours after purification.

B. External Variables

Stuiver (1958) emphasized that the duration and rate of flow of inspired or injected air influenced the threshold markedly. When the duration was changed from 0.1 to 0.05 sec, about equal numbers of molecules were required for a sensation. Above the critical time, the minimum concentration thus remains almost independent of the stimulus duration. The variation in threshold with rate of flow of inspired or injected air can be explained by taking into account diffusion and absorption phenomena in the nasal cavity. Two opposite effects are operating when rate of flow increases: the concentration of the odorous compound entering the olfactory slit increases (because fewer molecules are lost on the mucous membrane before reaching the olfactory region) while the fraction of molecules diffusing to the olfactory epithelium decreases. Tucker (1961) criticized Stuiver's equation because it did not take into account the decrease with time of the number of molecules striking and being effectively trapped on the mucous surface.

Reduction in olfactory acuity in the presence of prolonged noise has been noted. Mitchell (1957a) found more correct responses in beer testing when only one person was in the tasting room than with two or more.

The contrast between humid external and dry interior conditions leads to increased sensitivity, according to Guillot (1959). This increased sensitivity decreases normal appreciation of the quality of perfumes. The possibility of humidity changes modifying olfactory acuity was also considered by Stone (1963).

Pangborn *et al.* (1964) demonstrated that the method of presentation of samples greatly influenced the results. They used the constant-stimulus procedure, requiring 80% correct response. When a sequential procedure using increasing concentrations was used, a lower threshold was obtained (due to the error of anticipation, Chapter 5, Section III), and when a sequential procedure using decreasing concentrations was used, the threshold was higher—error of habituation (see Chapter 5, Section III). Their five judges differed greatly in sensitivity. In these tests one subject had a significant error of the first kind and on the basis of all responses, more errors of the second kind were made (Chapter 10, Section I).

C. Effect of Hunger and Chemicals

The influence of food on olfactory acuity was studied with the Elsberg technique, by Goetzl and his colleagues (see Goetzl and Stone, 1947, 1948; Goetzl *et al.*, 1949, 1950, 1951; Irvin *et al.*, 1950, 1953; Margulies *et al.*, 1950; Stone and Goetzl, 1948). In general, those researchers reported an increase in sensitivity during the morning and a rapid decrease after a meal. Alcohol, sugar, and amphetamine (10 mg) decreased olfactory sensitivity, and tannic, tartaric, or acetic acid ingested with the meal prevented the postcibal (after eating) decrease in acuity. Bitter tonics and dry red wines also prevented this decrease. With sugar, 20 g/135 cc (15%) was equivalent to no lunch, yet 20 g/100 cc (20%) did increase the threshold about half as much as a meal did. Goetzl's results have been criticized (Furchtgott and Friedman, 1960) for having no controls, for incomplete reports of findings, for use of the Elsberg technique, and for using coffee rather than a pure chemical as an odor stimulus. Hammer (1951) observed an increase in olfactory acuity in the morning, and a decrease after lunch. Sensitivity increased throughout the day if no lunch was given. Hammer also measured flicker-fusion frequency, which followed the olfactory and taste data except that the frequency after lunch was the same as if no lunch had been eaten. Hammer attributed this observation to homeostatic factors. The phenomenon seems to represent a complex mixture of fatigue effects and specific and nonspecific effects of food intake on chemoreception. Using an olfactometer presentation of 2-heptanone, Berg *et al.* (1963) observed greater

olfactory sensitivity after lunch than before. The difference was significant at the 0.1% level of probability. Furchtgott and Friedman (1960)
concluded that a mild degree of hunger lowers the olfactory thresholds—
but only slightly and not in all individuals. This subject variability, they
conclude, might explain earlier ambiguous results of Janowitz and Grossman (1949), Meyer (1952), and Zilstorff-Pedersen (1955). Pangborn's
(1959) results show trends, although the differences were not significant.

Before investigations on the relationship between food intake and
sensory acuity are to be meaningful, hunger, appetite, and satiety must
be defined in measurable physiological terms. Ginsberg *et al.* (1948)
reviewed the psychic effects of odors on gastric motility in dogs. In controlled experiments with man, appetite was affected by odors whereas
gastric motility (or tone) was not. Mancioli (1921) found, after meals, a
decrease in olfactory sensitivity which he attributed to excessive stimulation of the olfactory region (during eating).

In beer testing, Mitchell (1957b) found the best performance between 11 A.M. and 2:30 P.M., which would not indicate an after-lunch
decrease in olfactory acuity. Further data are needed, with new and
better techniques, particularly since the data from neurophysiological
studies suggest that the potentials are independent of nutritional needs
(Pfaffmann and Bare, 1950).

Using the Elsberg technique, Skouby and Zilstorff-Pedersen (1954)
found that acetylcholine in small amounts, 0.1–10 μg per milliliter, decreased the olfactory threshold for coffee. Larger amounts, 1 mg per
milliliter, increased the threshold. Menthol had similar effects. Sodium
chloride (0.9%) produced increases of up to 400% in all the 22 experiments. Strychnine, 1–10 mg per milliliter, decreased the threshold in all
experiments.

D. INDIVIDUAL VARIATION

Individual variation in odor thresholds not only is a matter of definition and technique but may be related to differences in the physiological
state of the nose, i.e., to the degree of vasoconstriction. Schneider and
Wolf (1960) pointed out that, since a large number of factors, by direct
or reflex action, may influence turgescence, blood flow, and secretion of
the nasal membrane, it is not surprising that olfactory acuity varies
greatly. Kuehner (1954) showed that extreme variations in sensitivity
made it necessary to "standardize" a subject from day to day in odor
tests. Recent work (Berg *et al.*, 1963; Stone, 1963) also revealed wide
day-to-day variations in thresholds, and some unexplained week-to-week
differences.

Engen (1960) demonstrated that olfactory thresholds obtained by sniffing were usually lowered by practice and by changes in the subject's criterion of discrimination. The practice effect was much greater for some odors than for others. If the subjects looked for "any" odor rather than the characteristic odor of the test material, the practice effect was even greater. Rosen *et al.* (1962) presented evidence that subthreshold concentrations of odors were not only additive but in some cases synergistic.

The effect of age on olfactory acuity was studied by Fortunato (1958a) and Fortunato and Niccolini (1958), who reported more degeneration in males of over 80 years than in females. Decreasing olfactory sensitivity was associated with hormonal imbalance. The decrease was very great with some compounds and much less for others; for acetic acid, for example, no decrease in sensitivity with age was noted. As with other studies of this nature, subjects of various ages were tested rather than the same subjects over a period of years. Weiss (1959) noted the contradictory nature of much of the data on the effect of age on olfactory sensitivity. Recently Kimbrell and Furchtgott (1963) showed significant increases in olfactory thresholds for age groups of 43–49, 50–59, 60–69, and 70–82 years. This agrees with Hinchcliffes' (1962) data.

Tanzariello (1958) reported many cases of occupational effects on olfactory acuity, including employees of cement, sulfur, pumice, coal, tobacco, and mining industries. Meurman (1948a,b) reported that lime and cement dust progressively impaired the sense of smell during 5 years' employment, after which no further diminution in acuity was noted.

E. TYPICAL VALUES

The usefulness of threshold values has been questioned by Kruger *et al.* (1955a), who point out that musk, despite its very low threshold, is not as intense in odor as many other substances with much higher odor thresholds.

The following data present an example of variation in thresholds reflecting differences in degree of control of the stimulus and the purity of the substance. The substance in all cases is methyl salicylate.

Author	Method	Threshold (M)
Jones (1954)	Controlled volume and rate	2.6×10^{-4}
Gundlach and Kenway (1939)	Sniffing	1.9×10^{-5}
Allison and Katz (1919)	Sniffing	11.5×10^{-5}

Laffort (1963a) has summarized the best available data on the olfactory threshold of 192 organic compounds. The results were expressed

in grams per liter, moles per liter and *p. ol* (potential of olfaction), calculated, in analogy to pH and pK, from the expression log (1/molar
concentration at threshold). The scale extends from 2 to 14 and is
roughly proportional to the strength of the odor (Fig. 38). The differences in thresholds were assigned to differences in technique and in
method of giving responses, and to individual variations. These arise

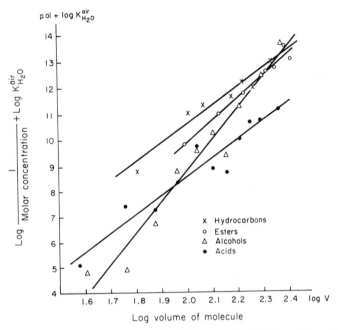

FIG. 38. Relation between potential of olfaction (*p. ol.*) log K and the log of
the molecular volume. Source: Laffort (1963b).

from the configuration of the nose, from failure to distinguish between
the presence of an odor and the presence of a "specific" odor, and from
the usual human differences: age, sex, hormonal balance, anosmia, etc.
The thresholds of different investigators were compared with those of
Schneider and Wolf (1955) and empirically "corrected." The final value
was the probable standard threshold. Some typical values, arranged in
order of the probable standard threshold are given in Table 36. We do
not have too much confidence in the values.

According to Jones (1953b), the International Critical Tables (Zwaardemaker, 1926), which contain a comprehensive collection of threshold
values, are in error by a factor of 100. Since the threshold values are
reported as $A \times 10^x$ molecules per cubic centimeter, increasing x by 2

TABLE 36
Olfactory Thresholds of Typical Compounds

| Compound | Threshold | | p. ol[a] | | Probable standard threshold |
	moles	g	Actual	Corrected	
Ethane	2.99×10^{-2}	8.99×10^{-1}	1.52	4.20	4.20
Ethyl alcohol	5.43×10^{-6}	2.50×10^{-4}	5.27	5.83	
	1.25×10^{-4}	5.75×10^{-3}	3.90	5.68	
	3.98×10^{-6}	1.83×10^{-4}	5.40	4.84	5.68
	2.00×10^{-4}	9.23×10^{-3}	3.70	6.38	
Formic acid	5.44×10^{-7}	2.50×10^{-5}	6.26	6.82	6.06
	1.36×10^{-5}	6.25×10^{-4}	4.87	5.30	
Butane	1.06×10^{-4}	6.16×10^{-3}	3.98	6.66	6.66
Ether	1.35×10^{-8}	1.00×10^{-6}	7.87	8.43	7.86
	7.86×10^{-5}	5.83×10^{-3}	4.10	7.71	
Acetaldehyde	9.09×10^{-8}	4.00×10^{-6}	7.04	9.05	
	2.72×10^{-9}	1.20×10^{-7}	8.57	9.42	8.90
	1.56×10^{-8}	6.88×10^{-7}	7.81	8.24	
Aniline	4.95×10^{-10}	4.61×10^{-8}	9.31	9.31	9.07
	1.04×10^{-8}	9.70×10^{-7}	7.98	8.83	
Benzaldehyde	4.01×10^{-8}	4.29×10^{-6}	7.40	10.21	
	2.83×10^{-8}	3.00×10^{-6}	7.55	9.56	9.61
	4.11×10^{-9}	4.36×10^{-7}	8.39	9.05	
	1.70×10^{-9}	1.80×10^{-7}	8.77	9.62	
Ethyl mercaptan	7.41×10^{-7}	4.60×10^{-5}	6.13	9.74	
	3.06×10^{-9}	1.90×10^{-7}	8.51	10.52	
	7.00×10^{-3}	4.35×10^{-11}	12.16	11.38	10.68
	5.78×10^{-11}	3.59×10^{-9}	10.24	11.09	
Thiophenol	5.63×10^{-10}	6.20×10^{-8}	9.25	11.26	
	1.09×10^{-11}	1.20×10^{-9}	10.96	11.81	11.54
Ionone	4.88×10^{-13}	9.38×10^{-11}	12.31	12.74	
	2.60×10^{-13}	5.00×10^{-11}	12.59	12.03	12.39
Trinitro-2,4,6-*tert*-butyl-3-toluene	2.65×10^{-14}	7.50×10^{-12}	13.58	14.14	
	1.41×10^{-10}	4.00×10^{-8}	9.85	13.46	
	3.53×10^{-14}	1.00×10^{-11}	13.45	13.45	13.24
	3.31×10^{-12}	9.38×10^{-10}	11.48	11.91	

[a] *p. ol.* = potential of olfaction.
Source of data: Laffort (1963a).

TABLE 37
Corrected Threshold Concentrations from International Critical Tables

Compound	Nature of odor	Threshold (mg/liter)
Methyl salicylate	Wintergreen	0.100
Amyl acetate	Banana oil	0.039
n-Butyric acid	Perspiration	0.009
Benzene	Kerosene-like	0.0088
Safrol	Sassafras	0.005
Ethyl acetate	Fruity	0.0036[a]
Pyridine	Burned	0.00074[a]
Hydrogen sulfide	Rotten eggs	0.00018
n-Butyl sulfide	Foul, sulfurous	0.00009
Coumarin	New-mown hay	0.00002
Citral	Lemon	0.000003
Ethyl mercaptan	Decayed cabbage	0.00000066[a]
Trinitro-*tert*-butyl xylene	Musk	0.000000075

[a] The lower values here compared to those in Table 38 are detection not recognition thresholds.

Source: Wenger *et al.* (1956).

TABLE 38
Recognition Threshold Concentrations of Various Odorous Materials

Substance	Boiling point (°C)	Milligrams per liter of air	Molar concentration[a]
Ethyl ether	35	5.833	7.8×10^{-5}
Carbon tetrachloride	76.7	4.533	3.0×10^{-5}
Chloroform	62	3.300	2.8×10^{-5}
Ethyl acetate	77.4	0.686	7.8×10^{-6}
Amyl alcohol	137.8	0.225	2.6×10^{-6}
Nitrobenzene	209.4	0.146	1.2×10^{-6}
Ethyl mercaptan	37	0.046	7.4×10^{-7}
Methyl salicylate	222.2	0.100	6.6×10^{-7}
Pyridine	115.2	0.032	4.0×10^{-7}
Amyl acetate	148	0.039	3.0×10^{-7}
Valeric acid	186.4	0.029	2.9×10^{-7}
Methyl isothiocyanate	119	0.015	2.1×10^{-7}
Butyric acid	162.3	0.009	1.0×10^{-7}
Isobutyl mercaptan	88	0.008	8.9×10^{-8}
Allyl isothiocyanate	151	0.008	8.0×10^{-8}
Propyl mercaptan	67	0.006	7.9×10^{-8}
Phenyl isocyanide	165	0.002	2.0×10^{-8}
Amyl thioether	95–98	0.001	5.8×10^{-9}

[a] Computed as the number of gram molecules in a liter of diluent or, more properly, in a liter of solution, but the concentrations are so low that a negligible error results from considering only the diluent.

Source: Allison and Katz (1919).

gives the correct value in each case. Grams per cubic centimeter $\times$ 6.06 $\times$ 10^{23}/molecular weight equals molecules per cubic centimeter. Some corrected thresholds from the International Critical Tables are given in Table 37. Other data, from Allison and Katz (1919), are given in Table 38.

Using a sniffing procedure, Jones (1955c) found median threshold values for 24 persons as follows: n-butanol, 2.86×10^{-9} M; safrol, 6.35×10^{-9} M; and n-butyric acid, 1.12×10^{-9} M. Using a syringe apparatus, Jones (1954) reported the following recognition thresholds for benzene and methyl salicylate: 1.5×10^{-4} M and 2.6×10^{-6} M. For m-xylene the average threshold in molecules for six normal subjects for five days in an eight-day period was ($\times 10^{13}$) 7.6, 6.1, 2.8, 8.0, 5.4, and 2.8.

Taking into account the molecules lost by absorption at low rates of flow, Stuiver (1958) calculated the following thresholds for five subjects (as molecules):

Compounds used	Subject				
	I	II	III	IV	V
Isobutyl mercaptan ($\times 4.4 \times 10^8$)	1	6.1	9.0	20.2	47.3
Allyl mercaptan ($\times 6.0 \times 10^7$)	1	0.7	1.0	2.7	5.3
Isopropyl mercaptan ($\times 2.0 \times 10^7$)	1	4.0	5.2	7.5	5.7
sec-Butyl mercaptan ($\times 1.3 \times 10^7$)	1	1.3	7.3	35.7	93.4

Assuming an inhaled volume of 500 cc per sec, the number of molecules striking the olfactory epithelium per second is about 5×10^7. If the normal inspiration stimulus time is considered, the number of molecules is about 9×10^6. If these strike a surface containing 2×10^7 sense cells and the molecules do not diffuse over a distance greater than the distance between two sense cells, it is obvious that every two sense cells get an average of one molecule. The probability that one or more receptors gets more than 10 molecules is 4×10^{-3}. Stuiver thus concluded that a receptor needs 9 or less molecules to respond. Assuming 20 receptor types, the number is 7 or less (assuming no losses on the olfactory epithelium). This approaches Neuhaus' (1953) calculation that only one molecule of butyric acid is necessary to activate the sense cell of a dog. For six fatty acids, dogs were much more sensitive than humans: 10^3 to 10^5 molecules per cubic centimeter for dogs, and 10^{10} to 10^{13} molecules for humans.

Stuiver (1958) calculated 9×10^6 molecules as the odor threshold for a mercaptan. Since there are 2×10^7 receptor cells, if only half are stimulated, about 9 molecules or less will produce a response. A minimum of 40 sensory cells were stimulated at threshold (see also Vries and Stuiver, 1961).

Piéron (1952) cited evidence for a response to as few as 200 molecules penetrating a sense cell. The ethyl mercaptan threshold of 5×10^{-8} mg per liter or 8×10^{-13} mole is perhaps the lowest recorded odor threshold.

Wright (1957a) stated that butylnitrotoluene can be perceived at a concentration of 5×10^{-15} g per milliliter of air. Guadagni et al. (1963) recently reported thresholds of 0.02 and 0.33 parts per billion for methyl mercaptan and dimethyl sulfide. For the n-alkanals the respective thresholds for C_3 to C_{12} were 9.5, 9, 12, 4.5, 9, 12, 4.5, 3, 0.7, 1, 0.1, 5, and 2 parts per billion.

Guadagni et al. (1963) also demonstrated additivity of sub-threshold concentrations of some odors, that is mixtures of odors at sub-threshold concentrations could be smelled. This was demonstrated over a wide range of combinations. In this case the effects were truly additive and not synergistic. In the case of Nawar and Fagerson (1962) there appeared to be synergistic effects (see also Chapter 3, Section I).

Stuiver (1958) reported a critical time of response of 0.16 to 0.20 sec. Thresholds, in numbers of molecules for various compounds tested, were: sec-butyl mercaptan, 2×10^9; m-xylene, 4×10^{13}; and o-nitrophenol, 8×10^{11}.

XI. Odor Intensities

The ratio of the olfactory threshold determined after sniffing the undiluted substance, to the threshold determined after sniffing the diluent, is termed the odor-intensity by Moncrieff (1957a). The thresholds found after smelling the undiluted substance were much higher than those obtained after smelling the diluent. The ratio ranged from 1.7 for benzylamine to 14,000 for 0.5% ethyl mercaptan. The odor intensities of some structural isomers differed considerably. Odor intensity measured thusly increases as the concentration of the "undiluted" substance is increased, but not after a certain point. Roughly, the odor intensity is proportional to the square root of the concentration of the solution.

The problem of defining and classifying olfactory intensity is complicated by the very wide olfactory spectrum and the change in intensity and quality with concentration. Kruger et al. (1955a) suggested a matching procedure analogous to one for sight and hearing. Arfmann and Chapanis (1962) were able to get subjects to quantitatively compare the intensity of vanilla odor to the taste. Just what the "taste" was is not clear.

The response of subjects to odor intensity is essentially the same according to Ough and Baker (1964). The relative differences between scale-point means is essentially the same. The major differences between subjects are the degrees to which they use the scale, the location of the central value, and in discriminating ability. An intensity rating procedure gave as much information in a shorter time than a paired comparison procedure.

Kruger *et al.* (1955a,b) tested several odorous compounds, using a sniffing procedure. Matching of unknowns to half and quarter positions between a reference of *n*-heptanal was accomplished. For the *n*-aliphatic alcohols (C_7 to C_{12}), the most soluble in polar and nonpolar solvents had the most intense odor. Odor intensity decreased with length of

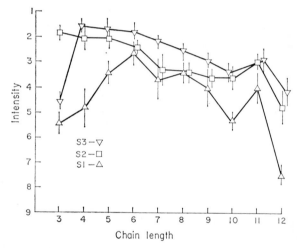

Fig. 39. Comparison of olfactory intensity with chain length for three subjects. Source: Kruger *et al.* (1955b).

molecule, except for C_{11}, which was higher than C_{10} or C_{12} (possibly because of its instability, due to its high rate of oxidation). In terms of vapor pressure, however, the longer molecules have more intense odors (see Fig. 39).

Jones (1958) was able to obtain subjective estimations of odor intensity for compounds as diverse as *n*-butanol, *sec*-butanol, isobutanol, ethyl acetate, cyclohexane, and pyridine. The relation of subjective magnitude to stimulus intensity was the same for polar and nonpolar compounds, i.e., it obeyed Steven's law for subjective intensities. Similar results were reported by Reese and Stevens (1960) with the intensity of coffee odor, and in general by Engen (1961) and Engen and Lindström (1963).

Engen and Lindström's (1963) data indicate that for amyl acetate in benzyl benzoate the response yields a function of the form $R = KS^n$, with n ranging from 0.39 to 0.57. Thus the intensity of smell appears to be a negatively accelerated function of stimulus intensity. Intensity of smell is on the prothetic continuum (see Chapter 5, Section IV,B). Analysis of subjective ratios as a function of stimulus ratios showed that the magnitude scale was a ratio scale and that the function corresponded to the power law. This agrees with Eisler (1963).

In odor investigations reported by the Arthur D. Little laboratory (Swain, 1960), there appeared to be 26 just-noticeable differences in concentration between threshold and strong odors when samples were compared directly. This observation held regardless of the material being examined. For the relation of odor intensity to Amoore's stereochemical theory (Chapter 3, Section V) see Johnston and Parks (1960).

Allison and Katz (1919) developed a scale to evaluate gas warning agents by matching the odor against a subjective, descriptive scale of 6 steps (0 = no odor; 5 = very strong odor). Kenneth (1927) demonstrated that odors are pleasant or unpleasant depending on concentration, chemical stability, and the subject's health and affective tone of association, and found no differences between the sexes for most odors. The reaction is partially due to previous experience with the same or a similar odor.

XII. Adaptation

According to Geldard (1953), adaptation, fatigue, and exhaustion are synonomous. It may exist in the end organ, in the nerves of the receiving centers, or in the central parts of the brain. Adaptation to odor may consist of: (1) the time during which a stimulus has to be supplied before the smell sensation disappears; (2) an increase of the threshold during adaptation as a function of time; and (3) the time of recovery of sensitivity of the sense organ after adaptation to a strong stimulus. Stuiver (1958) noted that measurement of adaptation time is complicated by accompanying sensations (especially of burning or heat). Stuiver believed that at a sufficiently high concentration, all odorous compounds stimulate the trigeminal nerve. Continuous excitation of the olfactory organ induces sensory adaptation, so that the given odor is no longer perceived. The rate of adaptation increases with increasing intensity of the stimulus. Recovery is slower than adaptation as detected by electrical response (Walsh, 1953). With prolonged stimulation there was, first, the usual spurt of activity, and then, three to five respiratory cycles later, adaptation occurred in the pause between exhalation and inhalation. There were also differences in the responsiveness to different odors. Adrian (1950) believes the olfactory bulb is of greater importance in determining sensory adaptation than the receptor. In the rabbit, he found two kinds of oscillations in the olfactory bulb: induced waves set up by strong olfactory stimuli, and intrinsic waves due to persistent activity of cells in the bulb. He suggested that the interference of the persistent intrinsic discharge swamps the transmission of olfactory signals and results in olfactory "fatigue." The failure of olfactory sensation after repeated stimuli "can be compared to our inability to pay continued attention to uninteresting sounds,' i.e., adaptation has a central origin.

Adaptation has also been tested by Cheesman and Mayne (1953), using a sniff test. When the stimuli were the same, the log-log plots versus adapting concentrations had a slope of +0.7. When the substances were different, the slopes varied from +0.2 to +0.1. In general, adaptation is proportional to the vapor pressure and hence to the molecular concentration in the nose. Mullins (1955a) believes that adaptation occurs because the concentrations necessary to excite some receptor types are more than sufficient to narcotize them.

Aronsohn (1886) reported adaptation times for nine odors of 2 to 11 minutes. Using a blast-injection technique, Elsberg and Levy (1935) found that adaptation for citral occurred within 150 seconds. When the injections were made every 20 seconds, the time for adaptation was 300 seconds. Stuiver (1958) obtained adaptation in 210 seconds for d-octanol at 100 times threshold concentrations.

The relation of adaptation time, t, and the adapting intensity, I, was reported by Woodrow and Karpman (1917) as $t = K + kI$. The formula is not valid at low concentrations, according to Stuiver, who proposed for d-octanol and m-xylene, respectively, the formulas $t = 20\sqrt{C - 1}$, and $t = 30\sqrt{C - 1}$, where C is the adaptation concentration. Following adaptation, the threshold after 30 seconds for d-octanol was increased by a factor of 6 in Stuiver's studies. A large adapting intensity raised the threshold slightly more than a small one. Thus, when adaptation is not complete, the threshold, after a few minutes' recovery, is determined mainly by the quantity of odorous substance used for adaptation.

When only one side of the nose is adapted, recovery is much more rapid in the unadapted side than in the other side. Stuiver asks why a sensation is perceived when adapted to a certain concentration if a slightly higher concentration is supplied. Adaptation would seem to be mainly in the central parts of the olfactory system. The formula for increase in threshold following adaptation was

$$1 + a(C - 1)\left[1 - \exp\left(\frac{-t}{15\sqrt{C - 1}}\right)\right]$$

where a is a constant that varies only slightly at different adapting concentrations, C. The adapting time is t.

During adaptation there are qualitative changes in the nature of the odor. Nitrobenzol, for example, changes from an odor of bitter almonds to one of tar or pitch. Trimethylamine smells fishy at first, and later like ammonia. It is believed that these changes are due to the differential adaptation rate of different components of the receptor mosaic. The effect was shown by Nagel (1897)—in a mixture of vanillin and coumarin, if the olfactory region is first adapted to vanillin, coumarin odor

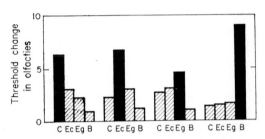

Fig. 40. The selective characteristic of olfactory adaptation. The ordinate indicates the threshold change in olfacties after adaptation by each of four substances (camphor, eucalyptol, eugenol, and benzaldehyde) in turn. Self-adaptation is indicated by the solid figure; threshold changes for the other substances, by cross-hatching. The threshold for each substance is most influenced by itself. In addition, camphor, eucalyptol, and eugenol all appear to show reciprocal adaptation effects. The sensitivity to benzaldehyde is little affected by these substances. Benzaldehyde has little effect upon their thresholds. Source: Ohma, in Skramlik (1926).

will be perceptible. Exposure to camphor raises the threshold for eucalyptol and eugenol, but the threshold for benzaldehyde is not affected nor does benzaldehyde affect the other three. Vanillin and terpineol affect each other's threshold but have little influence on the threshold for butyric acid. These data are summarized in Fig. 40. Gross adaptation to odors is best when the odorous substances are similar and odor is easily confused.

Using a modification of the Elsberg technique, Manci (1946) studied the possibility that the conditions at the surface of the olfactory region might modify the olfactory sensation. After application of 0.5% sodium bicarbonate or 0.5% potassium thiocyanate, the MIO was reduced, but after 0.5% tartaric acid or 0.25% aluminum acetate (all in 0.8% sodium chloride) the MIO was markedly higher. This was considered support for Niccolini's (1958) theory that "the nasal mucosa has a tendency to increase or decrease olfactory perception, according to the cases, through excitation of the negative charges of the substances which lend themselves to that particular action of a physico-chemical order during the transmission across the nasal mucosa."

In spite of its defects, the Elsberg technique continues to be used. Zilstorff-Pedersen (1962) recently employed the technique and noted that, for citral and coffee, fatigue effects lasted up to 2 min in most individuals, and in a few cases as long as 6 min.

It is frequently said that fatigue reduces olfactory acuity. However, there was no indication that olfactory thresholds varied with fatigue when the stream-injection method of determining minimum identifiable odor was used (Anonymous, 1952). See, however, Chapter 5, Section V. Fatigue is quicker at higher concentrations and varies among individuals. Earlier tests showed fatigue in about 2.5 to 11 min, and recovery in 1 to 3 (Parker, 1922). Using an olfactometer described by Ough and Stone (1961), Pangborn *et al.* (1964) observed no olfactory fatigue over a period of 1 hr during the presentation of 120 samples of 2-heptanone at near-threshold concentrations. Elsberg *et al.* (1935b) used the blast-injection technique and observed that the duration of olfactory fatigue is proportional to the length of time the odor affects the olfactory receptors and to the volume per unit time. If both passages are stimulated at the same time, fatigue lasts longer. Also, stimulation on one side affects the other. Elsberg believed that fatigue was due to temporary abeyance of function in the brain, *not* to a refractory state of the receptors or nerves. Most modern physiologists and psychologists reject this concept, as the following section suggests.

XIII. Theories of Olfaction

Any theory should accommodate all of the relevant facts and suggest new hypotheses. No present theory fits these requirements. Three main types of theories have been proposed: (1) direct radiation from the odor; (2) chemical activity as part of reception; and (3) a radiation mechanism in the olfactory region.

The first theory seems impossible since odors travel with the wind and are not transmitted through solids or reflected from mirrors. The others are discussed below.

Any theory for odor must explain a wide variety of conditions. Among these are: need for volatility, solubility of odorous material in the watery mucus and in the fatty or lipoid ends of the olfactory cells, and some idea of the chemical reactions in the cells. The possibility remains that the quality of an odor may be determined by its chemical properties. Volatility and solubility in fat solvents seem most important. All known odorous substances are gases or have a high vapor pressure, boiling below 300°C. Moncrieff (1951) lists twenty-four existing theories of odor,

none of which he finds satisfactory. He suggests the following requirements for any theory of odor:

(1) All normal people can smell.
(2) Anosmia occurs in people with obstructed nasal passages, brain
     lesions, or injured olfactory nerve.
(3) The possibility of preferential anosmia must be considered.
(4) Some substances are odorous, others are not.
(5) We can smell at a distance.
(6) Substances with different chemical compositions may have simi-
     lar odors.
(7) Substances with similar chemical composition *usually* have
     similar odors.
(8) High-molecular-weight substances are usually nonodorous.
(9) The quality and strength of the odor may change on dilution.
(10) The sense of smell fatigues rapidly.
(11) Fatigue for one odor has little effect on perception of dissimilar
     odors but interferes with the perception of similar odors.
(12) Odors can cancel each other out.
(13) Odor travels downwind.
(14) Many animals have keener senses of smell than man.

Guillot (1958) recently reviewed the proposed mechanisms for olfaction. He stresses the part that odors, even in subliminal concentrations,
may play in our actions. According to Guillot (1956), the character of an
odorous material is due to molecules, not to ions.

A. ADSORPTION

Moncrieff (1954b, 1957b) and Davies and Taylor (1957) noted that
the olfactory membrane adsorbed odorous materials. Moncrieff further
showed that there was a correlation between the odors of two materials
and their relative adsorbance on inorganic adsorbents. The amount of
adsorption was measured by the increase in temperature caused by the
adsorption of the odor. The sensitivity of Moncrieff's apparatus was equal
to that of the nose for acetone, but for vanillin, musk, etc., it was much
less sensitive. Moncrieff (1954a) prepared 5 adsorption columns. The
odor was forced through each column at an adjustable rate so that a
barely detectable odor was emitting. A quantity, called the critical contact time, was computed from the height of adsorbent in the column, the
cross-sectional area of the tube, and the rate of air flow. The different
contact times could be classified into 10 groups, from low to high values.
Thus, each odor could be classified into 5 numbers, respresenting the
adsorption times for the five adsorbents, i.e., 2,1,5,1,9 for amyl alcohol.

This is also a type of enzyme action theory. A test of this theory may be forthcoming since research on the structure of large molecules is very active at present, largely because of the use of electronic computers.

Moncrieff (1955) studied his theory with selective adsorbents. Subjects breathed air from the column filled with adsorbent until they could smell the odor (20–30 sec). By using a series of adsorbents—carbon, silica, alumina, attapulgus, and fat—on alumina, an odor profile was obtained. An air pump was used to supply odor stream at x cc (10–40) per second. The cross section of tube was ½ cm²: Therefore, the effective cross section of adsorbent tube is $n/2x$ sec, where n is the height of adsorbent in the tube. The air speed at which the "break" occurs was measured. Similar smells had similar profiles. Old fish had higher critical times than fresh fish. Applied to different coffees, the differences obtained were small. Ough and Amerine (1959) tested this theory with wines and found that the odor profiles differed, but no significant chemical data could be predicted from the results, because of the many variables involved.

As Davies and Taylor (1957, 1959) and Moncrieff (1954b) noted, several physical properties of chemical compounds can be roughly correlated with their odor. Davies and Taylor showed that olfactory thresholds depended on the adsorption energy of the odorous molecules passing from air to the lipid-aqueous olfactory membranes and on the dislocation of the membrane which is caused by these adsorbed molecules (which depends on shape, size, and flexibility of the odorous molecules). In other words, their basic concept is that odor molecules initiate the nervous impulse by causing localized changes in the cell membrane. Molecular shapes and sizes are also important (Timmermans, 1954; Mullins, 1955a). This appears similar to Pauling's (1946) hypothesis for antibody formation. Davies and Taylor (1957) derived the following general equation for calculating olfactory thresholds (OT):

$$\log \text{OT} + \log K_{\text{O/A}} = \frac{-4.64}{p} + \frac{\log p!}{p} + 21.19$$

where p is the adsorbed odorous molecules, and $K_{\text{O/A}}$ is the adsorption coefficient for the odor at the lipid/water interface. In order to have a strong odor, a substance must have a large $K_{\text{O/A}}$ and a small p. Adaptation, according to this theory, would be due to inability of the cell to build up "equilibrium" ion concentrations in the periods between successive inspirations. From their data they calculated the "active" area for one olfactory cell assuming a very odorous compound. If each site is 64×64 Å, then there may be 44,000 sites on each nerve cell! They found straight-line plots between $1/p$ against molecular volume and against molecular cross-sectional areas. Davies and Taylor noted that there are exceptions to the rule, i.e., spherical molecules have camphorous odors (see also Amoore's theory, Chapter 3, Section V).

Various theories are based on the assumption the olfactory stimulation results from penetration of the olfactory cell membranes. Davies and Taylor (1954) studied the influence of odors in accelerating hemolyses of red blood cells. A plot of the log of accelerating power against log olfactory thresholds showed a direct relation between the two. Weak odors had a low accelerating power. They believed their data supported the idea that penetration of the cells is a part of the olfactory stimulus. Much more elaboration of the mechanism is needed.

Davies (1962) further elaborated this theory, noting that as the olfactory substance penetrates the olfactory nerve cell a small region of the wall is dislocated. This dislocation allows potassium and sodium ions to move across the membrane, thus initiating the nervous impulse. He calculated that as many as 44,000 regions of the cell could be dislocated. He tested his theory by analogy: an odorant's acceleration power is a measure of the extent to which the cell wall is weakened by the odorant. Substances of high olfactory thresholds (weakly odorous) were poor accelerators. More direct evidence is needed.

While it is true generally that odor intensity rises as chain length increases (Chapter 5, Section V), for the homologous series of fatty acids one or more deviations occur. Moulton and Eayrs (1960) have reviewed this work. They tentatively concluded that, in the rat, olfaction involves an equilibrium process for medium- and long-chain alcohols but may not for shorter-chain alcohols. Solubility characteristics apparently play an important role in determining their olfactory stimulating efficiency, according to Ottoson (1958) and Moulton and Eayrs (1960).

B. PHYSICOCHEMICAL

Mullins (1955b) and Timmermans (1954) considered that olfaction is related to two molecular parameters: cohesive energy density (defined as the energy of vaporization of liquid per unit volume) and molecular shape. Mullins data were based on the odor of the three homologous series (n-paraffins, n-alcohols, and n-aldehydes). Thresholds were lowest for 4 to 5 carbon atoms, and higher for large or smaller numbers. The general criticism of such theories is that one cannot be sure that the parameters selected are the critical ones.

Mullins (1955a,b) suggested that the olfactory membrane is formed of macromolecular cylinders arranged in a regular hexagonal pattern with pores at the junctions between any three cylinders. Such a membrane should show considerable specificity in terms of interaction between the walls of the pores and the molecules in contact with the membrane. Eaton *et al.* (1954) believed surface tension was one of the parameters, but no general correlation was established.

Because of the obvious relation of molecular weight to odor in a homologous series, this approach has proven very tempting. Consider the following odor intensities for aliphatic compounds:

Compounds	Minimum	Strongest	Maximum
Alcohols	C_4	C_8	C_{14}
Aldehydes	C_1	C_{10}	C_{16}
Ketones	C_8	C_{11}	C_{16}
Acids	C_1	C_5	C_{14}
Ethers	C_6	C_8	C_{17}

Molecular weight, vapor pressure, lipoid solubility, thermodynamic activity, and other physical parameters have a correlation with the olfactory effectiveness of some compounds, but not of all. Mullins (1955a) suggested that it is the ability of the molecule to produce a local disorder in the oriented molecular structure of the cell membrane that leads to olfaction. The nature of the disorder is not specified, so the theory does not help us very much. Since adaptation to paraffins did not influence thresholds for alcohols, and vice versa, he suggested that at least two, and probably more, types of receptors are present in the olfactory epithelium. These types are believed to differ in "cohesive energy density" or in the internal attractive forces holding the molecules of the membranes together. Data on olfactory responses of the land tortoise to amyl acetate were fitted to Beidler's equation (Chapter 2, Section XII,B) by Tucker (1961), who found that similar processes of weak binding of stimulant molecules to receptor sites were involved.

There are many theories of olfaction; however, most are based on incomplete or inconclusive data (Jones and Jones, 1953). Pfaffmann (1956) does not believe that, with such a diversity of physicochemical relations, any of the chemical senses will be found to depend on a single general stimulus dimension in a manner equivalent to vision (protons) or hearing (air pressure). As he says, "Chemical processes are rarely explicable in terms of a single parameter. There is less likelihood that this will be the case in the more complex biological systems."

Since many molecular characteristics are closely related, it is not strange that the properties of odorous molecules should be related to several parameters. The problem, then, is to be certain that one has selected the characteristic which is related to odor. Further experimentation is certainly needed to elucidate the relation of olfaction to structure.

C. ANALYTICAL

Engen and Pfaffmann (1959) determined that a human subject could identify about 5 stimulus intensities which, in informational analysis, yielded 1.9 bits. [The "bit," a measure of information, provides an index of the maximum number of single-stimulus categories that can be discriminated without error by the absolute-judgment method (Garner and Hake, 1951).] Unpracticed subjects could identify three levels of odor intensity, and well-practiced individuals identified four. For odor quality, Engen and Pfaffmann observed that a subject's channel capacity was twice as great. The information analysis from identification of 16 different odors yielded approximately 4 bits of information. Later (1960), they reported about 1.5 bits of information for judgments of odor intensity. For combined judgments of odor intensity and odor quality they found 0.3 and 3.5 bits, respectively. They attribute the high value for quality to the fact that quality is a multidimensional stimulus. The low value for intensity in this case may be due to the fact that the judgments of intensity were made equivalent in physical dilution terms, not in terms of intensity. Thus, multidimensional stimuli transmit more information, although at the cost of less information per dimension. Jones (1958) showed that subjective intensity was related to stimulus magnitude by a power function. The exponent was about 0.5 and did not vary with the type of odor used.

Jones (1957) determined absolute olfactory thresholds for 20 compounds. Factorial analysis yielded four group-factors which were not readily interpreted in terms of the chemical or physical properties of the stimuli. Jones concluded that the individual differences were systematic, that the results indicate a variety of receptors, and that no existing scheme of odor classification fitted the data. See also Wright (1964) and Woskow (1964). The latter believed the most important factor in odor classification to be pleasantness.

Hainer et al. (1954) classified theories of odor perception into three groups: (a) chemical stimulation of the receptor by the bombardment of odorous molecules; (b) vibratory stimulation of the receptor by the presence of the odorous molecules; and (c) wave or photon stimulation of the receptor by radiation from or to the odorous molecule. Discarding all these, Hainer et al. (1954) developed an ingenious "information" theory of odor based on the subjective olfactory experience that most individuals can differentiate between a large number of odors at near-threshold concentrations, that memory for the odor may be permanent, and that perception of intensity appears to be a logarithmic function of the internal chemical concentration. They also noted that the neurophysiology of the olfactory system is favorable. A neuron is either "on" or "off" in a given interval. An overstimulated neuron fails to respond, but does recover with time. They note that 10,000 different odors, but only about 30 levels of intensity, can be discriminated. They calculate that there are 1900 glomeruli in the nose, each sending messages by 24 neurons at a rate of 10 pulses per second, so that 16 million distinct patterns can be differentiated! In order not to interfere with each other, there must be some sort of memory hold arrangement. They postulated that the "granular" cells have this function, receiving the pulse from the end organ and delaying it just the right time before releasing it. More experimental data are needed.

The kind of odor depends on the pattern, and the strength depends on how many of the 1900 bundles and 24 neurons react. Intensity thus depends on the fraction of fibers activated, and this is not the best information for learning or complete storage. Hence, odor quality, which is registered discretely, is retained more precisely than the more continuous odor intensity pattern. An odor is represented by six digits on a 24-digit code.

A	0	X	0	X	0	X	Fatigue for A will also fatigue B
B	0	X	0	X	0	0	but not C. A will cancel C. A
C	X	0	X	0	X	0	and D will enhance B but not C.
D	X	X	X	X	0	0	Anosmia can be partial.

D. Enzyme

Examples of such single-parameter theories are those of Heusghem and Gerebtzoff (1953), who postulated that the lipids of the olfactory mucosa were a part of the receptor mechanism, and Lauffer (1954), who stressed the importance of enzymes and believed that adsorption of the stimulant on the enzyme surfaces of the sensory cell might be a factor. Lauffer (1950) suggested enzyme activity since enzymes are macromolecules and form addition compounds. The more active proponents of enzyme theories have been Kistiakowsky (1950) and Baradi and Bourne (1951a,b). They assume that odorous (or taste) compounds inhibit the activity of one or more of the enzyme systems in the olfactory (or taste) regions. This selective inhibition alters the relative concentration of various compounds at the receptor and thus initiates neural response. Alkaline phosphatase, found in the olfactory and gustatory epithelia, was inhibited by vanillin, coffee oil, and aniseed, whereas sugar, salt, and quinine did not inhibit it. Esterase was inhibited by quinine but not by sugar or salt. Sumner (1954) criticized the enzyme signal concept because enzymes are seldom inhibited by a specific inhibitor. Further, the concentrations we smell are too small to trigger enzyme action, and a whole series of new enzymes would be needed. Sumner also objects to the idea that alkaline phosphatase is important in perception of vanillin, since the enzyme is widely distributed in the body and its inhibition by vanillin is not surprising. Many nonodorous substances also inhibit enzymes. Although Bourne (1948) and Baradi and Bourne (1951a,b) have shown that certain enzymes are localized in the olfactory region, their relation to olfaction has not been demonstrated. However, Coumétou (1959) still considered the enzyme theory tenable. If optically isomeric pairs of substances have similar odors, as Wright (1964) believes, it is difficult to accept an enzyme theory which presupposes high stereospecificity.

Even if the enzymes are not concerned in the olfactory process, Ottoson (1963) suggests that they may be important in the elimination of odorous material. Since the olfactory receptors may respond to a given odor for up to an hour, there must be some efficient method for removing the odor after each stimulation. While some may be removed by the vascular method, Ottoson believes enzymes in the mucosa may also be important.

Another speculative theory is that of Dravnieks (1962), who postulated that adsorption on ferroelectric substrates provides the triggering mechanism for olfaction.

Bartalena (1959) subjected 30 normal individuals to prolonged olfactory stimulation with coffee or citral while 30 controls received odorless air. The thiocyanate concentration of the nasal mucus of the controls was 108.8% after 5 min of stimulation, and 97.9% after 10 min; that of the individuals receiving coffee or citral was 84.3 and 78.1%, respectively, after 5 min, with a slight rise, 85.1 and 95.1%, respectively, after 10 min of stimulation.

E. ABSORPTION

Beck and Miles (1947) revived the old concept that the infrared absorption of a compound was related to its odor. Again, no broad correlation has been secured. Stereoisomers with identical infrared absorption spectra and differences in odor are known. Forrester and Parkins (1951) noted that a gas at body temperature should have no smell. In a test, cloves had a smell up to 42.4°C. The results with β-phenylethyl alcohol were less conclusive. Not all substances that absorb radiation in the infrared region possess an odor, and the theory, therefore, still remains unproven.

Shkapenko and Gerebtzoff (1951) reported no odor sensation when a closed polyethylene tube filled with odorized air was inserted in the nose. Ottoson (1956) obtained no odor if the olfactory membrane was covered with a plastic membrane that transmitted infrared radiation within the range supposedly involved. It seems established, then, that odorant particles must come into direct contact with the olfactory receptors.

The similarity of smell of a homologous series of compounds emphasizes that chemical structure is important. Odor theories based on chemical reactivity, oxidizability, or vibrational characteristics usually

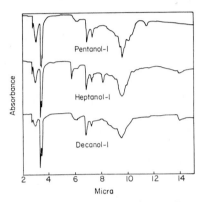

Fig. 41. Infrared absorption spectra of samples of three alcohols whose odors were distinctively different. Source: Kruger *et al.* (1955b).

fail to account for this. These characteristics may vary considerably between substances in a homologous series which all have essentially the same odor. Thus, a theory which ascribes odor to unsaturation is erroneous because many saturated substances have pronounced odors. Figure 41 illustrates the difficulties of such theories with respect to the infrared adsorption spectra.

Dyson (1928a,b, 1937) was convinced that the atomic vibrations within the molecule stimulated the nerve endings directly. Raman shifts of 1400 to 3400 units were believed to account for all distinctive odors. A 2500-unit-line spectrum should smell like mercaptan, a 2700-unit line like ether, and a 3300-unit line like pyridine. Gerebtzoff (1953), Hallam (1954), and Thompson (1957) criticized the molecular vibration theory on both theoretical and experimental grounds. For example, Hallam found the spectrum of ethyl carbonate to resemble that of Dyson's "almond-like" group, but it has no trace of such an odor.

The theory that the odor is related to the Raman shift has been revived by Wright (1954a,b) and Wright and Serenius (1954), emphasizing the shorter wavelengths. Later (Wright and Serenius, 1956), a central role was assigned to the olfactory pigment; their unproved theory "requires that the olfactory cell walls, and particularly the olfactory 'hairs,' shall contain pigment or other molecules having low vibrational frequencies associated with that part of the molecule which has a low-lying electronic level. The pigment must consist of several chemical species, probably of a single basic type but tuned to different vibrational frequencies by substituents of varying mass or position." Wright (1957 a,b, 1964) used mechanical models to illustrate the molecular vibration theory. Since the pigment is located mainly in the gland and supporting cells with little in the receptor cells, the pigment vibration theory appears difficult to support.

F. PHYSIOLOGICAL

Adrian (1948) concluded that olfaction is a "patterned" sense of restricted repertoire. Different loci of impingement of odorous particles on receptor cells, varying rates of nervous discharge, and variable latencies all provide pattern differentiation. Perhaps "specific" receptors are not present in great abundance. Adrian (1948, 1951) anesthetized animals, placed an insulated wire into the olfactory bulb until it was in contact with the nerve fibers, and then recorded the activity of individual nerve impulses. A discharge occurs with respiration. At first, Adrian thought that the pressure of inspiration invalidated olfactory electrical data obtained when there was a pressure variable. However, it was possible to distinguish between these two effects. When odors were given to the animal, well-defined responses were obtained. From these data, Adrian obtained characteristic patterns from different substances, at two levels of response, one immediate and one delayed, the latter where diffusion was a factor. Thus, substances of low molecular weight were more reactive than those of high molecular weight. Organic solvents such as xylol, gasoline, and ether did not always have an intense smell, but they reached the olfactory receptors more quickly and started an electrical discharge which was almost continuous. Adrian believed the particular structure of the olfactory apparatus (folded membranes, etc.) explains why substances of different diffusion rates reach different parts of it at different times, and thus elicit different responses. This does not, of course, explain different odors. Furthermore, different receptors may come into operation at different times according to their chemical affinities and their position on the olfactory surface. As they come into play, like different instruments in the orchestra, they lead to varying olfactory patterns. Others have noted the change in odor quality with time; however, fatigue (adaptation) may be a factor. See also Chapter 5, Section V.

Results of Nováková and Dlouhá (1960) seem to indicate that the olfactory mechanism may be related to maintenance of water balance.

G. Present Status

Sumner (1954) objects to theories assuming that the energy for olfaction arises from modification of atomic bordering angles within a molecule at the time the molecule goes into solution. The energy for other physiological processes comes from adenosine triphosphate (ATP).* Sumner's theory, expressed in his own style, is worth quoting:

> Freely admitting that far too little is known about the olfactory process to permit one to construct a complete theory, nevertheless, against my better judgment I am going to propose the following admittedly sketchy and incomplete scheme:
> Chemical No. 1 reacts with receptor A and displaces molecules from A. These displaced molecules stimulate the nerve to send an impulse to the brain.
> Chemical No. II reacts with receptor B and displaces molecules of B. Chemical No. II reacts with receptor C and displaces molecules of C, and so on.
> Large amounts of these chemicals displace more molecules than do small amounts of these chemicals.
> Chemical No. I reacts more readily with receptor A, but also reacts to a slight extent with receptor B and with receptor C.
> When chemical No. I has displaced molecules of receptor A there is a dearth of these molecules available and fatigue results until the supply can be replenished.
> Some individuals possess a greater number of receptors A than of receptors B, or C, or *vice versa*. This would explain preferential anosmia.

As a first approximation, Beets (1957) proposed that olfaction be considered a physical or chemical process of the type $I \rightarrow II \rightarrow III$:

$$A + xB \rightarrow [A \ . \ . \ . \ x \ . \ . \ . \ B] \rightarrow Ax + B$$
$$\text{I} \qquad\qquad \text{II} \qquad\qquad \text{III}$$

A and Ax represent odorous molecules; xB and B represent the nasal receptor before or after the creation of the odor impression; and II represents a transition state. The term x may symbolize any change in the molecule and receptor taking place during the olfaction process and may represent energy, electric charge, solvation, etc.

Beets (1957) summarized theories regarding the transition state and concluded that most odor theories stress the importance of the general structure or the functional group. Ruzicka (1920, 1957) considered that

---

* Sumner also differs with several of Moncrieff's statements: that carbon monoxide has an odor; that hydrocyanic acid, benzaldehyde, and nitrobenzene smell differently; that brass has an odor; that palmitic and stearic acids have an odor; and that pigmentation is not important to olfaction. Others also have failed to relate pigmentation to olfaction, for example, Ottoson (1963).

both have an influence—functional groups on variety of odor, and the rest of the structure on the type of odor.

Naves (1957) summarized a variety of evidence on the relationship between stereochemistry and the odorous properties of organic substances.

The result of modern studies was summarized by Beets (1957) as follows:

> I. Molecules enter the nose and approach the nasal receptor up to 'transition state distance.'
>
> II. (1) If their concentration is high, crowding of the receptor surface with multimolecular layers takes place, leading to a decrease in the sensitivity of the receptor and consequently in the intensity and specificity of the odour impression.
>
> II. (2) If their concentration is favourable, a transition state is achieved in which the molecules may be arranged in a chaotic or in an organized way. Decisive in this alternative is the tendency of orientation. This tendency will be absent or weak in molecules containing no functional groups or in molecules containing two identical functional groups in identical positions, stronger in molecules containing two similar functional groups or two identical functional groups in structurally different positions, and strong in molecules with one functional group or with more than one functional group of widely different character.
>
> II. (3) In such cases where the transition state involves orientation of a molecule, a single functional group determines the direction of the orientation of that molecule.
>
> II. (4) The nature of the odour impression caused by a molecule is determined by the separate influences of two structural details of the transition state:
>
> (a) the functional group responsible for the orientation of the molecule and
>
> (b) the profile, i.e., the bulk and the form of the rest of the molecule.
>
> III. The energetic or material consequences of these influences cause a stimulus which is translated by the brain into an odour impression. This part of the process falls outside the scope of this paper.

This speculative model Beets called a "profile-functional group concept." The functional group with the highest solvation tendency is believed to be responsible for the orientation of the molecule at the receptor surface. Thus the nature of the odor is decided by the functional group with the highest hydration tendency, and by the profile of the rest of the molecule. Beets concluded that data are lacking to accept or reject this model.

Thompson (1957) doubts if any satisfactory theory of the mechanism of smell exists. He criticizes theories based on molecular vibration, primarily because odorous materials have characteristic vibration frequencies in several parts of the spectrum. He specifically criticizes

Wright's theory because many compounds have intense Raman frequencies in the same region but do not have similar odors. As he states, "Many of the recent physical theories about the actual mechanism contain errors of fact, and also some misleading conceptions about the nature of molecular dynamics." In studies on cross adaptation to aliphatic alcohols, Engen (1963) showed that no single-stimulus dimension could account for the complex olfactory system. We believe this to be correct.

The explanation of the mechanism of smell will depend, Thompson states, on the following:

> (1) more detailed knowledge is needed about the receptor cells and olfactory pigments, their absorption spectra, the adsorbability of odour molecules upon them, and the chemical reactions which occur between pigments and odour molecules;
> (2) the mucous membranes should be examined and the nature of any enzymes present should be determined;
> (3) the biochemical processes concerned should be studied, possibly using tracer isotope techniques;
> (4) the effect of inhibitors or catalytic effects of odour molecules upon the likely biochemical reactions should be examined. Known enzymic poisons could indeed, as a cruder experiment, be sprayed upon the olfactory organs to test their effect upon smell;
> (5) the threshold concentrations of different odour molecules need further examination: and indeed, a less subjective and more quantitative measure of odour is required than that obtained by human perception;
> (6) comparative studies of the smell of isotopic molecules are needed, especially with hydrogen-deuterium molecules where the vibrational frequency changes are greatest;
> (7) the full infra-red spectra of all kinds of odour molecules from 1 to 50 μ should be measured, although it is doubtful whether this will reveal any correlations of the types which have been suggested.

Kalmus (1957) feels that progress in the field will depend on the production of a variety of pure and well-defined organic substances, the development of adequate quantitative methods for the measurement of gaseous and vaporous stimuli, and a more imaginative and less narrow approach.

Jones (1962) has correctly suggested to us that olfactory theory must account for the excitation process and also for the odor quality. These are not completely separable, but nevertheless are somewhat different.

XIV. Summary

The sense of smell is extraordinarily sensitive in differentiating odorous materials. Since the response is so subjective, we communicate our sensations poorly to each other. Systems for classifying odors are thus not of much help. Even the definition of odor has to be on a phenomenological basis. However, there is no doubt as to the importance of odor to the food industries, both as an esthetic quality factor and as an indicator of soundness.

The relation of odor quality to molecular weight, volatility, and chemical structure is an intimate one, but no precise rules have been formulated. Amoore's classification that odor quality is based on the size, shape, and electronic status of the molecule appears promising and merits further investigation.

The relation of nasal anatomy and air flow to olfactory acuity has been neglected. Only a small fraction of the odorous molecules reach the olfactory region. The number of, and the differences between, the odor receptors are not known. Partial or complete anosmia is rare, but recent suggestions that odor sensitivity is modified by various diseases and by the use of certain drugs is most interesting and may prove useful in selecting subjects for studying olfaction.

Several satisfactory olfactometers have been constructed recently. These should permit greatly expanded investigations on odor threshold, intensity, and quality, and the factors which influence these. The deficiency of the Elsberg technique and the importance of controlling adaptation should especially be noted.

No present theory can explain all the relevant facts concerning odors. Certainly some physical process of a weak binding of stimulant molecules to receptor sites appears attractive. Also some differential pattern of receptor stimulation (or adaptation) is required to explain odor quality and intensity.

In spite of the lack of unifying theories there are many problems of odor measurement and classification in the food industry which could be solved by appropriate psychophysical research.

REFERENCES

Adey, W. R. 1959. The sense of smell. *In* "Handbook of Physiology," Vol. 1, 779 pp. (see pp. 535–548). Am. Physiol. Soc., Washington, D. C.

Adrian, E. D. 1948. The sense of smell. *Advance. of Sci.* 4, 287–292.

Adrian, E. D. 1950. The electrical activity of the mammalian olfactory bulb. *Electroencephalog. and Clin. Neurophysiol.* 2, 377–388.

Adrian, E. D. 1951. Differential sensitivity of olfactory receptors. *J. Physiol. (London)* 15, 42P.

Adrian, E. D. 1955. Potential oscillation in the olfactory organ. *J. Physiol. (London)* 128, 21–22.

Adrian, E. D. 1956. The action of the mammalian olfactory organ. *J. Laryngol. and Otol.* 70, 1–14.

Adrian, E. D. 1957. Problems of the modern physiology of the nervous and muscle systems. *Acad. Sci. Georgian S.S.R.* 1956, 13–19.

Allison, A. C. 1953. The morphology of the olfactory system in vertebrates. *Biol. Revs.* **28**, 195–244.

Allison, V. C., and S. H. Katz. 1919. An investigation of stenches and odors for industrial purposes. *J. Ind. Eng. Chem.* **11**, 336–338.

American Society for Testing Materials. 1954. Symposium on odor. *ASTM Spec. Tech. Publ.* **164**, 1–81.

American Society for Testing Materials. 1960. "Manual on Industrial Water," 2nd ed., ASTM Committee D-19, 653 pp. Philadelphia, Pennsylvania.

American Society for Testing Materials. 1961. Measurement of odor in atmospheres (dilution method). *ASTM Standards* **10**, 1603–1606 (Designation: D1391–57).

Amici, A., and D. Raschella. 1958. Sulla opportunità di ricerche sistematiche relative a un trascurato aspetto dei rapporti tra i sensi chimici. *Riv. biol.* (*Perugia*) **50**, 237–245.

Amoore, J. E. 1952. The stereochemical specificities of human olfactory receptors. *Perfumery Essent. Oil Record* **43**, 321–323, 330.

Amoore, J. E. 1962a. The stereochemistry theory of olfaction. 1. Identification of seven primary odors. *Proc. Sci. Sect., Toilet Goods Assoc. Spec. Suppl. to No.* **37**, 1–12.

Amoore, J. E. 1962b. The stereochemical theory of olfaction. 2. Elucidation of the stereochemical properties of the olfactory receptor sites. *Proc. Sci. Sect., Toilet Goods Assoc. Special Suppl. to No.* **37**, 13–23.

Amoore, J. E. 1963. Stereochemical theory of olfaction. *Nature* **198**, 271–272.

Amoore, J. E., J. W. Johnston, Jr., and M. Rubin. 1964. The stereochemical theory of odor. *Sci. American* **210**, 42–49.

Anonymous. 1950. Perception and measurement of odor. *Nature* **165**, 394–395.

Anonymous. 1952. The effects of general activity and extended diurnal variation on olfactory sensitivity. *Office Surgeon General Tech. Rept.* No. 11 (U. S. Army Med. Research Dev. Bd., Project DA-49-077-Md-222, 0.1. 19–52).

Arfmann, B. L., and N. P. Chapanis. 1962. The relative sensitivities of taste and smell in smokers and non-smokers. *J. Gen. Psychol.* **66**, 315–320.

Aronsohn, E. H. 1886. Experimentelle Untersuchungen zur Physiologie des Geruchs. *Arch. Anat. u. Physiol.* (*Physiol. Abt.*) **1886**, 321–357.

Baradi, A. F., and G. H. Bourne. 1951a. Localization of gustatory and olfactory enzymes in the rabbit, and the problems of taste and smell. *Nature* **168**, 977–979.

Baradi, A. F., and G. H. Bourne. 1951b. Theory of tastes and odors. *Science* **113**, 660–661.

Barail, L. C. 1952. Measurement of odors. *Drug and Allied Inds.* **38**, 18–19.

Bartalena, G. 1958a. Diagnostica funzionale: acutezza, finezza, fatica; metodi olfattometrici subiettivi. *In* "Olfatto e sue Correlazioni" (V. Fortunato and P. Niccolini, eds.), 699 pp. (see pp. 135–217). Tipografia dell'Università, Catania.

Bartalena, G. 1958b. Iposmie, parosmie, anosmie. *In* "Olfatto e sue Correlazioni" (V. Fortunato and P. Niccolini, eds.), 699 pp. (see pp. 437–463). Tipografia dell'Università, Catania.

Bartalena, G. 1959. Sulle variazioni del KSCN del muco nasale nelle fatica olfattoria. *Boll. mal. orecchio, gola, naso* **77**, 1–18.

Bartley, S. H. 1958. "Principles of Perception," 482 pp. (see pp. 348–354). Harper, New York.

Baten, W. D. 1946. Analyses of scores from smelling tests. *Biometrics Bull.* **2**, 11–14.

Battiston, M. N. 1962. Setting of an olfactometer. *Phys. Med. Biol.* **7**, 93–104.

Beck, L. H., and W. R. Miles. 1947. Some theoretical and experimental relationships between infrared absorption and olfaction. *Science* **106**, 511.

Bedichek, R. 1960. "The Sense of Smell," 264 pp. Doubleday, Garden City, New York.

Beets, M. G. J. 1957. Structure and odour. *Soc. Chem. Ind.* (*London*) *Monograph* **1**, 54–90.

Beets, M. G. J. 1961. Odor and molecular constitution. *Am. Perfumer* **76**, 54–63.

Beidler, L. M. 1954. Physiological problems in odor research. *Ann. N. Y. Acad. Sci.* **58**(2), 52–57.

Beidler, L. M. 1961a. The chemical senses. *Ann. Rev. Psychol.* **12**, 363–388.

Beidler, L. M. 1961b. Mechanisms of gustatory and olfactory receptor stimulation. *In* "Sensory Communication" (W. A. Rosenblith, ed.), 844 pp. (see pp. 143–147). M.I.T. Press, Massachusetts; Wiley, New York.

Berg, H. W., R. M. Pangborn, E. B. Roessler, and A. D. Webb. 1963. Influence of hunger on olfactory acuity. *Nature* **157**, 108.

Bhargava, I. 1959. Palato-epiglottic overlap in relation to the sense of smell. *J. Anat. Soc. India* **8**, 7–11.

Bienfang, R. 1946. "The Subtle Sense," 157 pp. Univ. of Oklahoma Press, Norman, Oklahoma.

Bloom, G., and H. Engström. 1952. The structure of the epithelial surface in the olfactory region. *Exptl. Cell Research* **3**, 699–701.

Boring, E. G. 1928. A new system for the classification of odors. *Am. J. Psychol.* **40**, 345–349.

Boring, E. G. 1942. "Sensation and Perception in the History of Experimental Psychology," 644 pp. (see pp. 437–449). Appleton, New York.

Borsanyi, S. J., and C. L. Blanchard. 1962. Psychogalvanic skin response olfactometry. *Ann. Otol., Rhinol. & Laryngol.* **71**, 213–221.

Borsanyi, S. J., C. L. Blanchard, and F. J. Baker. 1962. Psychogalvanic skin response as a method of objective olfactometry. *Bull. School Med. Univ. Maryland* **47**, 10–11, 13.

Bourne, G. H. 1948. Alkaline phosphatase in taste buds and nasal mucosa. *Nature* **161**, 445–446.

Bozza, G., C. Calearo, and G. P. Teatini. 1960. On the making of a rational olfactometer. *Acta Oto-Laryngol.* **52**, 189–209.

Bravo, J. 1592. "De Saporum et Odorum Differenitis, Causis et Effectionibus," liber unus, 166 pp. J. P. Ciottum, Venice.

Brunn, F. A. W. von. 1892. Beiträge zur mikroskopischen Anatomie der menschlichen Nasenhöhle. *Arch. mikroskop. Anat.* **39**, 632–651, also pp. 651–652.

Buddenbrock, W. von. 1958. "The Senses," 167 pp. (see pp. 107–123). Univ. of Michigan Press, Ann Arbor, Michigan.

Calingaert, G., and D. S. Davis. 1925. Pressure-temperature charts. Extended ranges. *Ind. Eng. Chem.* **17**, 1287–1289.

Castello, R. 1958. Olfatto e psichiatria. *In* "Olfatto e sue Correlazioni" (V. Fortunato and P. Niccolini, eds.), 699 pp. (see pp. 351–405). Tipografia dell'Università, Catania.

Cheesman, G. H., and H. M. Kirkby. 1959. An air dilution olfactometer suitable for group threshold measurements. *Quart. J. Exptl. Psychol.* **11**, 115–123.

Cheesman, G. H., and S. Mayne. 1953. The influence of adaptation on absolute threshold measurements for olfactory stimuli. *Quart. J. Exptl. Psychol.* **5**, 22–30.

Cheesman, G. H., and M. J. Townsend. 1956. Further experiments on the olfactory thresholds of pure chemical substances using the "sniff-bottle method." *Quart. J. Exptl. Psychol.* **8**, 8–14.

Ciurlo, L. 1934. Sulla funzione olfattoria nel neonato. *Valsalva* **10**, 22–34.

Cloquet, H. 1815. "Dissertation sur les Odeurs, sur le Sens et les Organes de l'Olfaction" [2nd ed., 1821 (title varies)], 758 pp. Mequignon-Marvis, Paris.

Cohn, G. 1915. "Geschmack und Konstitution bei organischen Verbindungen," 100 pp. Enke, Stuttgart. (See also *Pharm. Zentralhalle* **55**, 735–747; 763–767; 1914.)

Coumétou, M. 1959. "Les Examens Sensoriels," 189 pp. Presses Universitaires de France, Paris.

Crocker, E. C. 1945. Volatility in food flavor. *Ind. Eng. Chem.* **37**, 214–216.

Crocker, E. C., and L. F. Henderson. 1927. Analysis and classification of odors. *Am. Perfumer Essent. Oil Rev.* **22**, 325–327, 356. (See also *Proc. Sci. Sect., Toilet Goods Assoc. No.* **6**, 24–26, 1946.)

Daniels, F., and R. A. Alberty. 1955. "Physical Chemistry," 671 pp. Wiley, New York.

Darkis, F. R., E. J. Hackney, W. W. Bates, and L. Leiserson. 1954. The problem of odor in the cigarette industry. *Ann. N. Y. Acad. Sci* **58**(2), 22–26.

Davies, J. T. 1962. The mechanism of olfaction. *Symposia Soc. Exptl. Biol.* **16**, 170–179.

Davies, J. T., and F. H. Taylor. 1954. A model system for the olfactory membrane. *Nature* **174**, 693–694.

Davies, J. T., and F. H. Taylor. 1957. Molecular shape, size and adsorption in olfaction. *Proc. 2nd Intern. Congr. Surface Activity (London)* **2**, 329–340.

Davies, J. T., and F. H. Taylor. 1959. The role of adsorption and molecular morphology in olfaction: the calculation of olfactory thresholds. *Biol. Bull.* **117**, 222–238.

Davis, D. S. 1925. Pressure-temperature charts for organic vapors. *Ind. Eng. Chem.* **17**, 735–736.

Deininger, N., and R. W. McKinley. 1954. The design, construction, and use of an odor test room. *ASTM Spec. Tech. Publ.* **164**, 23–30.

Dorn, H. W. 1954. The problems of controlling odors in processing protein foods. *Ann. N. Y. Acad. Sci.* **58**(2), 27–33.

Dravnieks, A. 1962. Possible mechanism of olfaction. *Nature* **194**, 245–247.

Duncan, R. B., and M. Briggs. 1962. Treatment of uncomplicated anosmia by vitamin A. *Arch. Otolaryngol.* **75**, 116–124.

Dyson, G. M. 1928a. Odour and constitution among the aromatic mustard oils. *Perfumery Essent. Oil Record* **19**, 3–5, 88–91.

Dyson, G. M. 1928b. Some aspects of the vibration theory of odour. *Perfumery Essent. Oil Record* **19**, 456–459.

Dyson, G. M. 1937. Raman effect and the concept of odor. *Perfumery Essent. Oil Record* **28**, 13–19. (See also *Chem. & Ind. (London)* **16**, 647–651, 1938.)

Eaton, J. R., J. E. Christian, and J. A. Campbell. 1954. Surface phenomena related to odor measurements. *Ann. N. Y. Acad. Sci.* **58**(2), 239–249.

Ehrensvärd, G. 1942. Ueber die Primärvorgänge bei Chemorezeptorenbeeinflussung. *Acta Physiol. Scand.* **3** (Suppl. 9), 1–151.

Eisler, H. 1963. How prothetic is the continuum of smell? *Scand. J. Psychol.* **4**, 29–32.

Elsberg, C. A. 1935. The sense of smell. VIII. Olfactory fatigue. *Bull. Neurol. Inst. N. Y.* **4**, 479–495.

Elsberg, C. A., and I. Levy. 1935. The sense of smell. I. A new and simple method of quantitative olfactometry. *Bull. Neurol. Inst. N. Y.* **4**, 5–19.

Elsberg, C. A., E. D. Brewer, and I. Levy. 1935a. The sense of smell. III. The relation between olfactory coefficients and boiling-points of odorous substances. *Bull. Neurol. Inst. N. Y.* **4**, 26–30.

Elsberg, C. A., E. D. Brewer, and I. Levy. 1935b. The sense of smell. VII. The odorous substances to be used for tests of the olfactory sense. *Bull. Neurol. Inst. N. Y.* **4**, 286–293.

Engen, T. 1960. Effect of practice and instruction on olfactory thresholds. *Perceptual and Motor Skills* **10**, 195–198.

Engen, T. 1961. Direct scaling of odor intensity. *Psychological Laboratory, Univ. Stockholm Rept.* **106**, 1–13.

Engen, T. 1963. Cross-adaptation to the aliphatic alcohols. *Am. J. Psychol.* **76**(1), 96–102.

Engen, T., and C. O. Lindström. 1963. Psychophysical scales of the odor intensity of amyl acetate. *Scand. J. Psychol.* **41**, 23–28.

Engen, T., and C. Pfaffmann. 1959. Absolute judgments of odor intensity. *J. Exptl. Psychol.* **58**, 23–26.

Engen, T., and C. Pfaffmann. 1960. Absolute judgments of odor quality. *J. Exptl. Psychol.* **59**, 214–219.

Fauvelle, L. J. 1888. Notes. *Am. J. Psychol.* **1**, 357–358.

Fischer, E., and F. Penzoldt. 1886. Ueber die Empfindlichkeit des Geruchssinnes. *Sitzber. physik.-med. Sozietät Erlangen* **18**, 7–10. (See also *Ann. Chem. Liebig's* **239**, 131–136, 1887.)

Forrester, A. T., and W. E. Parkins. 1951. A test of the infrared absorption theory of olfaction. *Science* **114**, 5–6.

Fortunato, V. 1958a. Olfatto nelle varie età. *In* "Olfatto e sue Correlazioni" (V. Fortunato and P. Niccolini, eds.), 699 pp. (see pp. 519–575). Tipografia dell'Università, Catania.

Fortunato, V. 1958b. Fisiologia dell'apparato recettore periferico. *In* "Olfatto e sue Correlazioni" (V. Fortunato and P. Niccolini, eds.), 699 pp. (see pp. 119–134). Tipografia dell'Università, Catania.

Fortunato, V., and G. B. Catalano. 1958. La struttura dell'apparato olfattivo nell'-uomo. *In* "Olfatto e sue Correlazioni" (V. Fortunato and P. Niccolini, eds.), 699 pp. (see pp. 5–51). Tipografia dell'Università, Catania.

Fortunato, V., and P. Niccolini. 1958. "L'Olfatto; Cognizioni Antiche e Recenti," 694 pp. Istituto Farmacoterapico Italiano, Rome.

Foster, D., and K. M. Dallenbach. 1948. The olfactorium, an apparatus for odor research. *Am. Psychol.* **3**, 253–254.

Foster, D., and E. H. Scofield. 1950. Odor mixtures. *Am. Psychol.* **5**, 244–245.

Foster, D., E. H. Scofield, and K. M. Dallenbach. 1950. An olfactorium. *Am. J. Psychol.* **63**, 431–440.

Furchtgott, E., and M. P. Friedman. 1960. The effects of hunger on taste and odor RLs. *J. Comp. and Physiol. Psychol.* **53**, 576–581.

Garner, W. R., and H. S. Hake. 1951. The amount of information in absolute judgments. *Psychol. Rev.* **58**, 446–459.

Gasser, H. S. 1956. Olfactory nerve fibres. *J. Gen. Physiol.* **39**, 473–496.

Gavaudan, P., H. Poussel, G. Brebion, and M. P. Schutzenberger. 1948. L'étude des conditions thermodynamiques de l'excitation olfactive et les théories de l'olfaction. *Compt. rend.* **226**, 1395–1396.

Geldard, F. A. 1953. "The Human Senses," 365 pp. (see pp. 270–294). Wiley, New York.

Gerebtzoff, M. A. 1953. L'olfaction; structure d'organe olfactif et mécanisme de l'olfaction. *J. Physiol.* (*Paris*) **45**, 247–283.

Gerebtzoff, M. A., and E. Philippot. 1957. Lipides et pigment olfactifs. *Acta oto-rhino-laryngol. Belgica* **11**, 297–300.

Gesteland, R. C. 1961. Action potentials recorded from olfactory receptor neurons. Approx. 104 pp. Ph.D. Thesis. M.I.T., Cambridge, Massachusetts.

Ghirlanda, M. 1958. Olfatto nelle disendocrinie. *In* "Olfatto e sue Correlazioni" (V. Fortunato and P. Niccolini, eds.), 699 pp. (see pp. 407–436). Tipografia dell'-Università, Catania.

Ginsberg, R. S., M. Feldman, and H. Necheles. 1948. Effect of odors on appetite. *Gastroenterology* **10**, 281–285.

Goetzl, F. R., and F. Stone. 1947. Diurnal variations in acuity of olfaction and food intake. *Gastroenterology* **9**, 444–453.

Goetzl, F. R., and F. Stone. 1948. The influence of amphetamine sulfate upon olfactory acuity and appetite. *Gastroenterology* **10**, 708–713.

Goetzl, F. R., M. Goldschmidt, P. Wheeler, and F. Stone. 1949. Influence of sugar upon olfactory acuity and upon the sensation complex of appetite and satiety. *Gastroenterology* **12**, 252–257.

Goetzl, F. R., M. S. Abel, and A. J. Ahokas. 1950. Occurrence in normal individuals of diurnal variations in olfactory acuity. *J. Appl. Physiol.* **2**, 553–562.

Goetzl, F. R., A. J. Ahokas, and M. Goldschmidt. 1951. Influence of sucrose in various concentrations upon olfactory acuity and sensations associated with food intake. *J. Appl. Physiol.* **4**, 30–36.

Graf, K. 1961. Die Geruchs- und Geschmacksstörungen nach Schädelunfällen. *Pract. Oto-Rhino-Laryngol.* **23**, 104–114.

Gruber, C. W. 1954. Odor pollution from the official's viewpoint. *ASTM Spec. Tech. Publ.* **164**, 56–65.

Guadagni, D. G., R. G. Buttery, and S. Okano. 1963. Odour thresholds of some organic compounds associated with food flavours. *J. Sci. Food Agr.* **10**, 761–765. (See also *Nature* **200**, 1288–1289, 1963.)

Guillot, M. 1956. Aspect pharmacodynamique de quelques problèmes liés à l'olfaction. *Actualités pharmacol.* (*Paris*) **9**, 21–34.

Guillot, M. 1958. Sur les mécanismes psycho-physiologiques de l'olfaction. *J. Psychol. Norm. et Pathol.* **55**, 1–20.

Guillot, M. 1959. Sur quelques variations de la sensibilité. *Recherches* **9**, 23–31.

Gundlach, R. H., and G. Kenway. 1939. A method for the determination of olfactory thresholds in humans. *J. Exptl. Psychol.* **24**, 192–201.

Hainer, R. M., A. G. Emslie, and A. Jacobson. 1954. An information theory of olfaction. *Ann. N. Y. Acad. Sci.* **58**(2), 158–174.

Hallam, H. E. 1954. Odor and molecular vibrations. *Nature* **174**, 134.

Haller, A. von. 1763. "Elementa Physiologiae," Vol. 5, pp. 125–185. Lausanne.

Hammer, F. J. 1951. The relation of odor, taste, and flicker-fusion thresholds to food intake. *J. Comp. and Physiol. Psychol.* **44**, 403–411.

Hassler, W. W. (ed.). 1947. "Taste and Odor Control in Water Purification," 164 pp. Industrial Chemical Sales, New York.

Henkin, R. I., and G. F. Powell. 1962. Increased sensitivity of taste and smell in cystic fibrosis. *Science* **138**, 1107–1108.

Henkin, R. I., J. R. Gill, Jr., and F. C. Bartter. 1962. Effect of adrenal insufficiency and of cortico-steroids on smell threshold. *Clin. Research* **10**, 400.

Henning, H. 1916. "Der Geruch," 1st ed., 533 pp. Verlag Barth, Leipzig.

Henning, H. 1924. "Der Geruch," 2nd ed., 434 pp. Verlag Barth, Leipzig.

Heusghem, C., and M. A. Gerebtzoff. 1953. Résultats concordants des analyses biochimiques et histochimiques des lipides de la muqueuse olfactive. *Compt. rend. soc. biol.* **147**, 540–541.

Hinchcliffe, R. 1962. Aging and sensory thresholds. *J. Gerontol.* **17**, 45–50.

Hoeven-Leonard, J. van der. 1908. Riechschärfen- und Farbensinnabweichungen. *Umschau* **12**, 367–369.

Hofmann, F. B., and A. Kohlrausch. 1925. Bestimmung von Geruchsschwellen. *Biochem. Z.* **156**, 287–294.

Irvin, D. L., A. J. Ahokas, and F. R. Goetzl. 1950. Influence of ethyl alcohol in low concentrations upon olfactory acuity and sensation complex of appetite and satiety. *Permanente Foundation (Oakland) Med. Bull.* **8**, 97–101.

Irvin, D. L., A. Durra, and F. R. Goetzl. 1953. Influence of tannic, tartaric, and of acetic acid upon olfactory acuity and sensations associated with food intake. *Am. J. Digest. Diseases* **20**, 17–22.

Jackson, R. T. 1960. The olfactory pigment. *J. Cellular Comp. Physiol.* **55**, 143–147.

Janowitz, H. D., and M. I. Grossman. 1949. Gusto-olfactory thresholds in relation to appetite and hunger sensations. *J. Appl. Physiol.* **2**, 217–222.

Joergensen, M. B., and N. H. Buch. 1961. Studies on the sense of smell and taste in diabetics. *Acta Oto-Laryngol.* **53**, 539–545.

Joergensen, M. B., and N. H. Buch. 1962. Sense of smell and taste in pregnant diabetics. Clinical Studies. *Pract. Oto-Rhino-Laryngol.* **24**, 111–116.

Johnston, J. W., Jr. 1960. Current problems in olfaction. *Georgetown Med. Bull.* **13**, 112–117.

Johnston, J. W., Jr., and A. B. Parks. 1960. Odor-intensity and the stereochemical theory of olfaction. *Proc. Sci. Sect., Toilet Goods Assoc.* No. 34, 4–7.

Johnston, J. W., Jr., and A. Sandoval. 1960. Organoleptic quality and the stereochemical theory of olfaction. *Proc. Sci. Sect., Toilet Goods Assoc.* No. 33, 3–9.

Johnston, J. W., Jr., and A. Sandoval. 1962. The stereochemical theory of olfaction. 4. The validity of muskiness as a primary odor. *Proc. Sci. Sect., Toilet Goods Assoc. Spec. Suppl.* to No. 37, 34–45.

Jones, F. N. 1953a. A test of the validity of the Elsberg method of olfactometry. *Am. J. Psychol.* **66**, 81–85.

Jones, F. N. 1953b. Olfactory thresholds in the International Critical Tables. *Science* **118**, 333.

Jones, F. N. 1954. An olfactometer permitting stimulus specification in molar terms. *Am. J. Psychol.* **67**, 147–151.

Jones, F. N. 1955a. A comparison of the methods of olfactory stimulation: blasting vs. sniffing. *Am. J. Psychol.* **68**, 486–488.

Jones, F. N. 1955b. Olfactory absolute thresholds and their implications for the nature of the receptor process. *J. Psychol.* **40**, 223–227.

Jones, F. N. 1955c. The reliability of olfactory thresholds obtained by sniffing. *Am. J. Psychol.* **68**, 289–290.

Jones, F. N. 1957. An analysis of individual differences in olfactory thresholds. *Am. J. Psychol.* **70**, 227–232.

Jones, F. N. 1958. Scales of subjective intensity for odors of diverse chemical nature. *Am. J. Psychol.* **71**, 305–310; also pp. 423–425.

Jones, F. N. 1962. Personal communication.

Jones, F. N., and M. H. Jones. 1953. Modern theories of olfaction: a critical review. *J. Psychol.* **36**, 207–241.

Kalmus, H. 1957. Physiology and genetics of organoleptic perception. *Soc. Chem. Ind. (London) Monograph* **1**, 13–28.

Kenneth, J. H. 1927. An experimental study of affects and associations due to certain odors. *Psychol. Monograph* **37**(3), 1–64. (See also: "Osmics, the Science of Smell," 42 pp. Oliver and Boyd, Edinburgh, 1922.)

Kenney, E. J. 1954. Hotel odor problems. *Ann. N. Y. Acad. Sci.* **58**(2), 44–46.

Kiesow, F. 1922. Über bilaterale Mischung von Licht- und Geruchsempfindungen. *Arch. néerl. physiol.* **7**, 281–284.

Kimbrell, G. M., and E. Furchtgott. 1963. The effect of aging on olfactory threshold. *J. Gerontol.* **18**, 364–365.

Kistiakowsky, G. B. 1950. On the theory of odors. *Science* **112**, 154–155.

Kruger, L., A. N. Feldzamen, and W. R. Miles. 1955a. A scale for measuring suprathresholds olfactory intensity. *Am. J. Psychol.* **68**, 117–123.

Kruger, L., A. N. Feldzamen, and W. R. Miles. 1955b. Comparative olfactory intensities of the aliphatic alcohols in man. *Am. J. Psychol.* **68**, 386–395.

Kuehner, R. L. 1954. The validity of practical odor measurement methods. *Ann. N. Y. Acad. Sci.* **58**(2), 175–186.

Laffort, P. 1963a. Essai de standardisation des seuils olfactifs humains pour 192 corps purs. *Arch. Sci. Physiol.* **17**, 75–105.

Laffort, P. 1963b. Mise en évidence de relations linéaires entre l'activité odorante des molécules et certaines de leurs caractéristiques physicochimiques. *Compt. rend.* **256**, 5618–5621.

Lauffer, P. G. I. 1950. Odor and olfaction. I. II. *Drug & Cosmetic Ind.* **64**, 694–695, 775–779; **67**, 326–327, 410–417.

Lauffer, P. G. I. 1954. Odor and olfaction-biochemical approaches. *Drug & Cosmetic Ind.* **75**, 182–184, 270–273. (See also *Proc. Sci. Sect., Toilet Goods Assoc.* No. **21**, 28–35, 1954.)

Lawson, E. 1954. Odor modifiers. *Ann. N. Y. Acad. Sci.* **58**(2), 37–39.

Le Gros Clark, W. E. 1956. Observations on the structure and organization of olfactory receptors in the rabbit. *Yale J. Biol. and Med.* **39**, 83–95.

Le Magnen, J. 1948. Un cas de sensibilité olfactive se présentant comme un caractère sexuel secondaire féminin. *Compt. rend.* **226**, 694–695.

Le Magnen, J. 1952a. Les phénomènes olfacto-sexuels chez l'homme. *Arch. Sci. Physiol.* **6**, 125–160.

Le Magnen, J. 1952b. Les phénomènes olfacto-sexuels chez le rat blanc. *Arch. Sci. Physiol.* **6**, 295–331.

Le Magnen, J. 1953. L'olfaction; le fonctionnement olfactif et son intervention dans les régulations psycho-physiologiques. *J. Physiol. (Paris)* **45**, 285–326.

Le Magnen, J. 1956. Rôle de l'odeur ajoutée ou régime dans la régulation quantitative à court terme de la prise alimentaire chez la rat blanc. *Compt. rend. soc. biol.* **150**, 136–139.

Le Magnen, J., and A. Rapaport. 1951. Essai de détermination du rôle de la vitamine A dans le mécanisme de l'olfaction chez le rat blanc. *Compt. rend. soc. biol.* **145**, 800–803.

Linnaeus, C. 1752. "Amoenitates Academicae." II. "Lugduni Batavorum." Also 1762.

Luvarà, A., and M. Maurizi. 1961. Ricerche di olfattometria in gravidanza. *Boll. mal. orrecch, gola, naso* **79**, 367–375.

McCord, C. P., and W. N. Witheridge. 1949. "Odors: Physiology and Control," 405 pp. McGraw-Hill, New York.

Manci, F. 1946. Modificazione della acuitá olfattoria determinata per mezzo di spostamenti dell'equilibrio ionico del muco masale. *Riv. Clin. Med.* (*Suppl. 1, Margin. otolaryngol.*) **5**, 367–378.

Mancioli, T. 1921. Fisiopatologia delle cavitá nasali. Relaz. al XVIII Congr. Soc. Ital. Laringol. Otol. e Rinol., Parte I, Milano, 1921. *Policlinico* (*Rome*) *Sez. prat.* **28**, 1653–1660.

Margulies, N. R., D. L. Irvin, and F. R. Goetzl. 1950. The effect of alcohol upon olfactory acuity and the sensation complex of appetite and satiety. *Permanente Foundation* (*Oakland, Calif.*) *Med. Bull.* **8**, 102–106.

Mateson, J. F. 1954. The olfactory area and the olfactory receptor process. *Ann. N. Y. Acad. Sci.* **58**(2), 83–95.

Meurman, O. H. 1948a. Studies of the effect of lime and cement dust on the upper respiratory tract and the sense of smell. *Acta Oto-Laryngol. Suppl.* **73**, 1–111.

Meurman, O. H. 1948b. Do lime and cement dust impair the sense of smell? *Acta Oto-Laryngol. Suppl.* **73**, 111; *Suppl.* **74**, 313–317.

Meyer, D. R. 1952. The stability of human gustatory sensitivity during changes in time of food deprivation. *J. Comp. and Physiol. Psychol.* **45**, 373–376.

Michels, K. M., D. S. Phillips, R. H. Wright, and J. Pustek, Jr. 1961. "Odors and Olfaction, a Bibliography, 1948–1960," 179 pp. Purdue Univ., Lab. of Physiol. Psychol., Lafayette, Indiana. (See also *Perceptual and Motor Skills* **15**, 475–529, 1962.)

Miner, R. W. 1954. Basic odor research correlation. *Ann. N. Y. Acad. Sci.* **58**, 13–260 (also published separately).

Mitchell, J. W. 1957a. Problems in taste difference testing. I. Test environment. *Food Technol.* **11**, 476–477.

Mitchell, J. W. 1957b. Problems in taste difference testing. II. Subject variability due to time of the day and day of the week. *Food Technol.* **11**, 477–479.

Moncrieff, R. W. 1951. "The Chemical Senses," 538 pp. (see pp. 32–41, 89–130, 220–227, 355–401). Leonard Hill, London.

Moncrieff, R. W. (1954a). The characterization of odours. *J. Physiol.* (*London*) **125**, 453–465.

Moncrieff, R. W. 1954b. The odorants. *Ann. N. Y. Acad. Sci.* **58**(2), 73–82.

Moncrieff, R. W. 1955. Classification and identification of odorants. *Food* **24**, 154–157.

Moncrieff, R. W. 1957a. Olfactory adaptation and odor-intensity. *Am. J. Psychol.* **70**, 1–20.

Moncrieff, R. W. 1957b. The sorptive nature of the olfactory stimulus. *Proc. 2nd Intern. Congr. Surface Activity* (*London*) **2**, 321–328.

Moncrieff, R. W. 1961. An instrument for measuring and classifying odors. *J. Appl. Physiol.* **16**, 742–749.

Morimura, S. 1934. Untersuchung über den Geruchssinn. *Tôhoku J. Exptl. Med.* **22**, 417–448.

Moulton, D. G., and J. T. Eayrs. 1960. Studies in olfactory acuity. II. Relative detectability of *n*-aliphatic alcohols by the rat. *Quart. J. Exptl. Psychol.* **12**, 99–109.

Moulton, D. G., E. H. Ashton, and J. T. Eayrs. 1960. Studies in olfactory acuity. IV. Relative detectability of *n*-aliphatic acids by the dog. *Animal Behavior* **8**, 117–128.

Mozell, M. M. 1958. Electrophysiology of the olfactory bulb. *J. Neurophysiol.* **21**, 183–196.

Mullins, L. J. 1955a. Olfaction. *Ann. N. Y. Acad. Sci.* **62**, 247–276.

Mullins, L. J. 1955b. Olfactory thresholds of some homologous series of compounds. *Federation Proc.* **14**, 105.

Nader, J. S. 1958. Current techniques of odor measurement. *A.M.A. Arch. Ind. Health* **17**, 537–541. (See also *Am. Ind. Hyg. Assoc. J.* **19**, 1–7, 1958.)

Nagel, W. A. 1897. Über Mischgerüche und die Komponentengliederung des Geruchssinnes. *Z. Psychol. Physiol. Sinnesorg.* **15**, 82–101.

Naves, Y. R. 1957. Relation between stereochemistry and odorous properties of organic substances. *Soc. Chem. Ind. (London) Monograph* **1**, 38–53.

Nawar, W. W., and I. S. Fagerson. 1962. Direct gas chromatographic analysis as an objective method of flavor measurement. *Food Technol.* **16**(1), 107–109.

Neuhaus, W. 1953. Über die Riechschärfe des Hundes für Fettsäuren. *Z. vergleich Physiol.* **35**, 527–552.

New York Academy of Sciences. 1964. Recent advances in odor: theory, measurement, and control. *Ann. N. Y. Acad. Sci.* **116**, 357–746.

Niccolini, P. 1958. Il complesso fenomenologico iniziale del processo olfattorio. *In* "Olfatto e sue Correlazioni" (V. Fortunato and P. Niccolini, eds.), 699 pp. (see pp. 53–118). Tipografia dell'Università, Catania.

Noferi, G., and S. Guidizi. 1946. Le variazioni della sensibilità gustativa in particolari situazioni fisiologiche ed in alcuni stati morbosi. IV. *Riv. Clin. Med.* (*Suppl. 1, Margin. otolaryngol.*) **5**, 89–100.

Nováková, V., and H. Dlouhá. 1960. Effect of severing the olfactory bulbs on the intake and excretion of water in the rat. *Nature* **186**, 638–639.

Ogasawara, N. 1954. Histological study of olfactory bulb in man. *Tôhoku J. Exptl. Med.* **59**, 357–369.

Ottoson, D. 1956. Analysis of the electrical activity of the olfactory epithelium. *Acta Physiol. Scand.* **35** (Suppl. 122), 1–83.

Ottoson, D. 1958. Studies on the relationship between olfactory stimulating effectiveness and physico-chemical properties of odorous compounds. *Acta Physiol. Scand.* **43**, 167–181.

Ottoson, D. 1963. Some aspects of the function of the olfactory system. *Pharm. Rev.* **15**, 1–42.

Ough, C. S., and G. A. Baker. 1964. Linear dependency of scale structure in differential odor intensity measurements. *J. Food Sci.* **29**, 499–505.

Ough, C. S., and M. A. Amerine. 1959. Odor profiles of wines. *Am. J. Enol. and Viticult* **10**(1), 17–19.

Ough, C. S., and H. Stone. 1961. An olfactometer for rapid and critical odor measurement. *J. Food Sci.* **26**, 452–456.

Pangborn, R. M. 1959. Influence of hunger on sweetness preferences and taste thresholds. *Am. J. Clin. Nutrition* **7**, 280–287.

Pangborn, R. M., H. W. Berg, E. B. Roessler, and A. D. Webb. 1964. Influence of methodology on olfactory response. *Perceptual and Motor Skills* **18**, 91–103.

Parker, G. H. 1922. "Smell, Taste and Allied Senses in the Vertebrates," 192 pp. Lippincott, Philadelphia.

Parker, G. H., and E. M. Stabler. 1913. On certain distinctions between taste and smell. *Am. J. Physiol.* **32**, 230–240.

Parkes, A. S., and H. M. Bruce. 1961. Olfactory stimuli in mammalian reproduction. *Science* **134**, 1049–1054.

Paschal, G. 1952. "Odors and the Sense of Smell, A Bibliography, 320 B.C.–1947," 342 pp. Airkem, Inc., New York.

Passy, J. 1892a. Sur les minimums perceptibles de quelques odeurs. *Compt. rend. soc. biol.* 114, 306–308, 786–788.

Passy, J. 1892b. Les propriétés odorantes des alcools de la série grasse. *Compt. rend. soc. biol.* 114, 1120–1143. (See also *Mem. Soc. Biol. Paris* 44, 447–449, 1892.)

Patterson, P. M., and B. A. Lauder. 1948. The incidence and probable inheritance of smell blindness to normal butyl mercaptan. *J. Heredity* 39, 295–297.

Pauling, L. 1946. Analogies between antibodies and simpler chemical substances. *Chem. Eng. News* 24, 1064–1065.

Paulsen, E. 1892. Experimentelle Untersuchungen über die Strömung der Luft in der Nasenhöhle. *Sitzber. Akad. Wiss. Wien, Math. Naturwiss. Kl., Abt. III* 85, 353–373.

Pfaffmann, C. 1948. Studying the senses of taste and smell. *In:* "Methods of Psychology" (T. G. Andrews, ed.), 716 pp. (see pp. 279–285). Wiley, New York.

Pfaffmann, C. 1951. Taste and smell. *In* "Handbook of Experimental Psychology" (S. S. Stevens, ed.), 1436 pp. (see pp. 1143–1144, 1158–1168). Wiley, New York.

Pfaffmann, C. 1956. Taste and smell. *Ann. Rev. Psychol.* 7, 391–408.

Pfaffmann, C., and J. K. Bare. 1950. Gustatory nerve discharges in normal and adrenalectomized rats. *J. Comp. and Physiol. Psychol.* 43, 320–324.

Pfaffmann, C., W. R. Goff, and J. K. Bare. 1958. An olfactometer for the rat. *Science* 128, 1007–1008.

Piéron, H. 1952. "The Sensations; Their Functions, Processes and Mechanisms," 469 pp. Yale Univ. Press, New Haven, Connecticut.

Pilgrim, F. J., and H. G. Schutz. 1957. Measurement of the qualitative and quantitative attributes of flavor. *In* "Chemistry of Natural Food Flavors" (J. H. Mitchell, Jr., H. J. Leinen, E. M. Mrak, and S. D. Bailey, eds.), 200 pp. (see pp. 47–55). Quartermaster Food and Container Institute, Washington, D. C.

Portmann, G. 1951. "Diseases of the Ear, Nose, and Throat," 723 pp. Williams & Wilkins, Baltimore, Maryland.

Posvic, H. 1953. The odors of optical isomers. *Science* 118, 358–359.

Prince, R. G. H., and J. H. Ince. 1958. The measurement of intensity of odour. *J. Appl. Chem.* 8, 314–321.

Proetz, A. W. 1953. "Applied Physiology of the Nose," 452 pp. Annals Publ. Co., St. Louis, Missouri.

Reed, E. 1954. Odor problems in the paper industry. *Ann. N. Y. Acad. Sci.* 58(2), 34–36.

Rennes, P. 1945. Une méthode nouvelle d'olfactométrie. *Année. Psychol.* 41–42, 243–247.

Reese, T. S., and S. S. Stevens. 1960. Subjective intensity of coffee odor. *Am. J. Psychol.* 73, 424–428.

Reynolds, W. E. 1954. Odor problems in federal office buildings. *Ann. N. Y. Acad. Sci.* 58(2), 47–51.

Rosen, A. A., J. B. Peter, and F. M. Middleton. 1962. Odor thresholds of mixed organic chemicals. *J. Water Pollution Control Federation* 34, 7–14.

Rosenblith, W. A. 1961. "Sensory Communication," 844 pp. M.I.T. Press, Cambridge, Massachusetts; Wiley, New York.

Rubin, M., D. Apotheker, and R. Lutmer. 1962. The stereochemical theory of olfaction. 3. Structure and odor: 1,4-cyclohexane lactones and related compounds. *Proc. Sci. Sect., Toilet Goods Assoc. Spec. Suppl. to* No. 37, 24–33.

Ruzicka, L. 1920. Die Grundlagen der Geruchschemie. *Chemiker-Ztg.* 44, 93–94, 129–131.

Ruzicka, L. 1957. Fundamentals of odour chemistry: a summary. *Soc. Chem. Ind.* (*London*) *Monograph* 1, 116–124.

Sagarin, E. 1954. Odor: a proposal for some basic definitions. *ASTM Spec. Tech. Publ.* 164, 3–8.

Salis, B. 1959. Rilievi sulla soglia olfattiva in gravidanza. *Minerva otorinolaringol.* 9, 149–150.

Saunders, H. C. 1962. The stereochemical theory of olfaction. 5. Some odor observations in terms of the Amoore theory. *Proc. Sci. Sect., Toilet Goods Assoc. Spec. Suppl. to* No. 37, 46–47.

Schneider, R. A., and S. Wolf. 1955. Olfactory perception thresholds for citral utilizing a new type olfactorium. *J. Appl. Physiol.* 8, 337–342.

Schneider, R. A., and S. Wolf. 1960. Relation of olfactory acuity to nasal membrane function. *J. Appl. Physiol.* 15, 914–920.

Schneider, R. A., J. P. Costiloe, R. P. Howard, and S. Wolf. 1958. Olfactory perception thresholds in hypogonadal women: changes accompanying administration of androgen and estrogen. *J. Clin. Endocrinol. and Metabolism* 18, 379–390.

Schutz, H. G. 1964. A matching-standards method for characterizing odor. *Ann. N. Y. Acad. Sci.* 116, 517–526.

Semeria, C. 1958. Le alterazioni olfattive nei traumi cranici, nelle neoplasie craniche e nelle ipossiemie sperimentali. *In* "Olfatto e sue Correlazioni" (V. Fortunato and P. Niccolini, eds.), 699 pp. (see pp. 465–500). Tipografia dell'Università, Catania.

Sfiras, J., and A. Demeilliers. 1957. Tentatives de mesure de l'intensité de l'odeur. *Soc. Chem. Ind.* (*London*) *Monograph* 1, 29–37.

Shibuya, T. 1964. Dissociation of olfactory neural response and mucosal potential. *Science* 143, 1338–1340.

Shibuya, T., and S. Shibuya. 1963. Olfactory epithelium: unitary responses in the tortoise. *Science* 140, 495–496.

Shkapenko, G., and M. A. Gerebtzoff. 1951. Critique expérimentale de l'intervention des radiations dans le mécanisme de l'olfaction. *Arch. intern. physiol.* 59, 423–429.

Sjöström, L. B., S. E. Cairncross, and J. F. Caul. 1957. Methodology of the flavor profile. *Food Technol.* 11(9), 20–24.

Skouby, A. P., and K. Zilstorff-Pedersen. 1954. The influence of acetylcholine-like substances, menthol and strychnine on olfactory receptors in man. *Acta Physiol. Scand.* 32, 252–258.

Skramlik, E. von. 1926. Die Physiologie des Geruchs- und Geschmackssinnes. *In* "Handbuch der Physiologie der niederen Sinne," Vol. 1, 532 pp. (see pp. 1–345). Thieme, Leipzig.

Spealman, C. R. 1954. Odors, odorants, and deodorants in aviation. *Ann. N. Y. Acad. Sci.* 58(2), 40–43.

Stein, M., P. Ottenberg, and N. Roulet. 1958. A study of the development of olfactory preferences. *A.M.A. Arch. Neurol. Psychiat.* 80, 264–266.

Stirniman, F. 1936a. Le goût et l'odorat du nouveau-né. Une contribution à la connaissance des réactions du nouveau-né. *Rev. Franç. pédiat.* 12, 453–485.

Stirniman, F. 1936b. Versuche über Geschmack und Geruch am ersten Lebenstag. *Jahrb. Kinderheilk.* **146**, 211–227.

Stoll, M. 1957. Facts old and new concerning relationships between molecular structure and odour. *Soc. Chem. Ind. (London) Monograph* **1**, 1–12.

Stone, F., and F. R. Goetzl. 1948. Olfactory acuity and appetite: effects of bitter tonics on olfactory acuity in normal human subjects. *Federation Proc.* **7**, 120–121.

Stone, H. 1963. Some factors affecting olfactory sensitivity and odor intensity. 112 pp. Unpubl. Ph.D. Thesis. Univ. of Calif., Davis, California. (See also *J. Appl. Physiol.* **18**, 746–751, 1963.)

Stone, H., C. S. Ough, and R. M. Pangborn. 1962. Determination of odor difference thresholds. *J. Food Sci.* **27**, 197–202.

Stone, H., R. M. Pangborn, and C. S. Ough. 1965. Techniques for sensory evaluation of food odors. *Advances in Food Research* **14**, (in press).

Stuiver, M. 1958. Biophysics of the sense of smell. 99 pp. Thesis. Rijks Univ., Groningen, The Netherlands.

Stuiver, M. 1960. An olfactometer with a wide range of possibilities. *Acta Oto-Laryngol.* **51**, 135–142.

Sumner, J. B. 1954. Problems in odor research from the viewpoint of the chemist. *Ann. N. Y. Acad. Sci.* **58**(2), 68–72.

Swaine, R. L. 1960. Flavor methodology. Paper presented at the Canadian Inst. of Food Technol., Montreal Section, October 18, 1960. 13 pp.

Tanzariello, R. 1958. Olfatto e malattie professionali. *In* "Olfatto e sue Correlazioni" (V. Fortunato and P. Niccolini, eds.), 699 pp. (see pp. 643–698). Tipografia dell'Università, Catania.

Thompson, H. W. 1957. Some comments on theories of smell. *Soc. Chem. Ind. (London) Monograph* **1**, 103–115.

Timmermans, J. 1954. Odour and chemical composition. *Nature* **174**, 235.

Tucker, D. 1961. Physical variables in the olfactory stimulation process. *Dissertation Abstr.* **22**, 2858.

Turk, A. 1954. Odor control methods: a critical review. *ASTM Spec. Tech. Publ.* **164**, 69–80.

Ueki, S., and F. F. Domino. 1961. Some evidence for a mechanical receptor in olfactory function. *J. Neurophysiol.* **24**, 12–25.

Vries, H. de, and M. Stuiver. 1961. The absolute sensitivity of the human sense of smell. *In* "Sensory Communication" (W. A. Rosenblith, ed.), 844 pp. (see pp. 159–167). M.I.T. Press, Cambridge, Massachusetts; Wiley, New York.

Wagner, J. R., D. S. Titus, and J. E. Schade. 1963. New opportunities for flavor modification. *Food Technol.* **17**, 730–733, 735.

Walsh, R. R. 1953. Electrical activity in the mammalian olfactory bulb. *Federation Proc.* **12**, 150–151.

Walsh, R. R. 1956. Single cell spike activity in the olfactory bulb. *Am. J. Physiol.* **186**, 255–257.

Weiss, A. D. 1959. Sensory functions. *In* "The Handbook of Aging and the Individual" (J. E. Birren, ed.), 939 pp. (see pp. 503–542). Univ. of Chicago Press, Chicago, Illinois.

Wendt, G. R. 1952. Somesthesis and the chemical senses. *Ann. Rev. Psychol.* **3**, 105–130.

Wenger, M. A., F. N. Jones, and M. H. Jones. 1956. "Physiological Psychology," 472 pp. Holt, New York.

Wenzel, B. M. 1948a. Differential sensitivity in olfaction. 29 pp. Ph. D. Thesis. Columbia Univ., New York. (See also *J. Exptl. Psychol.* **39**, 129–143, 1949.)

Wenzel, B. M. 1948b. Techniques in olfactometry: a critical review of the last one hundred years. *Psychol. Bull.* **45**, 231–247.

Wenzel, B. M. 1954. The chemical senses. *Ann. Rev. Psychol.* **5**, 111–126.

Wenzel, B. M. 1955. Olfactometric method utilizing natural breathing in an odor-free "environment." *Science* **121**, 802–803.

Woodrow, H., and B. Karpman. 1917. A new olfactometric technique and some results. *J. Exptl. Psychol.* **2**, 431–447.

Woodworth, R. S., and H. Schlosberg. 1954. "Experimental Psychology," 948 pp. Holt, New York.

Woskow, M. H. 1964. Multidimensional scaling of odors. 72 pp. Ph.D. Thesis. Univ. of California, Los Angeles, California.

Wright, R. H. 1954a. Odour and chemical constitution. *Nature* **173**, 831.

Wright, R. H. 1954b. Odour and molecular vibration. I. Quantum and thermodynamic considerations. *J. Appl. Chem.* **4**, 611–615.

Wright, R. H. 1957a. Odour and molecular vibration. *Soc. Chem. Ind. (London) Monograph* **1**, 91–102.

Wright, R. H. 1957b. A theory of olfaction and of the action of mosquito repellents. *Can. Entomologist* **84**, 518–528.

Wright, R. H. 1963. Theory and methodology in olfaction. *Dissert. Abstr.* **23**, 2600.

Wright, R. H. 1964. "The Science of Smell," 164 pp. Basic Books, Inc., New York.

Wright, R. H., and R. S. E. Serenius. 1954. Odour and molecular vibration. II. Raman spectra of substances with the nitrobenzene odour. *J. Appl. Chem.* **4**, 615–621.

Wright, R. H., and R. S. E. Serenius. 1956. Odour and molecular vibration. III. A new theory of olfactory stimulation. *Chem. & Ind. (London)* **37**, 973–977.

Zilstorff-Pedersen, K. 1955. Olfactory threshold determinations in relation to food intake. *Acta Oto-Laryngol.* **45**, 86–90.

Zilstorff-Pedersen, K. 1962. Uebersichten die quantitative und qualitative Olfactometrie. *HNO* **10**, 97–102.

Zotterman, Y. 1963. "Olfaction and Taste," 396 pp. Macmillan, New York.

Zwaardemaker, H. 1895. "Die Physiologie des Geruchs," 324 pp. Engelmann, Leipzig.

Zwaardemaker, H. 1921a. A camera inodorata. *Perfumery Essent. Oil Record* **12**, 243–244.

Zwaardemaker, H. 1921b. Olfactometry. *Perfumery Essent. Oil Record* **12**, 308–310.

Zwaardemaker, H. 1925. "L'Odorat," 305 pp. Doin, Paris.

Zwaardemaker, H. 1926. *In* "International Critical Tables" (E. W. Washburn, ed.), Vol. 1, 358–361. McGraw-Hill, New York.

Chapter 4

Visual, Auditory, Tactile, and Other Senses

Taste and olfactory responses are of primary importance in the sensory evaluation of food, but other senses also influence discrimination and preference—and in some cases they may be paramount. Among these are the visual, auditory, tactile, kinesthetic, pain, and temperature senses. There are also a number of pressure nerves around the teeth, and in the tongue and jaws which indicate movement and tension on the teeth and in the muscles of the tongue and jaw. Psychologists and physiologists are undecided as to the exact number of true senses. We summarize here only those which clearly seem to have some importance in the sensory examination of foods. For basic physiological data on these senses, see Geldard (1953) and American Physiological Society (1959).

I. Vision

Color and other aspects of appearance influence food appreciation and quality, especially by the consumer. Man has subjective standards for the acceptable range and preferred optima for these qualities for almost every food.

A. COLOR

The importance of color in agriculture and to foods in particular cannot be overstressed (Judd and Wyszecki, 1963; Mackinney and Little, 1962). An important problem is discoloration or the fading of colors of various raw and processed fruits and vegetables. In some cases, color changes are accompanied by undesirable changes in texture, taste, or odor. Over-aged cheese, beer, meat, and fish all develop off colors which the consumer recognizes as being associated with poor flavor quality. The maturity of many fruits and vegetables is closely associated with color development or changes in color. In other cases a color change may not be actually detrimental but nevertheless reduces consumer acceptance. Consumers expect foods to have a certain color, and deviation from this color may introduce sales resistance. Many of these prejudices are altogether irrational. White oleomargarine, though it has the same taste and olfactory sensation as yellow, has a limited sales appeal. As noted by Johnson (1956), when natural carotene content is low, butter is artificially colored; mint-flavored ice cream is white before artificial green coloring is added; orange sherbet is also fortified with artificial coloring. Maraschino cherries, oranges, syrups, jellies, and many types of candy are artificially colored.

Unfortunately, the psychological aspects of food colors have been studied by only a relatively small number of investigators. Moir (1936) noted that test subjects almost invariably identified fruit flavors incorrectly when jellies were atypically colored. Kanig (1955) found that few of 200 pharmacy students tested could identify flavorings presented in colorless syrups, and even fewer responded correctly when solutions were presented in unusual colors. The influence of previous experience upon color and taste was operative in a study by Dunker (1939) in which white chocolate was reported to taste less like chocolate than the customary brown product. The specific influence of previous experience or training was not measured in that study.

Schutz (1954) reported that 52 subjects preferred the appearance of orange-colored orange juice over juice of a distinctly yellow color, although preferences for taste were identical and both colors were within the range of color acceptability for orange juice. In the same experiment, he demonstrated that the flavor scores of an inferior-tasting juice could be raised by coloring it to resemble a juice of a better quality. He noted that "spurious conclusions about food preferences may be reached by considering color independently of flavor factors, and colors can be experimentally manipulated to serve as standards of good quality."

Hall (1958) described an experiment where sherbets in six flavors (lemon, lime, orange, grape, pineapple, and almond) were prepared in their natural or commonly associated color, in an inappropriate color, and white or uncolored. As might be expected, the sensory panel was highly successful in identifying flavors presented in their customary colors, less so with flavors presented in white or uncolored form, and very unsuccessful with sherbets colored deceptively. Except with the almond-flavored sherbet, properly colored sherbets were rated highest in flavor acceptability, and deceptively colored sherbets rated lowest.

Pangborn (1960) reported that sweetness discrimination was not influenced by red, green, or yellow coloring in unflavored aqueous solutions. In pear nectar, in contrast, there was a pronounced tendency to designate the green-colored samples as the least sweet. With another panel, Pangborn and Hansen (1963) did not find this to be true. Considerable differences in color-taste associations between individuals were demonstrated. Pangborn *et al.* (1963) also found that pink-colored table wines were thought to be sweeter than white, light red, dark red, or light brown-colored wines of the same composition, by an experienced panel of wine-tasters but not by a naive panel. However, color did not influence the subject's ability to differentiate 1.5 from 1.8 and 5.0 from 5.4% sucrose. Bengtsson and Helm (1946) noted that flavor differences were not detected as easily when beer was served in dark containers as when served in clear glass. Complex association influences probably account for the results. They illustrate a type of stimulus error (Chapter 5, Section III). Whether the error could be avoided by warning the panel beforehand is not known.

Malphrus (1957) showed that beef steaks with white fat were distinguished significantly from steaks with yellow fat. Of subjects noting the difference, a significant proportion preferred the steaks with the white fat. With roasts, no difference in preference was observed.

Foster (1956) listed five functions which should be considered in understanding human reactions to color in foods:

(1) *Perception.* Food selection or judgment of food quality would be extremely difficult if color discrimination were removed even though size, texture, shape, and other cues were left intact.

(2) *Motivation.* Food color and color of the environment in which the food is seen can significantly increase or decrease our desire or appetite for it.

(3) *Emotion.* Liking or disliking a food is conditioned by its color; attractive foods are sought out as pleasure-giving, while unattractive foods are avoided as painful.

(4) *Learning.* By the process of experience, we learn what colors to expect and consider "natural," and we predict rather precisely what properties a food or beverage will have from our memory of similar materials.

(5) *Thinking.* Our reaction to unusual properties or to new foods can be changed if they are explained to us.

Obviously, far too little is known about the significance of color perception in food acceptance. Observers do associate certain colors with acceptance, indifference, or rejection. Colored lights are used to mask color differences and reduce some influence of color on sensory evaluation, but the psychological effect of the colored lights has not been adequately measured. These effects may be direct—on the appeal of the food as a whole—or indirect—in influencing odor, taste, or texture thresholds. Various interrelationships suggest themselves.

The human eye has a remarkably fine qualitative discrimination for color, but it is not a quantitative instrument. Consequently, precise color measurement requires modern instruments (Chapter 11, Section I). This need is felt particularly where food products are blended to a certain standard from raw materials which differ somewhat in their color properties, e.g., with tomato catsup. The effect of climate and time of harvesting have a marked influence on the color of the raw material from which many processed foods are made.

B. COLOR DEFINITION

The visible spectrum lies in the range of 400 (violet) to 700 (red) millimicrons (mμ). Within this region the eye is most sensitive to differences in color in the green-yellow region (520–580 mμ). Color can be discussed in general terms of light stimuli, but for specifying color phenomena in foods we are most interested in the energy coming to the eye from the illuminated surface or, with transparent foods, through the material. The color perceived by the eye from an illuminated object depends on the spectral composition of the light source, the chemical and physical characteristics of the object, the nature of the background illumination, and the spectral sensitivity of the eye viewing the object.

Precise definition of color phenomena requires specification of the dominant wavelength, colorimetric purity, and intensity. Of these, the most important is the wavelength—the average color. The purity (saturation) relates to a more complex dimension, and may be thought of as the degree of gray mixed in. The intensity or brightness is the amount of color—it corresponds roughly to loudness in hearing.

The C.I.E. system (Commission Internationale de l'Eclairage) depends upon three primary colors: red, blue, and yellow. Matching an unknown color against a proper mixture of these gives a satisfactory color match providing that we conceive of a mixture of a series of grays from white to black being present. Thus, mixing blue and yellow gives a green color. Color mixing is not a mixture of sensations but a mixing of stimuli to give a unitary sensation. With certain pairs of complementary colors, however, we get, not intermediate hues, but some shade of one or the other of the pair or a new color (as the violet from mixing red and blue).

In physical terms the fundamental quantities are designated as dominant wavelength (or hue), purity (or saturation), and lightness (or luminance). The chromaticity diagram, used to calculate these quantities, is prepared from the spectral chromatic data (usually from an absorption curve) of the visible spectrum of the particular color. From this diagram the tristimulus values of the color are calculated and are plotted directly on the chromaticity diagram. The absorption curves are quite easy to obtain now that recording spectrophotometers are available.

Mackinney and Chichester (1954) noted that in some parts of the spectrum the ability of the human eye to detect a difference in color samples is at least equal to the discrimination given by the usual spectrophotometric system, where the absorption is measured at 10-mμ intervals or the 10 selected ordinate procedure is used for determining the tristimulus values. A number of abridged spectrophotometers have been devised to give colorimetric data comparable to those of the spectrophotometer without the labor involved in calculations of spectrophotometric data.

In addition to the spectrophotometric procedure are comparison procedures that involve color dictionaries or color standards. The Munsell system, in most common use in this country, has the advantage that its quantities are reported in terms of hue, value, and chroma. Since hue is equivalent to the dominant wavelength, value to the lightness, and chroma to the saturation (purity), this system provides a convenient comparison with spectrophotometric data.

The duration of the stimulus is important in determining visual threshold since, in the Bunsen-Roscoe law, $I \times T =$ a constant, where I is the luminance and T the time. Beyond some critical duration the luminance depends on some other constant. The observed brightness depends on the area. A small area appears less bright than a larger area, even though the two have the same brightness. This is a form of summation and is particularly important near the threshold.

Hue discrimination is dependent not only on wavelength but on intensity. If the intensity of a red light (660 mμ) is sharply reduced it is necessary to decrease the wavelength to maintain the original hue. Likewise, if the intensity of a green light (525 mμ) is reduced it is necessary to increase the wavelength to maintain the same hue. At 570 mμ (yellow), 503 mμ (green), and 478 mμ (blue), and in the purple region (mixture of long and short waves), intensity does not have this effect. Saturation in purity discrimination is also important. Purity, as stated above, is the relative absence of grayness in colors.

Color contrast is another phenomenon which needs to be considered in evaluating food colors. If a gray square is placed on a colored surface the gray appears to be tinged with the hue complementary to the background color. The degree of contrast is affected by the distinctness of the surfaces, by the distance from the eyes, and even by the intentness with which one studies the colors. These factors may be quite important in certain cases, but have not been systematically studied with regard to foods.

Glitter, gloss, sheen, and other visual properties are also important to food processors in special cases. In some fruits, the gloss (specular, or mirrorlike, reflection) and transparency are important. For many liquids, turbidity (caused by suspended particles) is an indication of changes during processing or aging. Gloss and transparency are not of great importance with most food products, but turbidity is of critical importance with certain beverages, e.g., beer. In certain cases it is possible to measure turbidity so that it can be controlled when necessary.

The human eye is subject to the same physiological limitations as the other senses. The most important of these for vision are: visual acuity, absolute threshold, differential threshold, duality of reception, adaptation, and hue and saturation discrimination.

Visual acuity can be measured accurately. It can be shown that acuity increases markedly as a function of illumination. Adaptation and the brightness of the field surrounding the object are also factors which affect visual acuity. The effective light energy at the absolute threshold is a few hundred billionths of an erg—or 5–14 quanta (average 7) (Hecht *et al.*, 1941). This means that if the eye were much more sensitive we could "see" the "shot effect" of photon emission and the "steady" light would not be steady. The efficiency of the eye is often measured by determining the fusion frequency—the frequency at which a flashing light just disappears into appearance of a steady light. The higher the frequency at which the individual can see the flicker, the greater the efficiency of his vision. Fusion frequency depends on several stimulus variables, however, and its exact significance from the theoretical point of view is not clear.

The increment of intensity necessary to produce a perceptible change in color (the Weber fraction, Chapter 5, Section IV,A) is roughly constant at moderate intensities of illumination. The eye sees somewhat differently under high-intensity light (called photopic, or daylight, vision) than under low intensity (called scotopic, or twilight, vision). Color differentiation is much less under low intensity. The low-intensity region covers perhaps thirty just-noticeably different (jnd) steps (Chapter 5, Section IV,A) whereas the high-intensity region covers as many as 500 such jnd steps. Nevertheless, a certain approximate color constancy of objects is well known. The observer seems to reach a judgment of the color and to eliminate differences of illumination to a certain extent. This problem has not been considered in correlations of subjective color evaluation and instrumental measurements.

Adaptation is not particularly noticeable unless sensitivity is measured after being in a dark room. There is a gradual decrease in sensitivity in the light. Presumably the visual pigment rhodopsin is broken down in the light and synthesized in the dark. Lack of vitamin A has been shown to increase light thresholds markedly. Normally adaptation is of little importance in subjective evaluation of food colors.

Afterimages are known to occur (motion pictures may depend on them). These are positive at first, i.e., with the same quantitative characteristics, but soon become negative, i.e., opposite in brightness and complementary in hue. They probably are of little importance in food evaluation.

Many people are afflicted with various deficiencies of color vision. Color blindness has not been much studied with respect to the color appreciation of food. If the visual impressions are important, the color-blind individual may substitute other parameters for color in his food appreciation. Also, many individuals with poor color perception have learned the socially approved color names for many objects. Birren (1963) has discussed the relation of color to appetite but no data or references are given. He believes "warm" colors (red, orange, yellow) stimulate the autonomic nervous system and "cool" colors (blue, green) retard it. Objective data would be desired. Dember (1961) quoted Russian reports that pleasant olfactory stimuli increased visual sensitivity and that unpleasant olfactory stimuli decreased it. Gustatory sensations also influenced the sensitivity of the fovea centralis (point of sharpest vision at back of retina). Visual-auditory interaction is also reported. This would seem to be a fruitful field of research, particularly visual-olfactory interaction.

We should also mention the particular problems of the perception of form such as the primacy of the figure perception over that of the background, memory, contour, etc. [see Woodworth and Schlosberg (1954) for further details]. The importance of these in food science has not been investigated, but they may be of significance in food packaging. Bartley (1948) stressed that with vision (as well as with the other senses) the observer is a contributor to the experimental end result. The individual's organization (attitude, etc.) influences the end results. Bartley emphasized how much remains to be learned about the basic features of the contact between the individual and the physical world.

Francis (1963) noted that the color problem differs between products where added color may be used and those where it cannot be used. But in both cases modern processors wish to standardize the color as much as possible. This involves statistical quality control over the raw material and the processes, and is best done by instrumentation. Francis gives a good review of the use of various instruments.

For a more thorough coverage of color and color measurement, the reader is referred to the texts by Judd (1952) and Judd and Wyszecki

(1963). A symposium on color in foods (comprising sixteen papers) covers color measurement in specific food products (Farrell *et al.*, 1954). In their book on quality control, Kramer and Twigg (1962) devoted a chapter to color and gloss. The most comprehensive coverage is that of Mackinney and Little (1962), who discuss vision and perception of color, the C.I.E., Munsell, and Lovibond color systems, color specifications, and color standards in foods.

As Yilmaz and Clapp (1963) pointed out, the eye and the brain receive color and form with amazing detail, far more efficiently than any device yet constructed by man. They have developed a general theory of perception based on a principle of relativity. For color the eye was evolved to meet human needs. It assumes that the perception mechanisms developed as a protective device during biological evolution and that we perceive differences, say in color, from relationships between wavelengths. This fulcrum shift theory is a mathematical formulation of the behavior of the senses in which the "fulcrum" of these faculties shifts so that recognition of, say, object color remains the same when light distribution changes.

II. Audition

The sounds of foods are familiar to all consumers who have heard the "snap, crackle, and pop" of some dry cereals upon the addition of milk, the "fizz" of champagne and carbonated beverages, and the "sizzling" of a hot steak. Sounds are associated with food preparation, such as the popping of corn, perking of coffee, simmering of liquids, bubbling of syrups, broiling of meats, frying of eggs, and cracking of nuts. Consumers have been known to prefer the sound of china and crockery tableware to that of plastic dishes.

Little has been written on the sounds of food or on the interrelationships of the chemical senses with sound. Rietz (1961) is of the opinion that eating blanched almonds concurrently with smoked finnan haddie reduces the fishy flavor of the latter through "an illusion caused by the dominance of the auditory sense over that of taste and smell generated by the kinesthesis of munching." No experimental evidence was cited. Fishy flavors may be reduced in the presence of crunchy foods, but it is doubtful if sound alone is responsible. (Chewing finely ground almonds would separate the taste factors from the auditory. Use of deaf persons in such experiments might yield interesting results.) Srinivasan (1955) reported less taste sensitivity with the ears closed, but controlled experiments on a variety of foods and taste stimuli with statistical analysis of the results are needed.

In sensory testing of beer, Mitchell (1957) observed that simple knowledge of the presence of another subject during a test provided enough distraction to lower sensitivity significantly; a noisy environment further reduced ability to discriminate. The effect of quiet and controlled sound (tape recording of clattering dishes and muffled voices at 80 decibels) on flavor preferences for tomato juice was tested by Pettit (1958). Neither the test location nor the background noise altered preferences significantly. Hodges (1962) reported that increased noise levels raised the absolute threshold for sucrose but lowered the threshold for tartaric acid. Woodworth and Schlosberg (1954) have summarized psychological evidence that reactions to distraction are highly individual. Therefore, experiments on the effect of noise or sound should be conducted with sufficiently large groups, and individual differences should be recorded. They noted: "If noise while you are trying to work makes you angry, this internal distraction is worse than mere noise." In our own experience we have noted some judges whose results were little affected by laboratory noise whereas others objected to even small distractions and were obviously handicapped by noise. Such reduction in efficiency may be important when differences between samples are small. It may be significant that Hernández-Peón *et al.* (1956) reported that auditory-evoked potentials were reduced when cats were attentive to visual, olfactory, or somatic stimuli.

The crispness of lettuce, the crackliness of celery, and the crunchiness of peanut brittle attest to the presence of auditory-kinesthetic interactions. Raw fish is said to be unattractive to Europeans because it "squeaks" when chewed; finding a small rock in a mouthful of cooked beans is very disturbing to the sense of hearing. In the foregoing two examples, however, factors of taste, kinesthetics, and esthetics are compounded with the sounds.

As a part of a study of vibrational properties of foodstuffs, Drake (1963) analyzed the amplitude, frequency, and duration of the sounds produced in chewing. A microphone, tape recorder, frequency analyzer, and strip-chart recorder were used to measure the sounds taken through the cheek during 2 sec of chewing. Characteristic patterns relating to specific foodstuffs, such as toasted and untoasted bread, were observed, as well as differences between experimental subjects. Further studies of this type are needed.

The sound of food alone may be seen to operate when the housewife relies on the "hollow" sounds derived from thumping a melon to determine its state of ripeness. In markets, shoppers may be observed shaking boxes of dry cereal products to estimate their fill, shaking cans of fruit to estimate the ratio of fruit to liquid, and agitating cans of frozen juices to determine whether they are still frozen solid.

III. Oral Perception Other Than Taste

The sense organs concerned with perception in the mouth, other than taste, pain and temperature, are: (1) those in the tongue, gums, and hard and soft palate—the tactile, or feel, sense; and (2) those around the roots of the teeth and in the muscles and tendons used in mastication— the kinesthetic sense. Of course, sensory responses, to chemicals for example, occur elsewhere than in the mouth.

The soft structures of the mouth have a network of free nerve endings plus encapsulated and unencapsulated organized nerve terminations. The free nerve endings respond to touch and light pressure, and probably to thermal, chemical, and mechanical stimuli, which, at sufficient intensity, cause pain. The organized structures are concerned with deeper pressures, distortion of the tissue by stretching, and to pain and cold. Pressure and touch receptors are arranged so that stretching or bending of the terminal filaments will discharge the nerve fiber. Most of the receptors are on the surface, but there are also deep pressure (Pacinian corpuscles) receptors.

According to Rose and Mountcastle (1959), pain, cold, warmth, and touch represent the four basic modalities of cutaneous sensation, and specific receptors could be assigned to each. They point out that some workers believe that the specific receptors are less important while others propose a duality of mechanisms—a generalized, more primitive (or protopathic) type at the periphery, and a more specific and advanced (or epicritic) system.

Mechanical stimulation of the skin and of some tissues beneath it results in tactile and kinesthetic sensations. Tactile sensations are caused by displacement of hairs or deformation of the skin without injury. Kinesthetic (or position or movement) sensations are the result of stimuli pressing upon or displacing, without injury, connective tissues, particularly those which cause displacement or compression of capsules of the joints.

Branches of the dental nerves terminate in the pulp of the tooth and also in the periodontal membrane. Pressure apparently displaces the tooth slightly in its socket, and the compression on the periodontal membrane is the stimulus detected. Pfaffmann (1939) showed that most of the nerve impulses resulting from touch or pressure on the tooth originate in the periodontal membrane. Adaptation times varied in a wide range. He also reported that dental nerves may respond to pressure in one direction and not in the other.

Mastication (chewing) exerts considerable force. According to Oldfield (1960), as early as 1681 Birelli estimated this force at 100 pounds.

The incisors exert a force of about 20 pounds and the molars about 100, but this depends on the type of food customarily eaten. The Eskimo, with his diet of tough foods, may attain forces of 300 pounds. The nervous mechanisms responsible for biting and chewing must be arranged in some sort of order. Opening of the mouth, chewing, tongue movement, and swallowing are all involved in an almost automatic sequence.

Chewing breaks up the food, increases the surface area available for enzymatic action, stimulates salivation, and mixes the food with salivary enzymes. Oldfield (1960) suggested that continued release of flavor as the food is chewed is important. If the flavor disappears or is exhausted before the chewing process is completed, as with a tough steak, an impulse to eject the food particle may be elicited. On the other hand, children and adults continue to masticate chewing gum long after its flavor and sweet taste have been exhausted. Oldfield suggested that to some people chewing appears to afford its own pleasure, and sometimes occurs compulsively and without awareness.

Tactile sensations were described by Ruch (1960) as touch-pressure, deep sensibility, vibratory sensibility, localization or topognosis, projection, two-point sensibility, etc. The receptor processes associated with these sensations have been studied very little, yet are very complicated since they are largely influenced by psychological factors of association (experience). When we see a piece of wilted lettuce, we already have some idea of its eating quality. Thus, before the food reaches the mouth the whole process of its appreciation or rejection has already been initiated. Once it is in the mouth, a second appraisal takes place—and may lead to chewing or to rejection.

Movement of the food over the surface of the tongue and sides of the mouth has a stimulatory effect. Adaptation of the cutaneous (touch) sense organ is partially prevented by movement of the material over the tongue's surface, across the gums and the hard and soft palates. The mechanoreceptors of the skin are subject to adaptation, but differences have been noted in the rate of adaptation of different fibers.

A. FOOD TEXTURE

The characteristic sense of feel of food products is often one of the most important aspects of their quality. Firmness, softness (yielding quality), and juiciness are measured in the mouth much as they would be measured by the finger. There are also factors, described as chewiness, fibrousness, grittiness, succulence, mealiness, stickiness, and oiliness, which influence the acceptance of different foods. Tenderness may be the most important sensory factor influencing the acceptance of meat (Bailey *et al.*, 1962).

Texture is a composite property. Undoubtedly it is related to the viscosity, elasticity, and other physical properties of foods, but the relationship is complex. Matz (1962) favors the following definition of texture: "The mingled experience deriving from the sensations of the skin in the mouth after ingestion of a food or beverage. It relates to density, viscosity, surface tension and other physical properties of the material being sampled." Kramer and Twigg (1962) classify texture characteristics as finger feel (firmness, softness, or yielding quality) and juiciness.

Szczesniak (1963) classified the textural characteristics of foods into mechanical and geometrical qualities and into properties related to moisture and fat content. The primary parameters of the mechanical characteristics are hardness, cohesiveness, viscosity, elasticity, and adhesiveness; the secondary parameters were brittleness, chewiness, and gumminess. However, foods are complex rheological systems and application of the principles of theoretical rheology is frequently difficult and too time-consuming for applied industrial research. For popular nomenclature of food texture and the above classification see Table 39.

Kramer (1964) has emphasized that there are different kinds of texture which require different instruments to measure. Thus, compression is the "yielding quality" of a peach or tomato. Tensile strength is the tearing of a slice of bread or the pulling apart of a piece of candy. The

TABLE 39

Relations between Textural Parameters and Popular Nomenclature

Primary parameters	Secondary parameters	Popular terms
Mechanical characteristics		
Hardness		Soft → firm → hard
Cohesiveness	Brittleness	Crumbly → crunchy → brittle
	Chewiness	Tender → chewy → tough
	Gumminess	Short → mealy → pasty → gummy
Viscosity		Thin → viscous
Elasticity		Plastic → elastic
Adhesiveness		Sticky → tacky → gooey
Geometrical characteristics		
Particle size and shape		Gritty, grainy, coarse, etc.
Particle shape and orientation		Fibrous, cellular, crystalline, etc.
Other characteristics		
Moisture content		Dry → moist → wet → watery
Fat content	Oiliness	Oily
	Greasiness	Greasy

Source: Szczesniak (1963).

toughness of the strings of canned green or wax beans are measured in this way. Cutting force is where the object is separated into two or more parts without changing the shape of the parts. Some compression, shearing, and perhaps even tensile strength is required for the cutting. The fibrousness of asparagus has been measured in this way. Shearing force is the force that causes two contiguous parts of an object to slide relative to each other in a direction parallel to their plane of contact. Thus, there is a separation, as in cutting, and a change in position. However, it is practically impossible to obtain shearing without some degree of compression or extension preceding the shear action. This resembles chewing and is the basis of the denture tenderometer and similar instruments. One problem of many instruments is that precision is poor because the rate of application of the force is not controlled. For several problems Kramer (1964) recommends a shear-press where a time-force curve is recorded. The different parts of the resulting curve can be interpreted in terms of compressibility, the force required to break, and the shearing properties. See also Chapter 11.

Matz (1962) feels that sensory tests are probably the only way to obtain meaningful information on texture. He suggested that, at the consumer level, geographical prejudices and traditions must be taken into account in the measurement of textural properties of foods. To study the problem of food texture in the laboratory, independent of the judges' experience, Oldfield (1960) suggested the use of artificial foods of known mechanical properties. Flavors and appearance characteristics could be incorporated and the response of human subjects studied. He further felt that anesthetic techniques that block off certain sensory systems would be helpful in separation and identification of the sense organs involved. We believe that results so obtained would have to be interpreted cautiously because of possible secondary effects of the technique.

The problems of subjective expression of firmness were studied extensively by Harper (1952). He noted fluctuations with time and between individuals. Even with a highly motivated (paid) subject there were pronounced daily fluctuations superimposed on a general upward trend. These fluctuations were attributed to factors of interest, motivation, general attitude, and emotional states. This subject's best performance was four times as sensitive as her original test. Harper also noted a subject who was very accurate in discriminating between soft samples but was poor with hard samples. These experiments suggest the necessity of using large panels in such experiments.

Using word-association tests, Szczesniak and Kleyn (1963) showed that laboratory "consumers" were highly aware of texture as a discernible characteristic of food. Women seemed to be more texture-conscious than men. The texture terms mentioned on questionnaires by their panel, in order of frequency, were: crisp (219), dry (117), juicy (104), soft (78), creamy and crunchy (67 each), chewy and texture (58 each), smooth (52), stringy (47), hard (41), light (37), flaky (36), moist (34), mushy (33), sticky (32), wet and tender (31 each), and fluffy and greasy (30 each).

Raffensperger *et al.* (1956) constructed a logical scale (based on a technique of rating word meanings) for grading toughness-tenderness in beef. With a trained panel the unstructured scale (only the two end points identified) was as useful as a structured scale (Chapter 8, Section II,A). In this case the structured scale was improved by eliminating the neutral (neither tough nor tender) category.

Szczesniak *et al.* (1963) developed rating scales for hardness, brittleness, chewiness, adhesiveness, and viscosity. For each, standards were developed. For example, the hardness scale is shown in Table 40, and the

TABLE 40
Standard Hardness Scale

Panel rating	Product	Brand or type	Manufacturer	Sample size	Temp.
1	Cream cheese	Philadelphia	Kraft Foods	1/2″	45°–55°F
2	Egg white	Hard-cooked, 5 min		1/2″ tip	Room
3	Frankfurters	Large, uncooked, skinless	Mogen David Kosher Meat Products Corp.	1/2″	50°–65°F
4	Cheese	Yellow, American pasteurized process	Kraft Foods	1/2″	50°–65°F
5	Olives	Exquisite giant size, stuffed	Cresca Co.	1 olive	50°–65°F
6	Peanuts	Cocktail type in vacuum tin	Planters Peanuts	1 nut	Room
7	Carrots	Uncooked, fresh		1/2″	Room
8	Peanut brittle	Candy part	Kraft Foods		Room
9	Rock candy		Dryden & Palmer		Room

Source: Szczesniak *et al.* (1963).

brittleness scale in Table 41. These scales offer a basis for sensory texture evaluation and should prove useful in developing descriptive texture scales of various foods.

Brandt *et al.* (1963) developed texture profiles using these scales. The procedure is indicated in Table 42. The results of studies on four chemically leavened biscuits are indicated in Table 43. These data indicate the complexity of the texture component of foods.

TABLE 41
Standard Brittleness Scale (Ratings at Room Temperature)

Panel rating	Product	Brand or type	Manufacturer	Sample size
1	Corn muffin	Finast	First National Stores	1/2″
2	Angel puffs	Dietectic, heated for 5 min at 190°F	Stella D'Oro Biscuit Co.	1 puff
3	Graham crackers	Nabisco	National Biscuit Co.	1/2 cracker
4	Melba toast	Inside piece	Devonsheer Melba Corp.	1/2″
5	Jan Hazel cookies		Keebler Biscuit Co.	1/2″
6	Ginger snaps	Nabisco	National Biscuit Co.	1/2″
7	Peanut brittle	Candy part	Kraft Foods	1/2″

Source: Szczesniak *et al.* (1963).

Matz (1962) subdivided his text on texture in foods into three sections: (1) the meaning and measurement of texture; (2) types of texture in foods; and (3) effects of processing methods on food texture. Kinesthetics and texture are covered in a recent text by Kramer and Twigg (1962, Chapter 7). In the monograph "Texture in Foods" (Society

TABLE 42
Procedure for Evaluating Texture

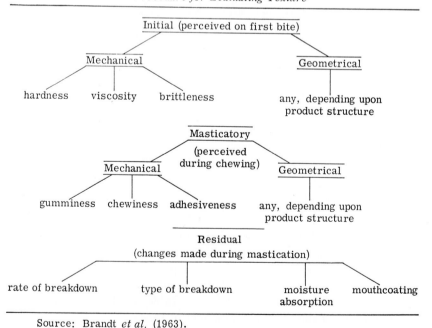

Source: Brandt *et al.* (1963).

TABLE 43

Texture Profile of Chemically Leavened Biscuits

	Raw dough	Freshly baked	Frozen at −10°F for 72 hr, thawed	Held at room temperature for 72 hr
Initial				
A. Mechanical characteristics				
Hardness (1–9 scale)	1.0	3.7	4.1	7.0
Brittleness (1–7 scale)	0	0	0	4.5
Adhesiveness (1–5 scale)	1.5	0	0	0
Masticatory				
A. Mechanical characteristics				
Chewiness (1–7 scale)	1.3 (12 sec)	2.5 (21 sec)	2.5 (20 sec)	2.5 (20 sec)
Gumminess (1–5 scale)	3.2	0	0	0
B. Geometrical characteristics	Soft lumps	Aerated	Aerated	Hardened and collapsed cell walls, uneven air pockets, hard grits
C. Degree of moisture	Moderately to very moist	Slight to moderately moist	Slightly moist	Very dry
Residual				
Breakdown characteristics	Breaks down quickly and evenly into a liquid	Absorbs saliva quickly and becomes very slightly gummy	Absorbs saliva somewhat slowly and becomes slightly gummy	Fractures into smaller, hard pieces that break down into small, mealy particles; absorbs saliva slowly

Source: Brandt *et al.* (1963).

of Chemical Industry, 1960), one paper discusses perception in the mouth, one describes scientific principles in relation to instrumental measurement of textural properties; and the remaining twelve papers describe the measurement of texture in selected food commodities.

Many problems of food structure and eating quality remain unsolved. Adjectives such as chewy, grainy, tough, creamy, crusty, smooth, slimy, viscous, soft, doughy, greasy, gritty, firm, mealy, stringy, crisp, watery, tangy, oily, are all related to the texture of foods and involve tactile sensations. Some of these have been well studied for certain foods, but many foods remain uninvestigated. Mouthfeel characteristics (chewiness, fibrousness, grittiness, mealiness, stickiness, and oiliness) may partially be true textural or kinesthetic factors .

B. KINESTHESIS

The receptors in and about joints control kinesthetic sensations. The receptor organs in articular tissue appear to be of three types, according to Rose and Mountcastle (1959). It is unnecessary to postulate a "muscle" sense to explain kinesthetic sensations. These receptors signal the steady position of the joint and the direction, rate, and extent of joint movement. Some adapt slowly, and others rapidly. The kinesthetic sense is difficult to study because it cannot be easily isolated for direct stimulation and measurement of sensation. Cocaine applied as an anesthetic makes possible a demonstration that the sensations come more from the joints than from the muscles. Four sets of receptors are involved—two in the muscle proper, one in the tendon, and one in the fascia associated with the muscle. There are also, of course, free nerve endings in the muscles. In foods where chewing is difficult, such as nuts, bones, and crackers, a sense of motion may be stimulated.

C. PAIN

The relation of pain to cutaneous (tactile) sensory impressions and to the common chemical sense has already been noted. Excessively hot or cold foods will also produce pain. Pain is difficult to define. Is it simply an unpleasant sensation? Furthermore, it is difficult to separate the initial sensation of pain from the individual's reaction to the sensation. That latter element—the psychological component—may be the more important aspect of pain to the individual.

In many cases pain certainly results from overstimulation of the sensations of heat, touch, sight, taste, or smell. However, the pain may be elicited by specific pain nerve pathways, at least for some areas. Armstrong et al. (1953) reported different rates of adaptation and recovery for various chemicals causing pain. In some cases, itching accompanied pain.

Hardy *et al.* (1952) believed that trained observers could distinguish 21 different degrees of pain arising from radiant heat, whereas Armstrong *et al.* (1953), using a chemical excitant, found 8, and possibly up to 16, levels of pain intensity.

The end organs for pain seem to be the same as those for touch at the great majority of all pain spots of the body. Different types of fibers of varying impulse speeds may, however, permit a differentiation of two or more qualities of pain, though Sweet (1959) believes this needs further study.

There is a wide variation in response to pain. Some people apparently derive pleasure from a certain degree of pain, as in the eating of excessively "hot" curries or chilis, drinking very hot coffee or distilled beverages "straight." A certain degree of adaptation to these foods is involved, besides psychological differences in the desirability of pain. There is also the possibility that pain is substituted for diminution in other sensory responses. No quantitative data are available on these phenomena.

D. TEMPERATURE

Receptors sensitive to temperature differences are located in many parts of the body, particularly in the mouth. Cold and warm spots that are specific for cold and warm sensations have been known for many years. Recordings of the spike activity of single thermal nerve fibers also indicate the specificity of cold and warm nerve endings. Krause end bulbs are generally believed to be the receptors for cold; the Ruffini end organ may be the receptor for warmth. In general, cold spots are more numerous than warm, and there is also a wide variation between areas in the density of temperature-sensitive spots. The eyelids and lips are particularly thermo-sensitive. Reaction time is slower for warmth than for cold, suggesting, according to Zotterman (1959), that the warm receptors should be located deeper in the skin than the cold receptors. Other evidence in favor of this is given by Woodworth and Schlosberg (1954). On the tongue the cold receptors are situated subepithelially, partly in the papillae but particularly at their base or just beneath them. Kenshalo and Nafe (1962) recently postulated that warmth and cold were signaled by constriction and dilation of small blood vessels. Morphological evidence for specific temperature receptors is indeed poor.

It is not known whether the stimulus of temperature sensations is the temporal differential quotient of temperature changes or absolute temperature levels. For a discussion of this question, see Zotterman (1959). The three factors governing the occurrence of a thermal sensation are: (1) the absolute intercutaneous temperature, θ; (2) the rate of change of θ, $d\theta/dt$; and (3) the area of the stimulated field, F.

The effect of temperature is important because of: (1) its own effect, e.g., in ice cream; (2) our expectation of certain temperatures with certain food; (3) its effect on the volatility of odorous substances; and (4) the change in sensitivity to the primary tastes with variation in temperature (Chapter 2, Section IX). The actual temperature of a food should be distinguished from the heat and cold sensations produced by certain materials in the mouth, sometimes called thermo-chemoreception.

E. THE COMMON CHEMICAL SENSE

The mucous membranes of the mouth, nose, eyes, etc., are responsive to a variety of irritants, especially in the nose, where such response was early recognized. True odors affect only the olfactory nerve, whereas irritants stimulate the free nerve terminals, served by the trigeminal nerve, and may result in sneezing. Stimulation of other free nerve endings may cause watering of the eyes (ammonia, onion, chlorine), choking, or pain. Apparently all of these sensations are some aspect of pain. Ammonia, for example, affects the nose and eyes and other mucous surfaces of the body. Pepper and ginger stimulate taste receptors and pain receptors in the mouth. An easy demonstration of odor and a common chemical effect is with a menthol nose inhalator. Upon inhalation, a cooling sensation (common chemical effect) and a menthol smell are apparent. If the nose is closed and the inhalator is placed in the mouth, a strong cooling effect but no menthol smell will be perceived. Elsberg et al. (1935), employing the stream injection method, found that many substances believed to be pure olfactory stimulants had trigeminal effects. Coffee, phenylethyl alcohol and musk ketone were reported to be pure olfactory stimulants, i.e., not to have trigeminal effects. Trigeminal fatigue was also demonstrated, but the reduction in degree of stinging or pain varied with time.

Parker (1922) pointed out that the receptors for the common chemical sense are distributed about the same in the lower vertebrates as in man, but that in amphibians and fishes a whole system of receptors covers their entire exterior. Even protozoa react to chemical irritants. Such receptors warn of danger and are not connected with nutrition. Parker postulated that air-inhabiting vertebrates have retained this capacity in a circumscribed and local way. Irritating substances are no longer effective when the nerve trunks to these free nerve endings are cut.

Since the free nerve endings for the common chemical sense are anatomically similar to those for pain, it must be a tactile sense. It may be different, however, for it can be shown with fishes that fatigue for nitric acid can be induced without affecting the touch responses and that touch fatigue can be induced without affecting the acid response. Furthermore, Crozier (1916) found that application of 2% cocaine on the dogfish abolishes the tactile response without affecting the chemical response (unless the cocaine treatment is prolonged). This response has also been demonstrated with frogs' feet. In man, pain is not so easily distinguished from the common chemical sense by applying narcotics. Using solutions of piperadine and needle pricks of the lips, one investigator could not find any differences in thresholds after cocaine treatments in 5 individuals. In two cases the chemical threshold was not increased after cocaine treatment. Pfaffmann (1951) criticized the experiment because the level of cocainization was not quantitatively controlled. Also, Pfaffmann feels that submersion of the whole frog's foot in acid may have caused spatial summation to make the chemical more effective. He concluded that pain and the common chemical sensitivity are mediated by the same nerve endings. Jones (1954) was also unable to distinguish the common chemical sense from cutaneous pain.

The common chemical sense differs from the gustatory in not having specialized nerve endings. Furthermore, the taste buds will respond to $3 M$ ethyl alcohol whereas 5–$10 M$ is necessary to stimulate the irritant receptors. The odor of ethyl alcohol is perceivable at a concentration of $0.000125 M$, according to Parker and Stabler (1913). If the olfactory nerve is cut, there is still a response to irritants even though the person is anosmic. The threshold for irritation is greater than that for gustation. Hydrochloric acid, which tastes sour, may elicit no response from a mucous membrane. Beidler and Tucker (1955) reported that the electrical responses of olfactory and trigeminal nerves of live rabbits to various stimulants were similar, suggesting that the two systems are also similar.

Using chloracetophenone (an early World War I war gas) as an eye and nose irritant, it can be shown that the eye is 2–3 times as sensitive as the nose. Even this powerful irritant, however, is only 1/160th as strong as powerful odors such as that of trinitro-*tert*-butyl xylene. Wenger *et al.* (1956) stated that for some substances the pain (common chemical sense) threshold is less than the olfactory threshold, although the opposite is more common.

The different sensations in the eye, mouth, nose, etc., from an irritant suggest that there are different aspects of the common chemical sense. Not all irritants are undesirable. Pepper, for example, is used because of its sweetish taste and its slight irritant action—which is greater if pepper gets in the nose. The active ingredients of pepper are piperine and chavicine. The amide linkage in the molecule seems necessary for pungency, but considerable modification of the piperine is possible without destroying its pungency. Moncrieff (1951) discusses the chemistry of these pepperlike substances. The problem is important since pepper is produced in a limited area of southeast Asia that could be inaccessible in time of war. Pepper substitutes could then be needed.

Ginger is another hot, spicy, pungent, sweet-tasting substance. The active principle is gingerol, which is readily hydrolyzed to zingerone (α-3-methoxy-4-hydroxyphenylethyl methyl ketone). Just what makes these pungent is not known. Zingerone has the structure

Shogaol is a related pungent compound found in the solution after zingerone is extracted. Capsaicin, the pungent ingredient of the hot varieties of red pepper, produces a very intense burning sensation. Vanillylamide is also intensely pungent. Vanillyl n-nonoylamide is the most intense of the series. Capsaicin is the amide of vanillylamine. Pungent and bitter compounds have also been isolated from water cress, from the roots of *Anacylus pyrethrum,* from the bark of *Fagara xanthoxyloides,* and from other plants.

Lachrymatories became important weapons in World War I. Chloracetone was used in March 1915, bromacetone in July 1915, ethyl iodoacetate in December 1915, and bromobenzyl cyanide and chloracetophenine later in that war. Sternutatories (sneezing gases) were also used in World War I, to force the gas mask wearer to sneeze and take off his mask. Diphenylchloroarsine and diphenylcyanoarsine were used beginning in September 1917. Adamsite, 10-chloro-5,10-dihydrophenarsazine, was a later development.

Moncrieff (1951) devoted 21 pages of his text to the common chemical sense, and concluded that any theory for the mechanism of the common chemical sense must cover the following facts: (1) the receptors are the free nerve endings, particularly of the trigeminal nerve; (2) receptors are usually confined to mucous surfaces; (3) fatigue is not as great as with taste or smell; (4) the stimulus may be solid, liquid, or gaseous; (5) overstimulation brings pain; and (6) there are differences in response of the mouth, eyes, and nose. Moncrieff suggested that irritants form a monomolecular layer on the surface. An additive compound is then formed by auxiliary valencies of the unsaturated element of the stimulant. The phenomenon of crying or rapid flow of mucous in involuntary attempts to remove the source of irritation probably suggested the monomolecular layer, but it certainly needs further study. Jones and Pyman (1925) believed that the shape of the molecule was an important factor in the pungency of capsaicin. Moncrieff (1951) postulated that the shape of the molecules as a whole, rather than the nature of the side chain, was perhaps the important factor in the pungency of these compounds (see Chapter 3, Section V).

Moncrieff also reviewed the toxophor-auxotox theory that an irritant must contain both groups. Toxophor groups are

$$>\!\!CO, \quad S\!\!<, \quad >\!\!C\!\!=\!\!C\!\!<, \quad -NO_2, \quad -NC, \quad -AS\!\!<$$

Auxotoxes are halogens, oxygen, $-NH_2$, benzyl, phenyl, methyl, etc. Not all compounds with these groups are irritants, and increasing the number of active groups does not always increase irritation to the extent it should, so the theory does not help us very much.

IV. Other Senses

Clark and Dodge (1955) reported on five patients whose olfactory nerves had been destroyed surgically, either by basofrontal brain tumors or by cranial trauma. They were blindfolded and given 31 different vegetables and fruits of different consistencies at room temperature. As each food was given, the subject was asked to identify it. If he could do this, he was asked whether he could perceive the flavor. Contrary to popular belief, several of the anosmic subjects were able to discern flavor. One normal control with complete dentures did poorly. Since olfaction was excluded in the anosmic subjects, it is apparent that extra-olfactory components must at times play the major role in identification of flavor. These are the somatic sensations experienced in the mouth, nasopharynx, and adjacent structures, as well as vision, hearing, memory, and the psychological state at the moment of eating. Clark and Dodge concluded that some undiscovered receptive mechanism in the mouth and nasopharynx may enter into the perception of flavor. This seems unnecessary in normal subjects. Furthermore, the role of learning and experience and use of other cues may play a role with subjects who have lost one of their senses.

V. Summary

Color and appearance are important attributes of food quality. The senses of hearing and kinesthesis are of minor importance in examination of foods. Texture is very important with some foods. Pain is a negative factor with some foods and a positive one with others. Temperature is important for its own sake as well as for its effects on the senses and on the physical properties of foods. These senses have been too little studied with respect to their influence on food acceptance and preference. However, there are many objective procedures which seem to correlate well with the subjective response of these senses, particularly color and texture (Chapter 11). More studies are needed correlating the two, and more precise definitions are needed of the meaning of terms such as tenderness and chewiness.

REFERENCES

American Physiological Society. 1959. "Handbook of Physiology," Vol. 1, 779 pp. Washington, D. C.

Armstrong, D., R. M. L. Dry, C. A. Keele, and J. W. Markham. 1953. Observations on chemical excitants of cutaneous pain in man. *J. Physiol. (London)* **120**, 326–351.

Bailey, M. E., H. B. Hedrick, F. C. Parrish, and H. D. Naumann. 1962. L. E. E.-Kramer shear force as a tenderness measure of beef steak. *Food Technol.* **16**, (12), 99–101.

Bartley, S. H. 1948. Studying vision. *In* "Methods of Psychology." (T. G. Andrews, ed.), 712 pp. (see pp. 189–222). Wiley, New York.

Beidler, L. M., and D. Tucker. 1955. Response of nasal epithelium to odor stimulation. *Science* **122**, 76.

Bengtsson, K., and E. Helm. 1946. Principles of taste testing. *Wallerstein Lab. Commun.* **9**, 171–180.

Birren, F. 1963. Color and human appetite. *Food Technol.* **17**, 553–555.

Brandt, M. A., E. Z. Skinner, and J. A. Coleman. 1963. Texture profile method. *J. Food Sci.* **28**, 404–409.

Clark, E. C., and H. W. Dodge. 1955. Extraolfactory components of flavor. *J. Am. Med. Assoc.* **159**, 1721–1723.

Crozier, W. J. 1916. Regarding the existence of the common chemical sense in vertebrates. *J. Comp. Neurol.* **26**, 453–461.

Dember, W. N. 1961. "The Psychology of Perception," 402 pp. Holt, New York.

Drake, B. K. 1963. Food crushing sounds. An introductory study. *J. Food Sci.* **28**, 233–241.

Dunker, K. 1939. The influence of past experience upon perceptual properties. *Am. J. Psychol.* **52**, 255–265.

Elsberg, C. A., I. Levy, and E. D. Brewer. 1935. The sense of smell. VI. The trigeminal effect of odorous substances. *Bull. Neurol. Inst. N. Y.* **4**, 270–285.

Farrel, K. T., J. R. Wagner, M. S. Peterson, and G. Mackinney, eds. 1954. "Color in Foods, a Symposium," 186 pp. Natl. Acad. Sci., Natl. Research Council, Washington, D. C.

Foster, D. 1956. "Psychological Aspects of Food Colors from the Consumer's Standpoint," 14 pp. U. S. Testing Co., Hoboken, New Jersey.

Francis, F. J. 1963. Color control. *Food Technol.* **17**, 546–550, 552–553.

Geldard, F. A. 1953. "The Human Senses," 365 pp. (see pp. 243–248). Wiley, New York.

Hall, R. L. 1958. Flavor study approaches at McCormick and Co., Inc. *In* "Flavor Research and Food Acceptance" (Arthur D. Little, Inc., ed.), 391 pp. (see pp. 224–240). Reinhold, New York.

Hardy, J. D., H. G. Wolff, and H. Goodell. 1952. "Pain Sensations and Reactions," 435 pp. Williams and Wilkins, Baltimore, Maryland.

Harper, R. 1952. Psychological and psychophysical studies of craftsmanship in dairying. *Brit. J. Psychol., Monograph Suppl.* **281**, 1–63.

Hecht, S., S. Shlaer, and M. H. Pirenne. 1941. Energy at the threshold of vision. *Science* **93**, 585–587.

Hernández-Peón, R., H. Scherrer, and M. Jouvet. 1956. Modification of electric activity in cochlear nucleus during "attention" in unanesthetized cats. *Science* **123**, 331–332.

Hodges, A. A. 1962. Environmental variables as they influence the absolute threshold of perception of taste. Paper presented at the Inst. Food Technologists, Miami, Florida, June 14, 1962.

Johnson, A. H. 1956. "Significance of Color in Dairy Products," 14 pp. Natl. Dairy Research Lab., Inc., Oakdale, Long Island, New York.

Jones, E. C. S., and F. L. Pyman. 1925. Relation between chemical constitution and pungency in acid amides. *J. Chem. Soc. (London)* **127**, 2588–2598.

Jones, M. H. 1954. A study of the common chemical sense. *Am. J. Psychol.* **67**, 696–698.

Judd, D. B. 1952. "Color in Business, Science and Industry," 401 pp. Wiley, New York.

Judd, D. B., and G. Wyszecki. 1963. "Color in Business, Science and Industry," (2nd ed.), 500 pp. Viking Press, New York.

Kanig, J. L. 1955. Mental impact of colors in food studied. *Food Field Reptr.* **23**, 57.

Kenshalo, D. R., and J. P. Nafe. 1962. A quantitative theory of feeling. *Psychol. Rev.* **69**, 17–33.

Kramer, A. 1964. Definition of texture and its measurement in vegetable products. *Food Technol.* **18**, 304–307.

Kramer, A., and B. A. Twigg. 1962. "Fundamentals of Quality Control for the Food Industry," 512 pp. Avi Publ. Co., Westport, Connecticut.

Mackinney, G., and C. O. Chichester. 1954. The color problem in foods. *Advances in Food Research* **5**, 301–351.

Mackinney, G., and A. C. Little. 1962. "Color in Foods," 308 pp. Avi Publ. Co., Westport, Connecticut.

Malphrus, L. D. 1957. Effect of color of beef fat on flavor of steaks and roasts. *Food Research* **22**, 342–350.

Matz, S. A. 1962. "Food Texture," 286 pp. Avi Publ. Co., Westport, Connecticut.

Mitchell, J. W. 1957. Problems in taste difference testing. I. Test environment. *Food Technol.* **11**, 476–477.

Moir, H. C. 1936. Some observations on the appreciation of flavour in foodstuffs. *Chem. & Ind. (London)* **55**, 145–148.

Moncrieff, R. W. 1951. "The Chemical Senses," vii, 538 pp. (see pp. 172–193). Leonard Hill, London.

Oldfield, R. C. 1960. Perception in the mouth. *Soc. Chem. Ind. (London) Monograph* **7**, 3–9.

Pangborn, R. M. 1960. Influence of color on the discrimination of sweetness. *Am. J. Psychol.* **73**, 229–238.

Pangborn, R. M., and B. Hansen. 1963. The influence of color on discrimination of sweetness and sourness in pear nectar. *Am. J. Psychol.* **76**, 315–317.

Pangborn, R. M., H. W. Berg, and B. Hansen. 1963. The influence of color on discrimination of sweetness in dry table wine. *Am. J. Psychol.* **76**, 492–495.

Parker, G. H. 1922. "Smell, Taste and Allied Senses in the Vertebrates," 192 pp. Lippincott, Philadelphia, Pennsylvania.

Parker, G. H., and E. M. Stabler. 1913. On certain distinctions between taste and smell. *Am. J. Physiol.* **32**, 230–240.

Pettit, L. A. 1958. The influence of test location and accompanying sound in flavor preference testing of tomato juice. *Food Technol.* **12**, 55–57.

Pfaffmann, C. 1939. Afferent impulses from the teeth due to pressure and noxious stimulation. *J. Physiol.* (*London*) **97**, 207–219.

Pfaffmann, C. 1951. Taste and smell. *In* "Handbook of Experimental Psychology" (S. S. Stevens, ed.), 1436 pp. (see pp. 1144–1145). Wiley, New York.

Raffensperger, E. L., D. R. Peryam, and K. R. Wood. 1956. Development of a scale for grading toughness-tenderness in beef. *Food Technol.* **10**, 627–630.

Rietz, C. A. 1961. "A Guide to the Selection, Combination, and Cooking of Foods," Vol. 1, 395 pp. Avi Publ. Co., Westport, Connecticut.

Rose, J. E., and V. B. Mountcastle. 1959. Touch and kinesthesis. *In* "Handbook of Physiology," Vol. 1, 779 pp. (see pp. 387–429). Am. Physiol. Soc., Washington, D. C.

Ruch, T. C. 1960. Somatic sensation. *In* "Medical Physiology and Biophysics" (T. C. Ruch and J. F. Fulton, eds.), 1232 pp. (see pp. 300–322). Saunders, Philadelphia, Pennsylvania.

Schutz, H. G. 1954. Color in relation to food preference. *In* "Color in Foods, a Symposium," (K. T. Farrell, J. R. Wagner, M. S. Peterson, and G. Mackinney, eds.), 186 pp. (see pp. 16–21). Natl. Acad. Sci., Natl. Research Council, Washington, D. C.

Society of Chemical Industry. 1960. Texture in foods. *Soc. Chem. Ind.* (*London*) *Monograph* **7**, 1–184.

Srinivasan, M. 1955. Has the ear a role in registering flavour? *Bull. Central Food Technol. Research Inst. Mysore* (*India*) **4**, 136.

Sweet, W. H. 1959. Pain. *In* "Handbook of Physiology." Vol. 1, 779 pp. (see pp. 459–506). Am. Physiol. Soc., Washington, D. C.

Szczesniak, A. S. 1963. Classification of textural characteristics. *J. Food Sci.* **28**, 385–389.

Szczesniak, A. S., and D. H. Kleyn. 1963. Consumer awareness of texture and other food attributes. *Food Technol.* **17**(1), 74–77.

Szczesniak, A. S., M. A. Brandt, and H. H. Friedman. 1963. Development of standard rating scales for mechanical parameters of texture and correlation between the objective and the sensory methods of texture evaluation. *J. Food Sci.* **28**, 397–403.

Wenger, M. A., F. N. Jones, and M. H. Jones. 1956. "Physiological Psychology," 472 pp. Holt, New York.

Woodworth, R. S., and H. Schlosberg. 1954. "Experimental Psychology," 948 pp. Holt, New York.

Yilmaz, H., and L. C. Clapp. 1963. Perception. *Intern. Sci. and Technol.* **23**, 76–84.

Zotterman, Y. 1959. Thermal sensations. *In* "Handbook of Physiology," Vol. 1, 779 pp. (see pp. 431–458). Am. Physiol. Soc., Washington, D. C.

Chapter 5

Factors Influencing Sensory Measurements

This chapter considers some specific variables which influence the sensory evaluation of foods. The chapters that follow will apply these principles to practical problems.

I. Attitudinal Factors

Studies on individual differences in perception,[*] intelligence, or special intellectual abilities have been pursued since before the turn of the century (Tyler, 1956), but only since about 1950 has there been a systematic study to correlate perceptual differences with personality differences, such as those defined below.

"Constancy" is defined as the tendency to react to objects in space in terms of their *known* size, shape, or color. There are great individual differences in "constancy," and people who are object-oriented may not be stimulus-oriented. With visual and auditory responses, Tyler reported that a subject might apply any one of six attitudes toward the stimulus: (1) casual survey of stimulus objects; (2) inquiring survey; (3) critical survey of the observer of himself observing; (4) critical particularizing survey of objects for accurate description; (5) personal valuation, in terms of pleasantness or unpleasantness; and (6) impersonal valuation of objects in terms of some conventional standard. These attitudes can affect the observer's response to food. In one set of experiments the attitudes assumed may be independent of the instructions given. It would be valuable to know what percentage of a population assumed each of these attitudes in evaluating the quality of foods, and how each attitude affected the results.

Other ways of looking at the perceptual world have been postulated. None of the following can be completely substantiated, but all could prove useful in practice.

1. *Analytic versus synthetic.* The analytic observer concentrates on

---

[*] We agree with Dember (1961) that the distinction between perception and sensation is somewhat ambiguous and arbitrary, and we make no such differentiation in this text.

details and sees only the individual parts. The synthetic observer sees the integrated whole but misses details. Some sensory scoring techniques are designed to analyze, whereas most preference testing encourages the latter approach. These may be related to Duffendack's (1954) groups I and II.

2. *Objective versus subjective.* The objective judge moves slowly, getting every detail right before proceeding, whereas the subjective judge makes a broad inspection, usually emphasizing his own particular interpretation or his personal liking.

3. *Active versus passive.* The active person works rationally, trying to make hypotheses to solve a problem, whereas the passive approach is to proceed by trial and error, guided only by immediate impressions. These attitudes can be demonstrated more clearly with children than with adults.

4. *Confident versus cautious.* The confident observer sees all at a glance and reports it all at once, sometimes reporting more detail than he actually sees. The cautious person hesitates to report even the detail he does see. The confident observer is likely to commit more statistical errors of the first kind (i.e., reporting a difference when none exists) than of the second kind (i.e., overlooking actual differences). See Chapter 10, Section I. The reverse would be true of the cautious observer.

5. *Color reactors versus form reactors.* Some observers respond to color before shape. In fruit evaluation this difference may be a factor affecting results.

6. *Visual versus haptic.* The visually minded person sees the world primarily through visual stimuli, whereas the haptically minded person is responsive primarily to touch and kinesthesis. No studies of this difference applied to foods have come to our attention, but obviously these could be important in consumer studies.

Thurstone (1944) mathematically isolated eleven factors that might be significant to perception. Seven of these proved of importance in perception. Three factors were related to speed: reaction time, speed of perception (to recognize), and speed of judgment (to come to a decision on what has been perceived). Two factors represented kinds of experimental materials: illusions which affect some individuals more than others, and stimuli where alterations or reversals occur. The rate at which any of the alternating figures tends to reverse itself differs among individuals.

Finally, there are the so-called closure* factors. Speed of closure seems to facilitate grasping or retaining a clear, coherent pattern of

---

* A bounded or closed area is usually seen as a separate unit. If closure of a complete pattern is possible, it supersedes closure of subparts.

stimulus materials. Flexibility of closure may facilitate retention of a figure in a distracting field. These have been shown to be related to certain personality factors, but whether they influence judgments of food is not known.

If we look at personality from a functionalistic point of view, the individual's perceptions have adaptive properties. These perceptions are the means of fending off or admitting only selected stimulation from the world about us. Such stimulation, if freely admitted, might traumatize or overwhelm the individual. This attitude toward the world is known in psychology as "*Anschauungen.*" The three sets of *Anschauungen* identified by Klein and his associates at the Menninger Foundation, include: (1) leveling and sharpening; (2) resistance to or acceptance of instability; and (3) physiognomic and literal attitudes. Levelers tend to make a stimulus simpler and less differentiated if they can, either by reducing figure-ground distinctions or by assimilating new stimuli to a dominating organization. Sharpeners try to heighten distinctions and to exploit differentiation. Holzman and Klein (1954) differentiated levelers from sharpeners on the basis of ability to distinguish size judgments for wooden blocks. The extremes of each group (9 in each case) were then tested for comparing brightness levels when the standard and variable light stimulus was interposed with other light stimuli. The theory that levelers would be more confused than sharpeners by the intermediate lights proved to be statistically correct. In all tests, sharpeners made fewer errors (were more accurate) than levelers. The ability of food judges has not been matched against *Anschauungen,* but sharpeners should obviously be used where maximum differentiation is required. As Dember (1961) noted, sharpeners do perform in the predicted fashion with visual cues. Data on the effect of these personality traits on the performance of prospective food judges would be welcome.

Gregson (1963a,b) studied the influence of psychological expectations upon the perception of, and preferences for, a series of mixtures of grapefruit and lemon drinks. He concluded that the population differed fundamentally in their expectations and that this did indeed influence their perception. He suggested that this should be taken into account in selecting panels. We agree wholeheartedly with this.

II. Motivation

It has long been recognized that sensory perception can be and is influenced by motivational variables. One reason is that, out of the total stimulation, the individual apparently responds to only selected portions. It is believed, however, that suitable motivation could make the individual more selective in his response.

Various types of motivation may be considered. The value of the stimulus to the individual may influence his perception. According to Dember (1961), it is obviously useful to the organism to be sensitized to stimuli that are potential need-satisfiers or, vice versa, potentially unpleasant stimuli. At a low stimulus level, the attention of the individual is directed more to relevant than to irrelevant stimuli. Hungry persons should react to lower concentrations of sugar, for example. That they do not always do so (Chapter 2, Section VIII,A) may be due to experimental factors such as training and methodology, insufficient motivation, and physical fatigue effects.

Galanter (1962) noted that the outcome of a psychophysical experiment can be influenced by a payoff function, i.e., by meting out prizes for a "correct" response or penalties for an "incorrect" response. Motivation, however, is not simply a response to organic drives and instincts [see, for example, Young (1961)].

Motivation also operates at the suprathreshold level. Food panels are often given time off or are rewarded with presents. Professional food experts are often paid more than regular employees. Punishment, according to Dember (1961), does not produce as clear an effect unless it is rather strong. It has also been demonstrated that object value is related to perceived size. We can conceive of numerous food evaluation situations where this phenomenon might influence the results. The highly motivated person responds with a better vocabulary of terms. McClelland and Atkinson (1949) even reported that, when stimulated ambiguously, hungry subjects "saw" more food-related objects than control subjects.

Knowledge of results is a motivational factor, and has been shown by Pfaffmann et al. (1954) to increase efficiency of performance and also to decrease the training period required to reach a certain level of performance.

Dawson and Harris (1951) stated: "Successful conduct of taste panels is frequently as much a matter of human relations as a scientific problem. Panel members must have a keen interest in their tasting ability and these feelings must be sustained. Informal conferences should be held periodically and imagination and suggestion must be eliminated."

The influence of motivation cannot be answered categorically. Schmidt (1941) indicated that children who feel inferior are more highly motivated by praise than blame, and that the opposite is true for self-confident children. Discriminating use of praise was recommended, and was more effective with some subjects than others. On the other hand, the experiments of Hamilton (1929) indicated that when a constant stimulus was used as an incentive, "reward" and "punishment" were equally effective in improving performance [see also Young (1961)].

In general, success breeds success and failure breeds failure. Obviously, success develops attitudes of self-confidence and a desire to succeed. Success appears to be dependent on the desire to excel per se and the desire to do better than other subjects. Furthermore, self- (individual) motivation appears to be stronger than group motivation. As pointed out by Pangborn and Dunkley (1964), "The interpersonal relationship between the investigator and the judge can mean the difference between the eager and the reluctant participant."

III. Psychological Errors in Judgments

The error of habituation results from a tendency to continue to give the same response when a series of slowly increasing or decreasing stimuli is presented. In the method of "just-noticeable difference" (jnd), this error increases the distance from the standard, while in the "just-not-noticeable difference" (jnnd) method, this error decreases the distance from the standard (Chapter 5, Section IV,A). Usually the tendency is equally strong in both directions, and the error tends to be canceled if both tests are given.

The error of expectation induces the overly anxious observer to find a difference when none exists. From his previous knowledge of the test the observer anticipates that a difference should have developed before it actually occurs. In this case, the jnd procedure is smaller than it should be and the jnnd is larger than it should be. If both procedures are used, these errors should also be canceled.

A stimulus error results when a subject knows that the test is being given in a certain way, or when the containers used or the procedures followed suggest differences and therefore cause him to find them when they do not exist. Thus, whenever irrelevant criteria influence the observer's judgments a stimulus error may arise. For example, knowing that wines in screw-capped bottles are usually less expensive than those in cork-closure bottles, tasters served wine from bottles with screw caps may rate the wines lower than they should. Stimulus error is probably greater when individuals are judging unfamiliar sensory characteristics, for irrelevant cues may then assume larger importance.

The logical error occurs when two characteristics of a food which are logically associated in the minds of the observers, are rated the same. Interactions between the sensory properties may then occur, influencing the response to the characteristic under consideration. Knowing from previous experience that off-color corn probably tastes or smells poor, unappetizing visual impressions may cause judges to assign lower scores for taste and odor than they otherwise would. In certain tests this error can be reduced through as close control as possible of all stimuli except the stimulus under observation. In other tests, removal of this error may be very difficult. For example, judges have associated increased flavor with sweetness, and vice versa (Valdés et al., 1956a,b; Hall, 1958). This is, we believe, a form of stimulus error.

The error of leniency applies to ratings where bias in favor of some person or some object causes the observer to rate them higher than they should. Some observers may recognize this and may consequently over-compensate and rate too low. This error might apply in rating tests where the observer likes or dislikes the investigator. In rating tests, one frequently encounters "easy raters" and "hard raters." The positive leniency error is much more common than the negative (Guilford, 1954). Appropriate scales have been used to counteract the error, such as a rating scale consisting of terms "poor, fair, good, very good, excellent," i.e., a scale that contains only a single unfavorable term.

In the error of central tendency, arising in tests involving judgment, raters hesitate to use the extreme values on a scale. This error probably also applies in sensory evaluation of unfamiliar foods. To prevent this error, the numbers or adjectives assigned to the points on the scale should be clearly defined to each judge. Guilford (1954) suggested that greater differences in meaning should be introduced between steps near the end of the scale than between steps near the center. Helson (1948) believed that central tendency is a special case found only when the method of single judgment is employed.

The contrast error may be noted in sensory tests where the expected or preferred method of evaluation is not followed: foods may then be rated lower than with the expected or preferred method. Also, when a poor sample follows a good sample, the contrast appears greater than when they are judged separately. Effective contrast is the increased contrast when pleasant follows unpleasant. There is also an increase, though less great, when unpleasant follows pleasant. This phenomenon is reinforced by other common reactions: After an unpleasant smell, our absolute judgment of unpleasantness is reduced; similarly, after a pleasant sensation we get a less powerful sensation of pleasantness from a second smell. Kamenetzky (1959) tested to determine if the contrast error was present in comparisons of food quality. It was demonstrated that a "poor" sample following a "good" sample rated lower than if it followed another "poor" sample, but the rating of samples that were "good" in the food qualities investigated did not seem to be affected by whether a "good" or "poor" preceded. It was also found in a successive presentation of "poor" samples that the ratings increased unless a "good" sample intervened. The alternative hypothesis was not confirmed: that in a successive presentation of good samples the ratings should increase unless a "poor" sample intervened. On the basis of his tests Kamenetzky (1959) put forward the additional postulate that "presentation of a poor increases an individual's awareness of the presence of positive characteristics in a good." Use of these assumptions in predicting consumer reaction to food products of different quality appears to be logical and useful.

The proximity error, associated with judging scales, is attributed to the fact that adjacent traits tend to be rated similarly. Thus, simultaneous scoring of color, texture, odor, taste, and general acceptability on the same set of samples can give different scores from those obtained when each trait is judged individually. To eliminate this error, separate sets of the same samples can be presented for evaluation of each characteristic.

A time-error, or positional, bias, i.e., over-selection of one sample on the basis of its order of presentation, has been demonstrated in paired tests by Gridgeman (1958) and others. Expectedly, tasters with the highest taste acuity had the least bias. With a laboratory preference panel of 120 subjects, and whiskey as the test product, Mitchell (1956) found a significant positive time-error in paired presentation, i.e., a greater frequency of choice of the first sample. The magnitude of the effect was related to the amount of taste difference between the paired samples, being greater when the difference was small and least when the difference was large. Use of a conditioner sample similar to the two samples eliminated the time-error. Using a hedonic rating scale, Hanson *et al.* (1955) also found that judges rated succeeding samples lower than the first sample when the lapse of time between sample presentation ranged from 5 minutes to 2 days. To reduce the effect of such biases, balanced and randomized presentations should be used (see Chapter 6, Section III,F). On the other hand, Schwartz and Pratt (1956) demonstrated a greater preference for the last sample presented, with increasing effect for wider intervals of time when a preference-difference scale was used. The difference between the results of Schwartz and Pratt and of Hanson *et al.* has been attributed to the different methods employed. Schwartz and Pratt suggested that the greater preference for the first sample found in laboratory tests with small panels, compared to home testing situations, reflects the simultaneous presentation used in the laboratory. In the home, however, successive paired comparisons, which are vulnerable to order of presentation and become more so as the time between samples increases, yield less strong preferences.

The association error is a tendency to repeat previous impressions—a form of conditioned response. Reaction to a stimulus may be modified, increased, or decreased by previous associations. In the triangular test it is believed that two normal samples and one abnormal lead to far superior taste discrimination than two abnormal samples and one normal. It is not certain that this phenomenon is different from the effective contrast error.

A. Errors of the First and Second Kind

Failure to detect a stimulus that is actually present is called an error of the first kind. Reporting a signal when no stimulus is present is called an error of the second kind. These errors may be caused by expectation and can be influenced by motivation (see Chapter 5, Section II).

It is believed by some investigators that errors can be avoided or partially counteracted by telling the tasters about the errors to be expected and asking them to make a conscious effort to eliminate such errors. Of course, undue attention should not be focused on these potential errors, but they must be kept in mind and, where possible, eliminated or isolated so that they can be taken into account in analysis of the data. As suggested by Guilford (1954), the most effective method of improving ratings, and thereby reducing psychological errors, is to train judges carefully. Training that includes practice, followed by group discussion, has been recommended as being most effective. See also Chapter 7, Section III and Chapter 10, Section I.

B. Other Factors Influencing Response

The influence of memory is admittedly important, but the mechanism by which it operates is not clear. Does memory help the taster identify the elusive odor more quickly so that he can then concentrate on determining its intensity? Or does memory help directly in ranking the intensity in its proper order? The experience of the subject may lead him to expect certain procedures, patterns of presentation, and differences in concentration. The mere fact that in a paired comparison the subject knows that the order of presentation is being randomized may introduce a bias. See Galanter (1962) for the need for a study of payoff structures in difference threshold experiments.

Objective evidence that concentration is important is difficult to obtain, but Elsberg (1937) showed that olfactory sensitivity was greater when the subject was concentrating on the specific odor. This requires, of course, that the judges have previous knowledge of the odor. Dawson and Harris (1951), Caul (1956), and others have stated that sensitivity to taste is greater under conditions of repose, freedom from distraction, and maximum opportunity to concentrate on the test situation.

Attention is achieved by some temporal change in stimulation, according to Dember and Earl (1957). They assert that attention is a function not only of stimulus complexity but also of the individual's complexity. Thus, heterogeneity may be preferred because it secures attention. This may have some importance in quality evaluations of foods.

Explicit instructions, i.e., the set given prior to stimulation, have been found to give lower thresholds than when no instructions are given. A misleading set will raise thresholds. Dember (1961) indicated that linguistic structure and content may influence perception.

Other psychological factors should be considered; for example, with untrained or consumer panels, beer should not be tasted from a cup or hot coffee from a glass. This may be less important in tests with trained panels, where normal conditions of consumption are not utilized (see also Chapter 6, Section III,D).

Since the appreciation of quality is an integrated sensation, experience is especially important in making quality judgments. A particular experienced judge may be less sensitive than a particular inexperienced judge, and yet be able to respond more quickly and reliably to a given quality pattern because his past experience has caused him to limit and categorize the possible quality factors. Trained observers may also respond faster because they have learned to correlate visual or tactile factors with quality whereas the inexperienced may not. Slight dislikes are intensified with experience. This is important in consumer tests, where the experience of the panel may lead to decreasing ratings with time.

IV. Relation between Stimulus and Perception

Thus far we have considered the attitudinal factors which influence responses to sensory stimuli. Now we shall consider some of the relationships between the stimulus and perception. "Psychophysics concerns the functional relation between stimulus and response" (Stevens, 1958b). The three parameters are the task undertaken by the observer, the manner in which the stimulus is presented, and the statistical measure used to describe the data.

The task may be classification, order, intervals, ratios, or magnitudes. In classification the observer judges whether the stimulus is present or not. In some cases this may be identification or recognition. With order, the task is greater or lesser, etc. With intervals, the observer judges the apparent difference between two or more perceptions. This often means partitioning a continuum into apparently equal intervals. The task with ratios is simply to report the ratio of the magnitude of two or more perceptions. Finally, with magnitudes, the observer judges the apparent magnitude of a perception.

Two types of stimulus arrangement are commonly used: fixed stimuli, which are not varied during observation; and adjustable stimuli, which may be altered, usually by the experimenter, during the experiment. Statistical measures usually involve some measure of central tendency, such as the median, and measures of variability and confusion. For further details see Gulliksen and Messich (1960). Galanter (1962) defined four types of sensory response: detection, recognition, discrimination, and scaling. Each of these imposes certain constraints on the response.

Detection pertains to whether there is a stimulus—what was known as the absolute threshold in classical psychophysics. Detection is a function of the stimulus, of stimulus probability, of background effects, and of the observer's motives and expectations. When the stimulus is barely detectable, it can be shown that detection also depends upon the subject's ability to recognize (identify) the particular stimulus. It is more difficult to detect an unknown signal than it is to detect one that is known. Thus, anticipation of the kind of signal to be expected often affects the ability to detect it.

Ability to categorize stimuli depends on whether the observer does or does not know the elements of the set of possible stimuli. Recognition thus defines the stimulus. For a homogeneous stimulus, three to sixteen equally likely alternatives can be recognized. As further dimensions are added to a stimulus, more alternatives can be recognized, though at a decreasing rate as the number is increased. Further, as Galanter (1962) pointed out, the efficiency of response depends more on the number of response categories into which the observer can sort the stimuli rather than the number of stimuli. "Thus, twenty stimuli can be sorted into five categories without error, although twenty stimuli cannot be sorted into twenty categories without error."

Discrimination relates to how two stimuli differ from each other, whereas scaling considers how much of a stimulus is present. These are discussed in the sections which follow.

There is considerable confusion in the literature as to the terms used in the sensory examination of foods. The simplest, and most basic, tests are the discriminatory tests. These may merely be the recognition of a sensory quality versus its absence, i.e., a threshold test. In some cases, discrimination is required between two foods containing suprathreshold quantities, and in other cases the relative intensities of the stimuli are to be rated. These are clearly primarily physiological-observer problems, although in their measurement certain psychological errors may arise and require analysis. The problem of defining a threshold is a classical one in psychology. Whatever threshold is being measured, it is obvious that the response is subjective, that individuals differ, and that the results require some sort of statistical analysis.

Gridgeman (1959) distinguishes between perception and character-ization. In some cases a faculty of matching is postulated. If the con-trasted stimuli differ in magnitude, the probability of correct ranking has to be considered. Finally, there is the concept of probability of prefer-ence, of interest for its own sake or as a means of testing discriminability. In principle, sensations can be fully described in terms of quality, in-tensity, and hedonics (pleasure). The latter two can be partially quanti-fied with arbitrary scoring scales.

There are also problems of defining the dimensions of the sensation: quality, intensity, extent, and duration. As Gregson (1962) has noted, "Given that a zone of uncertain perception surrounds a change that is capable of precise chemical or physiological definition in theory—at any rate—then there are, psychologically, as many thresholds or as few thresholds as one is able to conceptualize statement-forms ordered over the zone of uncertain perception." Various texts (e.g., Dember, 1961) give a detailed discussion of threshold definition and measurement. In this text we shall assume that fluctuations in the value of the threshold are randomly distributed and thus described by the normal curve. Un-less otherwise stated, the stimulus (or stimulus difference) corresponding to 50% identification of the prescribed distinction is used as the particular threshold.

The true detection threshold implies only that a sensation is per-ceived; it does not imply identification of the difference noted. In most cases of sensory evaluation of foods, the detection threshold is really a difference or discrimination threshold—between a subliminal concentra-tion and a higher one that gives a difference in sensation. The absolute or true detection threshold, between zero background and a low stimulus, is seldom measured. At some greater stimulus, not only the difference but the nature of the difference can be specified, i.e., a recognition threshold. Finally, comparative thresholds or degree or extent of difference thresh-olds may be measured. It is in the area of degree of difference that ac-ceptance and preference judgments can be made most easily.

As will be seen, the method of measurement can influence the thresh-old. The "yes or no" response has been shown to be subject to a variety of motivational influences but is more rapid. Forced-choice procedures require the subject to respond—to demonstrate that he has detected the stimulus or has detected a difference between two stimuli, whether he actually has or not.

Gregson (1962) determined taste thresholds by a combination of ascending-series and rating-scale methods. The ascending-series method uses a series of solutions, each twice as strong as the preceding one. Thus, the sum of all stimulus intensities tasted is never greater than that of the next stimulus to be tasted (so that residual tastes should not mask the next taste), and the subjective intensity of taste is proportional to the log of the concentration strength (so that the scale is roughly a subjective equal-interval scale above threshold). The rating-scale method consists of having a series of statements corresponding to increasing taste sensations.

As Gregson noted, the usual "same" or "different" response is not always feasible for taste thresholds, for many "doubtful" answers may appear. For the ascending-series method, the subject used a rating card of the form "same as water; almost certainly the same as water; doubtful if water; very slightly different from water; slightly different from water; different from water; or certainly different from water." For the rating-scale method, the scale was "same as water; doubtful if pure water; a very faint taste, can't say what; a very faint sour (sweet) taste; a faint sour (sweet) taste; a weak sour (sweet) taste; or a clear sour (sweet) taste." The next-to-last or last category is taken as the threshold. Plotting cumulative proportions of thresholds on arithmetic probability paper against concentration strength, and locating each threshold-proportion midway between adjacent stimuli, gave a linear plot with absolute threshold at the fiftieth percentile.

The role of conditioned reflexes in the processes of perception has been stressed in Soviet research (Sokolov, 1963). Sokolov makes the special point that sensitivity to stimuli can be measured where signal significance is possible. Where no signal is possible, as for example in children, in animals and in the presence of pathological conditions, other methods must be used: primary cortical response, orientation of reflexes, special adaptation reflexes, defense reactions, and conditioned reflexes.

A. THE WEBER FRACTION

The two best known laws of psychophysics are Weber's and Fechner's, which are not always equivalent. The older is that of Weber, who stated: "In comparing magnitudes, it is not the arithmetic difference, but the ratio of the magnitudes, that we perceive." Nearly 130 years ago, E. H. Weber measured the difference threshold for weights, tone, and appreciation of length. One weight felt heavier than another when they were related 29:30. In another set of experiments, where muscle sense was also involved because the weights were actually lifted, the difference threshold was 39:40. This sensory phenomenon is now common knowledge. In lifting two bundles, one weighing 20 lb and the other 25 lb, it is the ratio of their weights that is noticed. If they differ in weight by only 2 ounces the difference will go unnoticed. With light objects, such as two envelopes, however, a 2-ounce difference in weight will be noticed readily. The principle applies to vision, touch, audition, and the chemical senses. This ratio, called the Weber fraction, is defined mathematically as K. $K = \delta S/S$, where δS is the amount necessary to produce the jnd (just-noticeable difference) and S is the stimulus. Since two stimuli are involved, the average of the two is taken as S and the difference between the two stimuli which can be just barely perceived is taken as δS. In fact, the Weber fraction is no longer considered a constant, but in the median range of concentration it does appear to be a good approximation of a complex relationship.

Discussion of the Fechner-Weber relationship requires some psychological background. The physical continuum refers to the ranges in magnitude of a series of physical phenomena, and the psychological continuum refers to the corresponding range in psychological response. For example, Fig. 42 presents, on the left, a range in concentration of sodium

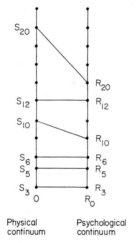

Physical
continuum

Psychological
continuum

FIG. 42. The relation between jnd and the concentrations needed to produce them. S_3 = stimulus limen; R_3 = absolute limen.

chloride solutions and, on the right, a range of sensory responses to the solutions. Note that there is a range in concentration where no sensory response occurs. The point R_0, or threshold limen, is where a response is produced 50% of the time. The difference limen is defined as that difference which is just noted 50% of the time above chance, and in psychophysics is taken as 1 psychological unit. The difference limen does not appear to have any relationship to the threshold limen, nor can we be sure how to evaluate these units in terms of the threshold.

Weber's law applies in relating these difference limens on the psychological continuum to the stimulus values on the physical continuum. ΔR_3,

ΔR_6, and ΔR_{12} are each just one psychological unit apart. They correspond, however, to physical units, S, of 2, 4, and 8 units. In other words, for equal increments on the psychological scale, there are larger and larger increments on the physical scale, or $\Delta S = KS$, where ΔS is any defined increment in a stimulus S corresponding to a defined unitary change in R. K is thus the ratio of the increment to S. K is constant for a given observer and a given stimulus. This is the equation of a straight line passing through the origin with a slope of K. Dividing by S, the equation becomes $\Delta S/S = K$, which states that the just-noticeable increment in any stimulus bears a constant ratio to that stimulus. *Or*, the stimulus must be changed in a certain ratio to produce equal-interval changes in R.

Various methods have been used to determine ΔS. In the method of constant stimuli one may start with two equal stimuli (one is the standard) and then change one by very small amounts above and below the standard until the observer just notices a difference (jnd) between them. Or one could start with two very different concentrations, approach one of them, the standard, by small steps, and require the observer to state when no difference was found (jnnd). It has been found that the difference limen is smaller with the jnnd procedure. The difference limen is not a fixed quantity, but an ideal calculated statistical value; it is usually determined from the average results from the methods of jnd and jnnd. In the method with complete knowledge, the subject is told ahead of time whether the stimuli are decreasing or increasing to find a difference, or are decreasing or increasing from an extreme concentration toward where there is no difference. The suggested advantage of this procedure is that the subject is able to keep his mind on the rate of change. His attention is especially fixed when he realizes that he is approaching the region where he should find a difference. At other times he can relax and not maintain maximum attention. However, the errors of habituation (Chapter 5, Section III) or of expectation (Chapter 5, Section III) may occur. The procedure of partial knowledge is where the stimulus is allowed to approach the standard so that no difference is found and is allowed to continue until a difference is found.

The point where a difference is found 50% of the time is usually taken as the jnd or jnnd. If the percent correct responses are plotted against the concentration of the stimulus it will be found that the comparison stimulus selected as equal is usually lower than the standard. This is the "time-order error."

It is generally agreed that the difference limen varies with the method employed. One of the objections to some data in the literature is that the effect of the method on the results was not evaluated. As Stevens

(1958b) pointed out, determination of the difference limen is a difficult "noisy" thing to measure and different procedures give different results. He favored the method of quantal increments, where a steady stimulus is present to which brief increments are added periodically. The observer signals when he notices the increment.

As indicated, Weber found for weights lifted by hand that the ratio ranged from 0.033 to 0.025. For brightness of light it varied from 0.017 to 0.005, depending on the observer. For pressure, K varied from 0.1 to 0.033. Kopera (1931) reported ratios of 0.33 for taste and smell. Gamble (1898), using Zwaardemaker's olfactometer (Chapter 3, Section IX), reported a Weber fraction for odor of about 0.33 in 36% of her subjects, 0.25 in 26%, 0.5 in 12%, 0.20 in 12%, 0.167 in 4%, more than 0.5 in 5%, and less than 0.162 in 5%. She believed that Weber's fraction applied to smell. Zigler and Holway (1935), however, again using the crude Zwaardemaker olfactometer and only themselves as subjects, showed that the fraction decreased as the stimulus increased. Stone *et al.* (1962) and Stone (1963), using modern equipment, reported a Weber fraction of about 0.2 for 2-octanone, *n*-heptanol, and ethyl-*n*-valerate. Wenzel (1949) calculated a Weber fraction of 0.15 at 84% threshold for the odor of phenylethyl alcohol. Individual differences were not notable, since one experienced subject did not differ from the others. Wenzel's data were criticized by Geldard (1950) because the Elsberg blast-injection technique was used. Since subjects may respond to the pressure, the Weber fraction should be slightly larger.

In studies on the salty taste, the Weber fraction decreased as the concentration increased (Holway and Hurvich, 1937). In Dahlberg and Penczek's (1941) work with sucrose, the Weber fraction was fairly constant over the range 10 to 20% sucrose, and decreased from 30 to 50%. Kopera (1931) reported fairly constant Weber fractions for fructose (0.104 for 3%), glucose (0.15 for 6%), and sucrose (0.12 for 3%). Sucrose values of 0.17 to 0.32 were reported by Nieman (1958). Bujas (1937) obtained fairly constant Weber fractions for citric acid, sodium chloride, and sucrose administered by a flow technique. Bujas believed that the Weber fraction changed because the whole tongue was being stimulated; specific areas of the tongue have different sensitivities. Even for electrical gustatory stimulation Bujas found that the Weber law held if he assumed a constant stimulus of low intensity in the mouth. Unfortunately, only one or two subjects were used in his study. Fodor and Happisch (1922–1923) found variable Weber fractions for salt, but sensations other than salty may have interfered. Saidullah (1927) found a Weber fraction of 0.14 for sodium chloride over the range 0.4 to 18%.

Schutz and Pilgrim (1957) have evaluated much previous work and contributed significantly to the problem of differential taste sensitivity. They noted a wide range in values for the Weber ratio for taste. Some of the variation was undoubtedly due to differences in methodology, especially in quantity and purity of sample. Using the method of single stimulus, Schutz and Pilgrim presented four solutions in randomized order, and required subjects to judge on an intensity scale of 1 to 4. The concentration interval between stimulus solutions was 0.15 from a hypothetical concentration midpoint (CM). The combined judgments

TABLE 44

Differential Sensitivity to Taste

Quality and compound	Concentration midpoint (%)	PSE[a]	ΔI	$\Delta I/I$
Salty, sodium chloride	0.150	0.150	0.0289	0.193
	0.400	0.396	0.0518	0.131
	1.10	1.10	0.133	0.121
	3.00	2.98	0.357	0.120
	8.00	7.80	1.81	0.231
Sweet, sucrose	0.500	0.496	0.150	0.303
	1.50	1.53	0.221	0.144
	3.00	3.07	0.481	0.157
	8.00	7.97	1.23	0.154
	20.0	19.8	2.87	0.145
Sour, citric acid	0.010	0.0100	0.0029	0.290
	0.030	0.0303	0.0069	0.228
	0.100	0.101	0.0235	0.232
	0.300	0.300	0.0510	0.170
	1.00	1.01	0.227	0.224
Bitter, caffeine	0.0315	0.0317	0.0122	0.385
	0.0600	0.0607	0.0206	0.339
	0.125	0.125	0.0332	0.265
	0.250	0.248	0.0715	0.288
	0.500	0.503	0.124	0.248
		For each quality over all levels of intensity		
Salty		0.993	0.152	0.153
Sweet		1.008	0.173	0.172
Sour		1.006	0.226	0.224
Bitter		1.003	0.303	0.302
All qualities		1.002	0.202	0.202

[a] Point of subjective equality.

Source: Schutz and Pilgrim (1957).

were converted to normal deviates. A line was fitted to the deviates by the method of least squares, and the point of subjective equality (PSE) and ΔI and $\Delta I/I$ were calculated. The ΔI calculated for PSE was not significantly different from that calculated for the CM. The data are given in Table 44. Analysis of variance was applied to the data, and curves were fitted by use of orthogonal polynomials to determine where the variation occurred at different ratio levels. For bitterness, the Weber ratio was constant, about 0.30. For sweet and sour, there was a linear relationship, owing to poor sensitivity at the concentration near the absolute threshold. The average values for $\Delta I/I$ for sweet and sour were 0.17 and 0.22, respectively. For salty there was a loss in sensitivity at the lowest and highest intensities. The average value was 0.30.

To adjust the Weber fraction to account for the discrepancies encountered, Miller (1947) suggested the equation $K = \Delta I/(I + Ir)$. The Ir was introduced to account for the stimulus greater than that required purely for activation of neural units. It may be considered as resulting from interfering stimuli, changes in neural sensitivity, shifts of attention, variability or equipment, and the like. Stone (1963) let $Ir = It$, the 50% threshold. Weber fractions by both formulae were as follows:

	$\Delta I/I$	$\dfrac{\Delta I}{1 + It}$
2-Octanone	0.24	0.20
n-Heptanol	0.27	0.21
2-Heptanone	0.23	0.20

For these compounds, but not for ethyl-n-valerate, the ratios, by either formula, were reasonably constant over the range of concentrations used. However, Miller's formula compensates for the fact that $\Delta I/I$ is larger for lower values of I and reasonably constant at higher values.

Pfaffmann (1959) summarized a wide variety of data on the Weber fraction, noting that high differential sensitivity for one taste quality is not correlated with high sensitivity for others, and that differences between subjects are great. In general, the Weber fraction for the primary tastes averages between 0.15 and 0.25. There were many deviations from Weber's law. Since all values are made on the stimulus scale (or physical continuum), it may be that Weber's law is not a true psychophysical law. However, ΔS does stand for some presumably constant psychological increment measured on the stimulus scale. Upon application, it can be seen that the Weber law is valid, if at all, only at medium stimulus values and over a relatively short range, since in many cases K changes with concentration of the stimulus. There is some relationship of ΔS to S, and ΔS is some function of S, but it is not a linear function, as Weber's law implies.

B. THE FECHNER EQUATION

Fechner, in 1860, drew the conclusion that the increment threshold, ΔS, of the stimulus S was a constant, and he carried out several series of experiments to establish the validity of this generalization: $\Delta S/S$ = constant. Fechner regarded the constant as a minute sensory unit, ΔR, which he defined as Weber's law:

$$\Delta S/S = k\Delta R \tag{1}$$

where k is a factor of proportionality. His next step was to suggest that ΔS and ΔR were true limiting values, dS and dR, such as required by the definitions of calculus, and that one therefore could rewrite Eq. 1 as a simple differential equation:

$$dR/dS = 1/kS \tag{2}$$

from which, by integration, one obtains

$$R = a \log S + b \tag{3}$$

in which the constant a also includes the factor for transformation into common logarithms, and b is an integration constant.

This is Fechner's law, which he also derived in other ways. It states that something in sensation that can be called its quantity, R, is proportional to the logarithm of the stimulus S (Fig. 43).

Fechner's law is derived mathematically from Weber's, but it need not refer to the same phenomena. In Weber's law, $\Delta S = kS$. In Fechner's

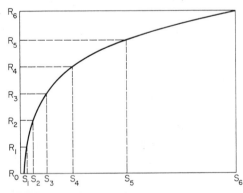

FIG. 43. The relation of response and stimulus according to Fechner's law. Source: Guilford (1954).

law, $R = a \log S + b$. Now, R is a psychological unit and was obtained by assuming that for each ΔS in stimulus there is a ΔR in response. The psychological procedure employed to demonstrate Fechner's law is not, usually, the jnd or jnnd procedure, but the method of equal-sense differences, in which the observer is asked what the midway point is between two stimuli.

To obtain Fechner's law from Weber's, Fechner *assumed* that all correspondingly small increments in S are psychologically equal. If ΔS increases, ΔR increases. Then $\delta R = C \delta S/S = K$, where C is a constant of proportionality between δR and $\delta S/S$. Since all the R increments are equal, we may integrate to get

$$R = C \log_e S + A \tag{4}$$

where A is the integration constant. It is necessary to get C in terms of S. Let S_0 (the absolute threshold) be the value of S when $R = 0$. Substituting ($R = 0$ and $S = S_0$), $0 = C \log_e S_0 + A$, or $A = -C \log_e S_0$. Substituting this in Eq. 4, we get:

$$R = C \log_e S - C \log_e S_0 = C (\log_e S - \log_e S_0), \text{ or } R = C \log_e S/S_0.$$

To convert to common logarithms requires a change in C to another constant, D. Then $R = D \log S/S_0$. To demonstrate this law, plot the data for a series of stimuli against the R values. The method of least squares is employed, and the test for goodness of fit will indicate whether the law fits the data. Plotting on semilog paper usually shows whether the regression is linear. For more detailed information, see Guilford (1954). For a modern and more correct derivation, see Luce and Edwards (1958).

Using coffee, naphthalene, and citral, and the method of critical fusion frequency, Blondal (1957) showed that the odors followed Fechner's logarithmic law of response, $N = k \log c + b$, where N is the critical frequency of olfaction for each concentration of the odor, c is the concentration, and k and b are constants which differ in numerical value for the two parts of the graph for each odor. The technique used may not be free of error.

Allen (1957) used DC and AC current; the former excited the sensations of sweet, bitter, and sour, and the latter those of sour and bitter. In some cases, sweet and sour or bitter and salty were excited together, but sweet and salty were never excited separately. When the data were plotted logarithmically, four linear graphs, conforming to the Fechner equation, were obtained (see, however, Chapter 2, Section III).

These laws are verified or not verified together when equally often noticed differences are equal psychologically. For Weber's law we determine small changes in S that are psychologically equal, i.e., $\Delta S/S$ is constant. Fechner's law is tested for supraliminal differences and with scaled values derived from ΔS. If the discriminal dispersions along the S scale are equal, then both laws apply. Fechner's law is not affected by the size of the dispersion, but Weber's is. Central tendencies establish Fechner's law, but ΔS in Weber's law is related to the spread of the discriminatory responses. If the dispersions for stimuli are not equal, responses are not equal.

There is an enormous literature dealing with Fechner's law—tests of its validity, criticism of the assumptions (which as mathematical propositions may be open to criticism), attempts to replace it with better expressions, epistemological difficulties, etc. As Galanter (1962) noted, the difficulty with Fechner's law is its unproven assumption that one jnd is subjectively equal to another. Stevens (1960b) criticized Thurstone's law of comparative judgment because it derived sensation magnitudes from variability measurements.

Lewis (1948) attempted to verify the validity of the Fechner relation by asking judges to choose a solution which "tastes the closest to one-half as strong." He found that the response to intensity was approximately directly proportional to the intensity of the stimulus rather than related logarithmically. Apparently the judges were trying to find a half-concentration or stimulus strength rather than a half-sensation. In our laboratory we have had students attempt to choose the half-concentration rather than the half-stimulus. In general, in magnitude estimation the results do not display the logarithmic form predicted by Fechner. When comparative rating scales are used to test the Fechner relation, Helson et al. (1954) noted that the scale must contain an odd number of categories, the central category must represent a "neutral" judgment, and the judgment-scale and the stimuli encountered must be equivalent in the sense that the scale must be broad enough to include judgments of all stimuli encountered and yet be so narrow that its extreme values do not fall outside the range of judgment elicited by any of the stimuli. The comparative rating scale has the advantage over the method of absolute judgment because it provides a stimulus standard which helps to standardize judgment of stimuli.

Stevens (1957, 1958a, 1959, 1960a, 1961a,b) re-examined Plateau's (1872) suggestion that sensation is related to stimulation by a power function, and claimed for it a wider range of validity than Fechner's law. Stevens (1960a) argued that Fechner's error lay in assuming that variability of judgment is constant up and down the psychological continuum. Further, Stevens believes that two kinds of continua may be distinguished: a prothetic, having to do with *how much;* and a metathetic, having to do with *what kind* or *where.* Both kinds of continua may be measured by at least three types of scales: discriminability (jnd, etc.), category (equal appearing intervals), and magnitude (estimates of apparent strength or intensity relative to a standard or modulus). Stevens considers that the primary difference between prothetic and metathetic continua is that the three kinds of scales are always nonlinearly related in the former and linearly related in the latter. In prothetic continua the magnitude scale is a power function, the discriminability (jnd) scale approximates a logarithmic function, and the category scale an intermediate form.

Stevens notes that, if psychological magnitudes, Ψ, are related to physical magnitudes, Φ, by the equation $\Psi = K\Phi^n$, the power function has the convenient feature that on log-log coordinates it plots as a straight line whose slope is equal to the value of the exponent. Reese and Stevens (1960) reported exponents on the prothetic continua of 0.55 for coffee odor, and 0.6 for heptane. Stevens (1960a,b) also reported exponents of 0.8 for saccharin, 1.3 for sucrose, and 1.3 for salt. Jones (1958) calculated an exponent of 0.59 for heptane. Stevens' (1960a) more complete version of the power law is: $V(\Psi) = c \, (I - I_o)^k$ where I_o compensates for the effects at low intensities.

As Pfaffmann (1959) noted, some studies find taste sensitivity to increase as an exponential function of stimulus concentration, but the exact relation between taste intensity and stimulus concentration is yet to be established.

The assumption that the sensation-stimulus relationship is logarithmic has also been questioned by Harries (1960). He gave a panel of judges plain pieces of paper marked with a straight line 6 inches long, labeled *A* at one end and *B* at the other. At each session, four samples of coffee, labeled *X, Y, A,* and *B* were presented. The judges were told that samples *A* and *B* correspond to the end of the line. The judge indicated by crosses the relative positions of *X* and *Y*, which were mixtures of *A* and *B.* The content of each ingredient in *X* and *Y* was varied from 10 to 90% in steps of 5%. Figure 44 gives the distance from *B* plotted by the subject against actual percentage of *B.* Note that the relationship is linear. Harries (1961) noted that the conditions of the test were unusual in that both ends of the scale were fixed. Nevertheless, in this case at least the differentiation proceeded in roughly equal steps and Harries suggested that sensory differentiation is logarithmic only when "seen from one end," like telegraph poles along a straight road.

Judgments can be made in terms of the adaptation-level, which is defined as a weighted geometric mean of present and past stimuli. Using a standard improves performance but, Helson (1947, 1948) stated, not as much as one might expect, because there are series stimuli and residual and background factors, and the standard affects the comparative-adaptation level (see also Michels and Helson, 1949). These proce-

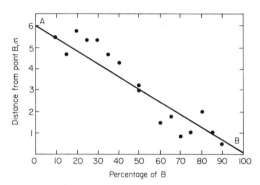

FIG. 44. Average scores given to mixtures of two samples. Estimates of mixtures of A and B were indicated on 6-inch paper marked A and B at the ends. These estimates were plotted against the actual percent B in the mixture. Source: Harries (1961).

dures facilitate the demonstration of apparent relationships but are subject to various biases, as Dember (1961) noted.

Much of the criticism directed against Fechner's law is valid, and the bulk of the evidence now favors Steven's interpretation or the similar one of Rosner (1962).

C. OTHER PROBLEMS

When we speak of the acceptance of, preference for, or quality of a food we are dealing with esthetics, and new and difficult psychological problems may be introduced. Harper (1962) called these "contingent influences," and noted the following: individual differences, effects of special knowledge and experience, sensory interaction, group differences, social influences, serial influence, systematic biases, etc. Some of the factors which influence quality evaluation have been summarized by Gregson (1960) and Amerine (1962).

Certainly, *de gustibus non est disputandum* is not wholly true. Furthermore, hedonic quality is not just pleasure. As Amerine (1962) stated: "Hedonic effectiveness, i.e., the degree of pleasure or displeasure, is not necessarily equivalent to esthetic worth since preference evaluations vary with the cognitive disposition of the observer."

Gregson suggested that the ability of subjects to discriminate depends on the rate at which their hedonic ratings change with respect to the physical variable with which their value judgments are associated. If the rate of change of value with departure from a physically defined standard is high, then discrimination should be facilitated over that range compared with discriminations over a similar range with no such hedonic change. This assumes that the value judgment is inseparable from discrimination and is not a separate subsequent process depending on prior discrimination. The value judgment thus would take its direction and magnitude not only from the stimulus materials but from the way they are encountered. Further experiments on the effect of methodology on preference would be most welcome (see also Chapter 9).

According to the theory of cognitive dissonance (Festinger, 1957), results which run counter to expectancies will be perceived as unpleasant. Carlsmith and Aronson (1963) showed that when solutions were presented that "disconfirmed", a subject's expectation, bitter was perceived as more unpleasant (i.e., more bitter), and sweet as less pleasant (i.e., less sweet). These results are not what would be predicted by affectual theories, which suggest that a positive effect follows a departure from an expected result (see also Chapter 5, Sections II and III).

V. Adaptation

When a stimulus is prolonged, sensory response declines, i.e., adaptation occurs. This applies not only to the direct sensory response but to electrical activity as well. In food psychophysics we are interested in the phenomenon because: (1) it may influence thresholds and other results, and (2) sensory response may be so changed by adaptation that the number of tests must be strictly controlled. Complete adaptation, i.e., no response, is possible but is certainly of little importance in the sensory examination of foods. Of more importance is partial or incipient adaptation. Helson (1947, 1948) defined adaptation level in terms of a stimulus invoking neutral or indifferent response. He did not restrict this to a constant stimulation with a consequently greatly reduced capacity for response, but defined it in terms of a function of all the stimuli acting upon the organism at any given moment as well as in the past.

When a stimulus is applied to a nerve, a wave of negative potential (the action potential) travels along the outer surface of the membrane. For a short time (about 0.001 sec) after the nerve discharge, the fiber is completely insensitive (the absolute refractory period). Then, sensitivity increases so that, after about 0.01 sec, the threshold is back to that of the resting state of the neuron. This assumes that only a single stimulus is applied. When, however, the stimulus is applied continuously, the insensitive period, naturally, lengthens. Adaptation appears to be due to some specific inhibition of the cell receptor membrane in the case of taste, rather than to exhaustion of some receptive substance in the cell. Furthermore, both peripheral and central adaptation may occur. Maximal subjective intensity does not occur for some seconds after the stimulus is applied, when the receptor sensitivity has already decreased through adaptation. As Pfaffmann (1959) noted, this indicates a process of central adaptation.

Because the study of adaptation is easier with the sense of taste, most of such studies have dealt with that sense. Using flowing solutions, the time of adaptation was shown by Hahn (1933) to be a function of stimulus concentration (Fig. 46). For example, at low concentrations

TABLE 45
Effect of Concentration on Adaptation Time

Sucrose					
Conc. (*M*)	0.066	0.131	0.246	0.737	1.260
Adaptation time (sec)	46.5	90.5	132.2	193.1	326.0
Sodium chloride					
Conc. (*M*)	0.84	1.66	2.44	3.11	—
Adaptation time (sec)	16.2	73.3	90.5	115.6	
Tartaric acid					
Conc. (*M*)	0.0022	0.0066	0.013	—	—
Adaptation time (sec)	78.6	129.6	194.8		
Quinine hydrochloride					
Conc. (*M*)	0.000013	0.000041	0.000083	—	—
Adaptation time (sec)	74.7	115.3	115.6		

Source: Abrahams *et al.* (1937) and Krakauer and Dallenbach (1937).

of sodium chloride, adaptation occurred in about 20 sec, but at higher concentrations it did not occur for nearly 2 min. Results were similar with other tastes, but with differing rates of adaptation.

Krakauer and Dallenbach (1937) reported that, in tests with four subjects, the time of adaptation for sucrose, tartaric acid, and quinine hydrochloride was gradual, and longer for more concentrated solutions (Table 45 and Fig. 45). These were "flowing" experiments, in which the tongue was kept still. Abrahams *et al.* (1937) studied adaptation to the salty taste. Pain may have interfered, but adaptation was relatively slow at the higher concentrations.

Adaptation and recovery are indicated in Fig. 46. The shapes of the recovery curves are similar for all concentrations. No cross adaptation for the salty taste has been found among many inorganic salts investigated, and little cross adaptation for sweet and bitter has been found among various compounds. For the sour taste, however, one acid cross-adapts for others. Furthermore, Dallenbach and Dallenbach (1943) showed that, following bitter adaptation, the threshold for the other tastes was lowered. Previous adaptation raises subsequently determined thresholds for the same taste.

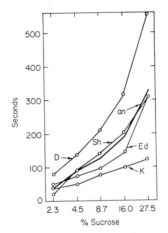

Fɪɢ. 45. Effect of sucrose concentration on adaptation time. The light curves represent individual subjects and the dark curve the average. Source: Krakauer and Dallenbach (1937).

In general, recovery from adaptation is rapid at first and slower thereafter. After adaptation, the measured threshold rises in a line which is approximately linear to the stimulus intensity.

If the electrical activity of neural response is used as a measure of adaptation, the rate of adaptation varies from one substance to another

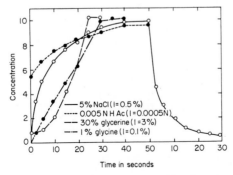

Fɪɢ. 46. Effect of adaptation and time on threshold. After 50 seconds, the tongue was rinsed for the number of seconds shown, and the threshold then determined. Source: Hahn (1963).

and from one concentration to another. With odor the magnitude of neural response activity as recorded electrophysiologically is constant at low levels of odor stimulation. Activity declines to a steady level with medium concentrations, and complete adaptation is observed at high concentrations. Adrian (1950) believes that the olfactory bulb is of greater influence than the receptor in determining olfactory adaptation. Adaptation is approximately linear to concentration. Recovery is rapid at first, and then slow. As determined by olfactory thresholds measured after adaptation, the rate of recovery is slower as the concentration of the adapting stimulus becomes greater.

In food testing there is evidence that adaptation is a factor with some foods but not with others. For example, Laue *et al.* (1954) reported an adaptation for maple syrup, Helm and Trolle (1946) reported adaptation for beer, and there are similar reports for other foods. Even so, in many tests adaptation appears to be, at most, a minor factor. Pfaffmann *et al.* (1954), for example, was able to continue tests with 50–75 samples of orange drink and tomato juice over a 40-min period without reduction of sensitivity. Bradley *et al.* (1954) showed that eight foods could be tasted with little fatigue. Adaption should be tested for each food product since efficiency in the use of panel personnel is greater if the number of tests per session period can be increased (see also Chapter 6, Section II).

A unique application of adaptation has been suggested by Cheesman (1960). He proposed that adapting different groups to different suspected off-odors might enable one to determine which suspected off-odor was responsible for an undesirable taint in a product.

While adaptation is the only physiological factor considered here, there are, of course, many others. These have been considered in the chapters on taste, odor, and the other senses, and some will be noted in the chapters on laboratory sensory studies.

VI. Summary

Attitudinal factors might be useful in connection with consumer acceptance and preference. Motivation influences our results at both threshold and suprathreshold concentrations.

Psychological errors in sensory examination have been emphasized. Especially important in food testing are errors of central tendency, time or position, and contrast. Memory, concentration, and explicit instructions may be important.

The differences between detection, recognition, discrimination, and scaling, and the factors influencing each, are outlined. The problems of defining the dimensions of a sensation, and hence of a threshold, are also considered.

Derivation of the Weber and Fechner relationships between stimulus and perception is outlined. The predictive value of the former is limited, and the Fechner relation appears to apply to only certain types of judgment.

Adaptation is a factor which must be taken into account in all subjective measurements.

REFERENCES

Abrahams, H., D. Krakauer, and K. M. Dallenbach. 1937. Gustatory adaptation to salt. *Am. J. Psychol.* **49**, 462–469.

Adrian, E. D. 1950. The electrical activity of the mammalian olfactory bulb. *Electroencephalog. and Clin. Neurophysiol.* **2**, 377–388.

Allen, F. 1957. The sensations of taste and the logarithmic law of response. *Z. Psychol.* **160**, 276–281.

Amerine, M. A. 1962. The importance of flavor. *Proc. 1st Intern. Congr. Food Sci. and Technol.* **3** (to be published in July 1965).

Blondal, H. 1957. Der Geruchssinn. *Z. Psychol.* **161**, 292–295.

Bradley, J. E., C. T. Walliker, and D. R. Peryam. 1954. Influence of continued testing on preference ratings. *In* "Food Acceptance Testing Methodology," 115 pp. (see pp. 92–100). Advisory Board on Quartermaster Research and Development, Committee on Foods., Natl. Acad. Sci., Natl. Research Council, Chicago, Illinois.

Bujas, Z. 1937. La mesure de la sensibilité differentielle dans le domaine gustatif. *Acta Inst. Psychol. Univ. Zagreb.* **2**(1), 1–18; also **2**(4), 1–12.

Carlsmith, J. M., and E. Aronson. 1963. Some hedonic consequences of the confirmation and disconfirmation of expectancies. *J. Abnormal Social Psychol.* **66**, 151–156.

Caul, J. F. 1956. The profile method of flavor analysis. *Advances in Food Research* **7**, 1–40.

Cheesman, G. H. 1960. Odour and chemical constitution—a new approach. *Proc. Roy. Australian Chem. Inst.* **27**, 70–73.

Dahlberg, A. C., and E. S. Penczek. 1941. The relative sweetness of sugars as affected by concentration. *N. Y. State Agr. Expt. Sta. Tech. Bull.* **258**, 1–12.

Dallenbach, J. W., and K. M. Dallenbach. 1943. The effect of bitter adaptation on sensitivity to the other taste qualities. *Am. J. Psychol.* **56**, 21–31.

Dawson, E. H., and B. L. Harris. 1951. Sensory methods for measuring differences in food quality. *U. S. Dept. Agr., Agr. Infor. Bull.* **34**, 1–134.

Dember, W. N. 1961. "The Psychology of Perception," 402 pp. Holt, New York.

Dember, W. N., and R. W. Earl. 1957. Analysis of exploratory, manipulatory, and curiosity behavior. *Psychol. Rev.* **64**, 91–96.

Duffendack, S. C. 1954. A study of non-sensory determinants of recognition thresholds. *Dissertation Abstr.* **14**, 1097.

Elsberg, C. A. 1937. The sense of smell. XIV. The relation of the cerebral cortex to the olfactory impulse and the areas of the brain involved in fatigue of the sense of smell. *Bull. Neurol. Inst. N. Y.* **6**, 118–125.

Festinger, L. 1957. "A Theory of Cognitive Dissonance," 291 pp. Harper & Row, New York.

Fodor, K., and L. Happisch. 1922–1923. Ueber die Verschiedenheit der Unterschiedesschwellen für den Geschmackssinn bei Reizzunahme und Reizabnahme. *Arch. ges. Physiol.* **197**, 337–346.

Galanter, E. 1962. Contemporary psychophysics. *In* "New Directions in Psychology" (R. Brown, E. Galanter, E. H. Hass, and G. Mandler, eds.), 353 pp. (see pp. 87–156). Holt, New York.

Gamble, E. A. M. 1898. Applicability of Weber's law to smell. *Am. J. Psychol.* **10**, 82–142.

Geldard, F. A. 1950. Somestheses and the chemical senses. *Ann. Rev. Psychol.* **1**, 73–86 (see pp. 80–81).

Gregson, R. A. M. 1960. Bias in the measurement of food preferences by triangular tests. *Occupational Psychol.* **34**, 249–257.

Gregson, R. A. M. 1962. A rating-scale method for determining absolute taste thresholds. *J. Food Sci.* **27**, 376–380.

Gregson, R. A. M. 1963a. The effect of psychological expectations on preferences for taste mixtures. *Food Technol.* **17**(3), 44.

Gregson, R. A. M. 1963b. Validation problems in interpreting preference responses to mixed food qualities. *Appl. Stat.* **12**, 1–13.

Gridgeman, N. T. 1958. Psychophysical bias in taste testing by pair comparison, with special reference to position and temperature. *Food Research* **23**, 217–220.

Gridgeman, N. T. 1959. Sensory item sorting. *Biometrics* **15**, 298–306.

Guilford, J. P. 1954. "Psychometric Methods," 597 pp. McGraw-Hill, New York.

Gulliksen, H., and S. Messich. 1960. "Psychological Scaling: Theory and Applications," 211 pp. Wiley, New York.

Hahn, H. 1933. Über die Adaptation des Geschmackssinnes. *Fortschr. Med.* **51**(20), 436–439.

Hall, R. L. 1958. Flavor study approaches at McCormick and Co., Inc. *In* "Flavor Research and Food Acceptance" (A. D. Little, Inc., ed.), 391 pp. (see pp. 224–240). Reinhold, New York.

Hamilton, H. C. 1929. The effect of incentives on accuracy of discrimination measured on the Galton bar. *Arch. Psychol.* **16**(103), 1–73.

Hanson, H. L., J. G. Davis, A. A. Campbell, J. H. Anderson, and H. Lineweaver. 1955. Sensory test methods. II. Effect of previous tests on consumer response to foods. *Food Technol.* **9**, 56–59.

Harper, R. 1962. The psychologist's role in food acceptance research. *Food Technol.* **16**(10), 70, 72–73.

Harries, J. M. 1960. The quality control of food by sensory assessment. *Soc. Chem. Ind. (London) Monograph* **8**, 128–137.

Harries, J. M. 1961. Some psychological aspects of taste testing. *Occupational Psychol.* **35**, 128–135.

Helm, E., and B. Trolle. 1946. Selection of a taste panel. *Wallerstein Lab. Commun.* **9**, 181–194.

Helson, H. 1947. Adaptation-level as frame of reference for prediction of psychophysical data. *Am. J. Psychol.* **60**, 1–29.

Helson, H. 1948. Adaptation-level as a basis for a quantitative theory of frames of reference. *Psychol. Rev.* **55**, 297–313.

Helson, H., W. C. Michels, and A. Sturgeon. 1954. The use of comparative rating scales for the evaluation of psychophysical data. *Am. J. Psychol.* **67**, 321–326.

Holway, A. H., and L. M. Hurvich. 1937. Differential gustatory sensitivity to salt. *Am. J. Psychol.* **49**, 37–48.

Holzman, P. S., and G. S. Klein. 1954. Cognitive system—principles of leveling and sharpening: individual differences in assimilation effects in visual time-error. *J. Psychol.* **37**, 105–122.

Jones, F. N. 1958. Subjective scales of intensity for three odors. *Am. J. Psychol.* **71**, 423–425.

Kamenetzky, J. 1959. Contrast and convergence effects in ratings of foods. *J. Appl. Psychol.* **43**, 47–52.

Kopera, A. 1931. Untersuchungen über die Unterschiedsempfindlichkeit im Bereiche des Geschmackssinns. *Arch. ges. Psychol.* **82**, 273–307.

Krakauer, D., and K. M. Dallenbach. 1937. Gustatory adaptation to sweet, sour and bitter. *Am. J. Psychol.* **49**, 469–475.

Laue, E. A., N. H. Ishler, and G. A. Bullman. 1954. Reliability of taste testing and consumer testing methods. I. Fatigue in taste testing. *Food Technol.* **8**, 387–388.

Lewis, D. R. 1948. Psychological scales of taste. *J. Psychol.* **26**, 437–446.

Luce, R. D. and W. Edwards. 1958. The derivation of subjective scales from just noticeable differences. *Psychol. Rev.* **65**, 222–237.

McClelland, D. C., and J. W. Atkinson. 1949. The projective expression of needs. I. The effect of different intensities of the hunger drive on perception. *J. Psychol.* **27**, 311–330.

Michels, W. C., and H. Helson. 1949. A reformulation of the Fechner law in terms of adaptation-level applied to rating-scale data. *Am. J. Psychol.* **62**, 355–368.

Miller, G. A. 1947. Sensitivity to changes in the intensity of white noise and its relation to masking the loudness. *J. Acoust. Soc. Am.* **19**, 609–619.

Mitchell, J. W. 1956. Time-errors in the paired comparison taste preference test. *Food Technol.* **10**, 218–220.

Nieman, C. 1958. Relative Süsskraft von Zuckerarten. *Zucker- u. Süsswarenwirtsch.* **11**(9), 420–422, 465–467, 505–507, 632–633, 670–671, 752–753, 791–792, 840–841, 878–879, 933–934, 974, 1051–1052, 1088–1089.

Pangborn, R. M., and W. L. Dunkley. 1964. Laboratory procedures for evaluating the sensory properties of milk. *Dairy Sci. Abstr.* **26**, 55–62.

Pfaffmann, C., H. Schlosberg, and J. Cornsweet. 1954. Variables affecting difference tests. *In* "Food Acceptance Testing Methodology," 115 pp. (see pp. 4–17). Advisory Board on Quartermaster Research and Development, Committee on Foods, Natl. Acad. Sci., Natl. Research Council, Chicago, Illinois.

Pfaffmann, C. 1959. The sense of taste. *In* "Handbook of Physiology," Vol. I, 779 pp. (see p. 526). Physiol. Soc., Washington, D. C.

Plateau, J. A. F. 1872. Sur la mesure des sensations physiques et sur la loi qui lie l'intensité de ces sensations a l'intensité de la cause excitante. *Bull. acad. sci. Bruxelles* **33**, 376–388; *Compt. rend.* **75**, 677–680.

Reese, T. S., and S. S. Stevens. 1960. Subjective intensity of coffee odor. *Am. J. Psychol.* **73**, 424–428.

Rosner, B. S. 1962. *In* "Psychology, a Study of a Science" (S. Koch, ed.), Vol. 4: Biologically Oriented Fields: Their Place in Psychology and in Biological Science, 731 pp. (see pp. 280–333). McGraw-Hill, New York.

Saidullah, A. 1927. Experimentelle Untersuchungen über den Geschmackssinn mit besonderer Berücksichtigung des Weber-Fechnerschen Gesetzes. *Arch. ges. Psychol.* **60**, 457–484.

Schmidt, H. O. 1941. The effects of praise and blame as incentives to learning. *Psychol. Monograph* **53**(240), 1–56.

Schutz, H. G., and F. J. Pilgrim. 1957. Differential sensitivity in gustation. *J. Exptl. Psychol.* **54**, 41–48.

Schwartz, N., and C. H. Pratt. 1956. Simultaneous vs. successive presentation in a paired comparison situation. *Food Research* **21**, 103–108.

Sokolov, Y. N. 1963. "Perception and the Conditioned Reflex," 309 pp. Macmillan (Pergamon Press), New York.

Stevens, S. S. 1957. On the psychophysical law. *Psychol. Rev.* **64**, 153–181.

Stevens, S. S. 1958a. Measurement and man. *Science* **127**, 383–389.

Stevens, S. S. 1958b. Problems and methods of psychophysics. *Psychol. Bull.* **55**, 177–196.

Stevens, S. S. 1959. The quantification of sensation. *Dædalus* **88**, 606–621.

Stevens, S. S. 1960a. The psychophysics of sensory function. *Am. Scientist* **48**, 226–253.

Stevens, S. S. 1960b. Ratio scales, partition scales and confusion scales. *In* "Psychological Scaling: Theory and Application" (H. Gulliksen and S. Messich, eds.), 211 pp. (see pp. 49–66). Wiley, New York.

Stevens, S. S. 1961a. To honor Fechner and repeal his law. *Science* **133**, 80–86.

Stevens, S. S. 1961b. The psychophysics of sensory function. *In* "Sensory Communication" (W. A. Rosenblith, ed.), 844 pp. (see pp. 1–33). M.I.T. Press, Cambridge, Massachusetts; Wiley, New York.

Stone, H. 1963. Some factors affecting olfactory sensitivity and odor intensity. 112 pp. Ph.D. Thesis. Univ. of California, Davis, California. See also *J. Exptl. Psychol.* **66**, 466–473 (1963).

Stone, H., C. S. Ough, and R. M. Pangborn. 1962. Determination of odor difference thresholds. *J. Food Sci.* **27**, 197–202.

Thurstone, L. L. 1944. Some new psychophysical methods. *In* "Food Acceptance Testing Methodology," 115 pp. (see pp. 100–104). Advisory Board on Quartermaster Research and Development, Committee on Foods, Natl. Acad. Sci., Natl. Research Council, Chicago, Illinois.

Tyler, L. E. 1956. "The Psychology of Human Differences," 2nd ed., 526 pp. (see pp. 221–244). Appleton, New York.

Valdés, R. M., E. H. Hinreiner, and M. J. Simone. 1956a. Effect of sucrose and organic acids on apparent flavor intensity. I. Aqueous solutions. *Food Technol.* **10**, 282–285.

Valdés, R. M., E. H. Hinreiner, and M. J. Simone. 1956b. Effect of sucrose and organic acids on apparent flavor intensity. II. Fruit nectars. *Food Technol.* **10**, 387–390.

Wenzel, B. M. 1949. Differential sensitivity in olfaction. *J. Exptl. Psychol.* **39**, 129–143.

Young, P. T. 1961. "Motivation and Emotion; a Survey of the Determinants of Human and Animal Activity," 648 pp. Wiley, New York.

Zigler, M. J., and A. H. Holway. 1935. Differential sensitivity as determined by amount of olfactory substance. *J. Gen. Psychol.* **12**, 372–382.

Chapter 6

Laboratory Studies: Types and Principles

Foods are submitted to sensory examination to provide information that can lead to product improvement, quality maintenance, the development of new products, or analysis of the market. This section summarizes the most important types of sensory problems encountered by food research groups and the main types of procedures used in solving them. This chapter covers the use of laboratory panels, as do Chapters 7 and 8. Consumer testing is discussed in Chapter 9, and statistical procedures for evaluation of the results of both types of panels are covered in Chapter 10.

Tests may be conducted to: (1) select qualified judges and study human perception of food attributes; (2) correlate sensory with chemical and physical measurements; (3) study processing effects, maintain quality, evaluate raw material selection, establish storage stability, or reduce costs; (4) evaluate quality; or (5) determine consumer reaction. Each of these purposes requires appropriate tests. In general, laboratory panels are used for the first three purposes, highly trained experts for the fourth, and large consumer groups for the last.

In this text we distinguish between two types of laboratory panels: (1) those which determine simple differences between treated samples; and (2) those which determine directional differences. Both are laboratory panels, and sometimes untrained judges are used, but it is the thesis of this book that trained subjects are more useful. The advantages of such panels are discussed in Chapter 7.

I. Types of Tests

The most important types of tests and their utilization are briefly described here. More detailed information of each procedure is given in Chapters 7, 8, and 10.

A. Difference Tests

The common true difference tests are referred to as single-stimulus, paired-stimuli, duo-trio, triangle, and multi-sample tests. In tests which do not reveal statistically significant differences between treatments, no further evaluation is needed. When differences are found, however, directional difference tests are used to establish the nature and magnitude of difference. After a significant difference has been established by a laboratory panel, consumers may be asked to express preferences.

Since most perceptual judgments are relative, *single-sample* presentation is used infrequently, except at the consumer level. Expert tasters of wines, beers, coffee, tea, and dairy products rate single samples, but they evaluate the quality of many samples at a time and compare them against their pre-established "memory standard." Occasionally a method called "A–not A" is used (Peryam, 1958), in which a standard, A, is presented followed by one or more coded samples. The judge indicates which one(s) *is* (are) A. This method may be classified as a paired comparison rather than single presentation since each coded sample is compared with the standard.

In the *paired-stimuli* procedure, judges simply specify whether there is a difference between two samples. When the judge also indicates what sensory characteristic distinguishes the two samples, we speak of the test as a *paired-comparison*. The samples are presented in a counter-balanced design, and a forced-choice is usually required. One half of the responses could be correct due to chance alone. The number of samples tested at a single session will depend on the commodity, the experience of the judges, and the amount of time and sample available. Paired testing is typically used in comparing new with old processing procedures, in quality control, and in preference testing at the consumer level.

The *duo-trio* is a modified paired presentation in which one sample is identified and presented first, followed by two coded samples, one of which is identical with the standard. The judge is asked which of the two is the same as the first sample. This method is primarily a laboratory tool for use with trained subjects. It lends itself to use for quality control and for selection of judges of superior discrimination.

In the *triangle test*, two identical and one different samples are presented simultaneously and the judge is asked to indicate the odd sample. Correct identification due to chance alone is one third. Like the duo-trio method, the triangle test should be used only by trained laboratory judges, and is suited to similar problems.

B. RANK ORDER

Ranking is used to determine how several samples differ on the basis of a single characteristic. A group of coded samples (which may contain a control, or standard) are presented simultaneously, and the judge is asked to rank them in order of the intensity of a specified characteristic.

This method is suitable for use by laboratory judges in product or process evaluation, by experts for selecting the best sample for a particular use, and by consumers for expressing relative acceptability among a limited number of samples. It is of importance that all judges use the same criteria. When necessary, one criterion (sweetness, for example) can be ranked, after which another criterion (sourness, viscosity, etc.) may be ranked in another set of the same samples.

C. Scoring Tests

The best use of *scoring* tests is in comparisons of a control sample with several experimental samples. The scoring may be expressed in terms of deviation from a reference—"no difference from control" to "very large difference from control." In other experiments, scores may be used on an absolute basis *if the scale is clearly defined and understood by all judges.* Although difference-from-control tests have been used widely by laboratory panels, the results may be meaningless if the judges change the basis of their scoring as the test proceeds, i.e., judges become experts. Thus, this method is best suited for use by experts. The test may be administered to consumers if it is clearly explained and the decisions required are simple.

Tests in which deviation from a control is measured are used for product or process evaluation and critical tests on basic perception of sensory attributes. Scoring tests are also used in new-product development, quality control, storage stability tests, screening of intensity levels, and measuring judge characteristics such as leniency, reproducibility, or central tendency (see Chapter 5).

D. Descriptive Tests

Descriptive sensory analyses are best conducted only by highly trained experts completely familiar with the product or the process. Such tests are used effectively in new-product development, in product or process improvement, for quality control, and for training judges for future testing. One type of descriptive test—hedonic—in which degree of liking is described, is suitable at the consumer level. Among the types of descriptive tests currently in use are scalar scoring of various types, hedonic ratings, semantic differential tests, and Arthur D. Little's "Flavor Profile" (see Chapter 8, Section V).

E. Hedonic Scaling

Scoring is called hedonic when the judge expresses his degree of liking by checking a point on a scale ranging from extreme disapproval to extreme approval. A five- to nine-point balanced scale is usually employed. Hedonic ratings are converted to scores and treated by rank analysis or analysis of variance. As indicated above, this test has been used both by experts and by untrained consumers, but we feel it is more effectively applicable to the latter.

F. ACCEPTANCE AND PREFERENCE

Distinction should be made between acceptance, which is a willingness to use or eat a product, and preference, which relates to a greater degree of acceptance of one product over another when a choice is presented. The acceptance or preferences of a laboratory panel are of very limited value except in gross screening of treatments. Some of the test methods described above can be adapted to measurement of consumer reaction (see Chapter 9).

G. OTHER METHODS

Dilution tests, described in Chapter 9, have been used for laboratory testing of selected treatments, employing methods of presentation described above, i.e., single, paired, and multiple samples. *Threshold* tests are seldom used except in studies where it is desirable to establish the minimum detectable difference of an additive or of an off flavor. Threshold and dilution tests have been used to a limited extent to select judges who can detect specific sensory properties. When so used, the test materials and their concentrations should be the same as those likely to be encountered in the actual test. Sequential analysis (Chapter 10) can be used to analyze the results.

It is our belief that laboratory judges should be carefully selected and screened on the basis of their sensitivity to the differences that may be encountered in the experimental samples. In this sense, all laboratory panels should consist of experts. It is recognized that in many organizations the time, money, and personnel necessary to achieve this goal are unavailable, but unless judges have had extensive training and experience, they should not be expected to make meaningful evaluations of quality, particularly of a descriptive nature. Neither should a laboratory panel, whether small or large, experienced or inexperienced, presume to predict consumer acceptance or preference. Preferences of a laboratory group are representative only of a limited and unknown portion of the consuming public. This concept is discussed in considerable detail in Chapter 9.

II. Panel Selection and Testing Environment

Systematic analysis of the sensory properties of foods involves the use of human subjects in a laboratory environment. The sensitivity and reproducibility of the analytical tool (in this case, the judge) greatly influence the direction and validity of the results. The environment under which the judgments are obtained also influences the data. Of additional importance are the time and labor and the supplies and equipment involved, for these factors materially control the cost of sensory analyses. We agree with Foster (1954) that more emphasis must be placed on controlling physical and psychological influences in sensory testing of foods. Unfortunately, the data available for a wide variety of food types are not adequate for the determination of the optimum ranges for all variables.

A. PANEL SELECTION

There is considerable controversy in the literature on the value of a sensory panel that has been selected and trained. Much of the confusion has arisen because discrimination or difference tests have not been distinguished from quality or consumer types of studies. In some cases a failure to find differences between trained and untrained panels in ability to discriminate has had its origin in methodological or statistical deficiencies. Tarver and Ellis (1961) believe the following considerations are important in selecting judges for flavor-difference tests: (1) precision or inherent ability to duplicate a difference judgment; (2) reliability or absence of bias in detecting a flavor difference; and (3) a tolerance level or inherent sensitivity to a particular flavor difference. According to Kramer *et al.* (1961), if the simulation of consumer reaction is the sole aim, a trained panel is not needed and should be avoided. In some cases it may be important to select individuals who are superior in their ability to detect differences. It is difficult, if not impossible, with our present lack of knowledge of consumer response, to select panels that will show good agreement with consumer evaluation. The problem seems to be our inability to define the difference and to train the panel to recognize the difference. Furthermore, the consumer uses many criteria other than sensory in evaluating foods.

Various procedures, based on intuition, rational judgment, or experimentation, have been applied in selecting people whose performance in sensory tests will be superior to that of an unselected population (Dawson *et al.,* 1963). These methods have been tested with varying degrees of success. One major problem is the amount of pretesting work required to establish reliable selection. A further difficulty may be an experimenter's inability to specify accurately the nature of the panel member's task. "Quickie" methods of panel selection, based upon only a few tests, have generally not been very satisfactory. On the other hand, although the tedious process of selecting subjects on the basis of sensitivity to the basic tastes is often recommended, the method is of doubtful value (Mackey and Jones, 1954; Peryam, 1958).

Since randomly selected and untrained individuals are variable in their judgments, large panels are needed for results that are stable and sensitive. By selecting the most stable and sensitive members and training them, one might expect to obtain a small but efficient panel. Selection is important since individuals differ considerably in sensitivity, interest, motivation, and ability to judge differences. Discriminatory skill need not be general; a good wine taster may not be a good judge of chocolates. Girardot *et al.* (1952) found that candidates who did well on some products often did poorly on others. Seldom is a judge equally proficient in testing all qualities and all flavors of foods. The skill of a connoisseur has been attributed to knowledge of what signs to look for and how to interpret them rather than to increased sensitivity to stimuli (Metzner, 1943). An ability or aptitude for flavor assessment could conceivably vary in three ways: between individuals, between products, and at different times for the same individuals and products (see Coppock *et al.*, 1952; Harvey, 1953). Thus it is evident that a general-purpose panel will be less useful than a specific panel selected for the product and method being tested. A general-purpose panel could be used for gross screening, however, when precision must be sacrificed to save time and expense. A sensory panel should be considered as a tool, and, as such, it can be compared to suitable chemical methods (Lowe and Stewart, 1947). Certain methods and tools may be used to show gross differences, but, as the measurements needed become more refined and precise, the methods and tools required for accurate sensory testing become more sensitive.

Moser *et al.* (1950) considered that selection and training of judges on the basis of sensitivities and consistencies are of extreme importance in evaluating edible oils. In selecting panels, those investigators used a double elimination test (see Chapter 6, Section II,C) based on acuity in oil evaluation. In scoring bitterness in orange juice, Coote (1956) illustrated the necessity of careful training and selection of panels for estimating the degree of bitterness. For beer-tasting tests, Helm and Trolle (1946) selected 20 out of 90 prospective judges. These 20 had the highest percentages of correct selections in triangle tests and were considered to compose a far more suitable taste panel than the original group. Kirkpatrick *et al.* (1957) showed the importance of panel selection for evaluation of milk and biscuits.

Any method of selection should include a preliminary training period designed to acquaint the tasters with the quality factors involved in the product to be tested. This should be followed by a blind test designed to show the individual's relative perception and discrimination (Harrison and Elder, 1950).

B. Screening

Most investigators employ some type of screening process for selecting panel members, including specific tests based on: (1) discriminating differences between solutions or substances of known chemical composition; (2) ability to recognize flavors or odors; (3) performance in comparison with other panel members; and (4) ability to discriminate differences in samples to be used later in the test. The pertinent question is the extent to which selection devices are reflected in superior performance in actual tests.

Kramer *et al.* (1961) reported that a single screening was insufficient for selecting panel members of continued superior ability in detecting flavor differences. After a first screening of 28 candidates, the 12 who performed best originally did not perform more efficiently than the average of the original 28 candidates. A second screening resulted in a more efficient group. Further screening and training would undoubtedly have resulted in a still more efficient panel.

A general approach may be summarized, stepwise, as follows: (1) use as test materials the same product that will be tested later; (2) prepare tests to obtain variations in the product similar to those which will be met with in the actual experiment; (3) adjust the difficulties of the test so that the group as a whole will discriminate between samples but some individuals will fail; (4) use test forms similar to those to be employed later; (5) start with as large a group of candidates as is feasible and with a selection test that is operationally simple if more than one stage is required; (6) screen on the basis of relative achievement, continuing until a top-ranking group of the size desired may be reliably selected; and (7) at each stage reject those who are obviously inadequate, but retain more people than will be required for the panel. This procedure is not a routine task; it requires judgment by the experimenter, particularly as to the criteria of achievement and as to how much data are needed for valid selection. According to Girardot *et al.* (1952), the multiple-stage selection assumes a good positive correlation between skills, but it will not be perfect.

It is felt that a person with previous experience might utilize some of the skill he has developed from a knowledge of techniques. Furthermore, he may note and detect differences which are unheeded by the inexperienced judge. He can often describe the sensory impressions more fully and usually has a better understanding of the particular terminology employed.

It would, however, be impossible to test independently for all of the characteristics or skills which may determine achievement. Christie (1956) believes it is not necessary. Various factors underline a unitary skill and they may be separated analytically, but in any given sensory test most of them will operate together. Realistic test situations may be set up to include acts of discrimination and judgment such as will be used later in definite experiments. Such tests will give each relevant factor its proper weight, so relative performance will be an adequate criterion for selecting the most useful panel members.

For selecting judges, Krum (1955) and Baker (1962) suggested that candidates fill out a questionnaire covering the following items: experience, availability, age, sex, health, smoking habits, quantity of particular foods habitually consumed, food prejudices, and asthmatic, physiocardiac, and respiratory behavior. It is doubtful whether this information will be of great value; conclusive evidence against the influence of some of these factors on perception has been noted in Chapters 2 and 3. Baker's (1962) suggestion is interesting—that individuals with a physiocardiac or asthmatic condition might be useful for certain panels since they seem to have lower thresholds for air pollutants—but the psychic attitudes of such individuals might be so unfavorable as to interfere with the tests.

Krum (1955) wrote: "It is believed that sensory ability decreases with age and that preferences change also." Therefore, he indicated, panel members should be between the ages of 20 and 50. The limiting factors are lack of experience in younger people and loss of perceptual ability in the older group. Panel members should be in good health and not physically fatigued or worried. They should not be overly susceptible to mouth and sinus infections or have frequent head colds. Persons should be eliminated who are allergic to the materials to be tested. For convenience and more accurate judging, Krum would eliminate all who do not like or refuse to eat a particular product. According to Overman and Jerome (1948), the members of the panel are frequently selected for their interest or their availability rather than for the acuity of their senses of taste and smell. In too many studies we have to "make do" with the available subjects.

C. Sensitivity Tests

In this section we discuss the many procedures that have been employed. In general, the screening tests use discrimination between solutions of known chemical composition for taste, ability to recognize odors, on-the-job performance in comparison with experienced panel members, and ability to discriminate actual differences that will be found in the samples to be used later in the tests. The experimental situation will dictate which, if any, of these should be used.

For general panel selection we recommend that of the Quartermaster group as outlined by Girardot *et al.* (1952). In the first stage, candidates are eliminated primarily on the basis of lack of sensitivity to the sensory attributes involved, and to a lesser extent because of poor memory, slow recovery from stimulation, and failure to understand the test. In the second stage the screening is done on the basis of ability to establish and use stable subjective criteria. This double testing screens out those who will do poorly because of lack of motivation, but it does not identify in advance those who may lose interest during the course of a lengthy experiment.

Threshold tests have been used as a basis of screening by many workers. This procedure is seldom justified since there is little evidence that sensitivity to the primary tastes is related to ability to detect differences in foods. At most it is only a single factor in discriminatory ability. As King (1937) and Hopkins (1954) demonstrated, thresholds vary greatly between individuals and, except in extreme cases, no consistent relation can be demonstrated between taste acuity and palatability and judges' responses. Hall *et al.* (1959) determined the thresholds of candidates for taste and flavors on two different days, and selected those sensitive to the lowest concentrations who could duplicate their sensitivity. Hanson *et al.* (1959) used ability to detect full-strength and dilute chicken broth in selecting a panel for studying chicken flavor. A similar approach was used by Tarver *et al.* (1959), who determined for each judge a bitterness tolerance level—the recognition threshold for bitterness. Repeatability (or precision) must also be determined by standard-to-standard comparison. Hall *et al.* (1959), using that procedure, found that success in distinguishing the odd sample in triangular testing of beers showed a good correlation with the bitterness tolerance level.

Mackey and Jones (1954) tested 22 individuals to determine thresholds for primary tastes in water solutions and their ability to arrange a series in the order of concentration. Also tested was their ability to arrange, in proper order, applesauce, pumpkin, and mayonnaise containing different levels of these same taste constituents. Both the water solutions and foods could be so arranged—but the ability to arrange one properly was not highly correlated with the ability to arrange the other properly. Further, a high sensitivity did not correlate significantly with ability to arrange foods in order of concentration of taste substances. The variability among the judges was high. This experiment should be repeated.

Similar conclusions were reached by King (1937), who found no correlation between excellence in judging pure solutions and ability to rate correctly samples of bread containing various quantities of sodium chloride, sucrose, lactic acid, and caffeine. He nevertheless suggested that the ability to identify the basic tastes at low concentration was valuable. Hopkins (1946) found a low but significant correlation between judges' ratings and the actual salt content of beef. Moreover, Krum (1955) also proposed that preliminary selection be based on sensitivity to the four primary tastes. From the results of such tests he would eliminate those who had low sensitivity. Knowles and Johnson (1941) classified judges on the basis of their sensitivity to the primary tastes but found no correlation between ability to identify the primary tastes and experience in judging foods. See also repeatability estimates of Sawyer *et al.* (1962).

Various selection tests were given to prospective panel members by Pfaffmann and Schlosberg (1952–1953), including: (1) a questionnaire designed to reveal habits, preferences, and interest in eating and drinking; (2) an odor recognition test consisting of 20 common odorous substances thought to measure interest in odors; (3) a low-odor recognition series approaching a threshold test; (4) a graded series of solutions to determine thresholds for the four primary tastes—salt, sweet, sour, and bitter; (5) use of the Elsberg blast-injection technique to determine threshold for oil of wintergreen, to detect gross departures from normal sensitivity, as from nasal obstruction; and (6) sixteen duo-trio tests on mayonnaise and thirty on an orange drink. The results failed to reveal clear evidence that any item on the questionnaire predicted performance in flavor discrimination. Selection scores on the battery of analytical tests described did not correlate well with the performance scores. The reliability coefficient (between test and retest) and the validity coefficient were very low.* Most noticeable was the rather unstable performance of the panel members for short-term work. No general clear-cut panel ability was evident, so that prediction of a given individual's later performance would be difficult. Those workers believe, however, that prediction of the relative ability of panel members is possible. They reported that, with the three panels tested, the score on a single discrimination session indicated who would do better on later tests: those who scored in the upper half of the total group. It is a gross measure, however, and its use might eliminate some persons who would be good performers.

---

* The words reliability and validity along with such terms as precision, accuracy, and relevance are often interpreted differently. A method of estimation which, on the average, gives the true value is called an unbiased method. Unbiased estimates are sometimes termed accurate or valid. The precision of a method refers to repeatability and is the ability of the method to produce estimates which are very close together (even if it is a biased method and is not actually measuring the true value). Thus accuracy (or validity) is related to lack of bias and precision to standard deviation.

Discrimination was measured by Morse (1954) in terms of the degree to which the individual or group can distinguish between two stimuli and communicate this distinction to investigators. Factors which affect discriminability are: (1) the individual's taste acuity at the time of the test; (2) the consistency or stability of this ability with time; (3) the distance or difference between the stimuli; (4) the design of the test, especially of its complexity and the premium it places on memory; and (5) the method of communicating the results from the subject to the investigator. Any conclusion on discriminability depends on the arbitrary standard set by the investigator of the number of correct versus incorrect judgments required. Morse required 10 correct judgments out of 12 trials for a judge to be declared discriminative, reasoning that such a ratio of judgments between equal stimuli could have occurred by chance in slightly less than 5% of similar repeated trials.

Many workers have used paired or duo-trio (Chapter 7, Section VI,A) tests for panel selection. Tarver *et al.* (1959) used a paired test for establishing bitterness tolerance levels. Byer and Gray (1953) used paired tests with beer samples, and applied x^2 for determining the consistency of the judges. In selecting a panel for coffee testing, Harrison and Elder (1950) presented candidates with six cups of coffee consisting of three sets of pairs over a period of 20 to 30 days. The candidates were then ranked in decreasing order of their successes in making the correct pairings, and only the top half was used. Bliss (1960) used replicate paired tests with each subject. Stability of preferences was used as the selection criterion. Lockhart (1951) noted that any of the binomial systems provides a means for rapidly selecting panel members whose sensitivities can be described in terms of probability levels. These systems can also be used for checking the sensitivities of the panel on a day-to-day or week-to-week basis.

The most common method of choice has been the triangle test (Chapter 7, Section VI,B). It was first used by Bengtsson and Helm (1946) and Helm and Trolle (1946) for selecting beer tasting panels. Beers of known differences were used first in simple tests and later in more difficult tests. Only the most sensitive individuals were used. Data from the tests were used to check panel performance. The Quartermaster group (Girardot *et al.*, 1952) used a triangle test in the first stage of selection. Simple tests were used first, but later the tests were of increasing difficulty. The judges were ranked on the basis of their percentages of correct judgments. All judges took about the same number of tests at each level of difficulty. Only the ranking near the cut-off point is critical.

Bradley (1955) recommended repeated triangle tests for selecting judges. Sequential methods (Chapter IV, Section III) can be recommended because of their efficiency and because they focus attention on the risk of accepting poor judges or of rejecting good ones. Using both paired and triangle tests, Schlosberg et al. (1954) found that a judge's relative performance during the first two days of testing "had a fair predictive value for his relative over-all performance during the following 20-day period." This was not true when preference for milk was measured, but that result will be discussed later (Chapter 6, Section II,F). Their experience was that ability for one panel did not carry over to another. Hening (1948) used the triangle test to select panels for distinguishing differences in flavor resulting from time and temperature of storage of various products. Amerine (1948) recommended it for selecting wine panels. Krum (1955) likewise used it, noting that each candidate should take the same number of tests. The cut-off point was determined by the number of panel members required and the precision required by the problem. Moser et al. (1950) found one experienced judge with an excellent record in testing oil but a poor record in detecting diacetyl by triangle tests. They attributed this disparity to confusion on the part of the subject. However, this judge may have been insensitive to low concentrations of diacetyl, even though reputed to have a keen sense of smell.

Dawson et al. (1963) showed that for taste thresholds the paired comparison resulted in lower thresholds than the triangular, and that the single-sample procedure was the least sensitive.

Various methods of scoring have been used in selecting panels. Hedonic scores were used by Girardot et al. (1952). Similar procedures have been used or reviewed by Sharp et al. (1936), Trout and Sharp (1937), Boggs and Hanson (1949), Harrison et al. (1954), and others. Used to evaluate performance have been average deviations between duplicate scores, the deviation from the score of a control sample introduced in series, or the deviations of scores between first and second tastings (with the samples coded and presented in different orders). Although these measure individual reproducibility, they do not relate reproducibility with one sample to ability to find differences between unlike samples. To rectify this, the correlation coefficient between the first score and duplicate scores for a series of samples of varying quality may be used. Bennett et al. (1956) used the standard error of the means to measure ability to reproduce judgments. Hopkins (1946) calculated both correlation coefficients and regression equations to relate each judge's assessment to the average of the panel. A range of sensitivity was demonstrable and the suitability of individuals for tests could be evaluated. The correlation coefficients were much higher for biscuits than for dried milk. Moser et al. (1950) likewise calculated the correlation coefficient and regression equation. Used for selection was the standard error of regression of the individual's scores with the average of the whole panel.

Overman and Jerome (1948) used scores and applied two tests: a comparison of the average range of a judge's scores and a comparison of the number of times a judge duplicated his score. The first, being rapid and easy to understand, was preferred for preliminary evaluation. Deviation from the mean was the statistical measure employed. A high deviation from an individual's mean indicates inability to duplicate judgments or marked changeability of opinion during the tests. A low deviation from his own mean indicates either a high degree of reproducibility or a lack of critical discrimination (as when all scores are very high or very low). Since the method of deviation from the mean may obscure discrimination, Overman and Jerome preferred analysis of variance for determining the consistency of the judges and their ability to discriminate. The variance ratios (F values) were used as an index of a judge's ability to duplicate his scores and can be used as an appropriate measure of the consistency of each judge. If members of the panel show marked differences in individual-error variances it is advisable to test the panel for homogeneity of variances before comparing individuals. Krum (1955), for his panel, also selected judges with highly significant F ratios (Chapter 10, Section V,A). Girardot *et al.* (1952) employed analysis of variance and demonstrated the superiority of the selected panels. Wiley *et al.* (1957) screened judges on the basis of F ratios. Those with a statistical significance at odds of 9:1 were retained. They were then retested, and only those were selected whose F values indicated significance at odds of 19:1. The quick method of "range ratio" of Tukey (1951) was also employed. In this method, if the ratio of (range among treatment) to (range within treatments $\times$ factor) = 1, then the difference is significant. (The factor depends on the number of treatments and is obtained from a table.)

Sawyer (1958) and Sawyer *et al.* (1962) based panel selection on repeatability—the interclass correlation of repeated measurements (a measure of the constancy of repeated observations by a given judge). This is a point estimate, and is estimated directly from variance analysis of discrimination test data. The proportion of judges whose sensitivity satisfies established specifications can be predicted. In these studies the average repeatability of performance was equivalent to or greater than the repeatability predicted by analysis of variance. "Thus, estimates of intraclass correlation appear to provide a reliable basis for predictions in the selection of panels" (Sawyer *et al.*, 1962).

Simple ranking of judges' scores often permits relative differentiation

of individual capabilities but does not ensure a specified level of pro-
ficiency.

Kramer (1955) recommended choosing judges on the basis of their
ability to detect differences at a given probability level. His procedure
involved matching concentrations, and the tables he published should be
useful whether or not duplicates are available for all samples.

Probably because of their extensive use in industry, control charts
have been used in selecting panels or maintaining level of performance.
A control chart is a statistical device used principally for the study and
control of repetitive processes. Such charts are based on the theory that
variations due to chance occur in a random pattern and that the frequencies approach those of the binomial distribution. To see whether a
process is out of control, past data are plotted on a control chart. If the
data conform to a pattern of random variation within the control limits,
the process will be judged as being in control. Reliability is indicated by
the narrowness of spread between control limits. Since pre-established
standards can be set up, the control chart also measures the validity of
the judge's results. For basic data, see Feigenbaum (1951) and Duncan
(1959).

Control charts have been recommended by Marcuse (1945, 1947),
Moser *et al.* (1950), Harrison and Elder (1950), Krum (1955), Coote
(1956), and Tarver and Ellis (1961). With them, not only an individual's
performance but that of an entire panel can be held to a given precision.

Harrison *et al.* (1954) defined the efficiency of a panel in terms of the
probability of the panel's acceptance of definite differences in the
samples. To eliminate the number of correct selections through chance
alone, the scores were corrected with the following formula:

$$S = \frac{100(R - C)}{100 - C}$$

where S is the percent score corrected for chance expectation, R the raw
percent score, and C the percent score expected by chance.

More elaborate mathematical procedures may be used in certain
cases: multiple-factor analysis, item analysis, discriminate functions,
product-moment correlation coefficients (Filipello, 1957), etc.

In most cases a simple test using some binomial procedure may be
used to eliminate insensitive judges. See Amerine *et al.* (1959) for detailed procedures used for wine panels. Analysis of variance or some
sequential procedure should be used for more complex situations or to
maintain the panel at some desired level of performance.

Variation among 30 judges in scoring scrambled eggs containing various amounts of added primary-taste compounds was described by Hop-

kins (1946). Significant variation ($p = 0.01$) was observed among judges. Some statistically significant discrimination among groups of samples containing different test substances and among concentrations of these substances was also found. Individual scores became progressively more erratic as quality deteriorated. Hopkins concluded that no consistent relation between taste acuity alone and palatability judgments should be anticipated. Quality evaluation includes visual, olfactory, and tactile sensations as well as taste sensitivity, and is further conditioned by the scoring methods used and the experience and frame of reference of the judges (see also Chapter 8).

Sensitivity to taste or odor appears to be only one factor influencing discrimination. In most cases, elaborate tests based on acuity seem unnecessary since absolute sensitivity to the basic tastes is not closely related to perceptual skills.

D. Panel Size

The number of judges needed in a given experiment will vary according to the variabilities of the individuals and of the product. A preliminary experiment will give information from which can be calculated the number of judges necessary to secure a given level of statistical significance. As quality decreases, variability among judges increases and panel size must be increased to obtain differences which are statistically significant (Boggs and Hanson, 1949; Kefford and Christie, 1960). A good example of this is found in work by Hopkins (1946, 1947) with biscuits, dried eggs, butter, dried milk, and bacon. He noted that, at low levels of acceptability, discrimination was very erratic, so that more judges were required for significance in results. Not enough information is available, however, on the interrelationship of acceptability and discrimination. In incomplete-block studies, Hanson *et al.* (1951) found, surprisingly, that the error of the panel means was greater for samples of intermediate quality.

Of course, the panels must be much larger in preference testing than in difference testing. Hopkins (1947) concluded that, with bacon varying in degree of saltiness, panels of 35 judges were necessary to discriminate sensory differences of 5% with intrapanel comparisons. For interpanel comparisons, 62 judges would be necessary. Girardot *et al.* (1952) preferred panels of 30 to 90 in food-development studies. Bengtsson and Helm (1946) preferred large panels (50 to 100) in testing for differences which might influence future work. For routine control, 10 to 30 judges were believed adequate. Krum (1955) found panels of 10 to 30 sufficient. When only three or four individuals were available he believed it possible to repeat the tests enough times to get a suitable number of results.

However, one judge tested 30 times is different from 10 judges tested three times or 30 judges tested once (Jones, 1958). Much classical theory is still based on the assumption that "the experiment may be repeated by the same judge or carried out by several judges independently" (see Trawinski and David, 1963). Judges vary greatly, however, and Baker et al. (1954, 1958, 1960), Mrak et al. (1959), and Ough and Baker (1961, 1964) have shown that the wide variation in response of individuals must be considered in evaluating sensory tests. Similar results are suggested by Duffendack (1954). Using replication of a small panel of judges to represent a larger group is valid only if one assumes homogeneous variance and similar preference patterns for all judges. The assumption appears to be more risky than is generally conceded.

The problem of individual variability is illustrated in the paper of Berg et al. (1955b). Here the minimum higher detectable concentration C_1, and the concentration being tested, C_0, were related: $C_1 = C_0 K + A$ where K was a constant and A the zero threshold. They suggested that K was free from panel characteristics. If plots were made for individuals, variations in both slopes and intercepts may have appeared. Obviously panels selected from homogeneous populations may have similar K values but if the panel is weighted heavily with individuals extreme in one direction and other panels with individuals extreme in another direction the curves for the two panels could vary. The point is that individuals are the ultimate units, not panels. Clements et al. (1954) also presented evidence that for orange juice there are at least two population groups. Mean scores are not meaningful in such situations.

Cartwright et al. (1952) noted that panel size is often limited by the costs of materials and training and the availability of acceptable panel members.

In any case, many workers favor fewer panel members. Peryam (1958) recommended difference panels with 16 to 20 judges. Brandt and Hutchinson (1956), Kefford and Christie (1960), Sheppard (1953), and Wiley et al. (1957) used relatively small panels of 3 to 12 members.

We agree with Boggs and Hanson (1949) that the panel should be large enough to counteract unusual variability or other factors which might influence day-to-day comparisons. However, small, highly sensitive panels would usually give more reliable results than large, less sensitive groups, assuming that repetitive ability is equal in each case. Harrison and Elder (1950) are probably correct that results obtained from some small panels are suspect, especially if the data have not been carefully analyzed statistically. For difference testing with trained laboratory judges, the panel should, in most cases, consist of 10 to 20 individuals, with at least three or four replications per judge per treatment. In order to achieve greater control of the panel, it is possible that 10 judges are better than 20. "Expert" panels of 5 to 10 are probably satisfactory. Consumer-type tests require at least 80 participants, and may need hundreds or thousands, depending on the problem (see Chapter 9).

In a guide prepared by the Committee on Sensory Evaluation of the Institute of Food Technologists (Anonymous, 1964) recommendations are given on the number of trained (3–10), semitrained (8–25), or untrained (80+) judges for various types of sensory methods.

E. Factors Influencing Sensitivity

Good health may be important to sensitivity since pain or discomfort interfere with judgment. However, Jones (1958) believed that extreme fatigue or even poor general physical conditions had little effect on sensory sensitivity.

Reports on the influence of age on acuity of sensory perception have been contradictory and/or incomplete (Boggs and Hanson, 1949). Harding and Wadley (1948) found that 23 high school students, 15 to 18 years old, were better able to evaluate orange juices than 39 adults, 19 to 70 years old (average 38). The population appears too small for conclusive results. Cooper *et al.* (1959) reported that sensitivity to basic tastes declined with age, especially after the late fifties (see Chapter 2, Section VIII,B). Helm and Trolle (1946) tested 90 individuals and found maximum sensitivity to differences in beer in the group aged 30 to 39 years. Bengtsson and Helm (1946) also found that acuity to differences in beer quality was optimum in a group aged 30 to 40 years. We believe that training, size of panel, type of product, and differences tested, as well as other factors, may have influenced those results. Morse (1954), for example, was able to illustrate discrimination ability and preference in citrus juices with children only 4 to 5 years old. Gustafson (1953) tested 28 pre-school children and found difficulty in securing discrimination between orange juices of similar flavor but was able to secure significant preference for orange over grapefruit juice, and between well flavored and insipid orange juices. Harvey (1953) believes that odor sensitivity is more strongly developed in adults than in children. Possibly memory and learning are responsible rather than sensitivity *per se.* Nevertheless, older, more experienced judges might be more valuable in some cases. Using only small numbers of judges, Bennett *et al.* (1956) reported that all age groups responded equally well to training. We agree with Bengtsson and Helm (1946) that the criterion of selection should be ability, not the age of the individual judge.

Pangborn (1959), in critical studies on taste, found that four college females had lower thresholds than four college males. Jones (1958) believed that the menstrual cycle might affect sensitivity, but admitted that more research was needed (see Schneider and Wolf, 1955). Bradley *et al.* (1954) reported that the preference ratings of women as a group did not differ significantly from those of men. Women's responses extended over a greater range than those of men, but individual women tended to be more consistent in their ratings than individual men. Studies such as this should be extended, not as a method of selecting the panel but as an indication of whom to select as prospective panel members so as to decrease the amount of testing required to secure a panel of adequate size.

Nonsmokers and smokers have been generally found equally useful for panels, according to Knowles and Johnson (1941) and Harvey (1953) (see, however, Chapter 2, Section VIII,C). Helm and Trolle (1946), Harding and Wadley (1948), Moser *et al.* (1950), Schlosberg *et al.* (1954), and Cooper *et al.* (1959) observed no significant differences in taste sensitivity between the two groups. Bennett *et al.* (1956) found no differences between the two in the effects of training. Boggs and Hanson (1949) found no conclusive evidence that smoking influences the ability of judges. However, Bengtsson and Helm (1946) believed it inadvisable for smokers to smoke within 1–2 hours of a test, and Kefford and Christie (1960) requested judges not to smoke for 30 minutes before judging. Jones (1958) also recommended against smoking.

The psychological effect on nonsmokers of smoke odors in the room does not appear to have been adequately investigated. It is recommended that participants on odor panels refrain from smoking for at least 30 minutes prior to the test so that they contribute no tobacco odor to the test environment. In addition, smokers' hands should be free of tobacco odors. Cosmetics may have similar interference effects.

There are a variety of psychological factors which may influence the sensitivity of judges (Chapter 5). Even after long training and experience, the possibility of bias must be considered, according to Kefford and Christie (1960). This is especially true if the investigator and/or his technicians participate as judges. Emotional factors appear to affect the ability of judges to concentrate, and thus may reduce their accuracy (Boggs and Hanson, 1949), but no reports are available on specific tests with foods.

Important factors in successful judging are interest, motivation, knowledge and comparison of results, adjustment to the test situation, memory, etc. Many investigators emphasize the importance of interest; see, for example, Moser *et al.* (1950), Girardot *et al.* (1952), and Peryam (1958). Participants who are bored are believed to have less repetitive ability than participants who are interested in the study. Although there do not seem to be any critical experiments in this matter, there appears to be no doubt that interest in the study is highly desirable. Methods of maintaining interest have therefore been of considerable importance to workers in this field.

It is generally agreed that panel members should be given as much information as possible on the purpose and necessity of the investigation (see Bengtsson and Helm, 1946; Krum, 1955; Helm and Trolle, 1946; Jones, 1958; Tompkins and Pratt, 1959). However, when such information might influence the subject's responses it must be withheld (Jones, 1958). An example of the undesirable influence of prior knowledge was detected by Sinsheimer (1959). In comparing an unknown with a range of concentrations the panel learned that two samples would be of lower intensity than the unknown, two of greater intensity, and one of an intensity approaching that of the unknown. The procedure had to be abandoned. Knowledge of the possible length of the experiment was considered desirable by Christie (1956).

Pfaffmann *et al.* (1954) noted the ways in which knowledge of one's results might improve performance. In addition to improvement through learning, knowledge could act as a reinforcer, verifying the cues for correct judgments and eliminating false cues. Knowledge might also result from an increase in general motivation in the test situation. Pfaffmann *et al.* concluded, "A subject who knows that he will find out, as the experimental session progresses, how well he is doing may be more motivated to do well from the start than one who knows he will get no information." A possible motivation resides in the competition that may result if all panel members know each other's results (see Helm and Trolle, 1946; Hanson *et al.*, 1951). In some situations where the level of discrimination of some judges is low, posting the results might be inadvisable. Both with experienced and inexperienced panels and with easy and difficult discriminations, Pfaffmann and co-workers found that discriminatory ability was significantly greater with knowledge of results than with no knowledge. The effect of this knowledge, a more significant level of discrimination, persisted even after this information was withheld. The improvement in performance is attributed to an increased motivational level rather than to greater ease of learning to discriminate. In very complex situations where many variables are present, learning might be a factor. No tests seemed to have been made where discrimination was very poor for some judges compared to others and where knowledge of the results might presumably prove discouraging to those doing poorly in the tests.

It also appears that when no differences can be detected the judges may grow discouraged and lose interest. Judges apparently like to find differences.

Discussion as a means of maintaining interest may also be useful, according to Boggs and Hanson (1949), Bennett *et al.* (1956), and Kefford and Christie (1960). However, discussions that might influence future results through some bias should be avoided. It is especially difficult to maintain interest where the judges find no difference between samples, as for example in the early stages of storage experiments.

A reward system for maintaining interest is frequently recommended (Pfaffmann *et al.*, 1954; Jones, 1958). This may take the form of special pay, time off, special privileges, providing refreshments after panel sessions, etc. Use of laboratory or technical employees is commonly believed to ensure a certain interest, but this is by no means universally true. It is said that panel members should be interested in foods. Again, we know of no critical experiments that would substantiate the statement, but the opposite situation should be tested.

Adjustment to the test situation appears to vary among judges, though we know of no experiment where this variation has been separated from differences in rate of learning. Filipello (1957) reported that when judges knew that five grades of wine were involved they showed a significant tendency to grade five unknowns on this basis even though they knew that the designs applied were being randomized. Sawyer (1958) and Sawyer *et al.* (1962) found a variation among judges relative to taste design: some did better with complex 9-sample arrangements, whereas others did better with simple designs. Filipello (1957) also reported that results with both experienced and inexperienced panels were significantly better when four samples were served in two incomplete blocks of three samples than when served in one set containing all four. He suggested that this may be a psychological factor where fatigue is reduced by serving the smaller blocks—even though the total number of samples is increased. This phenomenon was observed when the samples were graded on a 1- to 6-point scale but not when a 1- to 20-point scale was used. Harper (1949) also suggested that personal characteristics and temperamental differences may be important.

Memory (a form of retained learning) is important, if only in recognizing clues, but no experiments relating it to discriminatory sensory performance with foods have come to our attention. Memory may be more important in quality evaluations than in simple difference tests. For the importance of memory in judging wines, see Amerine *et al.* (1959).

F. TRAINING

Training should be distinguished from experience, according to Harper (1955). He defined training as the "steps which may be taken deliberately to increase the effectiveness and the rate at which the individual assimilates new knowledge or new techniques." Experience he considers to be the "cumulative effect of exposure to events or occurrences without any systematic attempt on the part of another person to focus attention upon what is most important." Harper stated that the "judgment of a properly trained person comes very near to the limiting errors of the physical measurement."

There is considerable controversy regarding the effect of training on sensory responses. In our opinion some of the confusion is due to differences in methods. In general we shall use "experienced" and "trained" interchangeably in this section (and likewise for "inexperienced" and "untrained"). However, the training of naive, inexperienced individuals may be different from the training of "expert," experienced judges. Pfaffmann *et al.* (1954) raised the question of how much training is simply familiarization with the laboratory type of situation. Training could be directed toward getting panel members to disregard their personal preferences, which should result in more objective decisions. It might also be directed toward securing recognition of small differences, or toward concentrating on obtaining more consistent results or toward a combination of these.

The effect of training may be due to a selection process or to improvement in familiarity with the product, according to Peryam (1958). Crocker (1945) believed that persons of ordinary sensitivity might become satisfactory in flavor discrimination tests if adequately trained, not through increased sensitivity but merely through the influence the training exerts on rapid and accurate description of flavor impressions. Moser *et al.* (1950) found that a planned training program could make most individuals acceptable panel members for testing edible oils. Krum (1955) used the same products and systems of evaluation in training as in the actual test. He believed in using samples illustrating various flavor components at various levels. Boggs and Hanson (1949) also favored using a series of samples differing in all the characteristics likely to be encountered in the actual investigation. Boggs and Hanson stated the amount of training may vary with the commodity, e.g., evaluation of tenderness of meat will require less training than judging milk flavors. Cartwright *et al.* (1952) also noted the differences between commodities in the amount of training required and that there was considerable transfer of ability and interest from one panel to another. Sawyer (1958), however, found that additional training was sometimes needed when the test method was changed.

One of the important aims of training is greater homogeneity of response. Overman and Jerome (1948) used Bartlett's test (Chapter 10, Section V,C) to determine the homogeneity of error variances. In their case the test showed that the variances of the panel were heterogeneous, that is, the judges were not homogeneous as far as consistency was concerned. Bennett *et al.* (1956) noted that the very process of selection results in a certain amount of training. The number of samples used per session seemed to affect efficiency less in a small trained panel than in a larger untrained panel (Kramer *et al.*, 1961).

It is universally recognized that sensitivity to basic tastes and odors increases with training, but whether this is due to increased sensitivity or to increased ability to recognize differences is not known. Cartwright *et al.* (1952) definitely believe that the purpose of training is to improve sensory acuity. Berg *et al.* (1955a) found experienced wine tasters more sensitive than inexperienced in recognition thresholds and difference thresholds for astringency (tannin), body (glycerol), and certain odors (acetic acid, acetaldehyde, and ethyl acetate), but there was no difference between the groups with regard to alcohol, acids, or sugars. Pangborn (1959) reported that the thresholds for the four primary taste qualities in aqueous solutions were lowered during a 2-week period of training. Degree of improvement varied greatly. Hall *et al.* (1959) noted that training of selected panels was necessary for evaluation of intensity of off-flavor so that all panel members would judge on the same basis. When the four basic tastes were incorporated in beer, Hopkins (1954) obtained much greater discrimination in all cases after the judges had undergone 12 days of training.

The importance of training in securing agreement on the meaning of descriptive terms is clearly evident in work of Ehrenberg and Shewan (1953) and Shewan *et al.* (1953). They also showed that training was effective in assigning scores to the descriptive terms. Training reduced differences in scoring levels between panel members and the error variances. They noted, however, that even with the best training the panel may occasionally "go out of control," and therefore recommended the use of control samples or standards. According to Bennett *et al.* (1956), when fresh and rancid beef were mixed in varying portions, scoring was inconsistent for the first week. Two weeks of training (with discussion) increased the differences between mean ratings, and also lowered sample variance. Degree of improvement in accuracy varied with the individual, but was greatest with the least rancid and most rancid samples. If no training period is used, Sheppard (1953) indicated, the first samples tend to be rated "average" whether they are or not (see also Chapter 5, Section III).

Training also helps judges learn to compare flavors and flavor strengths in spite of a time lag between samples. Amerine (1948) emphasized this in judging wines, as did Bengtsson and Helm (1946) and

Byer and Gray (1953) for beer. The latter particularly emphasized the importance of training in establishing uniform rating standards and in developing the degree of acuity desired for the panel. Cartwright *et al.* (1952) also emphasized that the purpose of training is not only to increase sensory acuity but to make certain that all members of the panel have substantially uniform understanding of the particular properties being evaluated, the criteria and the system of evaluation, the relationship between quality or intensity of sensory stimuli, the descriptive and numerical terms used in the rating system, and the precautions necessary to minimize the effects of irrelevant factors on the rating of each property. With descriptive sensory analysis, training is an integral part of the method (Cairncross and Sjöström, 1950). Judges may be trained for particular tasks: applying acuity to basic tastes or odors, making accurate descriptions, or improving scoring results. It may also be considered from the standpoint of the commodities to be tested.

Some effects of training with specific commodities will now be summarized. With edible oils, Moser *et al.* (1950) used 3 weeks of training but felt that a longer time would have been desirable. For judging sulfited mashed potatoes, Boggs and Ward (1950) trained their panels to recognize sulfite odor in sodium bisulfite solutions and then selected the best judges on the basis of reconstituted dehydrated mashed potatoes containing sulfite. With green beans, Kramer *et al.* (1961) found it advisable, because of great variation between panels, to use fewer well-trained judges with adequate replication. A similar result was reported by Murphy *et al.* (1957), who found that the number of tests required to detect differences between varieties of strawberries was 34 with eight trained judges, but was 234 with panelists selected at random. In meat testing, Naumann *et al.* (1957) preferred experienced (faculty) judges for tests of short duration, particularly those of an exploratory nature. For an extended series of tests, student panels seemed to exhibit less fatigue, possibly because of superior motivation. The explanation might be that even though students gain a great deal of training during an extended period of tests they may not be too sophisticated to place undue value on free samples of meat. Whether fatigue or the normal distractions of a busy faculty member interfered with the performance of the faculty group is not known.

With beer, Helm and Trolle (1946) found that performance in the last 12 triangles compared to the first 12 was better for experienced judges than for inexperienced judges. This result needs to be reinvestigated. The experienced judges obtained considerably better results than the inexperienced. The two groups showed varying reactions to different beers. Similar results have been obtained with wine by Amerine (1948), Baker and Amerine (1953), and Filipello (1957), who found experienced wine judges to be significantly better than inexperienced.

There are some reports that training is of little or no value in certain situations. Raffensperger and Pilgrim (1956) found that subjects with no prior experience in difference testing discriminated as well as experienced judges when appropriate instructions were given. Peryam (1958) noted the possibility that in a given instance only a small amount of training may be required. Kamen *et al.* (1960) believe that training and rigorous selection may not be worth the effort. King (1937) obtained as accurate results with 96 untrained judges as with 16 experienced judges.

In some cases training does not eliminate variability. Scott-Blair *et al.* (1941) found that experts had difficulty in judging the firmness of cheese, probably because they were influenced by other characteristics that they know to be important. Hopkins (1954) found that training did not eliminate individual differences in the sensitivity of milk judges. Bohren and Jordan (1953) were unable to train 20 girls to be satisfactory judges of dried eggs. They believed that large unselected panels would be better than small trained panels, because of the economics of less training and because comparability would be greater between unselected panels in different locations. They also preferred untrained panels because it was easier to replace a panel member or to increase the number of panel members. Statistically we find this difficult to reconcile with other results. Precision should not be sacrificed for expediency.

Schlosberg *et al.* (1954), using a homogeneous group of college undergraduates, found that selection and a training program did not affect difference or preferences for five types of milk. This report has been criticized on the basis that college undergraduates are quite familiar with milk and it would not be expected that training would cause them to change greatly in acuity or preference. The chief implication of Schlosberg's experiment seems to be that short training periods are unlikely to improve panel performance much.

We believe that the best results in difference tests will be obtained by using the most sensitive judges, and that careful selection and thorough training should be employed to obtain such judges. Failure to find differences may be due to method of presentation of samples, to confusion in specifying the sensory quality, or to other factors. We particularly agree with Ehrenberg and Shewan (1953) and Shewan *et al.* (1953), who found training and selection to be essential for securing internal panel consistency. When using rating systems that lend themselves to analysis of variance, judges and replications should be included among the main effects to determine internal panel consistency (see

Chapter 10, Section VI,A). Dawson *et al.* (1963) summarized as follows: "Variability in panel performance can be decreased by selecting sensitive individuals and training and checking their performance." In many cases this seems to involve training the panel to ignore variables that are *believed* unimportant by the experimentor. For details of such analyses, see Chapter 10, particularly as regards the proper error term for testing experiments.

G. Environment

Control of environmental factors and samples is universally recognized as being of value in sensory work with foods. Lowe and Stewart (1947) indicated that interruptions and distractions should be avoided during testing. Regularity, quietness, comfortable surroundings, orderliness, and smoothness of presentation of samples were emphasized by Bengtsson and Helm (1946), Moser *et al.* (1950), and Jones (1958). A special room that controls as many variables as possible is universally recommended (Dawson and Harris, 1951; Dove, 1947; Boggs and Hanson, 1949; Moser *et al.*, 1950; Byer and Gray, 1953; and Christie, 1956). Bennett *et al.* (1956) emphasized that conditions in the laboratory must be uniform for the sake of comparable performance not only over time but from panel to panel and from product to product. Independence of tasters, is of course, necessary. Not only must the judges record their results independently, but judges leaving the tasting room should not communicate their impressions of the samples to those entering later, either verbally or by facial expressions. The influence of one opinion on the whole group is described by Foster *et al.* (1955). For this and other reasons, the use of individual booths for sensory testing is now nearly universal.

Among the environmental factors to be considered are air conditioning, lighting, seating comfort, and distractions.

Important among the air-conditioning factors may be temperature, humidity, rate of flow, and air purity. Helm and Trolle (1946) used a room at 20°C, whereas Hopkins (1954) used 24.4°C and a relative humidity of 62%. At General Foods, Laue *et al.* (1954) specified proper control of ventilation and temperature. Boggs and Hanson (1949) further specified odor-free air. Where odors are to be manipulated, a special room, such as that of Deininger and McKinley (1954), would have to be provided. Certainly food preparation and laboratory odors should be absent (Byer and Gray, 1953). Smoking and cosmetic odors must be avoided in the test room.

Relative to illumination and color of the testing room, Dove (1947) and Jones (1958) preferred a neutral-gray background and adequate light. Boggs and Hanson (1949) quoted Eastmond that the light intensity should be 30–50 foot-candles at the table surface in the booth and should be diffused over an area so that several samples can be compared. The preferred light was similar in spectral character to that of a moderately overcast northern sky. Incandescent lights with special blue glass filters are more satisfactory. Eastmond specified a neutral-gray with a Munsell value of N/7, which reflects about 40 to 45% of the light.

In some cases, colored illumination has been used to mask differences in the color of samples (Dove, 1947; Laue et al., 1954; Cartwright et al., 1952; Kefford and Christie, 1960). In our opinion, the influence of changing illumination and/or color in the testing booth in order to minimize color differences between samples has not been adequately studied.

Judges should be provided with comfortable seating, a receptacle for expectoration, water for oral rinsing, and adequate space for the samples and for the score card. The facilities should all be thoroughly clean, especially after each subject leaves. This is often neglected when the booths are in constant use. Some individuals may undergo a possible claustrophobia effect from working in small booths, but this has not been adequately studied. Enggaard and Jul (1958) specifically mention that booths give a "shut-in" feeling, and they prefer seats and desks along a wall, schoolroom fashion. A system is necessary for the judge to indicate to the experimenter when he is ready for the next sample—usually an electric switch that turns on a light on the experimenter's side.

The booth should be quiet. Boggs and Hanson (1949), Andross (1961), and Trout and Sharp (1937) found that distractions influenced difficult judgments more than easy ones. Using duo-trio presentation of beer, Mitchell (1957a,b) compared results when: (A) only one person was in the tasting room; (B) two were present at the same time; and (C) one or more of the tasters caused some noise. Percent correct responses differed significantly between A and C, between A and B, and between B and C. That between A and B is apparently due simply to knowledge that another person is present. That between B and C is probably due to noise. This type of test should be repeated with other foods. Guthrie (1958) considered a quiet environment essential in judging dairy products. He also noted that the judges should not feel rushed.

H. TIME OF DAY

Among the most controversial questions in the sensory testing of food is the appropriate time of day for testing. Among those who found no effect or disregarded it were Helm and Trolle (1946), with beer; Baten (1946), with apples; and Overman and Jerome (1948), with various products. Bengtsson and Helm (1946) suggested that the tests be arranged for the time of day when the subjects felt best. This might be impractical in some situations. Byer and Gray (1953) recommended testing beer at least one hour after a meal. Kefford and Christie (1960) scheduled their tests at 10:15 and 11:45 A.M. and at 3:00 P.M. For sweet materials Harper (1949) preferred the period from 10:00 to 10.30 A.M. because the influence of breakfast had passed but the subject was not yet hungry enough to eat the samples. Christie (1956) recommended midmorning and midafternoon. She (1962) later noted that meat tasters seemed to perform better when slightly hungry. For a critical appraisal of Goetzl's work on thresholds and appetite, see Chapter 3, Sections IX and X.

The most extensive test was that of Mitchell (1957a,b). A group of seven subjects tested beers by a duo-trio system every 15 minutes during an 8-hour day. The results of the fourth, fifth, and sixth hours were significantly superior to all others, and the first and last hours gave the poorest results. Mitchell theorized that the subject is unable to concentrate in the early morning, is not yet fatigued in the middle of the day, and again becomes unable to concentrate toward the end of the day. Although eating may dull sensory receptiveness, physical and psychological factors seem to counteract this. Mitchell himself noted that the results do not necessarily mean that the middle of the day would be the best time when only one test was given. These results were obtained when an entire series of samples were being tested, and the results represent a combination of warming-up and fatigue effects.

As a corollary of this study, Mitchell tested subjects throughout the week. The level of performance was significantly better on Tuesday, with no significant difference among the other days, despite a seeming rise in level of performance on Friday. These results he interpreted as indicating a psychological effect of starting work on Monday. The rise on Tuesday may be due to a warming-up or training effect, whereas the rise on Friday could be due to the psychological lift of having nearly finished the week's work. Mitchell cautions that the results do not mean that Tuesday is the best day, only that in a series the second day seemed to give the best results.

Dawson *et al.* (1963) observed no significant differences in results between morning (11 A.M.) and afternoon (3 P.M.) sessions in a paired comparison study of bouillon reconstituted with different kinds of water.

I. SAMPLE FACTORS

Many factors—including inherent characteristics, preparation factors, and serving conditions—influence the conduct of sensory tests.

Foods differ from each other in intensity or quality levels, and these may influence the conduct of the test. Intensity of a specific taste or odor characteristic will also influence the design of the experiment. Boggs and Ward (1950) found that tasting a single portion of potatoes containing sulfur dioxide in 12 to 100 parts per million dulled the acuity of tasters for sulfur dioxide in subsequent samples, even when three portions of unsulfited potatoes were tasted after the first sulfited sample. Berg *et al.* (1955a) reported the same effect from sulfur dioxide and tannin in wines, and Boggs and Hanson (1949) for sulfur dioxide in dried apples. In scoring frozen orange juice, Carlin *et al.* (1956) found that samples containing 2% added sugar scored higher following samples with 5% added sugar than when following samples without added sugar. The 5% samples also received higher scores when tasted after the 2% samples than after the samples without added sugar.

It is frequently suggested that the higher the intensity level the fewer the samples that can be tested at a session, but that is not always true. Recovery appears to be rather rapid (see also Chapter 5, Section V). The number of samples permissible per session will vary from one food to another. Boggs and Hanson (1949) recommended a few breaths of air between samples to retain olfactory acuity. With biscuits in triangle tests there was no difference between the first triangle and the second in 3500 tests, according to Laue *et al.* (1954). Coffee, they reported earlier (1953), gave similar results. With dairy products Guthrie (1958) reported that 50 to 100 samples per session gave results as accurate as 5 to 10 samples per session. Pfaffmann *et al.* (1954), using single-stimulus, paired, duo-trio, and triangle tests with orange drink, brown bread, apple juice, V-8 juice, tomato juice, and milk, found but few cases where the last third of the samples tested gave less significant differences than the first third. Brandt and Hutchinson (1956), using the duo-trio test with alcoholic beverages, found no difference in performance with 3, 4, or 6 presentations per session. Tompkins and Pratt (1959) reported that up to seven samples of frozen orange juice concentrate could be tested successively without apparent fatigue. The panel of Kramer *et al.* (1961) could taste 18 samples of squash per session without appreciable decrease in efficiency. Pfaffmann *et al.* (1954) and Sather and Calvin (1960) gave evidence that rather extended testing is possible with a variety of food products. With tomato juice, Sather and Calvin noted even better discrimination after five samples. Ehrenberg and Shewan (1960) found no difference in accuracy of scoring and sensitivity in differentiating between rather similar samples of fish, whether six or 72 samples were tested on a given day. (The white fish used was non-fatty.)

Sawyer (1958) and Sawyer *et al.* (1962) found that 12 paired comparisons per session gave greater stability in olfactory performance than only two paired comparisons. In 2 to 36 consecutive triangle sets with vanillin in milk there was no indication that length of session influenced the results. While the nature of the product seems to be the chief factor involved in the number of samples possible per session, the influence of the design of the experiment can also be important, although no critical tests seem to have been made of this. For odor, Crocker (1945) indicated that a hundred samples could be tested per day. Pangborn *et al.* (1964) presented 100 samples of odorous material of low intensity without fatigue showing in the results.

In some cases the nature of the product reduces the number of samples which may be used at a session. Cartwright and Nanz (1948) reported that deviation of scores was greater for three spices per session than for two. In triangular tasting of beer (Helm and Trolle, 1946), the second set was inferior in results to the first set. Virden (1949) believed it difficult to express a valid opinion about more than six samples of beer per session. Bengtsson and Helm (1946) also would limit beer samples to two or three. The second set of a triangle test with maple syrup gave results significantly inferior to the first set (Laue *et al.*, 1954). With edible oils, Moser *et al.* (1950) preferred fewer than six samples at one session. Using a large untrained panel, Kramer *et al.* (1961) found three samples of applesauce or peaches per session to be superior to nine. Freeman (1956) limited apple tasters to four samples per session when detailed attention was required. Christie (1957) and Kefford and Christie (1960) recommended limiting the number of samples per session to three to eight, depending on the intensity of the flavor and the judges' capacity and interest. We agree with Cartwright *et al.* (1952) that simple boredom or inattention may sharply reduce the reliability of multiple evaluations. They recommend four to eight samples per session for a wide variety of foods, but for alcoholic beverages and highly seasoned foods would limit the number to three or four. For mild-flavored foods, Cartwright *et al.* (1952) and Krum (1955) reported recovery of efficiency in about 30 minutes; Bengtsson and Helm (1946), however, preferred one hour between tests.

Since the economic efficiency of sensory testing is increased by increasing the number of samples per session we agree with the suggestion of Pfaffmann *et al.* (1954) that the maximum number be determined by test. If interest can be maintained, panel members can evaluate rather large numbers of samples per session, especially with bland or mild-flavored foods (Kramer *et al.*, 1961). If samples are tasted but not swallowed, fatigue can be delayed. As Hanson *et al.* (1951) stated, the accuracy desired, the strength of the off-flavor, and the ability of the judges all influence the number of samples which can be evaluated. The psychological effect of as many as ten samples of dried eggs, if not actual fatigue, was considered to limit the number of samples. We have been unable to confirm the opinion of Kefford and Christie (1960) that consumer-type tests should be limited to two samples. Critical experiments need to be made with a variety of foods where the effect of panel experience can be evaluated against the number of samples which can be tested per session. Even short rest periods between sessions might add to the number of samples possible per session—but, again, assuming that interest can be maintained (see Peryam and Swartz, 1950).

J. MASKING

In sensory testing, "masking" refers to intentional minimizing of color, taste, or odor properties so that other differences between the samples can be evaluated with less interference from the variable which has been minimized (Boggs and Hanson, 1949). The influence of color-masking in flavor recognition has already been discussed (Chapter 4, Section I). As indicated by Harvey (1953), Moir's work suggests that, at least in some studies, normal visual appearance might well be allowed to function to give the judges the advantage of their established flavor memories.

A good example of the value of masking appears in work of Kramer et al. (1961) wherein off-flavors from pesticide treatment were easily detected in frozen peaches. When the samples were puréed, a coincidental change in color occurred in the untreated samples, and in some cases pesticide-treated samples were judged superior because of their superior color. Masking the color would be justified in such a case.

Christie (1956) used orange-colored tumblers for evaluation of carrots. Ruby-colored tumblers were used by Byer and Gray (1953) to cover color differences in beer. Amerine and Feduchy (1954) used green-colored wine glasses to cover color differences in wines of different ages. In the University of California laboratories at Davis, glasses painted black on the outside or black-lined china cups are often used. Bengtsson and Helm (1946) found, however, that judges found that detecting differences in flavor in alcoholic beverages was more difficult with opaque glasses than with clear glasses; in this case there was no actual difference in color between the samples. Clearly, there seem to be some visual factors which enhance taste responses. The effect may be simply psychological: the judges may be disturbed by, unaccustomed to, or resentful of the opaque glasses. Bohren and Jordan (1953) used coal-tar dyes rather than the usual commercial liquid food colors for masking color differences in dried eggs. Helm and Trolle (1946) used tasteless dyes to mask color differences in beers.

As Kefford and Christie (1960) stated, judges prefer foods in their normal state rather than as homogenized purées or otherwise modified. In order to mask effects of juiciness, texture, etc., Hanson *et al.* (1959) used a broth for comparisons of chicken flavors.

Blending may be justified to cover texture differences in some cases. With spices there is a strong negative attitude on the part of the observers to undiluted samples, so that flavor carriers are used almost universally. Peryam and Swartz (1951) have used tomato juice, hamburger, soup stock, white sauce, scrambled eggs, and mashed potatoes for this purpose. Water itself is a form of mask or diluent in dilution tests (Patton and Josephson, 1957). Swaine (1957) used water with natural and artificial food extracts and certain mint oils. Simple sugar syrups were useful in other cases. Spices may be mixed in a suspension of flour and water or with a bland liquid such as a simple white sauce, a cream sauce, sugar syrup, egg nog, pumpkin, cabbage relish, or even chopped beef or pork, according to Cartwright and Nanz (1948). Care must be exercised in such tests, because Mackey and Valassi (1956) have shown that some additives are more difficult to detect in gels than in liquids (see Chapter 2, Section IX). Method of preparation of foods cannot, therefore, be divorced from possible sensitivity levels.

K. Preparation

It is pertinent to discuss proper preparation of foods, cooking procedures, methods of detecting flavor pick-up, and the standards used. The normal procedure is to test the food under conditions approximately the same as those prevailing under normal consumption: bread should be dry, butter solid, vegetables whole, etc. As indicated above, when the material might have too intense an effect on the receptors, a departure from the normal is justified. Experiments need to be made on how the sensory properties of various foods are affected by serving them raw, cooked, whole, diced, sliced, puréed, or juiced.

Should a carrier be used when it is the normal method of presentation, i.e., bread with jelly, or catsup with hamburger? According to Kroll and Pilgrim (1961) this is not necessary. Thus, time and money can be saved by omitting the carrier, and, indeed, accuracy is increased thereby, for the non-uniformity of the carrier introduces a variable which is difficult to control. Similar observations were made by Pangborn and Luh (1964) in difference testing of tomato catsup.

McKinley (1957) and Sullivan (1958) have described a variety of techniques for estimating the possible effects that paper, textiles, rubber, and plastics may have on foods. In one, the material is sniffed when dry, and then is moistened and sniffed again. The materials can also be placed in small vials with distilled water and sniffed after 24 hours. Many fatty or oily materials such as chocolate, butter, or mineral oil, being especially receptive to certain odors, may readily pick up odors from package materials. These can be exposed and then compared with unexposed controls.

Method of cooking can certainly influence the results of experiments (Boggs and Hanson, 1949). A standard procedure is usually used—and all the variables should be controlled: meat temperature, time of boiling, quantity and composition of water, etc. Blending, of course, should be rigidly controlled.

The preparation and presentation of standards is important in many sensory tests. In many situations the memory of the judge is inadequate for providing a standard. Filipello (1957), for example, from a special case where the judges knew that there were five quality steps, reported that evaluation was best when all five grades of wine were presented simultaneously. When only one sample was served at a time, even experienced judges failed to make a good evaluation. Crocker (1945) also noted that judges needed standards in odor evaluation. He believed that experts differed from beginners because they occasionally compared the sample against their mental image of similar samples whereas the beginner did not. In the duo-trio test the standard is present and designated. In the paired-comparison and triangle tests it may be present but not designated. Standards are recommended to avoid conflict over what the taster is looking for, or to provide a more stable standard than memory provides. It may be true that judges usually make comparative, not absolute, assessments of flavor (Boggs and Hanson, 1949), but the presence of standards does improve accuracy. Sheppard (1953) favored standards in consumer studies. In the flavor-profile procedure, standards are essential, of course. The standards must be meaningful to the judges and to the experiment. Standards which change in an unknown fashion during the experiment could lead to very misleading results.

In some cases the presence of a standard may not improve results —as in studies of Sawyer (1958) and Sawyer et al. (1962) wherein vanillin was detected in milk by paired comparisons, although there was some evidence in that case that some judges may benefit from a reference. Carlin et al. (1956) found that sugar-level evaluation was not improved by judging stepwise or against a standard containing no sugar.

Within a set of samples, the standard should also be presented as an unknown. Frequently the hidden standard is slightly downgraded.

This appears to be a psychological effect. In theory, the presence of a standard reduces multiple-sample comparison to a series of paired comparisons. Mrak *et al.* (1959) found great variation in the individual's response when the order of presenting the standard in odor tests was varied. Hanson *et al.* (1951) noted another advantage of labeled standards: they prevented a tendency toward judging the better experimental samples too high. In their work with dried eggs the effect was greatest for samples with only a slight off-flavor. Samples with a pronounced off-flavor were graded about the same in the presence or absence of a control. Hanson *et al.* believed that standards of intermediate quality might be useful. Mixing the best and worst samples will give an intermediate quality standard, but some research may be necessary to find the correct proportions. In some cases the ratios of the different compounds causing deterioration may change at different stages of storage. Mixing good and bad samples would not duplicate such ratios.

Standards are not always easy to provide. Freshly prepared samples are usually best, but samples stored under conditions that minimize change in taste, odor, color, or texture often have to be used (Cartwright *et al.,* 1952). Samples previously scored or samples held under standard aging conditions are sometimes employed. Old, household-stored spices were used as a minimal standard by Cartwright and Nanz (1948). These were compared with a spice which the panel agreed was of high quality and to which was assigned an arbitrary score of 90 out of a possible 100. Fresh eggs from a small group of birds of one breed fed a special diet were used as standards in scoring dried eggs by Bohren and Jordan (1953). Maintaining standards without change for an extended period is often desirable—and frequently difficult. Ward and Boggs (1956) stored frozen peas at −30°F in hermetically sealed air packs for 13 months without change. One difficulty is whether the various compounds which account for the deteriorated flavor maintain the same ratios at all stages of storage.

III. Serving Procedures

Far too little information is available on how the serving procedure may influence the results of sensory tests. The general philosophy is that the samples presented must be exactly alike with respect to all of the factors under experimental control (Peryam and Swartz, 1950). The desideratum is uniformity of samples in all aspects and properties other than those to be evaluated. Among the factors to be considered are visual appearance, sample size, temperature, utensils, pouring, coding, order, instructions, and rinsing. The ability to taste may be affected by substances tasted prior to flavor evaluation. Dawson *et al.* (1963) showed that sodium chloride was discriminated significantly better after a pre-taste of distilled water, hot bouillon, hot coffee (1% level), or tomato juice (5% level), than after milk, apple juice, or raw apple. The temperature of the pretaste also appeared to have an effect: differentiation was better after hot pretastes than after cold pretastes.

A. APPEARANCE FACTORS

The requirement is universal that the samples be the same in form, consistency, color, and appearance. This is especially important where appearance is a prime factor of quality (Cartwright et al., 1952). For a discussion of masking see Chapter 6, Sections II,I and J.

B. SAMPLE SIZE

The size of the sample has been controlled in some experiments but not in others. Judges should be provided with sufficient sample to taste with confidence. Kefford and Christie (1960) noted that the judges seldom requested more than the minimal quantities served—normally only 1.5 ounces of a liquid. The duo-trio test in its original form controls this strictly. The variables are obvious; the amount of sample presented, the possibility of retasting, and the particular food being tasted. In the usual procedure the judge is presented with a sample which permits one or two sips. The amount sipped and the quantity swallowed are not specified or explicitly controlled. Certainly some control of this variable should be available within the limits of a reasonable quantity of the food which the panel members would normally consume. Sufficient sample to give a feeling of "mouthfulness" is often recommended. It has been suggested that the amount tested is sometimes the factor being judged. Artificial systems using a pipette or dropper are usually avoided in food testing. With beer, Gray et al. (1947) used one ounce (about 30 ml). Brandt and Hutchinson (1956) used 0.15 ounce (about 4 ml) of alcoholic beverages. Virden (1949) noted that in some situations the judges were permitted up to a half-pint of beer! Berg et al. (1955a) used one-ounce samples of wine and permitted retasting. With spices, control of quantity is clearly necessary. Cartwright and Nanz (1948) recommended that the judge use his own discretion as to the quantity tested. Guthrie (1958) noted that samples of dairy products should all be of the same size.

C. TEMPERATURE

Uniformity of temperature is generally agreed to be a necessary condition in sensory testing of foods (Peryam and Swartz, 1950; Cartwright et al., 1952). The mechanical problems of serving foods at a constant and uniform temperature are frequently not adequately considered.

The temperature should approximate that of normal serving (Laue *et al.*, 1954; Krum, 1955; Jones, 1958). Gray *et al.* (1947) served beer at 11°C, whereas Byer and Gray (1953) preferred 12–15°C and Helm and Trolle (1946) served it at 12°C. Amerine *et al.* (1959) recommended 13–16°C for white wine and 18–20°C for red and dessert wines. Hopkins (1954) served milk at about 15°C. Tompkins and Pratt (1959) evaluated frozen orange juice concentrates at 10–13°C and 23–24°C. There was little difference in relative scores at the low and high temperatures, although the absolute scores changed. Kefford and Christie (1960) obtained the same ratings for canned peas at normal serving temperatures as at room temperatures. Moser *et al.* (1950) served edible oils at 55°C, a rather high temperature but nevertheless preferred because odors and flavors were detected more easily and because the "mouthfeel" was better. The samples were maintained at this temperature by placing the beakers holding the oil in temperature-regulated aluminum blocks. Both a psychological and physiological factor may be involved.

Obviously there is greater odor at higher temperatures (Chapter 4, Section III,D) and the effect of temperature varies with the taste quality, but serving foods at too high or too low a temperature may result in undesirable psychological reactions. The general principle must be that the temperature used should be optimum for detecting the differences that are under study. The influence of temperature on the foods and on the tasters has not been adequately studied. Dove (1947) indicated that the responses to the texture and juiciness of different foods from different tasters could be expected to vary as temperatures are varied. In dairy product judging, all the samples should be served at the same temperature (Guthrie, 1958).

D. Utensils

It is generally agreed that all the samples should be served in containers of the same size and color. The containers should not impart a taste or odor to the samples (Bengtsson and Helm, 1946; Boggs and Hanson, 1949; Cartwright *et al.*, 1952).

Cleaning utensils is often difficult. Many detergents leave an odor unless the utensil is thoroughly rinsed. If towels are used for drying, those which leave lint on the containers should be avoided. In pouring samples into beer glasses, Byer and Gray (1953) recommended that the glasses be filled in a random order to equalize difference in carbonation and foam life.

We believe it is desirable for the samples to be placed in the containers in which they are to be served not only in a uniform manner but in an esthetic manner. Gravy dripping off the sides of the plate is not the best way of serving a sample of meat.

E. CODING

All samples presented to the judges must be coded in such a way as to avoid giving information to the panel (Boggs and Hanson, 1949; Dawson and Harris, 1951; Jones, 1958). Brandt and Hutchinson (1956) used no code in a duo-trio test, the attendant recording the results at the time in the light of the information supplied. Use of codes in alphabetical order, as used by Laue *et al.* (1954), may cause bias, according to Kefford and Christie (1960). Assignment of code markings by some method which ensures randomness is essential. We normally prefer three digits selected from a table of random numbers. The portion of this table that is to be used should be inspected to ensure that duplicate numbers do not occur. In triangle tests, to partially avoid a bias toward the middle sample, the containers can be served in a circular arrangement and the code markings can be placed on the under side of the utensils so that they are not seen by the taster. The attendant notes the code number of the sample that the judge identifies as the odd one.

F. ORDER OF SERVING

Order of serving has already been discussed as a problem (Chapter 5, Section III). Some investigations have found no effect from order of serving, as, for example, Bliss *et al.* (1953), with potatoes, or only an effect on scoring as compared to ranking, as found by Filipello (1957), with wines, but there is too much evidence for position bias and first-sample bias to neglect random serving. See Virden (1949) and Byer and Gray (1953) for typical examples. A related problem not previously discussed is the effect of serving two samples at intervals of 1, 2, 7, or 10 days. With two soups, Schwartz and Pratt (1956) showed that simultaneous presentation yielded stronger hedonic preferences.

IV. Instructions to Judges

It may not be necessary to give detailed instructions in difference tests with experienced judges, but that is not the case with many panels. Questions arise as to method of swirling the glass, chewing, smelling, to swallow or not, how many samples to warm up, to rinse between tastings or not, and the time allowed for each of these. Pettit (1958) obtained better preference judgments when the tasters were permitted to swallow the tomato juice than when they were not allowed to swallow, and also when they had at least 1.5 ounce available as compared to lesser amounts.

One school of thought believes that the taster should use his own judgment about swallowing the food, rinsing between tastes, and time between tastes. Exponents of this *laissez faire* procedure are Tompkins and Pratt (1959), Laue *et al.* (1954), Pfaffmann *et al.* (1954), and Pettit (1958). In difference tests it seems wise to prevent swallowing, so as to avoid fatigue and post-ingestion effects and to standardize the procedure. In flavor quality studies, chewing and swallowing may increase the release of odors.

There seems to be no objection to offering the tasters ample water or crackers as a palate-clearing procedure. Kefford and Christie (1960) make the point that if a judge clears his palate after one sample, he should do so after every sample. Peryam and Swartz (1950) also recommended that water used for rinsing be at room temperature for foods served at room temperature, and at or slightly above body temperature for warm foods. They also noted that the distilled water available in some laboratories may not be as satisfactory for rinsing as the tap water. Certainly the rinse water should be as neutral as possible. Depledt (1961) indicated that he had not been able to secure a neutral water for rinsing.

Some instructions seem useful. Crocker (1945) taught judges not to sniff too deeply until the intensity of the odor was known, and cautioned panel members against smelling one sample with one nostril and the other sample with the other. In tasting he felt that natural saliva flow was the best preparation for the next sample. Harries (1956) found that advising the tasters to "take their time" was effective in minimizing variance due to fatigue. To prevent adaptation, Schutz and Pilgrim (1957) required rinsing in determining thresholds and difference thresholds. Cartwright and Nanz (1948) and Peryam and Swartz (1950) found that rinsing with water between spice tests reduced the variability of scores. Moser *et al.* (1950) found warm water useful in removing the carry-over effect of edible oils. Baten (1947) used crackers and water, apples and water, cookies and water, bread and water, and water only, between tests with tomato juice and apple juice. The best all-around combination, he found, was crackers and water. Wöger (1952) recommended chewing bread between beer samples to remove the bitter taste. He preferred rest periods to too frequent rinsing.

Use of a warm-up sample to avoid bias in favor of the first sample has been favored by many investigators (see, for example, Boggs and Hanson, 1949; Hopkins, 1954; Mitchell, 1956; Kefford and Christie, 1960). In the duo-trio test, Peryam and Swartz (1950) gave a warm-up sample which was the same as the control sample. In threshold tests, Schutz and Pilgrim (1957) offered the judges the complete series of solutions in an identified ascending order before unknowns to acquaint the panel with their range and relative strength.

As for the time between samples, Peryam and Swartz (1950) noted that this should be long enough to permit recovery from adaptation— but not too long, lest the taster forget the flavor of the sample. They believed that 10 to 30 seconds was generally satisfactory but that the time might vary with the degree of adaptation induced by the food being tasted and with the skill of the observer. Jones (1958) expressed a similar opinion. In threshold tests, Schutz and Pilgrim (1957) allowed 30 seconds for each test. Peryam and Swartz (1950) noted that in the dual standard test for odor evaluation, inexperienced judges tended to alternate too rapidly between samples and that instructions as to the time interval should be emphasized during training. With relatively weak odors such as normally encountered in foods, a recovery period of one minute was found adequate, but strong odors might require more time. Crocker (1945) recommended only one strong odor in a 5-minute period. In order to reduce variability, Metzner (1943) recommended that the time between samples and per sample should be constant. We tend to agree with this conclusion if it does not slow down individual tasters too much. Certainly different foods may require different recovery times. The conclusion of Boggs and Hanson (1949) that in most cases no time limit be imposed is more in line with general practice. With confections, Clendenning (1940) believed recovery might be a matter of minutes. Helm and Trolle (1946) allowed 15 minutes for evaluating a triangle set. This is more time than allowed in most laboratories. Bengtsson and Helm (1946) noted that more time between samples was desirable when bitterness was a factor, and Trout (1946) found that, in milk, the time to react to and assess flavor was longer for an off-flavor than for an excellent flavor.

Ough et al. (1964) reported an experiment in judging sweetness in white wines where the judges were allowed to taste at their own speed or were allowed only 7 seconds to taste and score. The standard deviations about the individual means did not differ significantly, but throughout the sweetness scale the mean scores obtained under conditions of hurried tasting were closer to the expected values than those without time limitation. Presumably when the tasters had ample time they "thought" more about the task. This was suggested by Brunswik's (1956) distinction between perception and thinking in cognitive processes. Thus, an "explicit reasoning" experiment resulted in more exactly correct responses but a much wider range of responses than did an experiment where perception alone was allowed to function. In Ough's experiment the judges were presumably using both perception and reasoning. The old saying is possibly correct: that "the impression from the first taste is the best one."

In summary, the best practice seems to be to allow the judge, when possible, to use his preferred method; however, to standardize procedures, the same technique should be used by all the judges. This is in line with the results of Pfaffmann *et al.* (1954) with rinsing, and seems to be generally true for the variables discussed above.

Reports. Written reports are usually required in sensory tests. This prevents second-guessing, but there may be situations where tape recording of the judge's reactions might yield more information.

V. Summary

The various types of sensory tests are briefly described. The main purpose of the chapter is to identify the factors which influence the efficiency of laboratory sensory panels.

Careful selection of judges is essential in order to achieve maximum discriminability. Selection on the basis of sensitivity to the basic tastes or to general odors is not likely to be very successful in identifying the best judges. However, some form of screening will eliminate the least sensitive judges. Training we believe to be essential in all or nearly all laboratory situations.

The size of panel needed varies with the sensitivities of the judges and the range in acceptability of the product. Small expert panels of 3 to 10 are preferred for laboratory studies. For consumer studies, hundreds or thousands may be needed.

The influence of health, age, sex, and smoking on panel performance does not seem to be critical. However, emotional factors, interest, motivation, knowledge, comparison of results, adjustment to the test situation, and memory do seem to influence results.

Environmental conditions need to be controlled during testing. These include reducing distraction and providing air conditioning, proper lighting, and comfortable seating. The best time of day for testing has not been established, but we prefer the midmorning period.

Control of sample variability and number of samples is very important but varies with different foods. Less acceptable and more variable foods generally reduce the number that can be efficiently tested at one sitting. Masking, usually of color, can be used to eliminate judgments on unimportant criteria. However, the possibility should be borne in mind that artificial lighting may influence judgment.

Samples should be prepared so as to standardize conditions and avoid flavor pick-up. Special methods of preparation are justified in many cases of non-homogeneous materials. The use of a standard is indicated in many situations.

The effect of serving procedure on panel performance has been better studied. Control of appearance, sample size, temperature, utensils, coding, order of serving, instructions to judges, and reports have clearly indicated benefits.

REFERENCES

Amerine, M. A. 1948. An application of "triangular" taste testing to wines. *Wine Rev.* 16(5), 10–12.

Amerine, M. A., and E. Feduchy. 1954. Los resultados de la cata del vino y del análisis químico. *Bol. inst. nacl. invest. agron.* (*Madrid*) 14(31), 353–375.

Amerine, M. A., E. B. Roessler, and F. Filipello. 1959. Modern sensory methods of evaluating wine. *Hilgardia* 28, 477–567.

Andross, M. 1961. Flavour and flavour acceptance. *Proc. Nutrition Soc.* (*Engl. and Scot.*) 20, 40–46.

Anonymous. 1964. Sensory testing guide for panel evaluation of foods and beverages. *Food Technol.* 18(8), 25–31.

Baker, G. A., and M. A. Amerine. 1953. Organoleptic ratings of wines estimated from analytical data. *Food Research* 18, 381–389.

Baker, G. A., M. A. Amerine, and E. B. Roessler. 1954. Errors of the second kind in organoleptic difference testing. *Food Research* 19, 206–210.

Baker, G. A., V. Mrak, and M. A. Amerine. 1958. Errors of the second kind in an acid threshold test. *Food Research* 23, 150–154.

Baker, G. A., M. A. Amerine, E. B. Roessler, and F. Filipello. 1960. Non-specificity of differences in taste testing for preference. *Food Research* 25, 810–816.

Baker, R. A. 1962. Subjective panel testing. *Ind. Quality Control* 19(3), 22–28.

Baten, W. D. 1946. Organoleptic tests pertaining to apples and pears. *Food Research* 11, 84–94.

Baten, W. D. 1947. Material for removing taste effects in organoleptic tests. *J. Home Econ.* 39, 30–32.

Bengtsson, K., and E. Helm. 1946. Principles of taste testing. *Wallerstein Lab. Commun.* 9, 171–180.

Bennett, T., B. M. Spahr, and M. L. Dodds. 1956. The value of training a sensory test panel. *Food Technol.* 10, 205–208.

Berg, H. W., F. Filipello, E. Hinreiner, and A. D. Webb. 1955a. Evaluation of thresholds and minimum difference concentrations for various constituents of wines. I. Water solutions of pure substances. *Food Technol.* 9, 23–26.

Berg, H. W., F. Filipello, E. Hinreiner, and A. D. Webb. 1955b. Evaluation of thresholds and minimum difference concentrations for various constituents of wines. II. Sweetness: the effect of ethyl alcohol, organic acids and tannins. *Food Technol.* 9, 138–140.

Bliss, C. I. 1960. Some statistical aspects of preference and related tests. *Appl. Stat.* 9, 8–19.

Bliss, C. I., M. L. Greenwood, and M. H. McKenrick. 1953. A comparison of scoring methods for taste tests with mealiness of potatoes. *Food Technol.* 7, 491–495.

Boggs, M. M., and H. L. Hanson. 1949. Analysis of foods by sensory difference tests. *Advances in Food Research* 2, 219–258.

Boggs, M. M., and A. C. Ward. 1950. Scoring technique for sulfited foods. *Food Technol.* 4, 282–284.

Bohren, B. B., and R. Jordan. 1953. A technique for detecting flavor changes in stored dried eggs. *Food Research* 18, 583–591.

Bradley, J. E., C. T. Walliker, and D. R. Peryam. 1954. Influence of continued testing on preference ratings. *In* "Food Acceptance Testing Methodology," 115 pp. (see pp. 92–100). Advisory Board on Quartermaster Research and Development, Committee on Foods. Natl. Acad. Sci., Natl. Research Council, Chicago, Illinois.

Bradley, R. A. 1955. Statistical designs for taste test panels. *Trans. Am. Soc. Quality Control Conv.* 9, 621–626.

Brandt, D. A., and E. P. Hutchinson. 1956. Retention of taste sensitivity. *Food Technol.* 10, 419–420.

Brunswik, E. 1956. "Perception and Representative Design of Psychological Experiments," 154 pp. Univ. of California Press, Berkeley and Los Angeles, California.

Byer, A. J., and P. P. Gray. 1953. Some considerations in applying systematic taste testing to beer. *Wallerstein Lab. Commun.* 16, 303–312.

Cairncross, S. E., and L. B. Sjöström. 1950. Flavor profiles—a new approach to flavor problems. *Food Technol.* 4, 308–311.

Carlin, A. F., O. Kempthorne, and J. Gordon. 1956. Some aspects of numerical scoring in subjective evaluation of foods. *Food Research* 21, 273–281.

Cartwright, L. C., and R. A. Nanz. 1948. Comparative evaluation of spices. *Food Technol.* 2, 330–336.

Cartwright, L. C., C. T. Snell, and P. H. Kelley. 1952. Organoleptic panel testing as a research tool. *Anal. Chem.* 24, 503–506.

Christie, E. M. 1956. Some theoretical and practical aspects of the planning and conduct of tasting tests. *Food and Nutrition Notes and Revs.* 13, 21–30.

Christie, E. M. 1957. Tasting tests on foods. *C.S.I.R.O. Food Preserv. Quart.* 17, 38–41.

Christie, E. 1962. Conduct of tasting tests. *Food Technol. in Australia* 14(2), 77; (3), 124–125; (4), 161–162, 165, 169, 171.

Clements, F. E., J. A. Bayton, and H. P. Bell. 1954. Method of single stimulus determinations of taste preference. *J. Appl. Psychol.* 38, 446–451.

Clendenning, T. 1940. Flavor in confections. I. The physiological aspects. II. Methods of evaluation. *Mfg. Confectioner* 20(1), 17–19; (2), 23–25.

Cooper, R. M., I. Bilash, and J. P. Zubek. 1959. The effect of age on taste sensitivity. *J. Gerontol.* 14, 56–58.

Coote, G. G. 1956. Analysis of scores for bitterness of orange juice. *Food Research* 21, 1–10.

Coppock, J. B. M., J. H. Hulse, J. P. Todd, and A. Urie. 1952. Some organoleptic studies on bakery products. *J. Sci. Food Agr.* 3, 433–441.

Crocker, E. C. 1945. "Flavor," 172 pp. McGraw-Hill, New York.

Dawson, E. H., and B. L. Harris. 1951. Sensory methods for measuring differences in food quality: review of literature and proceedings of conference. *U. S. Dept. Agr. Inform. Bull.* 34, 1–134.

Dawson, E. H., J. L. Brogdon, and S. McManus. 1963. Sensory testing of differences in taste. I. Methods. II. Selection of panel members. *Food Technol.* 17(9), 45–48, 51; (10), 39–41, 43–44.

Deininger, N., and R. W. McKinley. 1954. The design, construction, and use of an odor test room. *ASTM Spec. Tech. Publ.* 164, 23–30.

Depledt, M. 1961. Les "panels" de dégustation. *In* "Mesure et control des produits finis," Conferences données au cours du 2ᵉ cycle 1961 au Centre de la Biscuiterie, Paris, pp. 51–74.

Dove, W. F. 1947. Food acceptability—its determination and evaluation. *Food Technol.* 1, 39–50.

Duffendack, S. C. 1954. A study of non-sensory determinants of recognition thresholds. *Dissertation Abstr.* 14, 1097.

Duncan, A. J. 1959. "Quality Control and Industrial Statistics," 663 pp. Richard D. Irwin, Inc., Homewood, Illinois.

Ehrenberg, A. S. C., and J. M. Shewan. 1953. Objective approach to sensory tests of food. *J. Sci. Food Agr.* 4, 482–490.

Ehrenberg, A. S. C., and J. M. Shewan. 1960. The development and use of a taste panel technique—a review. *Occupational Psychol.* 34, 241–248.

Enggaard, V., and M. Jul. 1958. The Danish meat products laboratory. *Food Mfg.* 33, 290–292.

Feigenbaum, A. V. 1951. "Quality Control; Principles, Practice, Administration," 443 pp. McGraw-Hill, New York.

Filipello, F. 1957. Organoleptic wine-quality evaluation. II. Performance of judges. *Food Technol.* 11, 51–53.

Foster, D. 1954. Approach to the panel studies of foods and the need for standardization. *Food Technol.* 8, 304–306.

Foster, D., C. Pratt, and N. Schwartz. 1955. Variations in flavor judgments in a group situation. *Food Research* 20, 539–544.

Freeman, G. H. 1956. The selection and use of a panel for taste sensitivity tests with fruit. *Ann. Rept. East Malling Research Sta. Kent* 1955, 86–88.

Girardot, N. F., D. R. Peryam, and R. Shapiro. 1952. Selection of sensory testing panels. *Food Technol.* 6, 140–143.

Gray, P. P., I. Stone, and L. Atkin. 1947. Systematic study of the influence of oxidation on beer flavor. *Wallerstein Lab. Commun.* 10, 183–194.

Gustafson, E. 1953. Exploratory methods for the study of children's taste preferences and discrimination. 43 pp. M. S. Thesis. Florida State Univ., Tallahassee, Florida.

Guthrie, E. S. 1958. Scoring of dairy products. *In* "Flavor Research and Food Acceptance" (Arthur D. Little, Inc., ed.), 391 pp. (see pp. 83–87). Reinhold, New York.

Hall, B. A., M. G. Tarver, and J. G. McDonald. 1959. A method for screening flavor panel members and its application to a two sample difference test. *Food Technol.* 13, 699–703.

Hanson, H. L., L. Kline, and H. Lineweaver. 1951. Application of balanced incomplete block design to scoring of ten dried egg samples. *Food Technol.* 5, 9–13.

Hanson, H. L., A. A. Campbell, A. A. Kraft, G. L. Gilpin, and A. M. Harkin. 1959. The flavor of modern and old-type chickens. *Poultry Sci.* 38, 1071–1078.

Harding, P. L., and F. M. Wadley. 1948. Teen-age students vs. adults as taste judges of temple oranges. *Food Research* 13, 6–10.

Harper, R. 1949. Food grading and its study. *Food* 18, 207–210.

Harper, R. 1955. Fundamental problems in the subjective appraisal of foodstuffs. *Appl. Stat.* 4, 141–160.

Harries, J. M. 1956. Positional bias in sensory assessments. *Food Technol.* 10, 86–90.

Harrison, S., and L. W. Elder. 1950. Some applications of statistics to laboratory taste testing. *Food Technol.* 4, 434–439.

Harrison, S., N. H. Ishler, and E. A. Laue. 1954. Note on the selection of a panel of judges so as to maximize panel efficiency. *Psychometrika* 19, 79–88.

Harvey, H. G. 1953. Flavour assessment. *Chem. & Ind.* (*London*) **1953**, 1163–1167.

Helm, E., and B. Trolle. 1946. Selection of a taste panel. *Wallerstein Lab. Commun.* **9**, 181–194.

Hening, J. C. 1948. Flavor evaluation procedures. *N. Y. Agr. Expt. Sta. Tech. Bull.* **284**, 1–20.

Hopkins, J. W. 1946. Precision of assessment of palatability of foodstuffs by laboratory panels. *Can. J. Research* **24F**, 203–214.

Hopkins, J. W. 1947. Precision of assessment of palatability of foodstuffs by laboratory panels. II. Saltiness of bacon. *Can. J. Research* **25F**, 29–33.

Hopkins, J. W. 1954. Some observations on sensitivity and repeatability of trial taste difference tests. *Biometrics* **10**, 521–530.

Jones, F. N. 1958. Prerequisites for test environment. *In* "Flavor Research and Food Acceptance" (Arthur D. Little, Inc., ed.), 391 pp. (see pp. 107–111). Reinhold, New York.

Kamen, J. M., F. J. Pilgrim, N. J. Gutman, and B. J. Kroll. 1960. Interactions of suprathreshold taste stimuli. *Quartermaster Food and Container Inst. Rept.* **14–60**, 1–26.

Kefford, J. F., and E. M. Christie. 1960. Sensory tests for colour, flavour, and texture. *C.S.I.R.O. Food Preserv. Quart.* **20**, 47–56.

King, F. B. 1937. Obtaining a panel for judging flavor in foods. *Food Research* **2**, 207–219.

Kirkpatrick, M. E., J. C. Lamb, E. H. Dawson, and J. N. Eisen. 1957. Selecting a taste panel for evaluating the quality of processed milk. *Food Technol.* **11**(9), 3–8 (supplement).

Knowles, D., and P. E. Johnson. 1941. A study of the sensitivities of prospective food judges to the primary tastes. *Food Research* **6**, 207–216.

Kramer, A., E. F. Murphy, A. M. Briant, M. Wang, and M. E. Kirkpatrick. 1961. Studies in taste panel methodology. *J. Agr. Food Chem.* **9**, 224–228.

Kramer, C. Y. 1955. A method of choosing judges for a sensory experiment. *Food Research* **20**, 492–496; also **21**, 598–600, 1956.

Kroll, B. J., and F. J. Pilgrim. 1961. Sensory evaluation of accessory foods with and without carriers. *J. Food Sci.* **26**, 122–124.

Krum, J. K. 1955. Sensory panel testing. *Food Eng.* **27**, 74–83.

Laue, E. A., T. Zlobik, and N. H. Ishler. 1953. Reliability of taste testing and consumer testing methods. (Abstr.) *Food Technol.* **7**, 14.

Laue, E. A., N. H. Ishler, and G. A. Bullman. 1954. Reliability of taste testing and consumer testing methods. I. Fatigue in taste testing. *Food Technol.* **8**, 387–388.

Lockhart, E. E. 1951. Binomial systems and organoleptic analysis. *Food Technol.* **5**, 428–431.

Lowe, B., and G. F. Stewart. 1947. Subjective and objective tests as food research tools with special reference to poultry meat. *Food Technol.* **1**, 30–38.

Mackey, A. O., and P. Jones. 1954. Selection of members of food tasting panel: discernment of primary tastes in water solution compared with judging ability for foods. *Food Technol.* **8**, 527–530.

Mackey, A. O., and K. Valassi. 1956. The discernment of primary tastes in the presence of different food textures. *Food Technol.* **10**, 238–240.

McKinley, R. W. 1957. Odor- and taste-transfer testing. *Coffee and Tea Inds.* **80**, 55–56. *Also in* "Flavor Research and Food Acceptance" (Arthur D. Little, Inc., ed.), 391 pp. (see pp. 94–96). Reinhold, New York.

Marcuse, S. 1945. An application of the control chart method to the testing and marketing of foods. *J. Am. Statistical Assoc.* **40**, 214–222.

Marcuse, S. 1947. Applying control chart methods to taste testing. *Food Inds.* **19**, 316–318.

Metzner, C. A. 1943. Investigation of odor and taste. Psychological principles. *Wallerstein Lab. Commun.* **6**, 5–18.

Mitchell, J. W. 1956. Time-errors in the paired comparison taste preference test. *Food Technol.* **10**, 218–220.

Mitchell, J. W. 1957a. Problems in taste difference testing. I. Test environment. *Food Technol.* **11**, 476–477.

Mitchell, J. W. 1957b. Problems in taste difference testing. II. Subject variability due to time of the day and day of the week. *Food Technol.* **11**, 477–479.

Morse, R. L. D. 1954. Exploratory studies of preschool children's taste discrimination and preference for selected citrus juices. *Proc. Florida State Hort. Soc.* **66**, 292–301.

Moser, H. A., H. J. Dutton, C. D. Evans, and J. C. Cowan. 1950. Conducting a taste panel for the evaluation of edible oils. *Food Technol.* **4**, 105–109.

Mrak, V., M. A. Amerine, C. S. Ough, and G. A. Baker. 1959. Odor difference test with applications to consumer preferences. *Food Research* **24**, 574–578.

Murphy, E. F., M. R. Covell, and J. S. Dinsmore. 1957. An examination of three methods for testing palatability as illustrated by strawberry flavor differences. *Food Research* **22**, 423–439.

Naumann, H. D., V. J. Rhodes, D. E. Brady, and E. R. Kiehl. 1957. Discrimination techniques in meat acceptance studies. *Food Technol.* **11**, 123–125.

Ough, C. S., and G. A. Baker. 1961. Small panel sensory evaluations of wines by scoring. *Hilgardia* **30**, 587–619.

Ough, C. S., and G. A. Baker. 1964. Linear dependency of scale structure in differential odor intensity measurements. *J. Food Sci.* **29**, 499–505.

Ough, C. S., V. L. Singleton, M. A. Amerine, and G. A. Baker. 1964. A comparison of normal and stressed-time conditions on scoring of quality and quantity attributes. *J. Food Sci.* **29**, 506–519.

Overman, A., and C. R. L. Jerome. 1948. Dependability of food judges as indicated by an analysis of scores of a food tasting panel. *Food Research* **13**, 441–449.

Pangborn, R. M. 1959. Influence of hunger on sweetness preferences and taste thresholds. *Am. J. Clin. Nutrition* **7**, 280–287.

Pangborn, R. M., and B. S. Luh. 1964. Storage stability of tomato ketchup with various sweeteners. I. Sensory properties. *Food Technol.* **18**(4), 576–579.

Pangborn, R. M., H. W. Berg, E. B. Roessler, and A. D. Webb. 1964. Influence of methodology on olfactory response. *Perceptual and Motor Skills* **18**, 91–103.

Patton, S., and D. V. Josephson. 1957. A method for determining significance of volatile flavor compounds in foods. *Food Research* **22**, 316–318.

Peryam, D. R. 1958. Sensory difference tests. *Food Technol.* **12**, 231–236.

Peryam, D. R., and V. W. Swartz. 1950. Measurement of sensory differences. *Food Technol.* **4**, 390–395.

Peryam, D. R., and V. W. Swartz. 1951. Methodology for sensory evaluation of imitation peppers. *Food Technol.* **5**, 207–210.

Pettit, L. A. 1958. Quantity of sample, swallowing, and rinsing factors in flavor preference testing of tomato juice. *Food Technol.* **12**(1), 1–4.

Pfaffmann, C., and H. Schlosberg. 1952–1953. An analysis of sensory methods for testing flavor: The selection of discrimination panels. *Quartermaster Project No. 7-84-15-007, Rept.* **7**, 1–21.

Pfaffmann, C., H. Schlosberg, and J. Cornsweet. 1954. Variables affecting difference tests. *In* "Food Acceptance Testing Methodology," 115 pp. (see pp. 4–17).

Advisory Board on Quartermaster Research and Development, Committee on Foods, Natl. Acad. Sci., Natl. Research Council, Chicago, Illinois.

Raffensperger, E. L., and F. J. Pilgrim. 1956. Knowledge of the stimulus variable as an aid in discrimination tests. *Food Technol.* **10,** 254–257.

Sather, L. A., and L. D. Calvin. 1960. The effect of number of judgments in a test on flavor evaluations for preference. *Food Technol.* **14,** 613–615.

Sawyer, F. M. 1958. Methodology in sensory analysis of food; problems involved in selection and training of judges. 72 pp. Ph.D. Thesis. Univ. of California, Davis, California.

Sawyer, F. M., H. Stone, H. Abplanalp, and G. F. Stewart. 1962. Repeatability estimates in sensory-panel selection. *J. Food Sci.* **27,** 386–393.

Schlosberg, H., C. Pfaffmann, J. Cornsweet, and R. Pierrel. 1954. Selection and training of panels. *In* "Food Acceptance Testing Methodology," 115 pp. (see pp. 45–54). Advisory Board on Quartermaster Research and Development, Committee on Foods. Natl. Acad. Sci., Natl. Research Council, Chicago, Illinois.

Schneider, R. A., and S. Wolf. 1955. Olfactory perception thresholds for citral using a new type olfactorium *J. Appl. Physiol.* **8,** 337–342.

Schutz, H. G., and F. J. Pilgrim. 1957. Differential sensitivity in gustation. *J. Exptl. Psychol.* **54,** 41–48.

Schwartz, N., and C. H. Pratt. 1956. Simultaneous vs. successive presentation in a paired comparison situation. *Food Research* **21,** 103–108.

Scott-Blair, G. W., F. M. V. Coppens, and D. V. Dearden. 1941. A preliminary study of the effects of varying pitching consistency and rate of scald on the physical and chemical properties of Cheddar cheese and on the firmness of the cheese as judged by cheese makers, bakers and others. *J. Dairy Research* **12,** 170–177.

Sharp, P. F., G. F. Stewart, and J. C. Huttar. 1936. Effect of packing materials on the flavor of storage eggs. *N. Y. Agr. Expt. Sta. Ithaca Mem.* **189,** 1–26.

Sheppard, D. 1953. Rating methods for assessing food qualities. *Food* **22,** 13–17.

Shewan, J. M., R. G. MacIntosh, C. G. Tucker, and A. S. C. Ehrenberg. 1953. The development of a numerical scoring system for the sensory assessment of the spoilage of wet white fish stored in ice. *J. Sci. Food Agr.* **6,** 283–298.

Sinsheimer, J. E. 1959. An intensity-response method for the measurement of flavor intensity. *Food Research* **24,** 445–450.

Sullivan, F. 1958. Presentation of odor samples. *In* "Flavor Research and Food Acceptance" (Arthur D. Little, Inc., ed.), 391 pp. (see pp. 100–102). Reinhold, New York.

Swaine, R. L. 1957. Experimental media for evaluating flavor. *Coffee and Tea Inds.* **80,** 93. *Also in* "Flavor Research and Food Acceptance" (Arthur D. Little, Inc., ed.), 391 pp. (see pp. 97–99). Reinhold, New York.

Tarver, M. G., and B. H. Ellis. 1961. Selection of flavor panels for complex differences. *Ind. Quality Control* **17**(12), 22–26.

Tarver, M. G., B. A. Hall, and J. G. McDonald. 1959. A statistical quality control approach to the selection of flavor panel members. *Trans. Am. Soc. Quality Control Conv.* **13,** 459–485.

Tompkins, M. D., and G. B. Pratt. 1959. Comparison of flavor evaluation methods for frozen citrus concentrate. *Food Technol.* **13,** 149–152.

Trawinski, B. J., and H. A. David. 1963. Selection of the best treatment in a paired comparison experiment. *Ann. Math. Statistics* **34,** 75–91.

Trout, G. M. 1946. Time required for making flavor judgments of milk. *J. Dairy Sci.* **29,** 415–419.

Trout, G. M., and P. F. Sharp. 1937. The reliability of flavor judgments with special reference to the oxidized flavor of milk. *N. Y. Agr. Expt. Sta. Ithaca Mem.* **204,** 1–60.

Tukey, J. W. 1951. Quick and dirty methods in statistics. II. Simple analyses for standard designs. *Proc. Conf. Am. Soc. Quality Control* **5,** 189–197.

Virden, C. J. 1949. The design and interpretation of tasting experiments. *J. Inst. Brewing* **55,** 228–233.

Ward, A. C., and M. M. Boggs. 1956. Development of a frozen pea reference standard for taste tests involving storage. *Food Technol.* **10,** 117–119.

Wiley, R. C., A. M. Briant, I. S. Fagerson, J. H. Sabry, and E. F. Murphy. 1957. Evaluation of flavor changes due to pesticides—a regional approach. *Food Research* **22,** 192–205.

Wöger, K. 1952. Geschmacksphysiologische Betrachtungen unter besonder Berücksichtigung der Kostprobe von Bieren. *Brauwelt* **6B,** 118–119.

Chapter 7

Laboratory Studies: Difference and Directional Difference Tests

Most information on human responses to physical and chemical stimuli has been obtained in laboratories under very specific conditions. These conditions, which are governed by the problem at hand, include the procedures established and enforced so that data will be reliable and the conclusions valid. The choice of methods and experimental design for a given situation depends on the type and precision of the information desired. Laboratory panels can provide answers to two general questions relative to the sensory properties of foods: Is there a difference between or among stimuli? And what is the direction and/or the intensity of any differences? These two aspects are frequently confused, as in the work of Helm and Trolle (1946). Peryam (1958) is much clearer in defining difference tests as those which determine a difference regardless of its nature or direction. In other words, the judge either discriminates or fails to discriminate. The statistical models are based on the theoretical distribution that would result from chance if the judge were completely unable to discriminate. In true difference tests, the subject's task is completely defined by the experimental situation.

I. Difference Tests

Difference testing is the most fundamental approach to sensory analysis of foods. There are three basic types of differences which may be sought: (1) simple difference; (2) directional difference of a defined criterion; and (3) quality-preference difference. Simple difference tests are used effectively for obtaining information in several fields of investigation. In physiology and psychology, basic information on human responses to stimuli, isolated and combined, is obtained through these procedures, as discussed in Chapters 2 and 3. In food science, difference

321

testing is used for detecting sensory variations in food resulting from chemical and physical alterations. Differences in the sensory properties of food may originate from genetic characteristics, horticultural or animal-husbandry practices, pre- and post-mortem treatments, methods and materials used in processing, types of packaging materials, and storage conditions. Information from these tests can be useful in developing quality standards and quality-control programs. Also, difference testing can be used to prepare and screen samples prior to tests for consumer preferences of foods (Chapter 9). For a general discussion, see Baker (1962), Boggs and Hanson (1949), Cartwright *et al.* (1952), Park (1961), Peryam (1958), Peryam and Swartz (1950), Pfaffmann *et al.* (1954), and Dawson *et al.* (1963).

Simple (true) difference testing requires the observer to respond in one of two ways: "there is a difference" or "there is no difference." This type of question provides the least equivocal approach. The objectivity is further increased by the fact that the results obtained can be easily adapted to quantitative statistical treatment, which in turn increases the reliability of the interpretation. Because of these characteristics, Pfaffmann *et al.* (1954) relate true difference testing in sensory analysis of foods to psychophysics, the relationship between physical stimuli and psychological response. Information from such testing is restricted by the fact that when a difference is established, there is evidence neither of the dimension of the difference nor whether each observer differentiated on the same basis.

II. Directional Difference Tests

In directional difference testing, the observer is required to state which sample is more intense in a predefined characteristic. This type is not quite as objective as true difference testing but has come to be accepted as a valid and useful variation of true difference testing. Peryam (1958) characterizes a directional difference test as one in which a reference is not immediately present but is brought to the test situation by the judge in the form of a "memory standard." In a true difference test, the judge brings only his sensory capacity. This criterion or predesignated standard must be similarly understood by, and receive the same reaction from, all of the judges; otherwise, the test becomes a vote and the results cannot be interpreted as failure or success in detecting a difference. Thus, the fact that a specified criterion is under test could very well increase the degree of interpersonal disagreement if selection and training of judges has been inadequate. With such familiar and common sensations as sweetness, hardness, or darkness, the degree of interpersonal disagreement is less than when flavor or "quality" are evaluated. Peryam and Swartz (1950) and Lockhart (1951) emphasized that the determination of whether a difference exists must precede questions related to direction or degree or preference.

Dawson *et al.* (1963) looked with suspicion on preference responses made along with difference decisions, because of bias when the difference was specified. Stone and Bosley (1964), however, postulated that bias against the odd sample in the triangle or duo-trio test should not be observed when no criterion of difference is specified, i.e., when the overall quality is being evaluated.

III. Analysis of Results

Byer and Gray (1953) suggested that useful "difference" information can be interpreted from two-sample preference tests by observing consistency in preference of individual observers upon repeated testing of two samples. Gregson (1960) postulated that in some circumstances, a preference judgment may be better evidence of discrimination than a judgment of difference. Subjects may be reluctant to commit themselves in borderline discriminations but are ready to express preference, confident that *de gustibus non est disputandum.* An experiment to demonstrate this would be welcome [see also Amerine (1963)].

The reluctance of subjects to make a decision can be overcome somewhat by disallowing "no-difference" responses, i.e., use of the forced-choice technique. Metzner (1943) stated that there is no reason for not asking the observers to guess, inasmuch as assumption of the normal curve of distribution of the data implies that any difference in stimulus magnitude produces a difference in relative proportion of judgments. Lockhart (1951) also agrees with this opinion. Only if identical paired stimuli are part of the test pattern should the observer be allowed the alternative of a "no-difference" response. In studies involving comparison of several controls (from different sources) against a variable, then a "no-difference" response could be omitted, and homogeneity among the controls could be determined as well as differences between the controls and the variable.

Difference testing is a very sensitive method of analysis, demanding precision in test design, in administration of the test, in the reaction of the observers to the test situation, and, of course, in analysis of the results. The experimenter has full responsibility for controlling the characteristics of the stimuli, test method, and details of administration. Preparation and administration of the stimuli are probably more important in true difference testing where subjects use all possible clues in the decision-making process. Except for the one variable being investigated, samples must be as identical as possible. As indicated in Chapter 6, there must be rigid control of the shape, size, color, temperature, flavor, and texture of the food samples. In many situations, the necessity for such control is a serious limiting factor. Many meats, vegetables, and fruits may be so inherently variable that control of these variables is very difficult.

Results of difference tests are interpreted simply, since the subject either does or does not recognize the difference. On the basis of the null hypothesis that the samples do not differ, the results may be analyzed statistically and the findings expressed in terms of probability levels or levels of significance, i.e., the expectancies that the results were obtained by chance alone. Thus, the smaller the assigned level of significance the greater is the confidence of the interpreter that an observed difference between the two stimuli is real. The levels of statistical probability commonly used in sensory tests are the 5, 1, and 0.1% levels.

There are two types of risks involved in use of the null hypothesis as applied to difference tests (Baker et al., 1954; Filipello, 1956; Gridgeman, 1955; Blom, 1955; Radkins, 1957): (1) concluding from the data that a difference exists when in fact there is no difference (commonly called "error of the first kind"); and (2) concluding that there is no difference when in fact a difference does exist ("error of the second kind"). These errors can be of great consequence, especially in applications to quality control. Errors of the second kind are minimized by using acute, reliable judges (Baker et al., 1954) and/or increasing the number of observations on which the conclusion is based (Blom, 1955). Errors of the first kind are reduced by selecting a more restrictive level of significance. The experimenter must decide what level of error risk he can or will tolerate at a predetermined significance level, then determine the number of observations needed to be in the region of his predetermined risk. Table 46

TABLE 46

Minimum Number of Tests Required for the Triangle Difference Test for Various Levels of α and β Risks[a]

Percent error risks		Predefined minimum percentage of correct odd-sample selections to be considered significant				
α	β	50	60	70	80	90
1	1	190	75	40	23	12
1	5	138	54	28	17	11
1	10	114	45	24	15	9
5	5	94	38	20	13	7
5	10	75	30	18	12	5

[a] α = error of the 1st kind; β = error of the 2nd kind.
Source: Blom (1955).

illustrates how the number of observations in the triangle (three-sample) difference test can vary.

The odds that a difference has been obtained through chance alone are influenced by three factors: the *real* stimulus difference, the number of observations on which the interpretation is based, and the variability from subject to subject and trial to trial. As the stimulus difference increases, the probability increases that the judges will detect this difference, and the occurrence of guesses or chance observations decreases. This phenomenon implies some quantitative characteristic in difference tests in that if the percentage of judges detecting a difference is greater

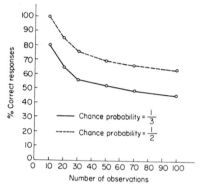

Fig. 47. Correct responses necessary for significance at 0.01 probability level when correct responses obtained by chance is ⅓ or ½.

with one set of samples than with another, the difference between the first set of samples is greater, providing the number of observations is equal for each set (Boggs and Hanson, 1949). The application of this inference is frequently the basis for panel selection, relating the differences in percent selections to differences in discriminability of the observers, i.e., by testing the significance of the difference of the two percentages. It should be clearly understood that an increase in the percent correct responses can legitimately be interpreted as indicating greater difference, but the higher statistical significance resulting from a larger number of responses with no change in percent correct responses cannot be so interpreted.

As the number of observations increases, the percent correct observations necessary for statistical significance decreases. However, this function is nonlinear, as illustrated in Fig. 47, for tests with two different chance probabilities (0.50 and 0.33), from tables published by Roessler *et al.* (1948, 1956). The formulas are based on the corrected normal-curve approximations to the binomial distributions. For convenience, there is, of course, a tendency to keep the number of judgments as low as possible; however, this fails to capitalize on the fact that the degree of difference will be reflected in the proportion of correct judgments of the difference. Note that above $N = 60$ the number of judgments has less effect.

Different chance probabilities are associated with the various test designs. In true and directional difference tests, there is only one possible correct answer, but the number of possible answers varies with the

TABLE 47

Probability of a Judge Making a Correct Separation by Chance of S Samples into Two Groups, Each Containing a and b Samples

	a equals:					
b	1	2	3	4	5	6
1	1	1/3	1/4	1/5	1/6	1/7
2	—	1/3	1/10	1/15	1/21	1/28
3	—	—	1/10	1/35	1/56	1/84
4	—	—	—	1/35	1/126	1/210
5	—	—	—	—	1/126	1/462
6	—	—	—	—	—	1/462

Source: Lockhart (1951).

number of stimuli a judge must examine to arrive at a single response. These chance probabilities are reproduced in Table 47.

Several methods of statistical analysis can be applied to data obtained from difference tests. Most common are adaptations of the binomial and chi-square distributions, from which tables have been prepared (National Bureau of Standards, 1950; Roessler *et al.*, 1948, 1956) to permit quick interpretation of data. Roessler *et al.* (1956) refer to true difference and directional difference tests as "one-tailed" because of only one possible correct answer, and refer to quality-preference applications of difference test designs as "two-tailed" because either response can be correct. A detailed discussion of these statistical procedures appears in Chapter 10.

It must be emphasized that statistics are essential to interpretation of results but will not correct erroneous data, improve a poor method or design, or compensate for lack of adequate control of experimental variables.

IV. Classification of Difference Tests

Difference implies comparison, either between two stimuli or among several stimuli. Each of these stimuli may be a single unit and/or a group of units. Since the number of units has a direct effect on the chance probability, it is reasonable to classify difference tests by the number of units a judge must evaluate before arriving at a single response, whether it be "yes or no" or "more or less."

Lockhart (1951) makes a broad classification of symmetrical and asymmetrical binomials. The symmetrical class consists of an equal number of each of the two samples being compared (AB, AABB, AAABBB, etc.). The asymmetrical class consists of unequal numbers of each (ABB, ABBB, AABBB, etc.). Fatigue, adaptation, memory span, and motivation limit the number of units presented. Wood (1949) discussed large numbers of units in theoretical systems which could be used in the sensory analysis of foods, but did not apply them to experimental situations. There are actually only a few reported studies where more than three units are presented to obtain a single response.

Several designs that have been classified as multistimuli or multisample difference tests are, nevertheless, actually difference tests in a single testing situation and should be classified as variations of their prototype. Most common is the "single-stimulus," which will be discussed under the two-sample classification.

Sensitivity is the criterion most frequently used in selection of a method for determining differences in sensory attributes of foods. However, the superior sensitivity of one design over another may become inferior with a different problem. What is meant by sensitivity? Peryam (1958) stated that a test should be considered better (more sensitive) if it will detect a smaller degree of difference with greater certainty, or with less effort. He frowns on the use of sensitivity per se as a useful criterion, and suggests the following criteria as being more useful: statistical and practical efficiency and appropriateness to the problem. Statistical efficiency is based on chance level; the lower the chance probability, the more efficient the design (Lockhart, 1951). Practical efficiency is related to the number of units evaluated to arrive at a single judgment (this Peryam defines as simplicity) as well as the probability of arriving at a correct response by chance. Lockhart (1951) used statistical efficiency as the criterion of choice because fewer tests are required to obtain statistically significant results in tests with the lowest chance probability. According to Peryam (1958), the appropriate test is influenced by the constancy of the panel, their level of motivation, amount of testing to be done, whether testing is to be continuous or intermittent, and whether the materials are uniform or varied. Important in addition may be variability among panel members in sensitivity to the designs, among facilities and conditions in the test environment, and among the quality of samples available. Since sensitivity is the main criterion for selection of a test design, factors of efficiency, simplicity, and appropriateness must be evaluated by the investigator in his test situation.

V. Two-Sample Tests

Comparison of two samples is commonly referred to as the paired-stimuli or paired-comparison test. In a true difference test, the judge is presented with two stimuli and asked to indicate whether there is a difference between them. In a directional test, two stimuli are presented for comparison and the judge must determine which of the two has the greater intensity of a specific, well-defined, and well-understood characteristic. In either test, the samples can be presented simultaneously or successively.

A. DIFFERENCE TESTS

Lockhart (1951) has stated that two-sample tests cannot be used to determine true difference or to measure discriminatory sensitivity, and should be used only for measuring quality judgments, consumer acceptance, or consumer preference. His justification for this statement is that "no-difference" answers are not permitted and that the question (is there or isn't there a difference) therefore is ambiguous and the test an absurdity. Pfaffmann *et al.* (1954), however, have shown that this system, allowing for "no-difference" answers, was comparable to others in discrimination of differences and did justifiably classify it as a difference test. We believe that their use in threshold determination clearly identifies them as difference tests.

When samples are presented successively, or singly, the term sometimes applied to this test is "single-stimulus," i.e., there is no direct intercomparison of the samples. It is actually a series of difference tests. Pfaffmann *et al.* (1954) also referred to this as the "A-not A" test. One of the two stimuli is designated as a standard. This standard is presented several times to acquaint the observer with its characteristics, and then the comparative stimulus and standard are presented randomly for a single response of "like A" or "not like A." The subject must be aware that the order is random and that the proportion of knowns (or standards) to unknowns may not be 50:50. To reacquaint the observer, the standard stimulus may be presented and identified from time to time during the series of trials in any one session. As described, this procedure seems to be somewhat casual, and there could be an effect on the number of correct responses obtained per trial, depending on the position of reintroduction of the standard stimulus. In an odor recognition study, Mrak *et al.* (1959) found that the number of correct responses when three successive unknowns followed the standard reference sample did not differ from that when only one unknown followed. Perhaps in some other test the result would be different, depending on the degree of difference between the two stimuli and on the variability among judges in memory spans.

Specific application of this procedure occurs in testing such as that by Mrak and co-workers in which an olfactometer was used and cross-comparison between two stimuli was physically impossible. It might also be applied where it is impossible to mask an uncontrollable sample characteristic which is detectable by the judges if the two samples are presented simultaneously but not if presented successively after a pre-determined lapse of time. The procedure can be used effectively to reduce adaptation by controlling the time span between stimuli. It might also be used when the quantities of test materials are limited. The procedure is well adapted to recognition studies, such as Yensen's (1959) work on determination of absolute thresholds for the basic tastes.

Since a response is obtained with each stimulus (except with the appearance of the identified A sample), one might say that this is the most economical difference test in that more information is obtained per stimulus, and that more trials can be made in a single test session because fatigue is reduced. It is also a simple test for the judge because he evaluates only one stimulus in obtaining his answer. The chance probability in the single-stimulus test is ½. This might appear to be inefficient statistically; however, such inefficiency could be overcome by the advantages just enumerated.

The presentation of two samples simultaneously (AA, AB, BA, or BB) is referred to as the paired-comparison method. The response in this case can be either "there is a difference" or "there is no difference." Requiring a "difference" response in all cases has been found to give better results than allowing "no-difference" responses in a paired test (Gridgeman, 1959). Figure 48 is an example of a record form. The paired-comparison procedure tends to minimize the memory effect associated with the single-stimulus procedure. Even so, if the time interval between stimuli is not controlled in paired-comparison tests of tastes or odors, there may be an increase in adaptation affect. Simultaneous presentation usually implies intercomparison (and may not be avoided in visual tests); however, in taste tests Pfaffmann *et al.* (1954) specified no retasting. Their procedure would simulate the single-stimulus except that the time lapse between samples would be regulated by the judge rather than by the experimenter.

Administration of the two-sample difference tests is most important. Judges must be informed of the probability of receiving identical or different stimuli. Complete randomness of presentation is essential so that the observer responds to each trial independently, and so that the probability of ½ in the statistical analysis may be justified. The procedures are limited in application because of the necessity of rigid homogeneity in sample characteristics.

Comparison of the same two stimuli in all trials at the same session is not necessary. Pangborn (1959) used the "choice" method of Richter and MacLean (1939) in threshold determinations for sucrose, sodium

	Apple Difference Study	
		Set_____
		Date_____
		Name_____
	Check one	
Pair	There is a difference	There is no difference
A		
B		
C		

Fig. 48. Record form for paired-comparison.

chloride, citric acid, and caffeine. Observers compared various concentrations of any one or all of these substances with distilled water at each session, and indicated whether the paired solutions were identical or different. If they indicated a difference, they then attempted to identify the taste. No statistical analysis was applied to the data obtained; thresholds were established when the observer made two successive correct identifications.

B. DIRECTIONAL TESTS

The paired-comparison test, adopted from psychophysical procedures (Guilford, 1954), is the two-sample directional test used most widely in laboratory studies. The judge is asked to designate the sample within each pair which is more intense in the predefined criterion under investigation (Fig. 49). If all other characteristics of the pair are not identical, response to the criterion may be subject to variations in interpretation among the panel of trained judges. Cognizance of this requirement of homogeneity was the basis upon which Cover (1936) applied the paired test to comparisons of tenderness in beef. The samples used in her studies varied in method of cooking: the two test materials presented to each judge were similar in that they were obtained from the same animal (right and left sides), same muscle, and same location within the muscles. Seeking homogeneity even to this extent cannot always eliminate unwanted differences in meat studies. Doty and Pierce (1961) reported that the ribeyes from the same position on the two sides of a carcass do not have exactly the same composition and properties.

SET_____

SWEETNESS DISCRIMINATION STUDY

NAME_____   DATE_____

CIRCLE SWEETER SAMPLE WITHIN EACH PAIR.

PAIR	SAMPLES
A	_____ _____
B	_____ _____
C	_____ _____
D	_____ _____
E	_____ _____

Fɪɢ. 49. Examples of paired-comparison directional test.

Tarver *et al.* (1959) adapted the two-sample difference test to measurement of the degree of difference between two samples. Test materials are compared with a standard, and the degree of difference between the two samples is indicated (0 = no difference; 5 = extremely large difference). Figure 50 is an example of a score card used for this type of test. A "chance" factor is determined from a standard-to-standard comparison. This factor is applied in the analysis of variance procedure in determining the observer's "real" difference response between the standard and the test-material comparison. Because it does require a quantity judgment, and therefore inherits subjective influences, it should not be classified as a true-difference test.

Difference tests applied to situations where homogeneity is difficult to attain are extremely subject to errors of both the first and second kinds. In such cases, for the data to be reliable and reproducible the number of replications must be greater than with more homogeneous materials.

Positional bias could be an important factor in two-sample dimensional tests, particularly when the criterion is such that adaptation is rapid and the time interval between the stimuli is short. As noted in

Chapter 6, difference thresholds of tastes have been reported to vary significantly with the order in which the stimuli are presented. This adaptation effect would be more pronounced in simultaneous presentation, and would bias the response toward greater intensity in the first

| | | | SET_____ |
| NAME_____ | | DATE_____ | |

Directions: Circle the sample within each pair with the greater FLAVOR, then indicate the degree of flavor difference within each pair.

Samples		Flavor Difference Within Pairs			
		Slight	Moderate	Large	Extreme

FIG. 50. Record form for paired test with degree of difference.

stimulus, i.e., would result in a positive time-error effect. In successive presentation, the time interval between stimuli could be such that a memory effect would bias the response inversely, as reported by Metzner (1943). Specific evidence of these effects is lacking in the literature.

In all such tests where different qualities of odors or flavors are presented, i.e., normal and abnormal flavors, it is essential that the judges be able to recognize the nature of the differences.

VI. Three-Sample Tests

Variations in the triad, or three-sample, test have been summarized by Gregson (1960), as follows:

1. Two stimuli, different from one another, are presented and followed by a third. The judge is asked to indicate which of the first two is the same as the third.

2. One stimulus, identified as a standard, is presented, followed by two unlike stimuli, and the observer is asked to indicate which of the two is the same as the labeled standard (the classical duo-trio test).

3. Three samples, two of which contain the same stimulus, are presented, and the observer is required to indicate the odd sample (the classical triangle test).

4. Three samples containing three stimuli are presented, and the

judge has a choice of three responses: all identical; two identical and one different; or all different. If the judge responds that one is different, he is asked to indicate which one.

Three-sample difference tests vary in psychological complexity and in the chance probability of a correct identification. In the first two variations, above, where there are set standards, the chance probability is $\frac{1}{2}$, and in the third variation, the triangle test, the chance probability is $\frac{1}{3}$. The last variation is considerably more complex, and, because of psychological and statistical implications, is rarely used. Ellis (1961) suggested that the "no-difference" and "all-different" responses be combined and split equally among the three possible odd-sample designations, but in view of the psychological complexities we do not recommend this procedure.

A. The Duo-Trio Difference Test

The duo-trio was described by Peryam and Swartz (1950) as first being applied in the Joseph E. Seagram Quality Control Laboratories, in 1941. In this triad design, the observer is first presented with a standard stimulus. After this sample is examined, it is removed and two unknown samples are submitted successively in random order. The judge is requested to indicate which of the two unknowns is the same as the first sample, with a chance probability of $\frac{1}{2}$. For a record form, see Fig. 51.

Tomato Juice

Duo Trio Design

Set_____   Judge_____

Taste the two samples of juice in each set and check the number of the coded sample which is the same as the reference sample, R.

Set	Samples	Same as R
_____	_____	_____
	_____	_____
_____	_____	_____
	_____	_____
_____	_____	_____
	_____	_____

Fig. 51. Record form for duo-trio test.

The time interval between the presentation of successive stimuli can be manipulated, depending on characteristics of the samples, i.e., whether they readily induce fatigue. The test also allows for control of the quantity of sample taken, because, as originally designed, no retasting is permitted. Normally, when the two stimuli are of an unknown characteristic difference, both samples are presented randomly as the standard. However, Peryam and Swartz (1950) and Mitchell (1956b) have found that discrimination is better when the weaker of the two samples or the one with the more typical or familiar characteristics is used as the standard. Dawson *et al.* (1963), however, reported better discrimination in the duo-trio when the stronger or more unusual flavor was the odd sample. Obviously further research is needed.

As with the other difference tests, the number of trials which can be evaluated by a judge at one session is dependent on the characteristics of the stimuli. Brandt and Hutchinson (1956) found that, for routine quality control of alcoholic beverages, a single duo-trio test per session was inefficient in use of the panel's time and ability. They found no loss in discrimination with four trials. Mitchell (1956a) obtained proportionately more correct responses with five trials of beer per session than with only two. He attributed this apparent increase in performance to the fact that a judge can learn from the first tests and profit from that knowledge in the succeeding tests. This philosophy might well apply to the other difference tests.

The duo-trio has not been used as extensively as the difference tests discussed previously. This may be attributable to its supposedly lesser discriminatory power than that of the triangle or two-sample design (Pfaffmann *et al.*, 1954; Gridgeman, 1955). However, Pfaffmann's tasters were allowed to retaste in the triangle tests and not in the duo-trio. Gridgeman's objections were largely statistical. What is needed here are a variety of experiments with different foods, comparing the two procedures. As pointed out by Peryam and Swartz (1950), the duo-trio has the advantage of controlled timing. It definitely helps the observer to remember the samples when he can place them in a visual-spatial frame of reference and can also recheck previous impressions. Those workers, however, recommend the duo-trio for tests involving simple flavors, but do not recommend it for testing differences in odor or appearance. It is believed to be most efficient when the labeled sample is always the control (normal) sample.

To date, there is little in the literature reporting use of the duo-trio design in directional difference testing. The disadvantages outlined above might not be present in such an application. Recently Boggs *et al.* (1964) used the duo-trio method as a modified directional difference test by asking the question "Which coded sample tastes more like the labeled sample?" and "Which coded sample tastes more like freshly cooked dried Lima beans of the same variety?" The control was always used as the labeled sample. Stone and Bosley (1964) also used the duo-trio as a directional difference test for quality of potato chips processed by two treatments. No characterization of the differences was possible. Because of possible odd-sample bias the orders of presentation should be balanced.

B. TRIANGLE TEST

The triangle test, first suggested by Bengtsson (1943), was used by Helm and Trolle (1946) as a method of selecting expert beer tasters. Peryam and Swartz (1950) reported that the triangle test had been developed independently in the laboratories of Joseph E. Seagram and Sons, in 1941, for quality control and research on whiskey. Since its appearance, the method has been used by most laboratories in measuring the sensory properties of foods. Because of its extensive application, the

Judge_____	Date_____

Two of these samples are identical and the other different. Please check the duplicate samples and score <u>all</u> samples for presence or absence of off-flavor. Please do not score for preference - only for off-flavor due to the treatment.

Scoring: Off-flavor present 1
Off-flavor absent   0

Sample No.	Duplicate samples (indicate by ✓)	Score
_____	_____	_____
_____	_____	_____
_____	_____	_____

FIG. 52. Report form for triangle test, including score.

test has been the most thoroughly studied and criticized of all test designs. It is applied as frequently for determining true differences as for determining directional differences. Although the three samples are usually presented simultaneously, allowing for intercomparison, they could also be presented successively. Figure 52 is an example of a report form for triangle tests. The triangle test was first applied to foods in true-difference tests. The judge is informed that two of the three stimuli are identical and one is different, and must select the odd sample. The two stimuli can be presented in six different arrangements (AAB, ABA, BAA, BBA, BAB, ABB), and the probability of selecting the odd sample by chance alone is ⅓.

The triangle test can be used in the same situations as the two-sample difference test when the samples are homogeneous and especially when the dimension of difference is not known or is too complex for all judges to comprehend alike. Pfaffmann *et al.* (1954) and Filipello (1956) found the power of difference discrimination quite similar in the two tests, and slightly in favor of the triad design. If fatigue and adaptation are not a problem, the triangle test might be more efficient from the statistical

TABLE 48

Illustration of Bias for the Middle Sample in Triangle Difference Tests When Three Samples Are the Same Stimulus

Test no.	Number of times identified as the pair		
	1 and 2	1 and 3	2 and 3
1	3	5	2
2	1	6	3
3	4	4	2
4	2	6	2
5	4	4	2
6	2	5	3
	16	30	14

Source: Harries (1956).

standpoint. However, several types of biases associated with the test could offset the statistical efficiency. The most obvious are positional and sample-characteristic biases. The positional bias of selecting the middle sample as the "odd" sample is referred to by Harrison and Elder (1950) as "psychological appeal of symmetry." These results were confirmed by Harries (1956), using triangle tests involving no stimulus variation. Harries' data, illustrated in Table 48, are from the same ten observers in six tests.

Harrison and Elder and Harries observed bias for the middle sample in total-panel observations. Hopkins (1954), on the other hand, found resistance to the same bias by individual judges. In his test, however, there were actual stimulus differences which may have been partially responsible for the reverse bias observed. The bias was not consistent within judges when the more or less intense stimulus appeared in the middle position, i.e., ABA or BAB. In the same study, Hopkins illustrated that stimulus characteristics had an effect on the judge's ability to discriminate in triangle difference tests. Some judges could discriminate better when the odd sample was of higher intensity, and others when it was of lower intensity. In beer tasting, when the comparison was between a "normal" and "abnormal" stimulus, the observers could make a correct response more frequently when the like-stimuli were the "normal" samples (Helm and Trolle, 1946). It has also been reported by Filipello (1956) and Pfaffmann *et al.* (1954) that in repeated testing, performance is better when the odd sample is kept constant. They attribute this to a learning effect, i.e., the observers became familiar with the odd sample, and once they identified it their work was complete.

Actually, keeping the odd sample constant reduces the triangle test to a paired test since any one comparison establishes the odd sample (if the taster knows that the odd sample is always the same). Thus p (the chance probability of the null hypothesis) is $\frac{1}{2}$ and it is easy to see why there is a greater degree of success. Even if the taster is not told that the odd sample is being kept constant he may so conclude after a series of tests.

It is questionable whether the triangle difference test should be applied for obtaining recognition threshold values for substances which can be unambiguously identified by judges without subjective inference. Several investigators have illustrated that the just noticeable difference (jnd) was significantly higher with the triangle test than with the two-sample directional difference test in measurements of simple bitterness and sweetness (Byer and Abrams, 1953; Filipello, 1956). On the other hand, Dawson and Dochterman (1951) and Pfaffmann *et al.* (1954) found the paired test to be superior for testing the flavor of chocolate fudge. Gridgeman (1955) found the tests about equal for measuring primary tastes in aqueous solutions, tomato juice, and ground beef. Dawson and Dochterman preferred the triangle method for selecting judges because of greater confidence in results: judges unable to identify duplicate samples could be eliminated. Filipello (1956) believes the superiority of the paired test results from the higher jnd of the triangle procedure. Thus, even though the triangle test may induce greater discrimination, the higher jnd overcomes its statistical advantage. Filipello noted at the subthreshold level of sucrose a significant lag in percent correct responses which did not appear with suprathreshold levels (Fig. 53). He suggested that this lag represented the judge's transition from noncognizance to recognition of the stimulus. It may be that at the subthreshold level the curve is sigmoid and that if the correct judgments were converted to probit values a straight line would result. The apparent straight line at the suprathreshold concentrations may be due to the large extrapolation of the triangular curve. More data would be useful.

As indicated in Chapter 10, application of the triangular procedure successively for difference and direction is not recommended. Some of the criticism might be eliminated if the directional differentiation were permitted only when the judge first successfully identified the odd sample. This would still include those who were correct by chance but

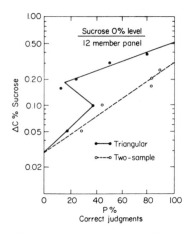

FIG. 53. Comparison of response for triangular and two-sample designs. Source: Filipello (1956).

would eliminate the judge's confusion of trying to identify the direction of the difference when the odd sample has not been correctly identified. However, removal of some of the judges confuses the statistical analysis.

For statistical considerations, see Chapter 10 and the tables referred to therein. When the number of judges is small, a multinomial rather than the binomial distribution may be useful (Roberts *et al.*, 1958).

C. TRIANGLE DIRECTIONAL TEST

Application of the directional variation of the triangle test requires the observer to identify the sample(s) which is (are) more intense in a predefined characteristic. Thus, the chance probability of a correct response is $\frac{1}{6}$, i.e., one of the six possible arrangements of the two stimuli (AAB, ABA, BAA, BBA, BAB, ABB). Requisites for this test are very similar to those for the two-sample directional test, i.e., homogeneity of the two stimuli in all characteristics but the specified criterion, and a completely consistent understanding of the criterion by the panel members.

The more common application of the triangle test in denoting direction of difference is a two-step or dual-answer test, i.e., the subject is first asked to identify the odd sample; then he is asked to designate the odd or duplicates in the defined criterion. There are two basic approaches to analyzing data from this procedure:

1. Use directional data only from the observations in which the odd sample was correctly identified. This assumes the basic triangle directional test chance probability of $\frac{1}{6}$. Bengtsson (1943) and Lockhart (1951) both recommended this procedure in analysis of results.

2. The other method of treating the data simulates the two-sample test procedure, with a $\frac{1}{2}$ chance probability. Byer and Abrams (1953) clearly illustrated that discrimination could be demonstrated better by applying this latter procedure of analysis (Table 50). They expressed results of their tests in σ units, or the number of standard deviations by which the correct selections exceeded expectation ($\frac{1}{2}$) of correctly identifying the odd sample by chance.

Several investigators indicated that, in triangle directional testing, the criterion of identification is not made randomly by the observers who do not identify the odd sample correctly (Helm and Trolle, 1946; Berg *et al.*, 1955; Pfaffmann *et al.*, 1954). This phenomenon is attributed to the presence of the third stimulus, which requires more than one comparison and consequently reduces observer efficiency by contributing to psychological error and/or physiological fatigue.

The adverse characteristic of applying the triangle as a directional test is clearly demonstrated by the data in Table 49 which indicate that it is not comparable in discriminating power to the two-sample directional test, where only one comparison is required of the observers. The results of Pfaffmann *et al.* (1954) showed less difference. Figure 54 is an example of a report form.

In 1954, Davis and Hanson published a system for analyzing test designs of two or more samples with only one level of difference, including the triangle directional test. Their approach takes more complete advantage of information obtained from such tests than those described above. The procedure provides for inclusion of weighted "intensity" values for partially as well as completely correct judgments in assignment of the direction of the criterion of difference. In their procedure, correct selection of the odd sample is incidental, and the analysis is based entirely on the number of samples identified correctly. We believe there is a fundamental difficulty in the use of such data. The philosophy of the triangle system rests on the ability to identify the odd sample. Use of data which fail to identify the odd sample thus seems inappropriate (see also Chapter 10, Section II,C). On the other hand, Bradley (1964) and Gridgeman (1964) argue that one can and should evaluate directional information based on data where the correct odd sample is not identified. White *et al.* (1964) utilized this procedure. The analysis can be somewhat arduous.

Positional biases which are inherent in the triangle difference test also operate in the directional test. With the added complexity of the criterion, additional biases may arise, particularly when the triangle test is applied to determine quality or preferences. Schutz and Bradley (1954)

TABLE 49

Comparison of Triangle and Two-Sample Procedures for Bitterness and Sweetness

	Total trials	No. correct selections	Percent correct selections Obtained	Expected	No. correct selections above chance expectancy, in σ units
Quinine sulfate: 0.0050% vs. 0.0075%					
Triangle					
Selection odd sample	50	25	50	$33\frac{1}{3}$	2.50**
Two-sample					
Selection more bitter	38	34	89	50	4.87***
Quinine sulfate: 0.0050% vs. 0.0060%					
Triangle					
Selection odd sample	46	21	46	$33\frac{1}{3}$	1.77*
Two-sample					
Selection more bitter					
Trial 1	64	47	73	50	3.75***
Trial 2	54	40	74	50	3.54***
Glucose: 1.19% vs. 1.40%					
Triangle					
Selection odd sample	45	21	47	$33\frac{1}{3}$	1.90*
Two-sample					
Selection sweeter					
Trial 1	45	33	73	50	3.13***
Trial 2	45	31	69	50	2.54**

*, **, *** Respectively significant at $p = 0.05$, 0.01, and 0.001.

Source: Byer and Abrams (1953).

suggested that when a sample is assessed as different from the other two, it may produce a bias in favor of the duplicate samples based on the analogy that things which are different are strange or not as good. They illustrate this point by use of a hedonic rating scale (Chapter 9, Section VII) whereby, in two different studies, samples judged to be the same were given average ratings of 7.63 and 6.87 and samples judged to be odd received average ratings of 6.90 and 5.79. In both studies, all three samples submitted to each observer as a test unit were identical. How-

TABLE 50

Quality Intensity Designations of Bitterness and Sweetness in Triangle Tests

	Total trials	No. correct	Percent correct[a]	No. correct above chance expectancy, in σ units
Quinine sulfate: 0.0050% vs. 0.0075%				
Odd sample selection correct	25	24	96	4.60***
Odd sample selection incorrect	25	20	80	3.00**
Total	50	44	88	5.37***
Quinine sulfate: 0.0050% vs. 0.0060%				
Odd sample selection correct	21	15	71	1.97*
Odd sample selection incorrect	24	17	71	2.04*
Total	45	32	71	2.83**
Glucose: 1.19% vs. 1.40%				
Odd sample selection correct	21	15	71	1.97*
Odd sample selection incorrect	26	21	81	3.14***
Total	47	36	77	3.65***

[a] Expected value = 50%.
*, **, *** Respectively significant at $p = 0.05$, 0.01, and 0.001.
Source: Byer and Abrams (1953).

ever, those workers also illustrated a bias *against* the odd sample when a real difference in hedonic rating existed as determined by single-sample evaluation. Further studies would be desirable to determine the extent of this effect under all conditions.

Although the triangle test has been demonstrated to be similar to the

				SET_____
NAME_____			DATE_____	

DIRECTIONS: Handle glass by stem. Swirl contents gently before sniffing. Indicate by a check:

1. Which sample is different.
2. Which sample(s) contain(s) the greater odor.
3. Whether the samples are pleasant or unpleasant.
4. A complete description of the odor of each sample.

SAMPLES	DIFFERENT SAMPLE	STRONGER ODOR	PLEASANT OR UNPLEASANT	DESCRIPTION OF EACH

Fig. 54. Report form for triangle test with directional information.

two-sample test in establishing significant directional or criterion differences, there are factors which should be considered before deciding to use it. The bias factors are greater in the triangle design, and could be effective in increasing the difference necessary for significant discrimination, particularly when analysis of the data is based on the binomial distribution or chi-square. In addition to the psychological effects, physiological fatigue may well be a critical factor. More practical considerations are the increased quantities of samples required and the additional details involved in administration for accuracy and thorough randomness in preparation of the sets of triads.

VII. Multisample Tests

Tests involving more than three stimuli are classified as multisample tests. They may have equal (symmetrical) or unequal (asymmetrical) numbers of each stimulus (Lockhart, 1951). When they are applied as

SET_____

NAME_____   DATE_____

Please answer the following questions concerning the samples presented.

SAMPLES _____   _____   _____   _____   _____

SAMPLE NUMBERS

Which are the sweetest samples?   _____

Which samples have more_____ flavor?   _____

Which samples do you like most?   _____

Which samples do you like least?   _____

Comments:

FIG. 55. Record form for multiple presentation of samples.

true difference tests, the judge is required to sort the samples into two groups of like samples. When they are applied as directional tests, the judge is requested to identify the groups of higher or lower intensity of a given criterion (Fig. 55).

Analysis can be based on the binomial or chi-square distributions when the data are classified as completely correct or incorrect, using the appropriate chance probability for the particular situation. Other methods of analysis have been recommended (Davis and Hanson, 1954) which would yield more information by considering partially correct responses. We agree with Lockhart (1951), however, that use of partially correct responses is not to be recommended and we favor the simpler procedures for testing purposes. However, he also recommended multi-sample testing and using partially correct responses for panel selection. Even this does not appear to be a good procedure. Difference-test designs involving more than three stimuli have had only limited use. As previously indicated, the limitation is based on the increase in psychological complexity and physiological fatigue which accompanies an increase in the number of stimuli. In addition, larger quantities of samples are required, and more time is needed for the observers to make a decision. If the judge cannot recognize the sensory attribute it is difficult for him to proceed; if he can recognize it then a paired comparison seems more appropriate. Under certain circumstances some of these disadvantages may be minimized. Peryam and Swartz (1950) found multi-sample tests applicable to odor evaluations, in which recovery from fatigue and adaptation are considerably more rapid than in taste analyses. The psychological complexity, however, still remains. These tests appear to be most applicable to visual discriminations, where the judge does not rely on memory, and fatigue is almost nonexistent. When applied to visual studies, the quantities of sample required are not necessarily increased greatly, since the samples are not consumed and more than one judge can evaluate the same set of stimuli. This may also be applicable to odor evaluations, if the stimuli are of such a nature as to allow for a number of observations on each set without contamination or loss of intensity.

As noted by Lockhart (1951), the statistical efficiency of a test increases with the number of stimuli per test unit, i.e., increasingly smaller chance probabilities with increase in numbers. However, the statistical efficiency is minimized by the previously mentioned psychological disadvantages. Gridgeman (1956) showed that small flavor differences were detected more efficiently when four two-sample directional tests were administered than when the same number of stimuli (eight) were presented as an octad (AAAABBBB) for the observers to group on the basis of a given criterion of difference.

The *dual-standard* test was adapted for odor tests by the Quartermaster Food and Container Institute (Peryam and Swartz, 1950). Both stimuli are presented as standards simultaneously, and after the judge develops a criterion of difference between the two, a second pair of unidentified stimuli is presented. The judge must match the unidentified samples with the standards, and the chance probability is ½ (Fig. 56). He may intercompare all four samples since they are all present simultaneously. The *multiple-standards difference* test was developed at the Quartermaster Institute for odor evaluation when a nonuniform standard was to be compared with an unknown. Any number of the questionable standards

---

MILK STUDY

SET_____

NAME_____   DATE_____

Directions: Taste each standard, then circle the number of the sample within each pair which is identical to STANDARD A. Indicate what criteria you are using to detect differences between A and B (flavor, odor, viscosity, sweetness, saltiness, aftertaste, etc.)

Standards: A = _____ Control _____

B = _____ Treated _____

Pairs   Pairs

1. _____   _____   4. _____   _____

2. _____   _____   5. _____   _____

3. _____   _____   6. _____   _____

Criteria of Difference Between A and B _____

Do not swallow the sample.

Rinse with distilled water between each pair.

Fig. 56. Paired test with dual standards. Source: Pangborn and Dunkley (1964).

are presented simultaneously with the unknown, and the judge is requested to designate the one which is most different. The chance probability of identifying the unknown correctly is one over the total number of samples involved.

VIII. Comparison of Procedures

Peryam (1958) ranked the various difference tests in terms of increasing complexity as follows: paired, single-stimulus, dual-standard, duo-trio, triangle, multiple standard, and multiple paired (where the judge sorts the samples into "A" and "not-A"). The paired-comparison test should not be used in directional tests unless the dimension and direction of difference can be clearly specified. The multiple standard test is infrequently used except in unusual situations where the standard is a family of materials rather than a single material.

For the same p (the chance probability on the null hypothesis), tri-

TABLE 51
Types of Difference Tests

Name	Method of presentation	Standard	Response	Probability
Single stimulus (A not A)	"A" or "B" A | ? ? ? ? ...	One present and designated at onset of test and can be reintroduced	"A" or "not A"; "like A" or "not like A"	1/2
Paired comparison	A B or A A or B B or B A ? ? ? ? ? ? ? ?	Subjective	"Different" or "Not different"	1/2
Paired comparison	A B ? ?	Subjective	Which is saltier?, Which is tougher, etc.	1/2
Duo-trio	A | A B | ? ?	One present and designated	Which is the different sample? or Which is the same as A?	1/2
Triangle	A A B or A B B ? ? ? ? ? ?	None designated; criterion is within test	Which is the odd sample?	1/3
Triangle	A A B or A B B ? ? ? ? ? ?	None designated; criterion is within test	Which is sweeter? More acid? etc.	1/6
Dual standard	A B | A B | ? ?	Two present and designated	Which is A and which is B?	1/2
Multiple standard[a]	B ? A A A ? ? ?	None designated; criterion is within test	Which is *most* different?	1/4 (or less)
Multiple pairs	A B A B ? ? ? ? B A B A ? ? ? ?	None designated; criterion is within test	Which are A and which are B?	1/35[b]

[a] Used where standard is nonhomogeneous; all samples presented simultaneously.
[b] As shown for all correct; various higher probabilities for partially correct responses.
Adapted from Peryam (1958).

angular tests have a statistical advantage over duo-trio or paired presentations, both per replicate and per aliquot. Byer and Abrams (1953) suggested that p is greater for paired comparison because fewer intercomparisons are required. It appears that such superiority in discrimination may sometimes offset the statistical advantages per aliquot in the triangular system.

Other factors are also important in selecting a system (Hopkins and Gridgeman, 1955). Scheduling, assembling, instructing, and return of the panel members to their normal occupations are operations that are largely independent of the number of samples tested. When the number of tests is small the relative power per man-hour for both methods may be intermediate between their relative powers per replicate and per aliquot. In large-scale testing and with scarce or costly materials, the relative power-cost ratios will resemble relative power per aliquot most closely.

Park (1961) noted that the triangular test is likely to be more vulnerable than the paired-comparison procedure to the complications arising from wide differences in treatments and interactions of judges × treatments. Thus it may be of limited applicability where treatments differ in kind rather than in degree.

IX. Summary

The various difference tests are summarized in Table 51. Further research is needed to evaluate the effect of various factors on the relative efficiency of the different procedures. Some of the problems that remain to be solved are the influence of time-stress in the duo-trio, the nature of the psychological decision when the triangle test is used as a directional test, the psychological complexity of multisample tests, and new procedures for special problems (such as storage tests).

REFERENCES

Amerine, M. A. 1963. Subjective aspects of flavor. *Proc. 1st Intern. Food Sci. Congr.* 3. In press.

Baker, G. A., M. A. Amerine, and E. B. Roessler. 1954. Errors of the second kind in organoleptic difference testing. *Food Research* 19, 206–210.

Baker, R. A. 1962. Subjective panel testing. *Ind. Quality Control* 19(3), 22–28.

Bengtsson, K. 1943. Provsmakning som analysmetod. Statistisk behandling av resultaten. *Svenska Bryggareforen Månadsblad* 58, 59–71, 102–111, 149–157.

Berg, H. W., F. Filipello, E. Hinreiner, and A. D. Webb. 1955. Evaluation of thresholds and minimum difference concentrations for various constituents of wines. I. Water solutions of pure substances. *Food Technol.* 9, 23–26.

Blom, G. 1955. How many taste testers? *Wallerstein Lab. Commun.* 18, 173–178.

Boggs, M. M., and H. L. Hanson. 1949. Analysis of foods by sensory difference tests. *Advances in Food Research* 2, 219–258.

Boggs, M. M., H. J. Morris, and D. W. Venstrom. 1964. Stability studies with cooked legume powders; flavor-judging procedure. *Food Technol.* **18**(10), 114–117.

Brandt, D. A., and E. P. Hutchinson. 1956. Retention of taste sensitivity. *Food Technol.* **10**, 419–420.

Bradley, R. A. 1964. Applications of the modified triangle test in sensory difference trials. *J. Food Sci.* **29**, 668–672.

Byer, A. J., and D. Abrams. 1953. A comparison of the triagular and two-sample taste-test methods. *Food Technol.* **7**, 185–187.

Byer, A. J., and P. P. Gray. 1953. Some considerations in applying systematic taste testing to beer. *Wallerstein Lab. Commun.* **16**, 303–312.

Cartwright, L. C., C. T. Snell, and P. H. Kelley. 1952. Organoleptic panel testing as a research tool. *Anal. Chem.* **24**, 503–506.

Cover, S. 1936. A new subjective method of testing tenderness in meat—the paired-eating method. *Food Research* **1**, 287–295 (see also **5**, 379–394, 1940).

Davis, J. G., and H. L. Hanson. 1954. Sensory test methods. 1. The triangle intensity (T-I) and related test systems for sensory analysis. *Food Technol.* **8**, 335–339.

Dawson, E. H., and E. F. Dochterman. 1951. A comparison of sensory methods of measuring differences in food qualities. *Food Technol.* **5**, 79–81.

Dawson, E. H., J. L. Brogdon, and S. McManus. 1963. Sensory testing of differences in taste. I. Methods. *Food Technol.* **17**(9), 45–48, 51.

Doty, D. M., and J. C. Pierce. 1961. Beef muscle characteristics as related to carcass weight and degree of aging. *U. S. Dept. Agr., A.M.S. Tech. Bull.* **1231**, 1–85.

Ellis, B. H. 1961. "A Guide Book for Sensory Testing," 55 pp. Continental Can Co., Chicago, Illinois.

Filipello, F. 1956. A critical comparison of the two-sample and triangular binomial designs. *Food Research* **21**, 235–241.

Gregson, R. A. M. 1960. Bias in the measurement of food preferences by triangular tests. *Occupational Psychol.* **34**, 249–257.

Gridgeman, N. T. 1955. Taste comparisons: two samples or three? *Food Technol.* **9**, 148–150.

Gridgeman, N. T. 1956. Group size in taste sorting trials. *Food Research* **21**, 534–539.

Gridgeman, N. T. 1959. Pair comparisons with and without ties. *Biometrics* **15**, 382–388.

Gridgeman, N. T. 1964. Sensory comparisons: the 2-stage triangle test with sample variability. *J. Food Sci.* **29**, 112–117.

Guilford, J. P. 1954. "Psychometric Methods," 597 pp. McGraw-Hill, New York.

Harries, J. M. 1956. Positional bias in sensory assessments. *Food Technol.* **10**, 86–90.

Harrison, S., and L. W. Elder. 1950. Some applications of statistics to laboratory taste testing. *Food Technol.* **4**, 434–439.

Helm, E., and B. Trolle. 1946. Selection of a taste panel. *Wallerstein Lab. Commun.* **9**, 181–194.

Hopkins, J. W. 1954. Some observations on sensitivity and repeatability of triad taste difference tests. *Biometrics* **10**, 521–531.

Hopkins, J. W., and N. T. Gridgeman. 1955. Comparative sensitivity of pair and triad flavor intensity difference tests. *Biometrics* **11**, 63–68.

Lockhart, E. E. 1951. Binomial systems and organoleptic analysis. *Food Technol.* **5**, 428–431.

Metzner, C. A. 1943. Investigation of odor and taste. Psychological principles. *Wallerstein Lab. Commun.* **6**, 5–18.

Mitchell, J. W. 1956a. Duration of sensitivity in trio taste testing. *Food Technol.* **10**, 201–203.

Mitchell, J. W. 1956b. The effect of assignment of testing materials to the paired and odd position in the duo-trio taste difference test. *Food Technol.* **10**, 169–171.

Mrak, V., M. A. Amerine, C. S. Ough, and G. A. Baker. 1959. Odor difference test with applications to consumer preferences. *Food Research* **24**, 574–578.

National Bureau of Standards. 1950. Tables of the binomial probability distribution. *Appl. Math. Ser.* **6**, 1–387. U. S. Govt. Printing Office, Washington, D. C.

Pangborn, R. M. 1959. Influence of hunger on sweetness preferences and taste thresholds. *Am. J. Clin. Nutrition* **7**, 280–287.

Pangborn, R. M., and W. L. Dunkley. 1964. Sensory discrimination of fat and solids-not-fat in milk. *J. Dairy Sci.* **47**, 719–726.

Park, G. T. 1961. Sensory testing by triple comparisons. *Biometrics* **17**, 251–260.

Peryam, D. R. 1958. Sensory difference tests. *Food Technol.* **12**, 231–236.

Peryam, D. R., and V. W. Swartz. 1950. Measurement of sensory differences. *Food Technol.* **4**, 390–395.

Pfaffmann, C., H. Schlosberg, and J. Cornsweet. 1954. Variables affecting difference tests. *In* "Food Acceptance Testing Methodology," 115 pp. (see pp. 4–17). Advisory Board on Quartermaster Research and Development, Committee on Foods; and Natl. Acad. Sci., Natl. Research Council, Chicago, Illinois.

Radkins, A. P. 1957. Some statistical considerations in organoleptic research: triangle, paired and duo-trio tests. *Food Research* **22**, 259–265.

Richter, C. P., and A. MacLean. 1939. Salt taste thresholds of humans. *Am. J. Physiol.* **126**, 1–6.

Roberts, H. R., C. H. McCall, Jr., and R. E. Thomas. 1958. Some statistical considerations for small sample evaluation in triangle taste tests. *Food Research* **23**, 388–395.

Roessler, E. B., J. Warren, and J. F. Guymon. 1948. Significance in the triangle taste tests. *Food Research* **13**, 503–505.

Roessler, E. B., G. A. Baker, and M. A. Amerine. 1956. One-tailed and two-tailed tests in organoleptic comparisons. *Food Research* **21**, 117–121.

Schutz, H. G., and J. E. Bradley. 1954. Effect of bias on preference in the difference-preference test. *In* "Food Acceptance Testing Methodology," 115 pp. (see pp. 85–92). Advisory Board on Quartermaster Research and Development, Committee on Foods; and Natl. Acad. Sci., Natl. Research Council, Chicago, Illinois.

Stone, H., and J. P. Bosley. 1964. Difference-preference testing with the duo-trio test. *Psychol. Repts.* **14**, 620–622.

Tarver, M. G., B. A. Hall, and J. G. McDonald. 1959. A statistical quality control approach to the selection of flavor panel members. *Trans. Ann. Convention, Am. Soc. Quality Control* **13**, 459–485.

White, E. D., H. L. Hanson, A. A. Klose, and H. Lineweaver. 1964. Evaluation of toughness differences in turkeys. *J. Food Sci.* **29**, 673–678.

Wood, E. C. 1949. Organoleptic tests in the food industry. III. Some statistical considerations in organoleptic tests. *J. Soc. Chem. Ind.* **68**, 128–131.

Yensen, R. 1959. Some factors affecting taste sensitivity in man. I. Food intake and time of day. *Quart. J. Exptl. Psychol.* **11**, 221–229.

Chapter 8

Laboratory Studies: Quantity-Quality Evaluation

A highly trained laboratory panel, besides measuring differences in sensory properties between treatments, is frequently used to establish the intensity of a sensory characteristic or the over-all quality of a food. Usually it is not difficult to assess intensity, but quality is more elusive and poses considerable difficulty in definition, measurement, and interpretation. Quality standards are dependent on the intended use of the product, the conditions of testing, and the frame of reference of the judge. Kramer (1959) defined food quality as "the composite of those characteristics that differentiate individual units of a product and have significance in determining the degree of acceptability of that unit by the user." Quality can be defined operationally, as a composite response derived from all the sensory properties of a specific food that cause it to be judged superior by users who have been exposed to a random selection of the product over a period of time. But the specific operations by which quality is "measured" are not always clear. Consistent and reproducible evaluations of quality can be made only by judges who have a complete frame of reference, derived from experience and prolonged exposure to the specific commodity. Quality evaluations made by groups of untrained judges are difficult to duplicate. Increasing the size of the group may or may not increase the reproducibility of the responses. Generally, absence of defects rather than a descriptive definition of quality is the criterion employed. *In all tests described in this chapter, unless otherwise specified, trained laboratory personnel or experts familiar with the product and procedures should be used.*

Lack of standardized procedures for measuring the quality of food has resulted in confusion, misuse of methodologies, and incorrect application of data. In order to provide a first step in the development of standardized sensory testing procedures, the Committee on Sensory Evaluation of the Institute of Food Technologists has published a guide outlining the types of sensory problems frequently encountered in research and industrial laboratories and suggested methods of evaluation (Anonymous, 1964).

This chapter describes methods reported in the literature and discusses their desirable and undesirable features. Development of an efficient and reliable evaluation procedure should be based on the fields of psychology, psychophysics, and statistics. The first explains and describes responses to sensory stimuli, the second quantifies the subject's response and describes the relationship between the stimuli and the response, and the third formulates the precision of the judgments (Tarver and Schenck, 1958). Among the methods that will be considered here are: ranking, scoring, hedonic scaling, dilution, descriptive analysis, and methods used less frequently. Some of the tests described in Chapter 7 have also been used for quantity-quality evaluation.

Excellent reviews of the literature on this subject have been presented by Boggs and Hanson (1949), Dawson and Harris (1951), Peryam *et al.* (1954), and Dawson *et al.* (1963). Pangborn and Dunkley (1964) have reviewed procedures for evaluation of the sensory properties of dairy products. Jellinek (1962b) reviewed a variety of procedures and has given useful cautions regarding descriptive analysis. Scoring of wines has been described in detail by Amerine *et al.* (1959) and Ough and Baker (1961). Procedures used in laboratories in the United States, Poland, England, Scotland, Australia, Canada, and Denmark are described in a series of articles published in the July and August issues of 1964 of the British journal, *Laboratory Practice.*

I. Ranking

Ranking tests require that judges arrange a series of two or more samples in an ascending or descending order of intensity of a specific characteristic (Fig. 57). In ranking tests for quality, the usual objective is to select one or two of the best samples rather than to test all samples thoroughly. Ranking is often used for screening inferior from superior experimental samples in product development, and occasionally in training judges.

As many as 20 samples have been ranked at one session; however, to avoid taste fatigue and loss of attention, a maximum of six samples is recommended. When many treatments must be ranked, presentation of samples in an incomplete block design may be used, as illustrated in a design described by Greenwood *et al.* (1951). Large treatment × block interactions, however, may necessitate the use of other procedures. Inclusion of one or more control samples or of standards of a designated quality can improve precision of ranks. The relative position of the standard within a test series may influence the judgment. In a study of reversion in hydrogenated soybean oil, judges ranked six samples, five of which were controls (Handschumaker, 1948).

Caul (1957a) classified dilution tests (Boggs and Hanson, 1949; Peryam *et al.*, 1951; Hanson *et al.*, 1954) and the disguising potential method (Purdum, 1942; Lankford and Becker, 1951a,b) within the category of recently developed, complex ranking tests. The ranking is achieved by comparing the dilution number derived from one sample with that of another.

Samples may be ranked in order of degree of acceptability or in order of general quality, or by specific attributes of color, volume, texture, or

---

Set No._____

Code_____

Product: <u>Pears</u>

Name_____   Date_____

<u>Directions</u>: Please rank these samples in order of increasing intensity of pear aroma, then in order of increasing firmness of texture.

Place the code number of each sample opposite the rank for each factor.

Sample Codes: _____   _____   _____   _____

	Aroma			Firmness	
	Rank	Sample Code		Rank	Sample Code
Least intense	1	_____	Least firm	1	_____
	2	_____		2	_____
	3	_____		3	_____
Most intense	4	_____	Most firm	4	_____

Fɪɢ. 57. Example of evaluation sheet used for ranking an intensity characteristic of canned pears.

---

flavor intensity. *Judges should be thoroughly familiar with all aspects of the sample characterizations under consideration* (Anderson, 1958). This may not be easily achieved in practice, for stimuli may vary along several dimensions simultaneously, complicating the interpretation of the criteria used to differentiate. This problem arises not only in ranking tests but in most methods (see Klingberg, 1941).

The ranking method is rapid, allows testing of multiple samples, is simple to administer, and lends itself to use of fixed scales with control or reference samples (Anderson, 1958; Caul, 1957a). Bliss *et al.* (1953) pointed out that as far as the judge is concerned, ranking sets its own standard in each test, the assigned scores being merely relative values. Although degree of difference is disregarded, ranking procedures reduce the effect of the judge who might assign a grade of 0 in the absence of a standard. In addition, ranking forces a relative decision since no two samples may be ranked identically. The effect of allowing ties appears not to have been investigated.

The main disadvantage of the ranking method is its disregard of the amount or degree of difference between samples. Excellent agreement among judges can be obtained in ranking tests if the differences among samples are relatively large (Caul, 1957a). When small differences are being compared, judges may feel they must distinguish between samples they consider identical and this leads to inconsistencies in ranking. In addition, because of the relative nature of the rank, ranked values from one set of data cannot be compared directly with values from another set of data.

Several investigators have compared ranking techniques with grading, scoring, paired comparisons, multiple comparisons, and checking of descriptive terms. In one case where ranking and grading were compared in rating samples of apple juice for acidity, results by the two methods did not differ significantly (Dawson and Dochterman, 1951). From tests for mealiness in six samples of potatoes, Bliss *et al.* (1953) concluded that ranking gave the greatest sensitivity of judgment, followed by scoring on a 10-point intensity scale, and that checking of seven descriptive terms gave the least sensitive judgments.

Ranking versus scoring, and ranking versus paired comparison, have been tested thoroughly by Murphy *et al.* (1954, 1957), using frozen strawberries as the test commodity. They applied analyses of variance using transformed scores for the ranked data, assigned scores for the descriptive-term data, and used a modified variance analysis for the intensity scale, and a specified chi-square analysis for the paired comparisons. According to those investigators, when the number of significantly different treatments, the significance level of the differences, and the sensitivity of the judges to flavor differences were used as criteria to appraise the adequacy or superiority of a technique, the paired comparison with eight replications was the most sensitive. Only by this method was there demonstrated a quality difference between two of the strawberry treatments. An attempt to rate precision by calculating the number of tastings required based on the sample number ratio, resulted in approximate efficiency ratings of ranks equally as efficient as the descriptive terms, and paired comparisons two or three times as efficient.

The ranking and descriptive-term methods require equal amounts of material and time. The time needed to judge three samples by the paired method was twice that required by the other two techniques and would be threefold for four samples and fourfold for five samples, but the fewer number of tastings required might compensate completely for the time expenditure. The panel used was "experienced but untrained" (presumably untrained with strawberries). Standards were not used. Further experiments of this type on a variety of foods with experts using standards would be welcome.

Ranking gave greater sensitivity of judgment than scoring on a 9-point hedonic scale of a 5-point descriptive "quality" scale in judgments of citrus drinks by Tompkins and Pratt (1959). They pointed out that the apparent superiority of the ranking technique is somewhat suspect because of underestimation of the error variance (Reimer, 1957). Tompkins and Pratt (1959) cautioned that, when various testing methods are compared, the method used first might result in training, thereby improving performance for the subsequent method, and added: "Furthermore, the statistical analysis of the results and the judges' understanding of, preference for, and experience with each technique and each rating sheet should be comparable before one method can be judged as better than another." Also, since each test method is designed to accomplish specific tasks, intercomparisons may be difficult and, in some cases, meaningless.

Ranking results can be summarized by enumerating the number of judges who gave each rank to the samples, or by averaging the total ranks. In evaluating off-flavors, Parks (1954) converted scores to ranks, applied the Bradley and Terry (1952) rank analysis, and concluded that the ranking method gave finer discrimination than scoring. Ranks have been converted to scores with Fisher and Yates (1948) conversion tables because the ranking distribution showed too great a departure from normal for direct use in analysis of variance (Bliss *et al.*, 1943; Aref *et al.*, 1956; Tompkins and Pratt, 1959). Kramer (1960) described a convenient procedure wherein ranks are summed and then compared to entries in a table (Table I in Appendix) of rank totals required for significance of differences. The number of treatments or samples ranked is compared against the number of replicates to give two figures—the lowest significant rank sum and the highest significant rank sum. In an example given by Kramer and Twigg (1962), ten judges ranked four treatments, giving rank sums of 33, 21, 25, and 21. The tabular entries are 17–33, and none of the observed rank sums is less than 17 or greater than 33; therefore no significant differences in treatments were obtained. In their text, Kramer and Twigg (1962) further describe the methods used for analyzing rank data: (1) comparing one treatment with the other; (2)

comparing treatments among themselves; (3) reranking to determine additional significant treatments; and (4) determining significance of interactions.

Ranking procedures have been combined successfully with other methods. Kirkpatrick *et al.* (1957) selected a panel on the basis of their ability to discriminate among evaporated milks, using a ranked, paired-comparison method. For statistical analysis of ranked data, see Chapter 10. Guilford (1954) gives a procedure for converting rank-order data into paired-comparison data.

II. Scoring

The most frequently used of all sensory testing systems is scoring—because of its diversity, apparent simplicity, and ease of statistical analysis. Scoring methods have been used extensively by the dairy industry since late in the 19th century. Crocker (1945) gave examples of scoring systems used by the dairy, egg, meat, and bread industries.

A. GENERAL

The fundamental supposition of any rational quality grading is that the number expressing the grade is proportional to the property to be measured (Plank, 1948). According to Anderson (1958), certain prerequisites must be met for a scoring system to be effective.

1. Development of a realistic score card with quality factors properly weighted to reflect their importance. Factors to be scored should be placed on the score sheet in logical order: first those estimated by sight, then odor, and finally those judged orally (Platt, 1931).

2. The scale should be such that a difference in score reflects a reproducible variation in the factors being scores (i.e., that the scale is not too large).

3. Agreement is necessary between judges as to standards of perfection so that the entire scoring range can be utilized and so that variability in scoring due to judges will be minimal.

4. The scaling system should lend itself easily to statistical analysis, but still recognizing that a complex, highly sensitive mathematical treatment does not and cannot overcome any deficiencies or lack of sensitivity in the original presentation or scoring of the samples. There is a tendency to be too arbitrary and to give a false sense of exactness in scoring food quality. Investigators often attempt to gather too much information from too many samples at one time.

5. Whenever possible, physical and chemical analysis of the commodity should be taken to supplement sensory evaluation.

To stimulate interest and foster uniform scoring of butter, cheese, ice cream, and market milk throughout the United States and Canada, the American Dairy Science Association and the Dairy Industry Supply Association sponsor judging contests among college student teams (Guthrie, 1958). Students are advised to rank samples according to quality, and score the best ones first. Guthrie feels that 50 to 100 samples of a dairy product can be scored more accurately than 5 to 10 samples, and bases this opinion on work by Trout and Sharp (1937) on the accuracy of ranking 1100 solutions of sodium chloride, sucrose, lactose, lactic acid, and quinine over a 2-hour period. Even though "warm-up" periods may help orient judges to flavor differences, the inference that large numbers of dairy products are as easy to score as large numbers of water solutions is misleading since this has not been tested directly. Ranking samples in order of increasing intensity is not necessarily a test of taste acuity; rather, the ability of a judge to detect small differences or to identify replicate samples would be a better measure of persistence of taste acuity over prolonged periods of testing. In the scoring of dairy products, the student often achieves recognition for his taste prowess on the basis of his ability to duplicate the opinions of experts. Thus, the established scoring method used in judging competitions tends to penalize students who have greater taste sensitivity than the experts (besides, of course, those who have less sensitivity).

As emphasized by Tarver and Schenck (1958), the main disadvantage of subjective sensory scales is their instability or tendency to drift in meaning with time and with judges, necessitating anchoring of the scale to known physical measurements or, if the product attribute is not measurable by physical means, correlating assigned quality scores directly with the subjective scale. Those investigators described the statistical development of an objective scoring system for color and clarity of a beverage, and recommended that when natural standards cannot be preserved, artificial standards may be developed and used to anchor the subjective scores. Ellis (1961) believed that numerical rating tests gave more complete information than either ranking tests or descriptive-rating tests, but the judges must be trained or the ratings will be of little value.

Miller (1956) showed that in general we can assign stimuli to only about 5 to 7 classes, although he did admit that superior individuals could identify accurately any one of 50 or 60 different tone pitches. This is for one-dimensional judgments. To improve accuracy, other dimensions may be added or the accuracy of the judgments be improved by making relative rather than absolute judgments, or by making a sequence of absolute judgments. The span of absolute judgment and the span of immediate memory impose severe limitations on the amount of information that we are able to receive, process, and remember. The process of recording—that is, grouping or organizing the input sequence into units or chunks—increases the amount of transmissible information.

Guilford (1954) made the following statement: "As compared with their nearest rivals, pair comparisons and the method of rank order, the rating-scale methods have certain definite advantages and results often compare very favorably with those from more accurate methods." Guilford listed advantages as follows:

1. Ratings require much less time than either paired comparisons or ranking methods.

2. The procedure is far more interesting to the observers, especially if graphic methods are employed.

3. Rating-scale methods have a much wider range of application.

4. They can be used with psychologically naive raters who have had a minimum of training. (We nevertheless question the use of rating scales with untrained judges who have had no opportunity to anchor their judgments.)

5. They can be used with large numbers of stimuli. However, both rating and ranking become difficult and irksome when there are more than 30 to 40 stimuli.

Descriptive terms accompanying numerical scores are aids in judging. The palatability rating scale, a variation of the hedonic rating scale, was developed by Peryam and Shapiro (1955) for use in quality control. The scale uses a form of descriptive terminology as follows:

Excellent	9
Very good	8
Good	7
Below good, above fair	6
Fair	5
Below fair, above poor	4
Poor	3
Very poor	2
Extremely poor	1

The above scale is very similar to that developed by Ramsbottom (1947), shown in Table 52. Between 15 and 20 trained judges rate each item for palatability, i.e., "the combination of those flavor qualities which tend to make the product pleasing to the consumer." Mean values of the assigned ratings are designated as the palatability rating, and the standard error is computed. Comparison samples of the same type, to be acceptable, are expected to fall within two standard deviations from the mean. This method suffers from at least three major disadvantages: (1) different palatability "norms" must be established for each product independently; (2) no allowance is made for shift in degree of liking with time or with

TABLE 52
Scales and Definitions Used in Scoring

Score	Term (Plank, 1948)	Term (Ramsbottom, 1947)	Score[a]	Term (Hopkins, 1950)
10	Perfect (fancy)	Excellent	+5	Gross excess
9	Excellent	Very good	+4	Very decided excess
8	Very good	Good	+3	Decided excess
7	Good	Slightly good	+2	Moderate excess
6	Slightly good	Borderline plus	+1	Slight excess
5	Average	Borderline	0	Ideal
4	Fair	Borderline minus	−1	Slight deficiency
3	Borderline	Slightly poor	−2	Moderate deficiency
2	Bad (defective)	Poor	−3	Decided deficiency
1	Very bad	Very poor	−4	Very decided deficiency
0	Inedible	Extremely poor	−5	Gross deficiency

[a] Applies to scales of both Ramsbottom (1947) and Hopkins (1950).

repeated exposure to the test commodity; and (3) with new product development, there is no control for purposes of comparison. The descriptive terms compared in Table 52 are used frequently.

Jakobsen (1949) recommended the following quality rating scale for use with untrained panels:

Excellent	10
Very good	9
Good	7
Medium	5
Poor	3
Very poor	1
Unacceptable	0

The Hopkins scale (Table 52), used in experiments with shortening containing varying amounts of odorous substances and with milk powder with graded additions of lactic acid, provided results of approximately calculable reproducibility related in a consistent way to the composition of the test materials. Although the Hopkins scale was designed for universal application, the findings are strictly valid only for the population of which the experimental subjects are representative.

For purposes of statistical analysis, the above-mentioned descriptive terms and those in Table 52 are assumed to represent equal sensory intervals, and the scales may be regarded as being linear. There is disagreement among investigators as to whether or not equally spaced grade numbers of arbitrarily ordered descriptive terms imply equal intervals of quality (Likert, 1932; Hicks, 1948; Plank, 1948; Ehrenberg, 1953; Sheppard, 1955). It was further stated by Sheppard that if scores and descriptive terms are used simultaneously, some judges may rate primarily by scores, thereby using a linear rating scale, while others may rate according to the descriptions and therefore may not be using a linear rating scale. It is the observation of the present authors that during the initial training period, judges orient themselves to the range of quality attributes of the commodity, use descriptive terms to anchor their own evaluations, then proceed to score numerically, thus utilizing a linear scale. This topic is treated further in a publication by Sheppard (1954). Much more evidence is needed as to the applicability of analysis of variance to scores assigned to descriptive words.

For wines, Ough and Baker (1961) suggested a balanced scoring scale with more points available in the middle range than the extremes: unacceptable, 1; average quality but with defects, 2 to 3; average quality, 4 to 6; above-average quality with some superior qualities, 7 to 8; and superior quality, 9. Although it was recognized that the degree of unacceptability or superiority of wine had a greater range than one scoring point, the preceding scale was very effective in establishing discrimination in the intermediate quality ranges, which were of more interest to these investigators. When provided with a 20-point scoring scale, the effective range of use for the same wine types tested on the 9-point scale was from 9 to 18.

Barylko-Pikielna and Metelski (1964) scored canned Polish ham on a 5-point scale and then computed contribution coefficients for eight quality factors: color, fatness, slice binding, odor, juiciness, tenderness, flavor, and saltiness. The statistical relationships provided information on the contribution of each factor independently and in the over-all score. It was emphasized that the coefficients would vary from panel to panel and from country to country in accord with individual preferences and acceptability.

In sensory scoring of any characteristic, there exists the psychological tendency called the "contrast error" (see Chapter 5, Section III), i.e., grading samples lower when they are presented in a series of high-quality samples, and grading them higher when compared with low-quality samples (Dove, 1943, 1947; Hopkins, 1950). Using a balanced, incomplete block design to establish flavor intensities in dried eggs, Hanson et al. (1951) observed that samples of intermediate quality were most susceptible to contrast errors. The use of one or two labeled standards of intermediate quality would tend to stabilize the scores assigned to unknowns.

The psychological error of "central tendency" (see Chapter 5, Section III) is frequently observed in scoring when the extreme values of a scoring scale are seldom used. Accuracy is not gained by using a scoring

scale that has a range of differences in excess of the number of gradations of quality or intensity that can be recognized. Conversely, a scale
that has fewer gradations than meet the scoring range of the judges
decreases the sensitivity of the scale (Lowe, 1955). Scoring scales consisting of 50 to 100 points have been largely abandoned in favor of scales
from 0 to 10 or 20, which are sufficient for most commodities when
trained judges are used.

The official scoring system for milk as adopted by the American Dairy
Science Association is based on 100 points, divided as follows:

Quality factor	Points
Flavor and odor	45
Sediment	10
Container and closure	5
Bacteria	35
Temperature	5
	100

Flavor is further subdivided:

Excellent:	40 and above; no criticism.
Good:	37 to 40; lacking special high flavor, flat, very slight feed, slight cooked.
Fair:	34 to 37; cooked, feed, salty, slight cowy, slight oxidized.
Poor:	25 to 34; strong feed, weedy, bitter, strong, musty, cowy, oxidized, very slight rancid.
Bad:	25 and below; rancid, strong cowy, high acid. 0; sour, putrid, or any flavor sufficiently strong to render the milk unfit for market purposes.

In practice, only five or fewer points are utilized (Downs *et al.*,
1954). In the opinion of the present authors, the above scoring system is
not suitable for laboratory use, because descriptive terms and intensity
scales are confounded. The judging and scoring of milk is described in
great detail by Nelson and Trout (1948), Fenton (1957), Guthrie
(1958), Jenness and Patton (1959), and Pangborn and Dunkley (1964).

Carlin *et al.* (1956), in tests of three sugar levels in orange juice,
used three scoring scales (0–5, 0–10, and 0–100) to determine whether
the scales had the same pragmatic value. The mean score over a group
of judges was related linearly between scales, so that the population of
judges could be assumed to be measuring the same attribute or combination of attributes on the different scales. Upon comparing the scales ac-

cording to coefficient of variation, standard deviation within judges, and sensitivity, those investigators concluded that the 0–10 and 0–100 scales were generally better than the 0–5 scale. (The "meaning" of a 0–100 scale with only three sugar levels is not clear to us.) In addition, scoring by paired tests gave consistent results.

Single samples may be presented for scoring; however, more precision is obtained by including a standard reference sample (Krum, 1955). Standards or controls may be presented in duplicate—one identified by a specific score and the other as a blind standard. Two different standards may be used—one a control and the other a high-intensity reference sample.

Unstructured and semistructured scoring systems have been used to a limited extent. Baten (1946) described an elastic system consisting of a horizontal line, 6 inches long, with "excellent" at the right end and "poor" at the left end. Judges expressed ratings by placing a vertical line across the horizontal one at the point representing their opinion. In addition, the same judges scored the samples on a numerical scale. The judges did not like the linear as well as the numerical form, but statistical analysis showed that they graded more accurately with the linear method. Raffensperger *et al.* (1956) measured tenderness in beef with the following structured and unstructured rating scales:

STRUCTURED:

Extremely tough	Very tough	Moderately tough	Slightly tough	Slightly tender	Moderately tender	Very tender	Extremely tender

UNSTRUCTURED:
Greatest   Greatest
toughness   tenderness

1	2	3	4	5	6	7	8

The range of grade means was almost identical for the two scales with two of the three cuts of beef, but with a sirloin strip cut was somewhat greater for the unstructured scale. A significantly greater amount of systematic error was found in the structured than in the unstructured scale, indicating that the former created confusion around the point of greatest variance. They therefore concluded that "with trained subjects a fully structured 9-point scale was apparently not superior to a 9-point unstructured scale."

Other structured and unstructured scales have been described by

Ellis (1961) and by Krum (1955). Further examples are given in Figs. 58, 59, 60, 61, and 62. These score cards are given as examples of those in current use with highly trained experienced judges. The complexity and length of the ballots would prohibit their use by judges inexperienced

Name_____ Sample No._____ Date_____

Each flavor characteristic increases in intensity on a scale from left to right. Rate flavor characteristics of sample on corresponding scale by placing an "x" mark in the appropriate place.

SWEETNESS
Unsweetened   Highly Sweetened

ACIDITY
No Acidity   High Acidity

FLAVOR STRENGTH
Low Flavor Strength   High Flavor Strength

CARBONATION
Uncarbonated   High Carbonation

AFTERTASTE
No Aftertaste or   Strong or Unpleasant
Pleasant Aftertaste   Aftertaste

ROUNDNESS OR
OVER-ALL BALANCE
Very Poorly Balanced   Well Balanced

IMPACT
Weak and Unsatisfying   Overpowering

REMARKS:

Fig. 58. Unstructured rating scale. Source: Hall (1958).

with evaluation systems and with the commodity being tested. Whether difference testing should be combined with hedonic rating of the same samples, remains a controversy which has not been resolved. See Chapter 10 for statistical consideration of this subject.

B. Quality Evaluations

In the opinion of Byer and Abrams (1953), multisample comparisons might obscure rather than reveal a judge's reactions. Therefore they developed a "trend-rating" procedure to measure changes in the opinion of

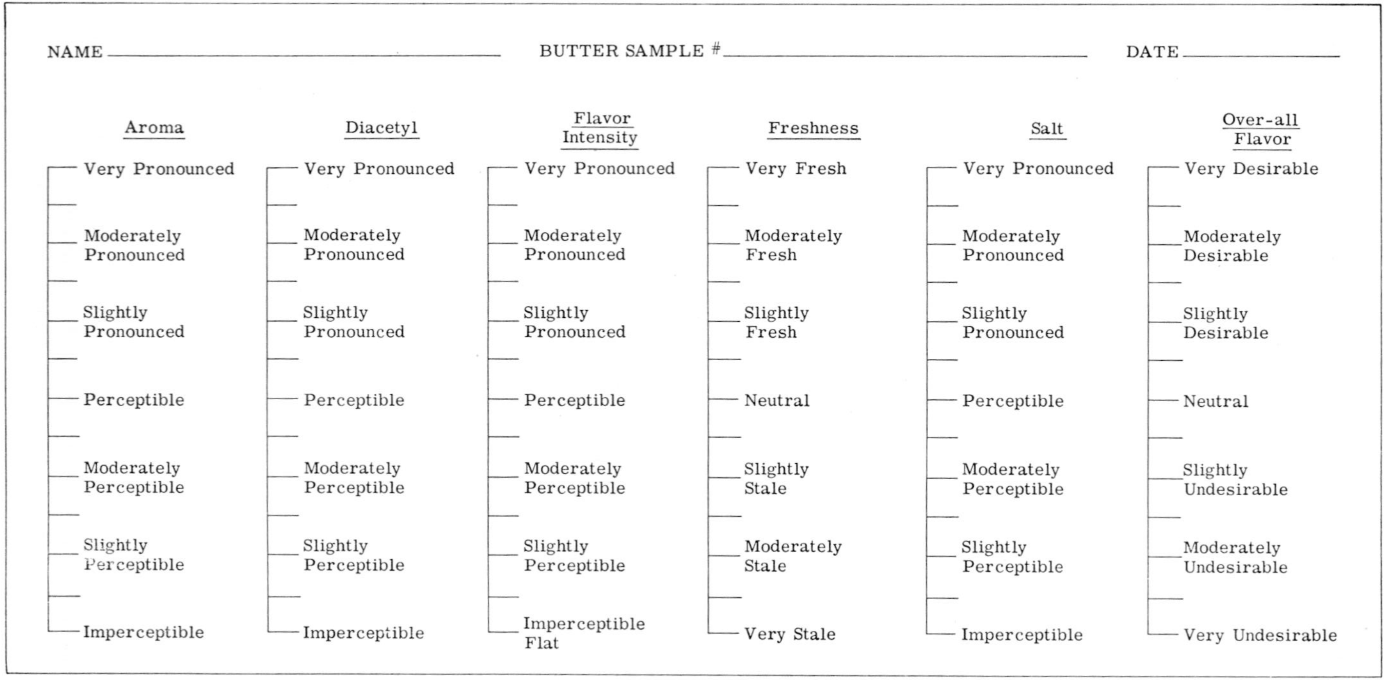

FIG. 59. Evaluation sheet illustrating the use of a structured, nonnumerical scoring method. (Points of the scale can be converted to scores ranging from 1 to 13 or 0 to 12.) Source: Day (1962).

LAMB SCORE CARD

Judge's Name _____

Date _____

QUALITY FACTOR	SCORING SCALE										SAMPLE CODES						
Color	10	9 Very desirable	8	7	6 Moderately desirable	5	4 Slightly undesirable	3	2 Very undesirable	1							
Juiciness	10	9 Very juicy	8	7	6 Moderately juicy	5	4 Slightly dry	3	2 Very dry	1							
Tenderness	10	9 Very tender	8	7	6 Moderately tender	5	4 Slightly tough	3	2 Very tough	1							
Texture	10	9 Very fine	8	7	6 Moderately fine	5	4 Slightly coarse	3	2 Very coarse	1							
Natural Flavor of Lean	10	9 Very full	8	7	6 Moderately full	5	4 Slightly weak	3	2 Lacking or masked	1							
Off-Flavor of Lean (Name off flavor)	None	9 Very slight	8	7 Slight	6	5 Moderate	4	3 Pro- nounced	2	1 Very pronounced							
Off-Flavor of Fat (Name Off-flavor)	None	9 Very slight	8	7 Slight	6	5 Moderate	4	3 Pro- nounced	2	1 Very pronounced							
General Acceptability	10	9 Very good	8	7 Good	6	5 Fair	4	3 Poor	2	1 Very poor							

Remarks: Doneness, other

FIG. 60. Evaluation sheet illustrating the use of a 10-point scoring method for judging quality factors, degree of intensity, and general acceptability. Source: Brant and Simone (1962).

Date_____   Product_____

Project_____   Treatment_____   Panel Replicate_____

Name of Judge_____   Code No. for Judge_____

TRIANGLE FLAVOR DIFFERENCE EVALUATION

Samples	Check Like Samples	Separate for Flavor Only Flavor Difference Between Odd and Like Samples	Did you Check By Guess?
(1)	(2)	(3)	(4)
_____	_____	_____ None _____ Slight	Yes _____
_____	_____		
_____	_____	_____ Moderate _____ Much	No _____

(5) If you checked a Moderate or Much in the flavor difference column (No. 3), then indicate below whether you consider either the odd sample or like samples to have an undesirable flavor.

   Odd Sample Yes___ No___   Like Samples: Yes___ No___

HEDONIC RATING SCALE

(6) RATE FOR FLAVOR ONLY. Place a check mark above either a short or long line on the scale below to indicate how you rate the like samples and the odd sample.

LIKE SAMPLES

   Very Poor   Poor   Fair   Good   Excellent

ODD SAMPLE

   Very Poor   Poor   Fair   Good   Excellent

(7) a. Did you detect any kind of difference, other than flavor, between the samples?

   Yes _____ No _____

   b. If "Yes," what kind of difference?_____

FIG. 61. Evaluation sheet utilizing triangle testing in combination with a hedonic-rating scale. Source: Hogue and Briant (1957).

a nonexpert panel upon repeated tasting of beer (Byer and Saletan, 1961). An unstructured scale was used with the upper point specified as "the best a beer could be," and the lowest point as "the worst a beer could be." One sample from each of two treatments was tested at a time, in random order until each treatment was tested a total of four times. Results were evaluated by constructing a trend-line graph for each judge, showing his rising or falling ratings for the four successive tastings. The trend line is obtained by connecting the mean of the first two ratings with the mean of the second and third and the mean of the third and fourth ratings. For each pair of beers, results were classified into one of

CODE _____

PICKLE STUDY

NAME_____ DATE _____

Please evaluate each pickle sample for the quality factor listed below, using the appropriate scale.

Texture	Quality of Pickling Flavor	Presence of Undesirable Flavor	Kind of Undesirable Flavor	Overall Reaction
+ 4 Hard	0 Poor	0 None	1 Astringent	1 Dislike extremely
+ 3	1	1 Slight	2 Bitter	2 Dislike very much
+ 2	2	2	3 Medicinal	3 Dislike moderately
+ 1	3 Fair	3 Moderate	4 Metallic	4 Dislike slightly
0 Optimum	4	4	5 Musty	5 Like slightly
- 1	5	5 Intense	6 Rancid	6 Like moderately
- 2	6 Good		7 Too acidic	7 Like very much
- 3	7		8 Unbalanced spicing	8 Like extremely
- 4 Soft	8		9 Soapy	
	9 Excellent		10 Salty	
			11 Other (please state)	

Sample	Color		Texture	Quality of Pickling Flavor	Presence of Undesirable Flavor	Kind of Undesirable Flavor	Overall Reaction
	Good	Poor					

Comments:

Fig. 62. Evaluation sheet illustrating the use of a combination of methods: negative and positive scoring, quality rating, intensity scoring, descriptive evaluation, and hedonic scaling. Source: Pangborn *et al.* (1958).

eight categories, depending on the signs of the slopes of the trend lines for the two beers, and which of the two beers showed the higher over-all mean rating. Figure 63 is an example of these eight categories. The same samples of beer were also rated differently with a triangular test procedure.

The trend-rating procedure permits comparison not only of samples but of learning effects of individual judges. Byer and Saletan suggested that the test may be used in selecting judges for laboratory panels. They listed the main advantages of their unstructured scale as: (1) it avoided the use of descriptive terms, which judges may tend to remember and reproduce; (2) it avoided hedonic terms, to prevent exclusive use of the lower part of the scale by a person not liking a product; (3) there was less chance for misunderstanding of the meaning of vocabulary or of a number system; and (4) most of the analysis is done geometrically rather than arithmetically. One could challenge some of these "advantages." For example, the anchor points at the extremes of the scale could be interpreted differently by different judges, and they additionally imply hedonic evaluations since "best" and "worst" are related directly to like

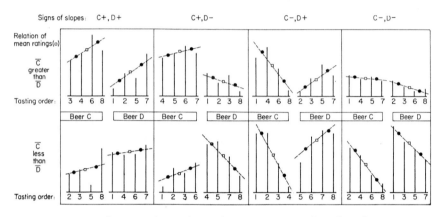

FIG. 63. Trend-rating charts for eight tasters; examples of eight categories. Source: Byer and Saletan (1961).

and dislike. In addition, visual acuity becomes a factor since the judge must gauge the physical distance from best and worst in placing his mark on the scale, and all judges may not use these "distances" similarly. Also, as used by Byer and Saletan, when two treatments are presented randomly until a total of four evaluations per treatment are obtained within a session, the psychological error of contrast could easily operate.

III. Hedonic Scaling

Hedonics relates to the psychology of pleasurable and unpleasant states of consciousness. In hedonic scaling, affective responses, i.e., psychological states of like and dislike, are measured on a rating scale. Essentials of the rating-scale method are: (1) the definition of a psychological continuum; and (2) the establishment of a series of successive categories of response. The value of the application depends on how meaningful the defined continuum and the successive categories are to the test subjects within the context of the problem. The essential features of the hedonic scale are its assumption of a continuum of preference and the direct way it defines the categories of response in terms of like and dislike (Peryam and Pilgrim, 1957). The role of hedonic processes in the organization of behavior has been discussed by Young (1952).

A. Classification

According to Guilford (1954), forms of rating scales in common use can be categorized as: (1) numerical; (2) graphic; (3) standard; (4) cumulated points; and (5) forced choice. These scales are alike in that they require the assignment of objects by inspection along an unbroken continuum or in ordered categories along the continuum, after which numbers are assigned. They differ in the operations of placement of objects, in the kind and number of aids or cues, and in the fineness of discrimination demanded by the rater.

Guilford gives the following example of a numerical rating scale used to obtain ratings of the affective values of colors and odors:

10 Most pleasant imaginable
9 Most pleasant
8 Extremely pleasant
7 Moderately pleasant
6 Mildly pleasant
5 Indifferent
4 Mildly unpleasant
3 Moderately unpleasant
2 Extremely unpleasant
1 Most unpleasant
0 Most unpleasant imaginable

Modifying the above scale, it is possible, instead, to assign a numerical value of 0 to the indifferent category, with positive integers above and negative integers below this point. Guilford (1954) does not recommend this, since he feels it would confuse unsophisticated subjects and might tend to suggest a break in the scale and thus destroy the continuity. We believe that negative and positive scoring scales can be used effectively with highly trained panels *if* the judges uniformly understand the points and terms used. The scale illustrated in Fig. 62 was appropriate for judging soft and hard texture in pickles (Pangborn *et al.*, 1958).

If only the terminal categories (0 and 10) in the foregoing scale had been anchored, these terminal points would serve to spread the entire distribution of ratings more toward the ends, thereby increasing dispersion (Hunt and Volkmann, 1937). As emphasized by Guilford (1954), subjects tend to avoid terminal categories, which means that if 0 and 10 were not included, then the new ends, 1 and 9, would be avoided, thereby shortening the range of rating. Similar observations have been made by several investigators, including Ough and Baker (1961) in tests with wines.

The choice of words or phrases to label the scale intervals is of great importance, since these verbal anchors not only convey the idea of the successive order of the intervals but also make clear to the respondents the meaning of the response continuum. The value of the scale will be reduced to the extent to which the words and phrases are ambiguous, or are not definitely in an order of meaning corresponding with the physical order of the scale intervals (Jones et al., 1955). Those investigators selected 900 soldiers on the basis of educational background representative of army enlisted men, and asked them to rate 51 descriptive terms according to what the words and phrases meant to them. The results are presented in Table 53. A scale value and a standard deviation were derived graphically for each word or phrase; the former was considered the "average meaning" of the phrase, and the latter a measure of its relative ambiguity. From these descriptive terms, nine scales were devised and tested with 20 food items by approximately 100 servicemen. The following criteria were established to determine the relative adequacy of the scales: (1) amount of time required for completion; (2) reliability, i.e., accuracy with which respondents duplicated results on an alternate-form retest; and (3) amount of information obtained about the relative preference values of the group of foods tested. No superior scale emerged from the nine tested, since the pretesting of the 51 descriptive terms had narrowed the alternatives. However, the study showed the following: (1) nine-interval scales tend to be more sensitive to differences among foods than shorter ones; (2) elimination of the "neutral" category is recommended; (3) an equal number of positive and negative intervals is not an essential feature of a rating scale.

The adequacy of quantitative descriptive terms in evaluation of the quality of various foods has been tested and discussed by Sheppard (1954, 1955).

Historical development of the use of hedonic scales for foods has been traced by Peryam and Pilgrim (1957). This scale was first used by the Quartermaster Food and Container Institute, in 1947, when a 7-point scale of like and dislike terms provided information on the preference of army personnel for menu items. The method used, first described by Peryam and Girardot, in 1952, was designed for use with observers entirely without experience in food testing, thus being applied consumer-type tests as used in Chapter 9. Figures 64 and 65 are examples (Peryam and Girardot, 1952) of the forms, respectively used in the laboratory and in the field. Instructions accompanying the test have two functions: (1) to inform the subject what he must know, or what the experimenter wants him to know, about the mechanics of the test; and (2) to encourage the subject to report immediate responses formed without exercising conscious effort to remember or to judge. The vertical scale on the form

TABLE 53

Scale Values and Standard Deviations for 51 Descriptive Terms

Phrase	Scale value	Standard deviation	Phrase	Scale value	Standard deviation
Best of all	6.15	2.48	Like mildly	0.85	0.47
Favorite	4.68	2.18	Fair	0.78	0.85
Like extremely	4.16	1.62	Acceptable	0.73	0.66
Like intensely	4.05	1.59	Only fair	0.71	0.64
Excellent	3.71	1.01	Like slightly	0.69	0.32
Wonderful	3.51	0.97	Neutral	0.02	0.18
Strongly like	2.96	0.69	Like not so well	−0.30	1.07
Like very much	2.91	0.60	Like not so much	−0.41	0.94
Mighty fine	2.88	0.67	Dislike slightly	−0.59	0.27
Especially good	2.86	0.82	Mildly dislike	−0.74	0.35
Highly favorable	2.81	0.66	Not pleasing	−0.83	0.67
Like very well	2.60	0.78	Don't care for it	−1.10	0.84
Very good	2.56	0.87	Dislike moderately	−1.20	0.41
Like quite a bit	2.32	0.52	Poor	−1.55	0.87
Enjoy	2.21	0.86	Dislike	−1.58	0.94
Preferred	1.98	1.17	Don't like	−1.81	0.97
Good	1.91	0.76	Bad	−2.02	0.80
Welcome	1.77	1.18	Highly unfavorable	−2.16	1.37
Tasty	1.76	0.92	Strongly dislike	−2.37	0.53
Pleasing	1.58	0.65	Dislike very much	−2.49	0.64
Like fairly well	1.51	0.59	Very bad	−2.53	0.64
Like	1.35	0.77	Terrible	−3.09	0.98
Like moderately	1.12	0.61	Dislike intensely	−3.33	1.39
			Loath	−3.76	3.54
			Dislike extremely	−4.32	1.86
OK	0.87	1.24	Despise	−6.44	3.62
Average	0.86	1.08			

Source: Jones *et al.* (1955).

used in the laboratory should suggest the idea of a continuum with equidistant points.

The scale is generally presented with the "like extremely" category at the top or left, but a reversal of both the horizontal and vertical scales did not appear to affect the results (Peryam and Girardot, 1952). Note that a single-stimulus presentation is always used when the scale is of this form.

The hedonic-scale rating reflects the attitudes of a group of people

Questionnaire

Instructions: You will be given three servings of food to eat and you are asked to say about each how much you like it or dislike it. Eat the entire portion which is served you before you make up your mind unless you decide immediately that it is definitely unpleasant. Rinse your mouth with the water provided after you have finished with each sample and then wait for the next. There will be approximately two minutes between samples.

Use the scales below to indicate your attitude. Write the code number of the sample in the space above and check at the point on the scale which best describes your feeling about the food. Also your comments are invited. They are generally very meaningful.

Keep in mind that you are the judge. You are the only one who can tell what you like. Nobody knows whether this food should be considered good, bad or indifferent. An honest expression of your personal feeling will help us to decide.

SHOW YOUR REACTION BY CHECKING ON THE SCALE

Code:_____	Code:_____	Code:_____
Like Extremely	Like Extremely	Like Extremely
Like Very much	Like Very much	Like Very much
Like Moderately	Like Moderately	Like Moderately
Like Slightly	Like Slightly	Like Slightly
Neither Like Nor Dislike	Neither Like Nor Dislike	Neither Like Nor Dislike
Dislike Slightly	Dislike Slightly	Dislike Slightly
Dislike Moderately	Dislike Moderately	Dislike Moderately
Dislike Very Much	Dislike Very Much	Dislike Very Much
Dislike Extremely	Dislike Extremely	Dislike Extremely
Comments:	Comments:	Comments:

FIG. 64. Questionnaire used by Quartermaster Food and Container Institute in laboratory evaluation by the hedonic-scale method. Source: Peryam and Girardot (1952).

toward certain foods under a given set of conditions. How well the observers and the test conditions represent any practical use situation will depend upon the adequacy of the test plan and the sampling procedures.

At the Quartermaster laboratories, the method is used primarily: (1) to detect small differences in the degree of liking for similar foods; (2) to detect gross differences in degree of liking of foods, even when time, subjects, and test conditions are allowed to vary (Peryam and Haynes,

QUESTIONNAIRE

FOOD ITEM	LIKE				INDIFFERENT	DISLIKE				
	Like Extremely	Like Very Much	Like Moderately	Like Slightly	Neither Like Nor Dislike	Dislike Slightly	Dislike Moderately	Dislike Very Much	Dislike Extremely	
Cream Gravy	Like Extremely	Like Very Much	Like Moderately	Like Slightly	Neither Like Nor Dislike	Dislike Slightly	Dislike Moderately	Dislike Very Much	Dislike Extremely	Not Tried
Bread Pudding	Like Extremely	Like Very Much	Like Moderately	Like Slightly	Neither Like Nor Dislike	Dislike Slightly	Dislike Moderately	Dislike Very Much	Dislike Extremely	Not Tried
Cheese	Like Extremely	Like Very Much	Like Moderately	Like Slightly	Neither Like Nor Dislike	Dislike Slightly	Dislike Moderately	Dislike Very Much	Dislike Extremely	Not Tried
French Fried Onions	Like Extremely	Like Very Much	Like Moderately	Like Slightly	Neither Like Nor Dislike	Dislike Slightly	Dislike Moderately	Dislike Very Much	Dislike Extremely	Not Tried
Lettuce Wedges	Like Extremely	Like Very Much	Like Moderately	Like Slightly	Neither Like Nor Dislike	Dislike Slightly	Dislike Moderately	Dislike Very Much	Dislike Extremely	Not Tried

FIG. 65. Questionnaire used by Quartermaster Food and Container Institute to study soldiers' responses in the field with the hedonic-scale method. Source: Peryam and Girardot (1952).

1957); (3) to reveal differences in group-preference attitudes toward foods in field questionnaire surveys. Subjects are urged to respond on the basis of their own immediate feeling, rather than to attempt to make a judgment of the quality of the food. The intent is to avoid, as much as possible, any reflective consideration of the problem, on the theory that it is the uncomplicated response which determines pleasure in eating and governs the formation of attitudes and future preference choices (Tuxbury and Peryam, 1952). Further study seems desirable on the "meaning" of the results of hedonic testing by laboratory panels.

At the Quartermaster Food and Container Institute, laboratory testers received a maximum of three or four foods at a test session. Judges were asked not to change a rating once it had been made, so that the foods were evaluated independently. Contrast effects, i.e., where an average quality is rated lower when preceded by a better-quality sample or rated higher when preceded by a poor-quality sample, are expected when samples are presented simultaneously (Kamenetzky, 1959). Presenting only one sample at a session would prevent this effect, but would be wasteful of laboratory and observer time. Even with single-sample presentation, judgments are relative since memory comparisons are being made.

In addition to contrast effects, Peryam and Pilgrim (1957) pointed out that "contamination" and "position" effects should be anticipated. In the contamination effect the rating for a sample of average quality tends to move in the direction of the quality of the samples with which it appears, as may occur in storage studies. In the position effect the first sample presented occupies the best position, relative to preference, while the later samples tend to be rated lower. With coffee, the drop in preference occurred after the first sample and was large; with fresh milk or orange juice, the effect was absent (Peryam and Pilgrim, 1957). Using a 9-point hedonic-rating scale for evaluating cherry beverage and beef broth, Kamenetzky (1959) was unable to show a "convergence" effect, i.e., a "good" sample was rated lower when preceded by a "poor" sample than when preceded by another "good" sample. As the poor samples were presented successively, the ratings increased if a good sample did not intervene; however, the converse was not observed. In addition, he found later samples were preferred more than the earlier ones.

Cover (1959) pointed out that hedonic scaling is useful for measuring consumer acceptance but is not designed for following quantitative changes in a food. Cover noted, for example, that hedonic responses to meat will differ between judges who like rare and those who like well-done steaks. Quantitative scales of juiciness and tenderness, however, can be used effectively by both groups of judges.

B. ANALYSIS

For analysis of data obtained with the hedonic method, numbers from 1 to 9 are assigned to the descriptive categories and the following are calculated: means, standard deviation, standard errors of the means, and the significance of difference between means. Both scores and means may be treated by analysis of variance.

The major advantages credited to the hedonic-rating scale are: (1) it is simple, which makes it suitable for use with a wide range of populations; (2) subjects can respond meaningfully without previous experience; (3) the data can be handled by the statistics of variables; (4) the results are, within broad limits, meaningful for indicating general levels of preference, which is in contrast to other methods (Peryam and Pilgrim, 1957). A caution, however. In a study of preference for orange juice at nine mess halls, Peryam and Gutman (1958) noted that the total range of variations was large, suggesting that a hedonic rating established in a single test can be quite unreliable.

For determining the acceptability of new or unusual foods where there are no similar products for comparison, the single-sample presentation, hedonic-rating method has proved successful (Seaton and Gardner, 1959). Since the variability in ratings from a group of observers tends to be high, the scale is not suited for use with small panels. It is generally believed that the hedonic rating of single samples is not as discriminating a test as the paired comparison, since degree of liking can be independent of acuity of detection of differences. The hedonic scale cannot be used for quality control in food production, because of two factors: (1) large test variations mean that a considerable number of observers are required for precision; and (2) the type of responses that are called for are expected to change with a number of conditions which cannot always be controlled, and correcting these would require more observers in each test than are generally available for quality-control work.

Eindhoven and Peryam (1959) tested the following rating scale to determine preferences for food combinations:

How well do French-fried potatoes go with:

Green peas	Extremely well	Very well	Moderately well	Slightly well	Slightly poor	Very poor	Extremely poor	Cannot decide
Sauerkraut	Extremely well	Very well	Moderately well	Slightly well	Slightly poor	Very poor	Extremely poor	Cannot decide

Results indicated that preferences for combinations were in large part independent of degree of liking for the individual components.

Hogue and Briant (1957) used a combination of triangle testing and hedonic-rating scale in evaluating the flavor differences of vegetables treated with pesticides. More validity could be placed on the degree of liking when it was established that judges could differentiate between treated and untreated samples.

IV. Dilution Procedures

The dilution technique, sometimes referred to as the extinction technique (Gelman, 1945), establishes the smallest amount of unknown that can be detected when it is mixed with a standard material. The method resembles the dilution procedures used for determining taste thresholds for sugars, salts, acids, and other compounds in water. Among the early uses of this principle were studies that developed sound-intensity units, the bel and decibel (Colby, 1938). The dilution principle was used by Fair (1933) to study odors in water, and by Trout and Sharp (1937) in studies of flavors in milk. In addition, the method has been used by some distillers in quality control (Peryam, 1950). Under carefully controlled conditions, the dilution test can be used to obtain an index of minimum acceptance. Various difference tests, such as the triangle and ranking procedures, may be used to differentiate the various dilutions.

Dilution of dried eggs was first mentioned in an abstract by Bohren and Jordan (1946), described in detail by Boggs and Hanson (1949), and then published in technical form by Bohren and Jordan (1953). The technique consisted of diluting experimental dried eggs into fresh shell eggs to the point where, after cooking, the mixture was just distinguishable from the undiluted fresh-egg control. Tests indicated that 20% decreases in the amount of experimental egg in the control fresh egg were detected consistently. Six different dilutions, based on a logarithmic scale, of dried egg in fresh egg were presented to judges, who identified them as fresh or experimental against a known fresh-egg sample. The percentage of correct judgments at each of the six dilution levels was then plotted against the percent dilution, and a regression line was plotted. The score was determined by a perpendicular line dropped from the point where the regression line intersects the 75%-correct horizontal line.

Established in the Quartermaster studies (Peryam et al., 1951) was an index of dried-milk quality called the "dilution number" (DN), defined as "percent of reconstituted dried milk in a mixture of that material with a fresh whole milk standard such that the difference in taste between it and the standard lies just above the threshold." The duo-trio test (see Chapter 7), with a total of 20 judgments from five to ten judges, was used to determine thresholds, involving only two milks at one session. Mixtures were tested for differences against fresh milk, start-

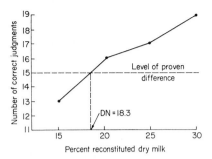

FIG. 66. Determining dilution number: Mixtures of reconstituted dry milk are compared against fresh milk by the duo-trio method. The DN is found by connecting the points (solid line) and interpolating (dotted line) to give a DN of 18.3, that point where 75% correct detection was made. Source: Peryam *et al.* (1951).

ing with low dilutions and proceeding until a test resulted in 15 correct judgments out of 20 trials, or at least 75% correct (see Fig. 66). Reproducibility was exceptionally good when the same samples were tested and retested 1 to 4 weeks later.

In studies on the flavor of roast beef, Kramlich and Pearson (1958) determined the threshold at which flavor could be detected in a series of water dilutions. Figure 67 gives an example of their results, expressed as "flavor threshold determinations." Descriptive terms were also used to characterize flavor.

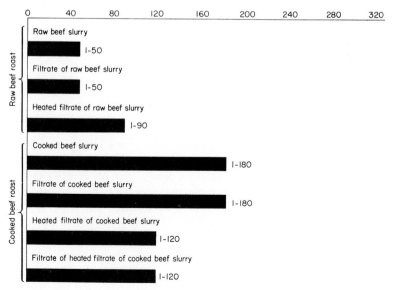

FIG. 67. Flavor thresholds for various raw and cooked beef fractions determined in water dilutions. Source: Kramlich and Pearson (1958).

A dilution index for margarine was described by Tilgner (1961). The method consisted of addition of the test margarine to prime butter until the ratio was such that the mixture was just distinguishable from the control sample of prime butter. The higher the dilution index (the ratio of percent margarine to percent butter) the better the quality of the margarine test sample. Thus the scoring is based on the flavor-difference threshold of the individual taster rather than on judgment of absolute flavors or on preference determination. A duo-trio, triangular test, or multiple comparison test can be utilized, with care taken to cleanse the palate with aged white bread or warm strong tea between tastings. Tilgner's dilution indices for margarine are shown in Table 54.

TABLE 54
Dilution Indices for Margarine

Dilution index	% butter in butter-margarine mixture	Quality description of test margarine
100 90	0 10	90–100 Excellent
89 80	11 20	80–89 Very good
79 60	21 40	60–79 Good
59 40	41 60	40–59 Medium
39 20	61 80	20–39 Poor
19 1	81 99	1–19 Very poor

Source: Tilgner (1961).

Previous publications of Tilgner (1954, 1957) and Tilgner and Barylko-Pikielna (1959) had also reported on use of the dilution index. Recently, Tilgner (1962a,b, 1965) summarized successful use of dilution tests with spices, syrups, coffee, tomato concentrate, and even fish. Juices, syrups, and other liquids are prepared for testing by diluting with distilled water, and solids and semisolids are comminuted to a standard sieve size and then decanted and filtered before dilution. Utilizing the principles of the flavor profile method of descriptive flavor analysis (see Chapter 8, Section V), Tilgner (1962a) obtained descriptive terms for the various dilutions of several commodities, and calls this combined method "dilution flavor profile." Tilgner feels that this combination of methods helps characterize the sensory properties of a food in three dimensions: qualitative, quantitative, and sequential. Diluting food samples may reveal components that are masked in the composite, preventing easy recognition by the judges. The technique may provide information on relative intensities at comparable dilution levels between treatments. In addition, dilution techniques may be used in quality control, usually in combination with other methods. It should be emphasized, however, that extreme care must be taken in interpreting the results since simple water dilution of sensory components may not give a true picture of the food in its normal concentration.

The main disadvantage of the dilution method is that it is based on a tenuous concept: that the effect of dilution is a straight-line function of concentration of the test product in a flavor-bearing vehicle and that all the test products, despite differences in flavor characteristics, will be affected identically by the vehicle (Caul, 1957a). As further indicated by Caul, the effect of the diluent and the test substance on each other is disregarded (even though the test substance may not be recognized, it may change the character of the standard). Also, visual and tactile properties of test products may give clues before flavor is detectable. However, experts may use other differences to place the samples in the correct order.

V. Descriptive Sensory Analysis

The best known method of descriptive sensory analysis is the flavor profile developed by the Arthur D. Little Co., Cambridge, Massachusetts. First described by Cairncross and Sjöström, in 1950, the technique provides a detailed, descriptive evaluation of the quantitative and qualitative attributes of a flavor complex. The profile approach is somewhat paralleled in the field of academic psychology by what is known as phenomenology.

In a comprehensive review of this method, Caul (1957a) explained that "The flavor profile was founded on the natural process of evaluating and comparing flavors by describing their impressions—either as a whole or by individual characteristics." Unlike difference testing, the profile method concentrates on the entire flavor of a product and the individual attributes of a flavor in relation to each other. Unlike difference testing, the profile method is not concerned with precision to the extent of considering single flavor judgments at a time in order to obtain results that can be analyzed statistically. Rather, the profile method's purpose is to record analysis in which all flavor components can be considered in perspective. It can be used to examine products separately or in groups (Caul and Swaine, 1959).

Workers at the Arthur D. Little flavor laboratory were already ponder-
ing the inadequacy of known methods of assessing flavor blends at the
time when they found that the carry-over taste of monosodium glutamate
precluded the use of multiple-sample evaluation. Boggs and Ward (1950)
had also reported on taste-transfer effects in the evaluation of sulfited
foods. In converting from a multiple- to a single-sample test, Arthur D.
Little established and refined a descriptive analysis in which, after smelling and tasting, the single sensory components were recorded in the
order of their appearance, the intensities defined, and the "amplitude,"
or over-all impression, determined. The method does not directly measure acceptance, and was not designed to do so (Sjöström and Cairncross,
1953). Neither is it applicable to testing of consumer preference.

A. PANEL SELECTION

Open-discussion panels of four to six highly *trained* judges are used.
Subjects are selected on the basis of several qualifications: (1) availability for panel work involving sessions up to one hour in length; (2)
interest in flavor and odor; (3) normal gustatory and olfactory sensitivity;
and (4) intellectual integrity. At the Arthur D. Little laboratories, prospective panelists are screened by three tests on: (1) taste sensitivity to
sucrose, citric acid, sodium chloride, and quinine; (2) perception of a
nonpungent odorous material administered with the Elsberg apparatus
(Elsberg and Levy, 1935); and (3) sensitivity in a timed odor-recognition
test consisting of a series of 15 common and 5 rare odors. In addition,
subjects are interviewed to establish their interests, education, experience,
and personality traits. Overly passive or dominant individuals should be
eliminated from open-panel flavor analysis. During a training period
extending from 6 months to a year, selected panelists are schooled in the
fundamentals of the profile method, of the physical and physiological
aspects of tasting and smelling, and of the chemical constitution correlated with taste and odor. Trained panel leaders organize, conduct, and
direct the panel sessions and interpret results. The job of panel leader,
which is usually full-time, requires not only normal sensory abilities but
meticulosity, understanding of people, patience, and the ability to plan
and execute flavor tests (Caul, 1957a). The panel leader serves as the
connecting link between the panel and the users of panel findings. In
formal profile sessions, each panel member independently examines his
sample, recording his findings, and then the group discussion is led by
the panel leader, who tabulates and later summarizes the discussion. In
this round-table period, language or vocabulary differences are resolved,
ideas are exchanged, and future panel sessions are planned. A partitioned
table designed for a modification of such analyses is shown in Fig. 68.

Between 1949 and 1957, the Arthur D. Little flavor laboratories have conducted formal training programs with panels from over 25 different companies in the general areas of foods, drugs, plastics, petroleum, paper, and rubber (Sjöström *et al.*, 1957). After selection of the panel members from the staff of the participating company, a 4-day basic course in flavor analysis is initiated, in which the following topics are covered: physiology of tasting and smelling, theories on taste and odor perception, odor and

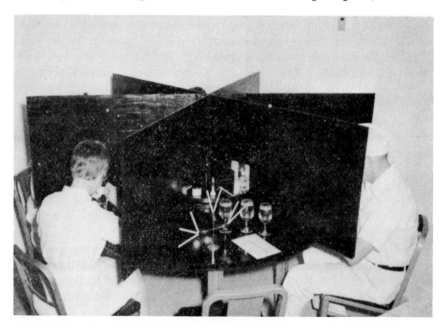

FIG. 68. Illustration of descriptive analysis panel. Reference compounds are available from the rotating "lazy susan" in the center of the round table. Subjects make individual judgments, after which portable partitions are removed for open discussion. Source: University of California, Davis.

chemical constitution, philosophy of flavor, definition of flavor terms, functions of panel leader, theory of odor masking, odor library and reference standards, and introduction to pertinent literature. Trainees participate in measurements of taste thresholds, determinations of odor thresholds via the Elsberg method, odor and flavor description, description of note intensities, and difference tests. Through lectures, and demonstrations, and by creating opportunities to participate, the course aims at developing: (1) familiarity with descriptive language; (2) some understanding of the chemical nature of odorous and flavorful substances; (3) facility for taste and odor perception and judging the quantitative aspects of flavor and odor concentrations; and (4) techniques and understanding of the disciplines and procedures required for reproducible tasting and smelling. During the first 6-month period, after adequate progress has been made through practice, the panel receives an advanced course including lectures, demonstrations, and participation —all aimed at broadening the scope of panel activities. Following is an outline of the topics covered in the advanced training course (from Sjöström *et al.*, 1957): critique of trainee panel's findings following basic course, problems of trainee panels, aids to odor and flavor analysis, methods for studying packaging materials, flavor compounding, effect of metals on odors, screening methods, consumer product testing, and physicochemical separation. Demonstrations and trainee participation include: the use of reference standards, complex flavor situations, temperature control, and independent participation in several profile panels. When the trainees return to their own laboratory, additional exercises in flavor analysis are taken up and the Arthur D. Little Company continues to supervise the monthly conferences for a period of one year. The plan costs the individual industry approximately $15,000 (Young, 1962).

B. PROCEDURE

The physical requirements for conducting profile panels do not differ from those needed for other sensory methods of evaluation (see Chapter 6) except that a table is needed to seat four to six people for the open discussion sessions. The test product is usually presented in the form that will yield the most information consistent with use of the product. However, as indicated in the discussion of dilution techniques, other methods and forms of presentation have been used in combination with conventional profile methods. A useful way of presenting a series of essential oils for preliminary evaluation has been to incorporate them into sugar wafers (Caul, 1957a). The number of samples tested at one session is governed by the odor and flavor characteristics of the commodity.

The dimensions of flavor analysis by the profile method include: (1) perceptible aroma, taste, flavor, and feeling factors (called "character notes"); (2) degree of intensity of each factor, graded on the following scale:

0	= not present
)(	= just recognizable or threshold
1 or +	= slight
2 or ++	= moderate
3 or +++	= strong

(3) order in which these factors are perceived; (4) aftertaste; and (5) amplitude or over-all impressions of aroma and flavor, graded on the following scale:

$$)(= \text{very low}$$
$$1 = \text{low}$$
$$2 = \text{medium}$$
$$3 = \text{high}$$

Unlike the intensity scale, the amplitude scale is not fixed but varies with the test product. Because of the complexity and intangibility of the concept of amplitude, it is necessary for the panel to establish a frame of reference for each type of product examined. Figure 69 is a typical

Test # _____ Date _____ Name _____

AROMA   Amplitude ___3___

                                           Intensity

Hop fragrance	2
Fruity (apple)	2
Sour	1.5
Yeast	)(
Malt	1
Phenylacetic acid (honey)	1

FLAVOR-BY-MOUTH   Amplitude ___1___

                                           Intensity

CO_2 tingle	High
Salt	1
Sweet	1
Sour	2
Fruity (winy)	1
Bitter (metallic)	3
Malt	)(
Yeast	1
Others:	
Astringent	

AFTERTASTE:

Bitter
Astringent
Dry throat

Fig. 69. Response sheet used for profiling a malt beverage (including the panel's composite profile of the beverage). Source: Caul (1957a).

response sheet developed for a malt beverage, including the intensities and amplitudes determined by a profile panel.

Since intensity levels are denoted by symbols (which cannot be added), an average intensity level cannot be obtained for a test product (Caul, 1957a). It is conceivable, however, that a scoring system could be developed for use with the open-discussion technique that would result in numerical averages which could be analyzed statistically.

Flavor-profile-panel results have been summarized by diagram. The diagram consists of a semicircle denoting threshold concentrations, with radiating lines for each individual character note (in order of appearance), the lengths representing intensities (Fig. 70).

Upon completion of the individual examinations, the findings are discussed in open panel, one person in the group acting as moderator and recorder. This discussion at the end of the closed panel, a unique feature of the flavor profile method, is intended to stimulate panel mem-

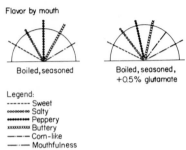

Flavor by mouth

Boiled, seasoned   Boiled, seasoned,
                           +0.5% glutamate

Legend:
------- Sweet
ooooooooo Salty
•••••••• Peppery
xxxxxxxx Buttery
——·—— Corn-like
——··—— Mouthfulness

FIG. 70. Diagrammatic representation of the flavor profiles of seasoned summer squash. Source: Cairncross and Sjöström (1950).

bers to increase their acuteness and reliability, and to foster interest and self-confidence. The moderator resolves differences about the intensity of notes by resubmitting samples (Cairncross and Sjöström, 1950).

C. ADVANTAGES

One of the major attributes of the flavor profile, according to its proponents, is its reproducibility. Caul (1957a) reported that a panel was able to obtain identical profiles from the same soup tested a year apart. In 1956, Sjöström stated that the 21 panels trained by the Arthur D. Little Company had all obtained profiles that agreed, but no details were presented on the nature of the commodity tested by these groups, nor on the degree of deviation in response to individual attributes. In our opinion, it is difficult to define reproducibility without some statistical test.

The Arthur D. Little Company has described successful use of profile techniques with milk and dairy products (Sjöström and Cairncross, 1951), cereals (Sjöström, 1951), beer (Swaine and Bell, 1951a,b), catsup and canned luncheon meats (Sjöström and Cairncross, 1953), pharmaceuticals (Caul and Rockwood, 1953; Sjöström, 1956), beef (Caul, 1957b), coffee (Sjöström, 1958), baked goods (Swaine, 1960), and packaging problems (Sjöström, 1950; Caul, 1961), and in flavor and odor titration studies (Sjöström et al., 1957).

D. DISADVANTAGES

There are several disadvantages in the flavor profile method: (1) selection of prospective panel members on the basis of responses to dilute solutions of the basic tastes has not been correlated with ability to judge foods (Mackey and Jones, 1954); (2) the Elsberg technique has been discredited as a sensitive olfactory measuring device (Jones, 1953); (3) selection, training, and conducting of profile panels is extremely time-consuming and therefore a very expensive method of analysis; (4) the results have not been analyzed statistically; (5) an intensity scale of 0–3 points lacks precision; (6) there is an inherent potential danger in exclusive use of open-discussion techniques; and (7) individual sensitivity to specific odors, tastes, or flavors cannot be quantified.

Relative to the first two points above, other methods of panel selection can be used (see Chapter 6, Section II,A) without minimizing the advantages of the profile approach to food evaluation. It is the opinion of the present authors that points 3 and 4 above might be remedied if difference testing methods were carefully combined with profiling methods. Depending on the test material and the sensitivity of the panel, one could expand the conventional scale of 0,)(, 1, 2, 3. Szczesniak and Farkas (1962) reported successful use of a 7-point intensity scale in profiling the texture of gum solutions.

Dangers of the group response have been studied by several investigators. As pointed out by Jones (1958), "A group-judgment is by no means the same as a group of judgments. At best a group-judgment may be expected to reflect unconscious signalling, and at worst, as when discussion is allowed, will result in the domination of the results by the loudest or most assured judge. During the 'hypothesis finding' phases of investigation this stricture need not hold, but if one wants valid judgments of, say, differences, he will be well advised to group his judges only statistically, not in reality."

Foster *et al.* (1955) compared round-table and individual testing of foods and demonstrated that the leader in the round-table session could readily sway the opinions of the group, especially when identical samples were being compared. This observation was demonstrated with three tests: evaluation of saltiness in tomato juice, preferences between brands A and B of baked beans, and sweetness of identical samples of crushed pineapple. Data from these three commodities, tested individually and in round-table sessions, are shown in Table 55. Thus, Foster *et al.* (1955) demonstrated that the round-table effect can create qualitative flavor differences and preferences where none exist. Although this biasing can be partially overcome by well-trained and sophisticated panels, the dangers inherent in round-table situations should be recognized by investigators. It is often difficult to determine whether a bias does exist.

In a similar experiment, Hall (1958) found that judgments from an experienced panel could be significantly influenced by the abnormal ob-

TABLE 55
Influence of a Leader on a Panel's Decisions on Three Food Items

Test materials	Individual Pair 1		Individual Pair 2		Round-table Pair 1		Round-table Pair 2	
	A	B	A	B	A	B	A	B
Tomato juice (which saltier)	8	21	7	25	10	26[a]	18[a]	16
Baked beans (which preferred)	11	21	9	23	15	21[a]	15[a]	18
Pineapple (which sweeter)	14	14	17	15	6	30[a]	13	20[a]

(The two upper spanning headers "Panel condition" covers all; "Individual" covers Pair 1 and Pair 2; "Round-table" covers Pair 1 and Pair 2.)

[a] Sample chosen by "leader."

Source: Foster *et al.* (1955).

TABLE 56
Average Profiles of a Mayonnaise Sample under Biased and Unbiased Influences

Characteristics	Type of group session Biased upward	No bias	Biased downward
Odor			
Acidity	—	0.98	0.74
Oily	1.55	1.05	1.12
Starch	0.75	0.23	—
Fruity ester	0.74	0.28	0.35
Metallic mustard	1.80	1.18	0.85
Oil inversion	0.59	0.35	0.09
Meaty	1.23	0.67	0.22
Total	6.66	4.74	3.37
Mean	1.11	0.68	0.56
Flavor			
Acidity	1.54	0.97	0.76
Oily	—	1.86	1.51
Sweetness	0.73	0.75	—
Mustard	1.49	1.01	—
Oil inversion	1.11	0.49	—
Salt	0.91	1.20	0.56
Lemon	0.66	0.17	—
Meaty	1.40	0.64	0.18
Fruity ester	0.67	0.43	0.31
Total	8.51	7.52	3.32
Mean	1.06	0.84	0.66

Source: Hall (1958).

servations of one person. Unknown to the other panelists, two members who sat alternately were chosen to vote a characteristic deliberately higher or lower than the value he would normally assign; each would introduce this bias only when he was the first or second judge to rate a given characteristic. In 22 out of 24 cases, an upward bias produced an upward shift of panel ratings; in 18 out of 20 cases, a downward bias caused a downward shift of panel results. Application of Student's *t*-test to the data obtained from upward bias versus no bias, and of the downward bias versus no-bias sessions, showed significantly different responses at $p = 0.01$. Table 56 shows the average intensity scores assigned to a sample of mayonnaise under the various biasing conditions. Hall concluded: " . . . errors in panel judgments can occur as an effect of extreme observations by an individual panel member. To say that they can occur, however, is not to say that they will. The hazard may remain potential rather than become real. Undoubtedly such errors can be minimized by panel education, by rigid selection and training procedures and by suspension of operations if potential bias appears."

E. OTHER DESCRIPTIVE PROCEDURES

The mechanics of open-discussion descriptive flavor analysis can and must be flexible and adapted to the requirements of each test situation. Jacobson *et al.* (1962) used descriptive flavor analysis to supplement scoring and difference testing of lamb, pork, and chicken. At McCormick & Co., for example, profiling methods are used to orient the panel, after which strictly personal ratings are made on the form shown in Fig. 58. As emphasized by Hall (1958), " . . . these modifications . . . involve an occasional change in mechanics, not a change in the philosophy of the profile method; nor has there been, by any means, a loss of confidence in the round-table procedure. We believe that there are many cases in which the round-table is by far the most effective and valid procedure. Particularly where the food in question changes constantly, where old flavor notes alter and new ones continually appear, round-table discussion is the quicker, more flexible approach. In these cases its advantages outweigh any potential dangers. In other cases, such as our beverage problem, where the flavor constituents are more clearly defined and less likely to change, the mechanics suggested here seem to offer advantages of precision and safety from bias."

Tilgner (1962a) criticized the flavor profile procedure as being too difficult, particularly because of compensation, superimposition, and masking phenomena in foods. He therefore proposed using an identification threshold, expressed as percent dilution, as a measure of the amount of odor or flavor of a food sample. A standard and a test material were treated in the same way so that a direct comparison was obtained. In addition, as the dilution increased the judges were asked to "profile" the odor, i.e., to identify the different sensory components. Various odor and taste characteristics disappeared at different dilutions. If applied to food evaluation, the method assumes that diluted foods have flavor properties directly related to those of the undiluted food.

Sjöström and Caul (1962) objected to this assumption and pointed out that flavor profiles should be conducted on a food product in its normal form, at its normal strength, and at its normal temperature of consumption. Tilgner's rejoinder (1962c) was that the dilution-profile method was the only technique he had found to characterize the sensory properties of the foods with which he was working. Dove (1962) made the useful suggestion that the flavor profile continue to be used as one of the methods of evaluating the quality of the final products and that Tilgner's procedure, which Dove prefers to call "scanning of the dilution scale," be used for research and development in food acceptance studies. Jellinek (1962a) agrees, but noted that, in materials such as perfumes, quality changes upon dilution. Dove (1962) also mentioned wide individual variation in hedonic response to sweetness on dilution and warned of the dangers of averaging sensory responses.

We conclude that descriptions based on dilution techniques should be accepted with caution if the purpose of the study is to evaluate food quality. We agree with Jellinek (1962b) that the most appropriate use of the profile techniques may be in developing specific descriptive flavor terms to assist in product development, quality control, and correlation with instrumental findings. In some cases, particularly with spices, the period over which a given taste or sensation persists is important. Neilson (1957) had her panel members face a clock with a piece of graph paper. The y axis had a scale of 0–4 for no sensation, threshold, slight, moderate, and strong. The x axis was marked in seconds and minutes. The tasters took the food and after swallowing marked the intensity sensation at intervals. The panel members might have to concentrate on a given flavor for as long as 10 to 12 minutes. The resulting graphs represent a time-intensity picture. Some compounds gave an immediate intensity peak and then declined, while others (for bitterness in beer, for example) did not reach their peak until 5 to 8 seconds after swallowing.

VI. "Contour" Method

The "contour" method was developed by Hall et al. (1959), at Continental Can Company, Chicago. A panel of 7 to 10 subjects, screened for sensitivity to quinine according to prescribed procedures, was presented with paired samples of a test substance, one member of each pair being

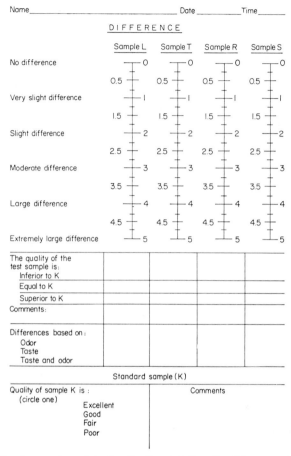

Name_____ Date _____Time_____

DIFFERENCE

	Sample L	Sample T	Sample R	Sample S
No difference	0	0	0	0
	0.5	0.5	0.5	0.5
Very slight difference	1	1	1	1
	1.5	1.5	1.5	1.5
Slight difference	2	2	2	2
	2.5	2.5	2.5	2.5
Moderate difference	3	3	3	3
	3.5	3.5	3.5	3.5
Large difference	4	4	4	4
	4.5	4.5	4.5	4.5
Extremely large difference	5	5	5	5

The quality of the
test sample is:
Inferior to K
Equal to K
Superior to K
Comments:

Differences based on:
Odor
Taste
Taste and odor

Standard sample (K)

Quality of sample K is :   Comments
(circle one)
Excellent
Good
Fair
Poor

Fɪɢ. 71. Scoring card used in the Continental Can Co. "flavor contour" method. (Samples *L, T, R,* and *S* are evaluated in terms of their deviation from the standard test sample, *K*.) Source: Hall *et al.* (1959).

designated as a standard, *K*. Using the scoring system shown in Fig. 71, deviation from the standard was determined for both odor and flavor characteristics. These differences were separated into several components, such as: (1) material factor, i.e., effect of test material other than bitterness upon the flavor of the food product; (2) differences in bitterness as measured by "quinine equivalents," calculated by the statistical method of correlation and regression from the predetermined bitterness sensitivity level of each taster; (3) difference in tasters, determined by standard-to-standard test for each medium; and (4) miscellaneous factors, those remaining after separation of the above components. The resulting information is plotted to form a so-called "contour," as shown in Fig. 72.

The contour method has been used successfully in selecting metal containers which will not affect the product. The primary purpose of the method is to determine flavor difference; the secondary purpose is to determine quality. Psychological factors are important in this method only insofar as they can be measured as a sum total (Ellis, 1960).

Hall *et al.* (1959) listed the following restrictions of the contour method: (1) the method does not analyze the over-all flavor of a food, but only that part which makes a test sample different from a control; (2) the test-sample medium and the standard-sample medium must be

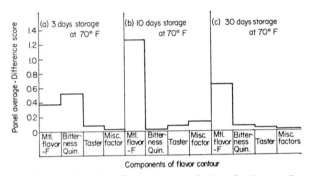

FIG. 72. Continental Can Co. "flavor contours." (Results from a flavor test on an experimental container material.) Source: Hall *et al.* (1959).

identical except for addition of a test material to the medium; (3) although the method can be used to analyze more than four components of a flavor difference, there is always a small component due to remaining or "unknown" factors. Other laboratories have made little use of the contour method because of its recent development and relative complexity.

VII. Other Procedures

A. DISGUISING-POTENTIAL METHOD

In the disguising-potential method, a series of samples containing increasing quantities of a distasteful drug in distilled water is compared with a corresponding series containing a selected disguising flavoring agent (Purdum, 1942; Lankford and Becker, 1951a,b; Reid and Becker, 1956). This method is used almost exclusively by the pharmaceutical industry in selecting appropriate flavor-masking agents. Usually only one characteristic is considered—off-flavor. Trained subjects are used in closed panel sessions. Determination of taste thresholds has been combined with the disguising-potential technique (Reid and Becker, 1956). For example, the mean threshold of 15 subjects for quinine hydrochloride was 5.2 ± 0.38 (between the fifth and sixth concentrations) in water and 16.3 ± 0.18 in Dutch-process cocoa with salt added. Therefore the mean disguising potential of the cocoa "vehicle" is calculated, by difference, as 11.1 ± 0.43. The concentrations were not quantified in the publication, so that the exact amount of the compound is unknown.

In Caul's (1957a) opinion the method is not practical, since it requires thousands of tastings for each test to give a negligible amount of information. Although the method as described above has only limited application, combining it with other methods of difference testing would perhaps increase its usability.

B. Dove's "D-Unit Scale"

In an attempt to standardize the measurement and reporting of taste responses, Dove (1953) developed a unified gustometric scaling device consisting of uniform dilution units regardless of stimulus or response, and called a "D-unit scale." The scale was designed for use with solutions of pure chemicals as well as natural foods, including dehydrated and concentrated foods, when a system of "C-units" is also used. For example, with sucrose (M.W. $= 342.296$), the following units were established:

$$1C = 342.2960 \text{ g/liter of solution}$$
$$1D = 171.1480 \text{ g/liter of solution}$$
$$2D = 85.5740 \text{ g/liter of solution}$$
$$4D = 21.3935 \text{ g/liter of solution}$$
$$8D = 1.3371 \text{ g/liter of solution}$$
$$\text{etc.}$$

For natural or processed foods and beverages, Dove proposed the scale in Table 57. The units can be further reduced to $\frac{1}{2}$ D's or $\frac{1}{4}$ D's.

TABLE 57

A Unified Gustometric Scale ("D-Unit" Scale) Consisting of Uniform Dilution Units Regardless of Stimulus or Response

Scale for dilutions $1/2^n$		Volume or weight		Scale for concentrations 2^n
1C	=	1000.000	=	1C
1D	=	500.0000	=	2C
2D	=	250.0000	=	4C
4D	=	62.5000	=	16C
8D	=	8.9063	=	256C
etc.				

Source: Dove (1953).

According to Dove, three scale intervals can be used: (1) "The Macro D-units of 1D (increments of 100 percent) are suitable to the scaling of taste thresholds, serve as loci for records of affective responses, and as levels for establishment of relative acuity of food judges and the extent of pathological change in taste or presence of genetic differences in taste ability"; (2) "The Micro D-units of ¼ C (increments of 18.9207 percent) serve as bench marks for taste matching, for food specifications, formulation, and establishment of levels for reconstitution of dehydrated foods"; (3) "The Ultramicro D-units, fractionated to ¹⁄₆₄ D (increments of 1.0889 percent), or smaller if necessary, mark off the degrees of fine taste discrimination and establish taste difference thresholds."

Dove's mathematical progression scale was designed to bring some order and universality to evaluation of sensory stimuli. It has met with limited use since it is still necessary to transpose the subjective responses into the standard reference D-unit before they can be used. Further refinement of the mode of expression of a response in no way increases the precision of measurement of either affective or discriminatory responses. Dove's proposal is really a plea for the use of geometric progression in dilution.

VIII. Summary

Methods were discussed that are used with laboratory panels to establish the intensity of a food characteristic or the over-all quality. Emphasized throughout is the importance of training and experience with each food commodity so that all judges understand the characteristic being evaluated and have similar quality standards.

In general, ranking procedures are rapid and simple to administer but give no information on relative differences between samples. Scoring, on the other hand, gives an indication of how much samples differ from each other qualitatively, but scoring scales need to be developed that reflect quality equally throughout the entire scoring range. Hedonic scales of like and dislike are useful if the assumption is correct that pleasure is directly related to preference. The choice of descriptive words or phrases for the scale intervals is important if the scale is to be meaningful. Dilution procedures are useful in revealing sensory components which may be masked in the original concentration, but their use for determining quality should be carefully tested before predictions can be made. Although descriptive sensory methods may require much time for training, and the round-table sessions are subject to serious psychological disadvantages, the method is useful in quality control and with certain flavor problems. Inability to express the judgments numerically precludes statistical analysis and limits its use in the research laboratory. The contour and trend-rating procedures are, as yet, too new to have been adequately tested with a wide variety of different foods and food products.

The importance of careful control of all testing conditions and procedures cannot be overstressed. No one method of evaluation can be used exclusively, for each has its strengths and weaknesses. It is necessary to determine what information is desired, and then select the appropriate method that will yield reliable and reproducible data. There is a great need for further development and testing of methods. Whenever possible, investigators should use more than one method in their sensory studies and publish their results, thereby contributing to our knowledge of sound, economical, and reproducible techniques of measurement of sensory properties.

REFERENCES

Amerine, M. A., E. B. Roessler, and F. Filipello. 1959. Modern sensory methods of evaluating wines. *Hilgardia* **28**, 477–567.

Anderson, E. E. 1958. Scoring and ranking. *In* "Flavor Research and Food Acceptance" (A. D. Little, Inc., ed.), 391 pp. (see pp. 75–82). Reinhold, New York.

Anonymous. 1964. Sensory testing guide for panel evaluation of foods and beverages. *Food Technol.* **18**(8), 25–31.

Aref, M., A. P. Sidwell, and E. M. Litwiller. 1956. The effects of various sweetening agents on frozen strawberries for preserve manufacture. *Food Technol.* **10**, 293–297.

Barylko-Pikielna, N. and K. Metelski. 1964. Determination of contribution coefficients.

Baten, W. D. 1946. Organoleptic tests pertaining to apples and pears. *Food Research* **11**, 84–94.

Bliss, C. I., E. O. Anderson, and R. E. Marland. 1943. A technique for testing consumer preferences, with special reference to the constituents of ice cream. *Conn. Univ. Agr. Expt. Sta. Bull.* **251**, 1–20.

Bliss, C. I., M. L. Greenwood, and M. H. McKenrick. 1953. A comparison of scoring methods for taste tests with mealiness of potatoes. *Food Technol.* **7**, 491–495.

Boggs, M. M., and H. L. Hanson. 1949. Analysis of foods by sensory difference tests. *Advances in Food Research* **2**, 219–258.

Boggs, M. M., and A. C. Ward. 1950. Scoring techniques for sulfited foods. *Food Technol.* **4**, 282–284.

Bohren, B. B., and R. Jordan. 1946. An objective technique for detecting flavor changes in dehydrated eggs. (Abstr.) *Poultry Sci.* **25**, 397.

Bohren, B. B., and R. Jordan. 1953. A technique for detecting flavor changes in stored dried eggs. *Food Research* **18**, 583–591.

Bradley, R. A., and M. E. Terry. 1952. The rank analysis of incomplete block designs. 1. The method of paired comparison. *Biometrika* **39**, 324–345.

Brant, A. W., and M. Simone. 1962. Personal communication. University of California, Davis, California.

Byer, A. J., and D. Abrams. 1953. A comparison of the triangular and two-sample taste-test methods. *Food Technol.* **7**, 185–187. (See also *Wallerstein Lab. Comms.* **16**, 253–259, 1953.)

Byer, A. J., and L. T. Saletan. 1961. A new approach to flavor evaluation of beer. *Wallerstein Lab. Comms.* **24**, 289–303.

Cairncross, S. E., and L. B. Sjöström. 1950. Flavor profiles—a new approach to flavor problems. *Food Technol.* **4**, 308–311.

Carlin, A. F., O. Kempthorne, and J. Gordon. 1956. Some aspects of numerical scoring in subjective evaluation of foods. *Food Research* **21**, 273–281.

Caul, J. F. 1957a. The profile method of flavor analysis. *Advances in Food Research* **7**, 1–40.

Caul, J. F. 1957b. Flavor study on development of beef flavor in U. S. Choice and U. S. commercial cuts of sirloin. *In* "Chemistry of Natural Food Flavors" (J. H. Mitchell, N. L. Leinen, E. M. Mrak, and S. D. Bailey, eds.), 200 pp. (see pp. 152–167). Quartermaster Food and Container Inst., Chicago, Illinois.

Caul, J. F. 1961. The American approach to odour in the packaging of food. *World's Paper Trade Rev.* June 22, 6 pp.

Caul, J. F., and E. L. Rockwood. 1953. A flavor panel study of the application of monosodium glutamate to the flavor of pharmaceutical products. *J. Am. Pharm. Assoc., Sci. Ed.* **42**, 682–685.

Caul, J. F., and R. L. Swaine. 1959. Definition of flavor and its evaluation by organoleptic properties. 11 pp. Mimeo. of paper presented at the 5th Ann. Seminar of Kurth Malting Co., Milwaukee, Wisconsin.

Colby, M. Y. 1938. "Sound Waves and Acoustics," 356 pp. Holt, New York.

Cover, S. 1959. Meat cookery from the scientific viewpoint. *Proc. Research Conf., Am. Meat Inst. Found.* **11**, 99–111.

Crocker, E. C. 1945. "Flavor," 172 pp. McGraw-Hill, New York.

Dawson, E. H., and E. F. Dochterman. 1951. A comparison of sensory methods of measuring differences in food qualities. *Food Technol.* **5**, 79–81.

Dawson, E. H., and B. L. Harris. 1951. Sensory methods for measuring differences in food quality. *U. S. Dept. Agr., Agr. Infor. Bull.* **34**, 1–134.

Dawson, E. H., J. L. Brogdon, and S. McManus. 1963. Sensory testing of differences in taste. I. Methods, II. Selection of panel members. *Food Technol.* **17**(9), 45–48, 51; (10), 39–41, 43–44.

Day, E. A. 1962. Personal communication. Department of Food Science and Technology, Oregon State College, Corvallis, Oregon.

Dove, W. F. 1943. The relative nature of human preference: with an example in the palatability of different varieties of sweet corn. *J. Comp. Psychol.* **35**, 219–226.

Dove, W. F. 1947. Food acceptability—its determination and evaluation. *Food Technol.* **1**, 39–50.

Dove, W. F. 1953. A universal gustometric scale in D-units. *Food Research* **18**, 427–453.

Dove, W. F. 1962. The dilution scale as a scanning device for food acceptance. (Letter to editor.) *Food Technol.* **16**(8), 7–8.

Downs, P. A., E. O. Anderson, O. J. Babcock, F. H. Herzer, and G. M. Trout. 1954. Evaluation of collegiate student dairy products judging since World War II. *J. Dairy Sci.* **37**, 1021–1026.

Ehrenberg, A. S. C. 1953. On Plank's rational method of grading food quality. *Food Technol.* **7**, 188.

Eindhoven, J., and D. R. Peryam. 1959. Measurement of preferences for food combinations. *Food Technol.* **13**, 379–382.

Ellis, B. H. 1960. Continental Can Company taste testing methods. 18 pp. Mimeo.

of paper presented at Research and Development Assoc., Food and Container Inst., Inc., Chicago, Illinois.

Ellis, B. H. 1961. "A Guide Book for Sensory Testing," 55 pp. Continental Can Co., Chicago, Illinois.

Elsberg, C. A., and I. Levy. 1935. The sense of smell. I. A new and simple method of quantitative olfactometry. *Bull. Neurol. Inst. N. Y.* **4,** 5–19.

Fair, G. M. 1933. Determination of odors and tastes in water. *J. New Engl. Water Works Assoc.* **47,** 248–272.

Fenton, F. A. 1957. Judging and scoring milk. *U. S. Dept. Agr. Farmers' Bull.* **2111,** 1–20.

Fisher, R. A., and F. Yates. 1948. "Statistical Tables," 112 pp. (see Table XX, pp. 66–67). Oliver and Boyd, Edinburgh.

Foster, D., C. Pratt, and N. Schwartz. 1955. Variations in flavor judgments in a group situation. *Food Research* **20,** 539–544.

Gelman, G. 1945. Psychometrics—a new quality control? *Food Ind.* **17,** 625.

Greenwood, M. L., M. Potgieter, and C. I. Bliss. 1951. The effect of certain pre-freezing treatments on the quality of eight varieties of cultivated highbush blueberries. *Food Research* **16,** 154–160.

Guilford, J. P. 1954. "Psychometric Methods," 597 pp. McGraw-Hill, New York.

Guthrie, E. S. 1958. Scoring of dairy products. *In* "Flavor Research and Food Acceptance" (A. D. Little, Inc., ed.), 391 pp. (see pp. 83–87). Reinhold, New York.

Hall, B. A., M. G. Tarver, and J. G. McDonald. 1959. A method for screening flavor panel members and its application to a two sample difference test. *Food Technol.* **8,** 699–703.

Hall, R. L. 1958. Flavor study approaches at McCormick and Co., Inc. *In* "Flavor Research and Food Acceptance" (A. D. Little, Inc., ed.), 391 pp. (see pp. 224–240). Reinhold, New York.

Handschumaker, E. 1948. A technique for testing the reversion properties of hydrogenated soybean oil shortenings. *J. Am. Oil Chemists' Soc.* **25,** 54–56.

Hanson, H. L., L. Kline, and H. Lineweaver. 1951. Application of balanced incomplete block design to scoring of ten dried egg samples. *Food Technol.* **5,** 9–13.

Hanson, H. L., L. Kline, and H. Lineweaver. 1954. A dilution method for the determination of relative flavor stability of egg solids. *In* "Food Acceptance Testing Methodology," 115 pp. (see pp. 20–24). Advisory Board on Quartermaster and Development, Committee on Foods; and Natl. Acad. Sci., Natl. Research Council, Chicago, Illinois.

Hicks, E. W. 1948. Tasting tests. *Food Preserv. Quart.* **8,** 1–5.

Hogue, D. V., and A. M. Briant. 1957. Determining flavor differences in crops treated with pesticides. I. A comparison of a triangle and a multiple comparison method. *Food Research* **22,** 351–357.

Hopkins, J. W. 1950. A procedure for quantifying subjective appraisals of odor, flavor, and texture of foodstuffs. *Biometrics* **6,** 1–16.

Hunt, W. A., and J. Volkmann. 1937. The anchoring of an affective scale. *Am. J. Psychol.* **49,** 88–92.

Jacobson, M., M. Weller, M. W. Galgan, and E. H. Rupnow. 1962. Factors in flavor and tenderness of lamb, beef and pork and techniques of evaluation. *Wash. State Coll. Agr. Expt. Sta. Tech. Bull.* **40,** 1–22.

Jakobsen, F. 1949. Rational grading of food quality. *Food Technol.* **3,** 252–254.

Jellinek, G. 1962a. Dilution flavor profile and flavor profile method. (Letter to editor.) *Food Technol.* **16**(10), 16, 18, 20.

Jellinek, G. 1962b. Flavor testing with the profile method. *In* "Recent Advances in Food Science" (J. Hawthorn and J. M. Leitch, eds.), Vol. II, 317 pp. (see pp. 287–292). Butterworths, London.

Jenness, R., and S. Patton. 1959. "Principles of Dairy Chemistry," 446 pp. (see pp. 360–390). Wiley, New York.

Jones, F. N. 1953. A test of the validity of the Elsberg method of olfactometry. *Am. J. Psychol.* **66**, 81–85.

Jones, F. N. 1958. Prerequisites for test environment. *In* "Flavor Research and Food Acceptance" (A. D. Little, Inc., ed.), 391 pp. (see pp. 107–111). Reinhold, New York.

Jones, L. V., D. R. Peryam, and L. L. Thurstone. 1955. Development of a scale for measuring soldiers' food preferences. *Food Research* **20**, 512–520.

Kamenetzky, J. 1959. Contrast and convergence effects in ratings of foods. *J. Appl. Psychol.* **43**, 47–52.

Kirkpatrick, M. E., J. C. Lamb, E. H. Dawson, and J. N. Eisen. 1957. Selecting a taste panel for evaluating the quality of processed milk. *Food Technol.* **11**(9), 3–8 (Supplement).

Klingberg, F. L. 1941. Studies in measurements of the relations among sovereign states. *Psychometrika* **6**, 335–352.

Kramer, A. 1959. Glossary of some terms used in the sensory (panel) evaluation of foods and beverages. *Food Technol.* **13**, 733–736.

Kramer, A. 1960. A rapid method for determining significance of differences from rank sums. *Food Technol.* **14**, 576–581.

Kramer, A., and B. A. Twigg. 1962. "Fundamentals of Quality Control for the Food Industry," 512 pp. Avi Publ. Co., Westport, Connecticut.

Kramlich, W. E., and A. M. Pearson. 1958. Some preliminary studies on meat flavor. *Food Research* **23**, 567–574.

Krum, J. K. 1955. Sensory panel testing. *Food Eng.* **27** (July), 74–83.

Laboratory Practice. 1964. Sensory food analysis. *Laboratory Practice* **13**, 596–641, 700–738.

Lankford, B. L., and C. H. Becker. 1951a. The use of some imitation flavors for masking distasteful drugs. I. Ammonium chloride. *J. Am. Pharm. Assoc., Sci. Ed.* **40**, 77–82.

Lankford, B. L., and C. H. Becker. 1951b. The use of some imitation flavors for masking distasteful drugs. II. Quinine hydrochloride. *J. Am. Pharm. Assoc., Sci. Ed.* **40**, 83–86.

Likert, R. 1932. A technique for the measurement of attitudes. *Arch. Psychol.* **140**, 1–55.

Lowe, B. 1955. "Experimental Cookery," 4th ed., 573 pp. (see pp. 34–47). Wiley, New York.

Mackey, A. O., and P. Jones. 1954. Selection of members of a food tasting panel: Discernment of primary tastes in water solution compared with judging ability for foods. *Food Technol.* **8**, 527–530.

Miller, G. A. 1956. The magical number seven, plus or minus two: some limits on our capacity for processing information. *Psychol. Rev.* **63**, 81–97.

Murphy, E. F., R. M. Bailey, and M. R. Covell. 1954. Observations on methods to determine food palatability and comparative freezing quality of certain new strawberry varieties. *Food Technol.* **8**, 113–116.

Murphy, E. F., M. R. Covell, and J. S. Dinsmore. 1957. An examination of three methods for testing palatability as illustrated by strawberry flavor differences. *Food Research* **22**, 423–439.

Neilson, A. J. 1957. Time-intensity studies. *Drug Cosmetic Ind.* **80**, 452–453, 534. *Also in* A. D. Little, Inc. "Flavor Research and Food Acceptance," 391 pp. (see pp. 88–93). Reinhold Publishing Corp., New York. 1958.

Nelson, J. A., and G. M. Trout. 1948. "Judging Dairy Products," 494 pp. Olsen Publ. Co., Milwaukee, Wisconsin.

Ough, C. S., and G. A. Baker. 1961. Small panel sensory evaluations of wines by scoring. *Hilgardia* **30**, 587–619.

Pangborn, R. M., and W. L. Dunkley. 1964. Laboratory procedures for evaluating the sensory properties of milk. *Dairy Sci. Abstr.* **26**, 55–62.

Pangborn, R. M., R. H. Vaughn, and G. K. York. 1958. Effect of sucrose and type of spicing on the quality of processed dill pickles. *Food Technol.* **12**, 144–147.

Parks, A. B. 1954. Ranking vs. scoring in palatability tests using small trained panels. *In* "Food Acceptance Testing Methodology," 115 pp. (see pp. 40–45). Advisory Board on Quartermaster Research and Development, Committee on Foods; and Natl. Acad. Sci., Natl. Research Council, Chicago, Illinois.

Peryam, D. R. 1950. Quality control in the production of blended whiskey. *Ind. Quality Control* **7**, 17–21.

Peryam, D. R., and N. F. Girardot. 1952. Advanced taste-test method. *Food Eng.* **24**, 58–61, 194.

Peryam, D. R., and N. J. Gutman. 1958. Variation in preference ratings for foods served at meals. *Food Technol.* **12**, 30–33.

Peryam, D. R., and J. G. Haynes. 1957. Prediction of soldiers' food preferences by laboratory methods. *J. Appl. Psychol.* **41**, 2–6

Peryam, D. R., and F. J. Pilgrim. 1957. Hedonic scale method of measuring food preferences. *Food Technol.* **11**(9), 9–14 (supplement).

Peryam, D. R., and R. Shapiro. 1955. Perception, preference, judgment—clues to food quality. *Ind. Quality Control* **11**, 1–6.

Peryam, D. R., D. V. Josephson, R. J. Remaley, and H. Fevold. 1951. New flavor evaluation method. *Food Eng.* **23**, 83–86, 167.

Peryam, D. R., F. J. Pilgrim, and M. S. Peterson. 1954. *In* "Food Acceptance Testing Methodology," 115 pp. Advisory Board on Quartermaster Research and Development, Committee on Foods; and Natl. Acad. Sci., Natl. Research Council, Chicago, Illinois.

Plank, R. P. 1948. A rational method for grading food quality. *Food Technol.* **2**, 241–251.

Platt, W. 1931. Scoring food products. *Food Inds.* **3**, 108–111.

Purdum, W. A. 1942. Method of evaluating relative efficacy of disguising agents for distasteful drugs. *J. Am. Pharm. Assoc., Sci. Ed.* **31**, 298–305.

Raffensperger, E. L., D. R. Peryam, and K. R. Wood. 1956. Development of a scale for grading toughness-tenderness in beef. *Food Technol.* **12**, 627–630.

Ramsbottom, J. M. 1947. Freezer storage effect on fresh meat quality. *Refrig. Eng.* **53**, 19–23.

Reid, A. W., and C. H. Becker. 1956. The use of cocoa syrups for masking the taste of quinine hydrochloride. *J. Am. Pharm. Assoc.* **45**, 151–152.

Reimer, C. 1957. Some application of rank order statistics in sensory panel testing. *Food Research* **22**, 629–634.

Seaton, R. W., and B. W. Gardner. 1959. Acceptance measurement of unusual foods. *Food Research* **24**, 271–278.

Sheppard, D. 1954. The adequacy of everyday quantitative expressions as measurements of qualities. *Brit. J. Psychol.* **45**, 40–50.

Sheppard, D. 1955. Descriptive terms and points systems for rating food qualities. *Food Research* **20**, 114–117.

Sjöström, L. B. 1950. Paper package odors. *Modern Packaging* **23**, 118–120.

Sjöström, L. B. 1951. Measuring cereal flavors by the flavor profile method. *Trans. Am. Assoc. Cereal Chemists* **9**, 96–103.

Sjöström, L. B. 1956. Flavor analysis. *Drug & Cosmetic Ind.* **78**(1), 28–31.

Sjöström, L. B. 1958. Flavor measurement as an industrial research tool. 13 pp. Mimeo. of paper presented at the 1st Ann. Meeting, Inter-American Food Congr., Bal Harbor, Florida.

Sjöström, L. B., and S. E. Cairncross. 1951. Flavor profiles, a method of judging dairy products. *Am. Milk Rev.* **12**, 42–44.

Sjöström, L. B., and S. E. Cairncross. 1953. What makes flavor leadership. *Food Technol.* **7**, 56–58.

Sjöström, L. B., and J. F. Caul. 1962. "Dilution flavor profile" reaction. (Letter to editor). *Food Technol.* **16**(4), 8.

Sjöström, L. B., S. E. Cairncross, and J. F. Caul. 1957. Methodology of the flavor profile. *Food Technol.* **11**(9), 20–25 (supplement).

Swaine, R. L. 1960. The use of the flavor profile panel in the baking industry. *Bakers' Dig.* **34**(5), 55–57, 86–87.

Swaine, R. L., and V. P. Bell. 1951a. The flavor profile—a method for measuring beer "taste appeal." *Modern Brewery Age* **45**(6), 41–42, 44, 100.

Swaine, R. L., and V. P. Bell. 1951b. The flavor profile—a method for measuring beer "taste appeal." *Modern Brewery Age* **46**(1), 25–26, 91.

Szczesniak, A. S., and E. Farkas. 1962. Objective characterization of the mouthfeel of gum solutions. *J. Food Sci.* **27**, 381–385.

Tarver, M., and A. M. Schenck. 1958. Statistical development of objective quality scores for evaluating the quality of food products. Development of the scoring scales. *Food Technol.* **3**, 127–131.

Tilgner, D. J. 1954. Organoleptyczny wskaźnik słoności (Organoleptic index of saltiness). *Przemysł Spożywczy* **8**, 14–22.

Tilgner, D. J. 1957. "Analiza Organoleptyczna Żywności" (Organoleptic analysis of food), 364 pp. Wydawnictwo Przemysłu Lekkiego i Spożywczego, Warsaw.

Tilgner, D. J. 1961. A sensory quality index for margarine. *Food Manuf.* **36**, 327–333.

Tilgner, D. J. 1962a. Dilution tests for odor and flavor analysis. *Food Technol.* **16**(2), 26–29.

Tilgner, D. J. 1962b. Anchored sensory evaluation tests—a status report. *Food Technol.* **16**(3), 47–50.

Tilgner, D. J. 1962c. Flavor analysis. (Letter to editor). *Food Technol.* **16**(7), 8.

Tilgner, D. J. 1965. Flavor dilution profilograms. *Food Technol.* **19**(1), 25–29.

Tilgner, D. J., and N. Baryłko-Pikielna. 1959. Poziom progu i minimum wrażliwości zymsłu smaku (Threshold and minimum sensitivity of the taste sense). *Acta Physiol. Polonica* **10**, 741–754.

Tompkins, M. D., and G. B. Pratt. 1959. Comparison of flavor evaluation methods for frozen citrus concentrates. *Food Technol.* **13**, 149–152.

Trout, G. M., and P. F. Sharp. 1937. The reliability of flavor judgments, with special reference to the oxidized flavor of milk. *N. Y. State Agr. Expt. Sta. Mem.* **204**, 1–60.

Tuxbury, G. P., and D. R. Peryam. 1952. The application of food acceptance methods and results to military feeding problems. *Proc. Research Conf. Am. Meat Inst., Chicago* **4**, 73–82.

Young, P. T. 1952. The role of hedonic processes in the organization of behavior. *Psychol. Rev.* **59**, 249–262.

Young, W. R. 1962. Cracking the secret riddle of flavor. *Life* **53**, 110–123.

Chapter 9

Consumer Studies

Although the fate of a food product has always rested on acceptance by the consuming public, formal studies of consumer preference are a comparatively recent development. Consumer reactions are difficult to measure (Hicks, 1948), but the necessity for such studies will continue to grow as competition for the consumer food dollar increases. The competitive aspects are readily visualized when it is considered that the daily per-capita caloric intake remains relatively constant in this country, so that a new food product succeeds to the extent that it replaces another food item or benefits by population increase. It has been estimated that grocery products purchased for the home totaled seventy billion dollars in 1960 in the United States, almost equal to the size of the federal budget (Strom, 1960). With a buying power of this magnitude it is obviously advantageous for the food industry to study the needs and desires of the consumer. In some cases, it is possible to create markets for certain foods where none existed previously. Well-established industries strive to maintain their sales by determining whether alterations in formulation, packaging, or diversification are advantageous. (The aspects of advertising that are influential in the area of food selection and acceptance are, of course, beyond the scope of this text.) It has been theorized that people do not know what they want and can be manipulated through psychoanalytically oriented promotion campaigns (Packard, 1957). Since "subliminal persuasion" is still in its infancy and no reliable statistics are available for comparison, the subject is not discussed here.

Demand by the time-conscious housewife for partially prepared foods and "convenience items" has increased rapidly, requiring alterations in raw-material selection, processing, packaging, distribution, and advertising. The acceleration of new-product development, emphasizes the need for reliable, efficient, and representative sampling of consumer opinion as well as continuous study of changes in food habits (Schaal, 1952).

398

The influence and magnitude of consumer opinion is recognized by such large consuming groups as the United States Army, which supports a very active food acceptance program (Peryam *et al.*, 1960). General Foods Corporation, the Kroger Foundation, and other private industries rely heavily on consumer reaction obtained by their preference surveys (Szczesniak and Kleyn, 1963; Elder, 1954; Garnatz, 1952). Private firms, government agencies, and various educational and research organizations are actively engaged in studies of techniques, methodologies, and application of results of consumer food surveys (Nicosia, 1962). Among the earliest publications on results of tests of consumer acceptance of food are those of Platt (1941), Cowan (1941), Arnold (1941), and Bogert (1941). Consumer psychology is reviewed by Twedt (1965).

One must distinguish carefully between studies of consumer preference and studies of consumer practice. Those who prefer may not be those who buy. *Preference* studies are designed to determine consumers' subjective reactions to external phenomena, and their reasons for having them. *Practice* studies are designed to determine what consumers actually *do* under given circumstances, such as the numbers of ripe and underripe peaches purchased when ripe peaches cost certain amounts more. The techniques for these two types of studies are usually quite different, although some approaches can be used for both types (Anonymous, 1949). Both acceptance and preference are primarily economic concepts. *Acceptance* of food varies with standards of living and cultural background, whereas *preference* refers to selection when presented with a choice (Harries, 1953). Preferences are frequently influenced by prejudice, religious principles, group conformance, "status value," and snobbery, in addition to the quality of the food. There is no denying that people have preferences, no matter how illogical they may appear to be.

The consumer expects to be favorably impressed with the food he selects, and expresses displeasure if the product does not measure up to his anticipations. Liebmann and Panettiere (1957) have shown that adverse impressions have a much greater influence on the consumer's reactions than do pleasant ones. Brady (1957) expressed a similar opinion, with specific reference to tenderness in meat.

I. Factors Influencing Acceptance and Preference

Many complex factors combine to influence the public's acceptance and selection of food, as indicated in the list on p. 400. The extent to which the sensory properties modify the selection and utilization of a food is difficult to ascertain since all of these factors interact and influence the consumer's decisions.

Appearance probably has the greatest initial influence, since visual

Attributes of the food product	Attributes of the consumer
1. Availability	1. Regional preferences
2. Utility	2. Nationality, race
3. Convenience	3. Age and sex
4. Price	4. Religion
5. Uniformity and dependability	5. Education, socio-economics
6. Stability, storage requirements	6. Psychological motivation
7. Safety and nutritional value	a. Symbolism of food
8. Sensory properties	b. Advertising
a. Appearance	7. Physiological motivation
b. Aroma and taste	a. Thirst
c. Texture, consistency	b. Hunger
d. Temperature	c. Deficiencies
e. Pain	d. Pathological conditions

properties significantly control selection of the item from the hundreds of choices on the grocer's shelves. Later, on the dinner table, appearance either succeeds or fails to stimulate appetite. To test the importance of color and appearance in food selection, the U. S. Testing Company (Foster, 1956) asked a large group of shoppers to wear specially tinted goggles while doing their normal food buying. When the glasses were removed prior to the checkout counter, every shopper was surprised at her selections of meats, cheese, fruits, vegetables, and even of strange brands. The experiment showed that removal of color discrimination slowed the shopper and altered her food selections. This experiment should have been replicated to test its repeatability and reliability.

Once the food has been tasted, color and texture become secondary to flavor. Flavor is mentioned by an overwhelming proportion of consumers as the reason for over-all preference and continued use of a product (Gould *et al.*, 1957; Pangborn and Leonard, 1958; Valdés and Roessler, 1956). The reason cited most often for disliking a given food is that "it does not taste good" (Hall and Hall, 1939). It is possible that degree of liking and flavor quality are synonomous in the minds of many consumers, but that would be difficult to measure.

A. PREFERENCE IN RELATION TO COST

Price is an important limitation on the freedom with which the consumer selects foods. Consumer buying behavior for canned pears indicated that 68% of 179 families said selection of a specific brand was made on the basis of flavor whereas 59% of the 128 families who purchased eight minor brands did so because of lower price (Pangborn and Leonard, 1958). In some surveys, hypothetical prices have been assigned to samples, and the participants asked to make selections

(Garnatz, 1952; Pangborn *et al.*, 1958; Pangborn and Nickerson, 1959; Hillman *et al.*, 1962). In the 1958 study, on cling peaches, consumers stated an unwillingness to pay 5¢ per can extra for the samples they preferred since all samples were within the range of acceptability. In the 1959 survey, on strawberry ice cream, however, most homemakers expressed a willingness to pay 5¢ more per pint for the ice cream the

QUESTIONNAIRE FOR HOUSEHOLD MILK PREFERENCE TEST

A. Prefer sample in: Container "A" _____; Container "B"_____
   (A preference must be indicated).

B. Why did you prefer the sample of your choice?
   (Check one or more)

   Preferred milk has:

   Richer taste _____

   Sweeter taste _____

   Smoother body _____

   More pleasing taste _____

   Less aftertaste _____

   Other: (Please write in) _____

C. If you had the choice of buying only these two beverages for regular consumption, how much more (if any) per quart would you be willing to pay for the sample marked as being preferred on this questionnaire?

   1 cent _____

   2 cents_____

   3 cents_____

   4 cents_____

   5 cents_____

   0 cents_____

Fig. 73. Example of questionnaire used to determine preference-price interrelationship for milk. Source: Hillman *et al.* (1962).

family preferred. Figure 73 shows a questionnaire used to determine the relationship between preference for milk and willingness to pay more for the preferred sample (Hillman *et al.*, 1962). All of the foregoing studies involve single-occasion testing, so that no information is available on whether the preference or the opinion on pricing would be sustained over a period of exposure.

Because the Homemakers Reference Committee of the Kroger Food

Foundation is a representative sample from the territory served by the Kroger grocery chain, information on the effect of price on acceptance collected from these homemakers can be verified by observation of buying behavior over relatively short periods in the Kroger stores (Garnatz, 1950, 1952). Products with the panel's approval have fared well at the hands of the consumer when such foods have gone through the normal channels of distribution.

Although the cost of a food item may be directly related to consumer preference, it cannot be assumed that these items will be purchased more frequently than other items. Rather, the prices of many foods are determined by the maximum amount the consumer is willing to pay, in addition to availability and costs of production and distribution. It is interesting that although a consumer opinion poll will show that oysters are generally disliked, the demand for oysters exceeds the supply, so that they are among the most expensive nutrition man can buy.

Benson (1955) developed a research model for analyzing and predicting consumer preference, then tested the preferences of 263 students for differentially priced appetizers (10¢–40¢), entrées ($1.10–$1.75), and desserts (15¢–45¢). The preference-cost curves for appetizers and desserts followed the expected principle of diminishing returns, whereas the curve fitted for the entrées was approximately linear. Benson also noted the role of price as a psychological attribute of an article, and reported, "The marginal preference for price is determined by observing how much the preference for a commodity changes when the price tag is altered, while its other qualities remain unchanged."

Meat preferences of military personnel (who received their meals free of charge) increased as the cost of the meat constituent increased; of 17 items, chili con carne at 8.8¢ per serving was least liked, whereas grilled steak at 56¢ per serving received the highest score (Benson and Peryam, 1958). When scores were plotted against cost per serving, the slope of the curve diminished with increasing cost, indicating that equal increments in cost did not produce equal gains in the soldiers' satisfaction.

B. REGIONAL PREFERENCES

Some regional food preferences exist for specific foods such as coffee (variations in roasts and blends), eggs [white vs. brown shells (Jasper, 1953)], weiners (red vs. orange casing), and the many interesting food items associated with nationality and ethnic groups. Cultural patterns of food consumption and induced changes in food habits are covered in an extensive bibliography by Gottlieb and Rossi (1961). The social, economic, cultural, and psychological factors influencing the formulation of food habits and facilitating the processes by which they are changed, are discussed in a book by Burgess and Dean (1962).

In an Iowa study (Eppright, 1950), Scandinavians differed from other groups in their food preferences and showed signs of adhering to customs and habits of their ancestors. Although some cultural influences are deeply embedded, it is generally believed that in the United States most regional or nationality preferences for specific food items are diminishing, because of:

1. Population mobility and intermarriage.
2. Standardization of processing.
3. Increased use of partially prepared foods and decreased consumption of dishes "prepared from scratch."
4. Greater availability—as a result of refrigeration, controlled ripening, development of different varieties, improved distribution.
5. Impact of national advertising via television, newspapers, radio, etc.

In a collaborative study between the Kroger Food Foundation, of Cincinnati, and the University of California (Pangborn *et al.*, 1958), preferences for canned cling peaches expressed by Californians were very similar to those indicated by families distributed throughout 19 Midwestern states.

C. Age

The age of the consumer has been reported to influence preferences for some food products. Gustafson (1953) made a review of the literature on hedonic and discriminatory responses of different age groups and reported on methods used for studying children's preferences for citrus juices.

Children under 16 and adults over 50 preferred sweeter canned fruit than did the participants in the middle-age group (Simone *et al.*, 1956; Valdés and Roessler, 1956; Pangborn *et al.*, 1957; Simone and Pangborn, 1957; Pangborn and Leonard, 1958; Weckel *et al.*, 1959). A definite preference for 3% sucrose over 1% sucrose in rosé wine was shown by all consumers tested, regardless of frequency of consumption, and the preference increased with the age of the consumer (Filipello *et al.*, 1958b). In contrast, Laird and Breen (1939) reported that with increasing age there was an increasing tendency to prefer less-sweet pineapple juice. According to Hansen (1958), although grammar school children represent a large segment of the confectionery market, they are generally avoided as test consumers in favor of adults because " . . . they (children) do not possess the degree of maturity necessary to bring about measurable reactions in taste tests" (see also p. 58).

D. SEX

Differences in personality, sensory acuity, and likes and dislikes are usually more pronounced between people of the same sex than between the two sexes as groups. There are, however, group differences between the sexes which can be used effectively in planning and conducting marketing campaigns (Alexander, 1947). Although Langwill (1949) reported that 46.7% of 242 men and 77.0% of 257 women distinguished among the four basic tastes, there is little relation between taste acuity and food acceptance. Eppright (1950) found that food dislikes were more prominent among older men and younger women. Hall and Hall (1939) pointed out that, through training and interest, women are familiar with a wider assortment of foods but have more food aversions than men. Bradley et al. (1954) found no significant differences in preference ratings between men and women but that women were more consistent in their ratings than men. In studies of canned fruit conducted in California, female consumers were more definite in their preferences than males, who gave less homogeneous responses as a group and preferred sweeter samples than did women (Simone et al., 1956; Valdés and Roessler, 1956; Pangborn et al., 1957; Simone and Pangborn, 1957; Pangborn et al., 1958). Similar observations had been made by Laird and Breen (1939). Simone et al. (1960) found that younger and older groups and females rated all bread samples higher than middle-age groups and males. Earlier, Bell (1956) had reported that preferences for breads of different formulation were unaffected by age and sex. A survey of consumer acceptance of sugar levels in canned corn and canned peas showed no consistent trend according to the age and sex of the participants (Weckel et al., 1960, 1961). The food attitudes of 51 children between 5 and 12 years of age differed considerably in responses of like, dislike, and indifferent, but no sex differences were found (Breckenridge, 1959). Baker et al. (1962) recently reported that males were much more sensitive to differences between varieties of almonds as well as to the circumstances surrounding tasting. In view of incomplete and inconclusive investigations, it is difficult to predict preference behavior of specific age groups, or of males versus females, for most food products (see also Chapter 6, Section II,E).

E. OTHER FACTORS

Interest, motivation, discrimination, intelligence, and many other attributes of the consumer undoubtedly influence responses to food. The role of the sensory stimulation of food is not completely understood; however, as stated by Lepkovsky (1959), the food industry is well aware of the nutritional value of food as well as sensory properties of appearance, flavor, texture, and "belly-filling" properties. According to Peryam and Seaton (1962), under conditions of dietary restriction, soldiers' average preference ratings of food increased significantly, and 97% of the available food was eaten. However, subjects on the low level of feeding (2400 calories/day) tended to reject the same food items rejected by men on the high level (4800 calories/day). Effects of menu combinations, frequency of serving, subjective satiety, and stability of food preferences were discussed by Pilgrim (1961).

Individual variation in sensory acuity influences responses at the consumer level as well as in the laboratory. As stated by Mrak *et al.* (1959), many consumers cannot detect differences which are critical for others. "The realization of this fact could well lead to a drastic reorganization of processing, advertising, and marketing of foods based upon extensive surveys of the olfactory and taste abilities of the potential consumers." The interrelationship of physiological, nutritional, and psychological factors influencing food acceptance has been reviewed by Gottlieb and Rossi (1961).

II. Objectives of Consumer Preference Studies

A. Determination of Market Potential

Whether consumers will purchase a product at a rate commensurate with the supply and at a price high enough to ensure a continuous flow of the product into the market, is of constant concern to the producer. An awareness of market conditions may be of greater interest to producers of convenience foods, specialty items, and new products than to distributors of standard staples and products, but all food producers benefit from studies of market potentials for their products. An example of a study of market potential is that of the Florida Citrus Commission, which engaged the Market Research Corporation of America to obtain, from a representative national sample of 6000 consumers, information on purchases, proportion of families buying, and average prices paid for frozen and canned fruit juices (Johnson, 1960). This, of course, was a market study, not a sensory study, although such statistics are related to consumer acceptance, and at times to consumer preference.

For the creation of foods that appeal to a specific population, knowledge is needed of the size, distribution, socio-economic make-up, and potential purchasing power of that population. In marketing baby food, for example, it is of value to know the number and distribution of infants in the country, as well as the food likes and dislikes of the mothers. Differentiating between total sales and repeat sales can yield useful information. Differentiation between food fads and food trends is difficult but may mean the difference between success and failure for an item.

Awareness of current health problems, such as obesity, atherosclerosis, and diabetes, prompt processors to collaborate with medical experts and nutritionists to formulate special dietetic items.

There is always an unpredictable amount of risk involved in applying results from market surveys. This is complicated by the time lapse between the survey and the actual marketing of the product. Among the advice extended to producers is the following guide compiled by Pettersen (1958):

1. Don't change a product until it has been product-tested, market-tested, and actively promoted.
2. Build a different feature into the product which can be promoted.
3. Pioneer new fields rather than imitate a successful leader.
4. Enter markets that are growing.
5. Seek rapid acceptance through products featuring convenience in preparation, performance, or packaging.
6. Design a reliable test program of ample sample size, adequate cross section, with proper collection and interpretation of the data.
7. Be patient; testing takes time.

B. INTRODUCTION OF NEW PRODUCTS

Years ago a manufacturer could maintain a loyal clientele for a product of acceptable quality through advertising and special services. Increased competition has infringed upon brand loyalty, necessitating development of new products to attract consumer attention and to meet

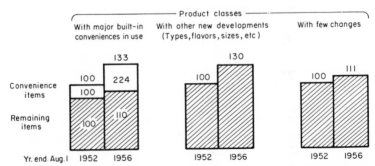

FIG. 74. Importance of new-product developments in comparative dollar sales. Source: Pettersen (1958).

the needs of a constantly changing society. The extent to which new-product development has influenced sales is illustrated in Fig. 74.

In addition to developing new products, progressive food processors develop new uses for established products; make innovations in flavoring, coloring, packaging, and distribution; and rely on consumer approval to determine a future course of action.

A combination of retail sales audit and a household survey was used effectively by the United States Department of Agriculture to establish consumer opinion of a new product, canned frozen grapefruit sections (Branson *et al.*, 1955). Opinions were obtained on uses of the product, taste, size of container, price, and frequency of purchase.

C. Quality Control of Existing Products

When a specific brand of food has enjoyed popularity as indicated by repeated sales over the years, there is reluctance to change the product unless the alteration increases sales. Consumer testing can serve as a quality-control measure to assure uniformity and to maintain standards. As a check on quality, a processor may have consumers compare his product against that of his nearest competitor in a test where the identity of the sample is not known to the consumer. A leading manufacturer of a popular condiment does not allow his product to be tested, lest the participants suspect that an alteration has been made and lose confidence in the company's name. Few examples of quality-control surveys are reported in the literature, for manufacturers keep these results secret in a highly competitive market.

D. Establishment of Specific Factors of Importance to the Consumer

A food product may sell well because of quality, price, size, packaging, promotion, availability, or a combination of all or any of these factors. The processor may wish to study consumer criteria for selection groups of foods in order to concentrate on influential characteristics. What is the maximum price the consumer will pay? What is the minimum quality the consumer will tolerate? How great a deviation in color, size, texture, uniformity, or flavor can a product have and still have good acceptance? How important are the sensory properties of a product in relation to other characteristics? Where will consumers purchase specific items, in what quantities, and how often? How often do consumers switch brands, and why? Which items are planned purchases and which are selected on impulse? How do changing socio-economic patterns influence food selection?

Agricultural economists have studied consumer buying behavior of fresh fruits and vegetables in surveys in Denver and Milwaukee on consumer demand for ripeness in Elberta peaches (Anonymous, 1952), and in Los Angeles, Cincinnati, and Kansas City on potatoes (Eberhard and Eke, 1951). The Home Makers Guild of America (1958) surveyed 1000 households, a cross section of age groups, income levels, family size, and geographic area of the United States, to determine buying and consumption patterns for pickles.

E. EFFECT OF ADVERTISING CAMPAIGNS AND EDUCATIONAL PROGRAMS

Survey research groups are actively involved in evaluating the effectiveness of promotional campaigns and programs by government and industry to educate consumers in wise use of their food dollar. Populations may be interviewed and oral and/or written responses obtained, or the behavior of consumers in the market is observed directly. Whenever possible, both the magnitude and duration of the influencing medium are measured. Producers may investigate market conditions to eliminate less popular food items.

F. EFFECT OF GROUP FEEDING

For adequate nutrition and proper morale, group eaters (as in the Armed Forces, hospitals, schools, and private eating establishments) must like their meals. Extensive research has been undertaken by these organizations to assure that proper nutrients are available and eaten. Adequate nutrition is not enough. During World War II it was evident that the "best-fed army in the world" would not always eat its rations. Effective group feeding involves close collaboration among dieticians, food processors, cooks, psychologists, and sometimes physicians. Several surveys have been reported on the food acceptance of members of the Armed Forces under peacetime conditions and during periods of environmental, physical, and psychological stress (Spector and Peterson, 1954; Peryam et al., 1960; Eindhoven and Kamenetzky, 1956; Wood and Peryam, 1953). In addition, the Quartermaster Corps has sponsored research to determine the food preferences of boys of pre-army age (Kennedy, 1952).

Extensive surveys on dietary habits and food likes and dislikes have given nutritionists important information on the type of educational campaigns most effective in improving the nutritional status of specific groups (Eppright, 1950).

A survey conducted by the Coffee Brewing Institute (1956) provided information on the coffee-drinking habits and motivations of restaurant customers, and also revealed the relationship of proper coffee-brewing techniques to the success of a restaurant.

G. Methodological and Statistical Studies

Consumers may be surveyed to test the adequacy of sampling methods, type of interview, and length and wording of the questionnaire, or to compare the opinions of laboratory panels with those of the public. Pilot testing, *i.e.* pretesting of the methodology prior to the distribution of samples, can orient the participants to the method and check on the clarity of the questions (Caul, 1958). A large number of reactions may be collected to test the sensitivity of various statistical methods of analyses. A survey of this nature is sometimes included as part of another study of food habits or preferences.

III. Information Obtained from Consumer Studies

A. Past Behavior of Consumers

Information may be obtained on food selection and preparation, meal planning, quantities consumed, use of leftovers, or amount of waste. A consumer may not be able to recall accurately the quality and quantities of food selected and consumed. The questionnaire must be carefully worded to avoid influencing the type of response, since many consumers will give what they consider to be the "correct" or "desirable" answer rather than describe the true situation (Payne, 1951). All survey methods are limited by the inability of the subject to remember, to generalize, or to identify motives; by biases; and by desire to please the interrogator (Alevizos, 1959).

B. Present Behavior of Consumers

The consumer's behavior in the grocery store may be observed, oral or written opinions may be recorded, or specific preferences obtained between two experimental food products. In each case the past experience of the consumer influences the response, and there is no assurance that retesting in the future will give the same response.

C. Estimates of Future Behavior

It would be presumptuous to state that consumer preferences of the future can be adequately predicted. Estimates of future consumption patterns are based on past behavior under known conditions, and extrapolations made to fit expected market conditions of the future. However, a more accurate estimate would be of great value to the food industry. Pilgrim and Kamen (1963) recently reported that three fourths of the variation in the number of military personnel who select foods in mess halls is predictable from knowledge of food preferences, the subjective satiety or "fillingness" of the food, and the amounts of two major nutrients, fat and protein. Conversion of fat and protein content to percentage of total calories reduced their predictive abilities.

IV. Factors Influencing Results from Consumer Surveys

A. POPULATION SAMPLED

The reasons for conducting a survey, of course, determine the methodology selected, the population sampled, and the type of questions asked. In evaluating results obtained by consumer sampling, it is well to consider what population the investigators used for their "consumer panel." Dryden and Hills (1957) established preferences for applesauce among 100 employees of their research laboratory. In a consumer study described by Hanson *et al.* (1955) test subjects were selected from among laboratory personnel who had no previous tasting experience, who had tasted the test product only once before, or who had not served on the consumer-type preference panel for the test product in the previous 18 months. Students living in sorority and fraternity houses made up a butter panel used by Hibbs (1960). Dunsing asked married university students (1959a,b,d) and university employees (1959c) to take beef steaks home for testing. Undergraduate students were used as ice cream testers by Bliss *et al.* (1943). Elder (1954) reported that General Foods Corp. invites the customers of New York department stores to test the company's products. The continuous consumer-preference panel used by Gould *et al.* (1957) consisted of 300 families selected from an area within a one-mile radius of Ohio State University and stratified on the basis of income. The Michigan State College Consumer Panel of 240 families, representative of a Michigan city of 100,000 population, has supplied detailed information on practices in purchasing ice cream and other commodities (Quackenbush and Shaffer, 1955).

People attending the 12-day California State Fair tasted wine for Berg *et al.* (1955) and Filipello *et al.* (1955), ice cream for Pangborn and Nickerson (1959), and peaches for Simone *et al.* (1956) and Simone and Pangborn (1957). A random sampling of telephone subscribers tested experimental food products for Pangborn and Leonard (1958), Pangborn and Nickerson (1959), and Simone *et al.* (1960). Carlin *et al.* (1954) tested visitors at a university open house. Preferences of service men were collected by Peryam *et al.* (1960).

B. AMOUNT OF PILOT TESTING

Pretesting of the questionnaire, the commodity, or the population can yield important information that can save time and money. Ambiguous and misleading questions can be eliminated from the questionnaire, antagonistic or apathetic participants can be determined from the sample, or the experimental samples may be modified in packaging, size, or method of presentation to accommodate unanticipated conditions of testing.

In pilot testing, the emphasis is on the inherent properties of the product—aroma, flavor, texture, shape, color, consistency. There is no effect of marketing factors such as brand, label, price, packaging, distribution, or advertising. One important use of pilot testing in the food industry is to provide an estimate of the relative importance of the flavor of the product in comparison with other properties such as convenience, storage stability, or brand identity. To test first impressions, the consumer may be given only enough of the sample for a single use—the single-exposure method. This method is a valuable tool when the amount of sample to be tested is limited, when time and money are limited, when few consumers are available, or when only an estimate of consumer preference is desired. Single-exposure tests can be given in supermarkets, mess halls, fairs, conventions, or other public gatherings. According to Caul (1958), the philosophy of the method is this: " . . . when discrimination is possible it can be measured through the use of a relatively small group of persons provided extraneous variables are controlled." Pilot testing of consumer acceptance after prolonged use of a food is usually done in the home, is more expensive and time-consuming, but is more typical of normal consumption than the single-exposure method.

C. Method of Sampling, Amount of Replication, Size of Statistical Error

Techniques employed in consumer preference studies are often deficient because of failure to define the universe sampled or the use of inadequate sampling methods which give immeasurable degrees of error. If the population is small, it is sometimes convenient to sample the entire population to obtain the desired information. Usually time and money can be saved by studying only a sample portion of the population.

There are many possible methods of selecting a sample from a population. Some of these depend on the judgment of people who claim to know the population; some merely define the sample as that part of the population which is most conveniently available; others are random, based on the theory of probability. Use of an expert's opinion is generally a relatively inexpensive method of obtaining information. There are situations where objective measurement is not possible and complete dependence must be placed on expert judgment. In the evaluation of estimates which rely heavily upon the opinions of experts, one must have faith in the validity of these opinions. Limitations of the procedure are the inability to evaluate this faith, and the lack of an objective basis for choosing between the varying opinions of two or more experts.

Methods which select for the sample that portion of the population which is conveniently available, offer no assurance that the sample is representative of its whole population. When the required information is more than a general survey, methods based on probability theory should be selected. For the laws of probability to be applicable, sampling methods must ultimately result in random samples from the population. These are the only methods which can provide valid precision measures, without which the confidence to be placed in an estimate cannot be assessed even though a high degree of accuracy is employed in obtaining the data. With sampling methods employing reasonably large samples, the precision of the results from a sample can be measured from the sample itself, and limits on the magnitude of possible sampling errors can be assigned so that the probability of exceeding these limits is very small.

The uses made of results from some surveys are sufficiently general that a sample selected by any method will yield satisfactory information. Certainly the simplest and least expensive method that fulfills the requirements of the survey should be used.

If little or nothing is known about the characteristics of the population being sampled, probability sampling methods may not be possible, and, certainly, if probability methods have not been employed in the sampling procedure, probability statements concerning precision of the survey should not be made. The application of such statements to nonprobability surveys can lead to confusion and misunderstanding.

In planning a sample survey, the size of sample needed to estimate the population value with a specific precision must be determined. Questions regarding size of sample, replication, and magnitude of sampling error vary with the type of material to be sampled, the degree of reliability desired, and the costs involved.

In designing a sample to serve a specific purpose, the following questions must be answered:

1. How large an error in the estimate is permissible before the inference drawn will be incorrect?
2. How great a risk is one willing to take that the conclusions drawn from the sample differ by more than the permissible error?

Before the size of the sample can be estimated, "error risk" limits must be established. In some cases the results of a survey might be acceptable if the chances were 19:1 that the sample estimate would be within 10% of the true value. In other cases, where an error could be more costly, greater accuracy might be required and higher odds demanded; that is, one might require that the sample estimate not differ from the true value by more than 5% in 99 out of 100 trials. See Chapter 5, Section III,A; Chapter 7, Section III; and Chapter 10, Section I.

Once a tolerable error and an acceptable significance level are established, a sample can be designed to meet these specifications. For example, in a normal population with variance σ^2, let a population characteristic under study be defined by its mean value, m, the best estimate of which, from a random sample of n measurements, is $\bar{X}$. Then the normal deviate, z, is:

$$z = \frac{\bar{X} - m}{\sigma/\sqrt{n}}$$

from which

$$n = \left(\frac{z\sigma}{\bar{X} - m}\right)^2.$$

In this expression, if $\bar{X} - m$ is replaced by the allowable error and if the value of z is assigned according to the levels of significance adopted, then the numerical value of n can be calculated. Application of the method depends on some knowledge about the variability of the population. After the sampling is completed, the variability of the sample may be used to verify the assumption about that of the population. If one has no knowledge of population variability, preliminary sampling can be used to provide a satisfactory estimate.

Having obtained the size of sample necessary to provide the required amount of precision and knowing the cost factors involved in the sample design, the cost of the survey can be estimated. If it is acceptable, the design can be used as specified; if, however, the cost is excessive, additional funds must be found or some balancing of precision against cost must be effected. Frequently, some relaxation of precision will still provide usable results and will permit development of the survey within available resources. If, however, it is impossible to design an acceptable survey within the budget allowance, then the survey must be abandoned.

Cost limitations often lead to the use of "cluster sampling," in which the population is first divided into groups which serve as sampling units. A sample is drawn from the groups to represent the population.

A population may be stratified according to a desired criterion (age, sex, socio-economic level, etc.), and the participants selected in proportion to their occurrence in the population. Stratification affords a method of using known information to increase precision in sampling estimates. From former surveys it may be possible to divide the population into groups such that the elements within each group are more homogeneous than are the elements of the population as a whole. If, by simple random selection from each group, a sample of size proportional to the size of the group is drawn, then each group has comparable representation, and the laws of probability apply to the sampling procedure.

Another type of sample selection which is widely used is systematic sampling, in which the design calls for selection from the population of every *R*th element or the use of some other specified pattern. An example is sampling by the selection of every 10th name from the telephone directory. This, of course, samples only the population with listed telephone numbers.

Although there are no set rules for selecting the best design among all possible ones, sampling theory is an exceedingly useful guide in choosing an appropriate and effective method. Excellent and complete discussions of sampling procedures have been given by Deming (1950), Hansen *et al.* (1953), Cochran (1953), and Sukhatone (1954).

There are investigators who disagree with the principles of sampling discussed above. For example, Caul and Sjöström (1959) emphatically believe that a consumer panel should not be a random sample of the population. Rather, it should consist of people who have particular qualifications, such as interest, discrimination, ability to communicate, and a higher than average intelligence. Their philosophy is based upon their assumption that "In this group of people are found the community leaders, the respected citizens, the triers of new products. If the product pleases them, it likely will please others whose quality standards may be lower and who are followers rather than leaders." In the opinion of the present authors, such a conclusion (without benefit of comparative data) may be applicable to only a few food products.

D. METHOD OF COLLECTING AND ANALYZING DATA

Discussion of the collection and analysis of data is deferred to later in this chapter, after more background material is presented.

E. RETESTING AND/OR FOLLOW-UP STUDIES

Retesting is advisable: (a) if a survey shows inconclusive results; (b) if the investigator suspects that the consumer misinterpreted the questionnaire; (c) if there is any question whether the samples may have been served or tested incorrectly; or (d) if there is a possibility that the sampling procedures may not have been adequate. A follow-up testing at a specific interval after the first survey can be used effectively for establishing the persistence of the preference over a given period and can measure the degree to which the preference has been affected by changes in the market or in the general economy. Miller *et al.* (1955) related that their panel of 600 consumers gave preferences of high statistical reliability for noodle soup, yet contradictory preferences were obtained in two successive trials. Those investigators concluded: " . . . one can scarcely hope to improve the precision of the verdict through an increase in panel size to 2,000 judges . . . [but] panels of this larger size might give a verdict closer to the truth and thus improve the accuracy of the judgment." In tests with various fruit drinks, Kramer *et al.* (1963) found that consumer preference could be determined accurately and with reasonably good precision by panels of 40 to 80 judges. Larger panels were needed only when unusually high precision was required. This should be investigated further, in different localities and with several food products.

F. INTERPRETATION OF RESULTS

As with any investigation, results are not necessarily valid except under the conditions of the study. The investigators should be conservative in projecting findings to other populations or to other commodities unless the prediction is adequately supported by the data obtained. There are always a number of consumers who, when approached, refuse to cooperate. Between 60 and 95% of those who agree to cooperate actually return their questionnaires. We know nothing about the preferences of the noncooperating consumers, but as the number of the noncooperators increases, conclusions reached on the basis of those who did cooperate become less reliable, and it is more difficult to estimate the way in which the opinions of the noncooperators might change the direction of the response.

Correct interpretation and projection of results requires that consumer opinion be viewed in its proper perspective. Undue importance should not be placed on selection of a specific food item on a single occasion, since the decision is but one of hundreds that the consumer makes each day.

G. PSYCHOLOGICAL CONSIDERATIONS

Allowances may have to be made for the "human element" in a food survey. Unexplainable inconsistencies in response are sometimes obtained. Careful reorganization of the data may reveal the causative factor, but there may be no effective way of measuring all factors that influenced the responses. Some of the psychological factors which influence laboratory panels can affect the consuming public also. Some of these apparent variations can be minimized or accounted for by close control and/or observation of all details of the testing procedure and the testing environment, and by interviewing a sufficiently large number of consumers to reduce the standard error of the mean.

V. Methods of Approach

A. HISTORICAL METHOD

Statistics of food distribution, sales records, and product turnover rate should be consulted to understand present market activities and to estimate future market events. In the food industry, where the mark-up on certain commodities is very low, it is essential that trends be observed accurately to assure achieving the volume of sales necessary for profit.

B. OBSERVATIONAL

A person trained to observe group behavior can gather quantitative and qualitative data on food habits and selection. Hidden observers have watched consumers in supermarkets to determine whether purchases are planned or impulsive, to establish what displays and packaging appeals to them, to determine whether certain food items are selected more often by men than by women. Merchandisers may be interested in knowing the effect of background music, product location, or other physical or psychological factors. Advertisers and producers are interested in how the consumer appraises the product—does she smell it, squeeze it, weigh it, read the label, study the instructions, or compare it with others on the shelf? Hidden cameras have taken photographs and movies of consumers; recorders have been used to record dialogues; observers have been stationed at the check-out stand to record brands and sizes purchased. The value of the observational method can be enhanced if the same customers are observed during a second or third shopping session and if they are interviewed in the home about preparation methods, serving, and food waste. Results obtained from observational studies may be difficult to interpret because of the complexity of the environmental factors influencing the behavior.

A combination questionnaire and observational technique was used by Fleishman (1951) to establish consumer preference for six brands of bottled beer. On each of seven days, families were provided with more beer than they needed so they could have an unrestricted choice of brands (identified only by code). Each day, the remaining bottles and empties were collected as well as the questionnaires, with preferences recorded.

Hobson and Schaars (1935) observed cheese preferences of college students by making unlimited quantities available to them at their regular meals for a one-week period and then calculating the average daily per-capita consumption. Three weeks elapsed before another kind and quality of cheese was placed on the luncheon table for one week. Processed American cheese had much greater popularity than natural Cheddar, brick, or Swiss cheese. The distribution of preferences was the same for 6770 retail store customers in six cities and 1137 farm residents, who expressed preferences between paired presentations. In those studies there was no measure of the variability of the response of the two groups of consumers.

With 4- and 5-year-old children, Morse (1954) served two one-ounce portions of citrus juice from identical pitchers and then asked the child, "Which juice would you like more of?", necessitating only that the child point to the pitcher containing the juice of his choice. The children consistently preferred orange to grapefruit juice on the basis of taste, not color differences. Morse concluded that children of pre-school age may be satisfactory experimental subjects if suitable methods are employed.

C. QUESTIONNAIRES

Carefully worded questionnaires are frequently used to obtain consumer reactions on a multitude of topics related to selection and use of commodities. The questionnaire may range from one short question to several hundred inquiries about past, present, and future behavior. The effectiveness of this method depends on the questionnaire and the degree of cooperative spirit elicited from the consumer, as well as the type of approach employed.

In a comprehensive, nationwide survey of household food consumption, made in the spring of 1955 by the United States Department of Agriculture (1955), a national stratified probability sample of 6000 households was polled. Trained interviewers used a detailed food list to help respondents recall quantities of foods used and amounts paid for purchased items—the recall-list method. Consumption figures reported refer to food used in an economic sense, i.e., eaten, thrown away as waste, or fed to pets. In surveys of this nature, the consumer may tend to report consuming foods of a high nutritional value in substantial quantities when this may not be the fact. In addition, the interviewer may influence the direction of the responses to an unmeasurable degree.

A newspaper survey group, called "Consolidated Consumer Analysis Newspapers," publishes yearly summaries of consumption patterns for food, clothing, drugs, and other household items. Over 60,000 families in 21 major U. S. cities provide information on subjects such as: (a) 3-year trends of product use, market-by-market; (b) relative position of leading brands; and (c) percentage of preference shown for leading brands in each market.

The Market Research Corporation of America has published a national menu census and a retail food audit to provide manufacturers with insight on consumer food habits. The detailed questionnaire covers conventional topics but also includes inquiries into more unusual aspects of food consumption such as the percent of the population eating cheese for breakfast, the characteristics of families who never serve canned meat, and food preferences of teenagers versus parents. Methods of approach by this organization are: (a) depth interviews; (b) word association; (c) sentence completion; (d) projective questioning; (e) role playing; (f) recorded group discussion; and (g) pretest questionnaire.

With the questionnaire method the four most common approaches are: telephone, mail, personal interview, and public test.

The telephone approach is economical provided no long-distance calls are made. It has the disadvantage of not reaching those in the population who are not telephone subscribers. Also, decisions made on the telephone may lack depth and sufficient thought, and questions can be misinterpreted by people with hearing defects or by those who are not fluent in the vernacular language.

Approach by mail has the advantage of economy and allows the respondent to answer at his leisure. However, the replies constitute only a percentage of the total number sent out, since not all people return their questionnaires. In addition, some recipients of the questionnaire may not be able to read, and many may misunderstand the questions.

Personal interview has the advantage of collecting observational data concomitantly but is more expensive and introduces the potential bias of the interviewer. The trained interviewer is alert, friendly, patient, and nonauthoritative, does not argue or give advice, and, insofar as possible, does not influence the consumer's response. This latter influence is always present and is difficult to measure. Often, mailing techniques and personal interviews are used together. At times the personal interview is the only reliable way of obtaining information on food preferences that need to be classified by race, age, education, religion, political affiliation, or income level.

In experimental studies, samples of the food product are tasted by the consumer, and opinions are obtained. The consumer may be approached in a public meeting place, such as a market or a country fair, at a private function, such as a meeting or dinner, or in the home. An example is the consumer wine analysis conducted at the University of California (1957) among 202 families to determine the effect of repeated tasting, over a relatively short period, on degree of liking of experimentally prepared wine samples. Also established was the correlation of degree of liking with buying behavior and the effect of familiarization with wine on buying behavior. Coleman (1964) gave a brief description of the consumer test methods utilized by General Foods Corp.

VI. Development of the Questionnaire

One of the most difficult aspects in measuring consumer response is wording of the questionnaire to obtain the exact information desired. Payne (1951) has written a helpful book on the practical problems of wording questions, covering semantic, sociological, and psychological aspects.

Among the general rules which help an investigator in wording questionnaires are the following:

A question should not be ambiguous. The inquiry "What kind of oil do you use?" does not indicate whether the oil is auto, fuel, mineral, salad, or hair oil. Even if the type was specified, the respondent might give the brand name, the weight, the color, or the price range. In each case, he would be answering the question but his answer might be useless to the researcher, depending upon the specific information desired.

Questions should be realistic. The respondent cannot be expected to recall specific details of meals consumed several weeks previously or to predict specific behavior accurately into the distant future. The average consumer cannot be expected to evaluate the sensory properties of a food as thoroughly, as rapidly, or as consistently as a highly trained judge can. In the example in Fig. 75, not only are too many detailed questions asked but it is assumed that the consumer considers the terminology on the left completely opposite to that on the right.

Use appropriate terminology. The wording should not appear to be above or below the intelligence of the population being sampled. Where necessary, terms should be defined and examples given. A pretesting of the level of understanding of the specific population would be useful, although expensive and time-consuming.

Avoid stereotype answers. Questions must be worded to elicit the participant's true opinion rather than the answer the participant thinks is the most "proper." To a question on belief in freedom of speech, 97% of a certain population indicated they believed in it. However, when asked specifically who was to be allowed the freedom, most of these same people thought it should be limited to certain individuals, which, of course, would not be freedom of speech at all.

Placement. Placement of questions on the ballot is important since, in long questionnaires, often only the first few are answered. Restaurants have long known that placement of selections on the menu can influence the frequency with which they are ordered. Arrange questions in logical

	Extremely (7)	Very (6)	Somewhat (5)	Neither or Both (4)	Somewhat (3)	Very (2)	Extremely (1)	
CONSUMER REACTION RATING SCALE CRACKERS								
Vegetable taste		†			X			Fruit taste
Crisp		X	†					Stale
Flat					X †			Sharp
Salty			†			X		Non-salty
Tasty		† X						Tasteless
Not spicy				† X				Spicy
Sweet			X		†			Bitter
Greasy			†				X	Not greasy
Aftertaste				†	X			Afterthirst
Snack use		†		X				Picnic use
Luncheon use	†				X			Cocktail use
Spread with cheese			†	X				Spread with jelly
Eaten by matron			†	X				Eaten by teen-ager
Baked by big firm		X	†					Baked by small firm
Eat with soup			†			X		Eat with tea
† = Test cracker X = Control cracker								

FIG. 75. Example of ballot used to determine consumer reaction to two crackers and the kinds of users that consumers would associate with the particular cracker. Source: Hansen (1960).

order, since one question can influence the response to the following question.

Allowance for no opinion. In planning the original experimental design, the investigator must decide whether he will allow a respondent to express a "no preference" or "don't know" opinion. Some participants may have a "don't care" attitude. A large percentage of "no preference" votes by the respondents may mean either that differences between the products were undetected or that there was no preferences between detectable differences (Nair, 1949). The questionnaire can be worded so as to distinguish between these two types of "no preference" responses. In many surveys it is of interest to allow for lack of preference, disinterest, and uncertainty. Such data can give useful information relative to the commodities being tested as well as to the characteristics of the consumer (Gridgeman, 1959). With the paired comparison presentation, the proportion of no-preference or tied votes is particularly dependent on the phrasing of the questionnaire or emphasis of the question (Ferris, 1958). Miller *et al.* (1955) reported that the no-preference votes in consumer evaluation of noodle soup decreased as the difference in flavor and/or appearance became greater and as the preference for one sample over the other increased.

Coding of responses and classification of data. For ease of handling data, questions should be planned so that the answers can be coded numerically or otherwise tabulated. Appropriate questions must be included if the data are to be subdivided by age, sex, race, occupation, national origin, socio-economic group, religious belief, geographic location, or other criteria.

VII. Types of Questionnaires

The types of questions asked when opinions are sought but no experimental samples are evaluated include the following general categories:

1. True-false response
2. Yes-no response
3. One-word answer
4. Multiple choice
5. Essay type
    (a) Why do you ....?
    (b) What do you think of ....?
    (c) What would you do if ....?

Selection of the questionnaire to be used when experimental food products are judged depends on the number of treatments, the sensory intensity of the food commodity, and the information desired. Following is a list of examples of presentation methods suitable for consumer survey purposes. (The advantages and disadvantages found with laboratory panels, described in the previous chapters, apply generally to consumer panels also.)

1. Single-sample presentation
    (a) Acceptable or unacceptable
    (b) Degree of liking

(c) Description (with or without suggested terminology)

(d) Numerical scoring

2. Paired-sample presentation

   (a) Identified-product paired comparison in which sample of known quality is compared against sample of unestablished quality

      (1) General preference

      (2) Degree of preference

      (3) Difference testing

      (4) Quality scoring or scaling devices

   (b) Blind paired comparison, in which the quality of neither sample has been established previously

3. Three-sample presentation

   (a) Triangle test

   (b) Ranking

Date_____

Consumer Rating Test for _____

Please place a check mark in the first column to indicate your rating of the product, as it is usually served to you. If you have never had it before, indicate by checking "Unfamiliar" below. In the second column rate the product as it is served today. Then comment on both favorable and unfavorable characteristics.

	How do you usually consider this item?	How do you rate today's item?
Acceptable Range		
10. Excellent	_____	_____
9. Very good	_____	_____
8. Good	_____	_____
7. Fair	_____	_____
6. Poor	_____	_____
Non-acceptable Range		
5. Slightly undesirable	_____	_____
4. Definitely undesirable	_____	_____
3. Unpleasant	_____	_____
2. Very unpleasant	_____	_____
1. Repulsive	_____	_____

Unfamiliar _____

FIG. 76. Example of ballot used to obtain consumer opinion of food samples in a cafeteria survey, using single-sample presentation. Source: Ac'cent International (1963).

Consumer Wine Survey

Instructions

We are leaving you 4 bottles of wine, two labeled "Des-Rose," and the other two labeled "Cal-Rose." Serve the wine cold, under any conditions you desire, such as with meals, between meals, etc. Please keep the wine in the refrigerator between uses. You may consume all or part of the wine. You may use it as often as you like. After you have consumed as much as you wish of these wines, please check below in the appropriate box which you prefer.

1. I prefer the following wine: (Check one)

HUSBAND   Prefer Des-Rose_____   WIFE   Prefer Des-Rose_____

            Prefer Cal-Rose_____   Prefer Cal-Rose_____

            No preference_____   No preference_____

2. Select the number or numbers at the right, which best describe your reaction to these wines:

HUSBAND   Descriptions

Des-Rose _____   1. Smooth
                                      2. Syrupy
Cal-Rose _____   3. Fresh, fruity
                                      4. Tart
                                      5. Sour
WIFE   6. Bitter
Des-Rose _____   7. Weak, watery
                                      8. Relaxing
Cal-Rose _____   9. Sweet
                                     10. Dry (not sweet)
                                     11. Acid
                                     12. Pleasant aroma
                                     13. Unpleasant aroma
                                     14. Stimulating
                                     15. Strong
                                     16. Harsh
                                     17. Salty
                                     18. Flat

FIG. 77. Example of a ballot used to measure consumer opinion of wine in a household survey, using a two-sample preference-description method. Source: University of California (1957).

    (c) Quality scoring or numerical scaling
    (d) Descriptive terms
    (e) Duo-trio
4. More than three samples
    (a) Ranking
    (b) Scoring or scaling
    (c) Degree of liking.

Examples of ballots used in consumer survey are given in Figs. 73, 75–80.

Because of its simplicity and flexibility, the hedonic-rating scale can be recommended for use at the consumer level. The language it employs is easily understood and the test requires only brief and simple instruc-

CONSUMER SURVEY

Please answer the following questions:

1. AGE: Under 16_____   16 to 25_____   25 to 50_____   Over 50_____

2. SEX: Male_____   Female_____

3. How often do you eat this food product?

    Several times a week   _____

    Several times a month   _____

    Several times a year or never   _____

TASTING PROCEDURE

You will receive two samples numbered "1" and "2." Taste both samples, then check the term which expresses your opinion of each sample.

SAMPLE 1		SAMPLE 2	
Like Extremely	_____	Like Extremely	_____
Like Very Much	_____	Like Very Much	_____
Like Moderately	_____	Like Moderately	_____
Like Slightly	_____	Like Slightly	_____
Neither Like Nor Dislike	_____	Neither Like Nor Dislike	_____
Dislike Slightly	_____	Dislike Slightly	_____
Dislike Moderately	_____	Dislike Moderately	_____
Dislike Extremely	_____	Dislike Extremely	_____

FIG. 78. Example of ballot used to determine consumer opinion of food samples in a mass survey, using paired-hedonic presentation. Source: Simone and Pangborn (1957).

tions. This method has been used successfully to determine consumer opinion of canned cherries (Weckel *et al.*, 1959), canned apricots (Valdés and Roessler, 1956), and canned peaches (Pangborn and Leonard, 1958). In order to establish the basis for the degree of liking in the latter two studies, two additional questions were asked of the consumers, "What did you like about this fruit?" and "What did you dislike about this fruit?" In another consumer survey, Simone and Pangborn (1957) found that paired-preference techniques were more precise in establishing significant preferences for canned peaches than were single-hedonic or double-hedonic presentations. The number of ballots discarded (because of confusion of the consumers) was greatest for the paired hedonic, followed by the single-hedonic, then the paired-preference method. Ratings were higher for all samples with the single-hedonic than with

CANNED PEACHES - TEST NO. 182

INSTRUCTIONS: You will receive two cans of cling peaches which we want you to submit to each member of your family ten years old and older. Please have each member take the test in such a way as not to be influenced by anyone else.

Both cans of peaches have been cubed to make it more convenient for you to divide into uniform portions and has nothing to do with the test. Place cans in the refrigerator so they will be chilled at time of serving. Everybody should taste the sample coded "red" first.

Family Member	SEX		AGE					Time of Serving		
	Male	Female	Under 16	16 to 24	25 to 39	40 to 59	60 and over	Morn-ing	After-noon	Even-ing
1										
2										
3										
4										
5										
6										

Family Member	APPEARANCE PREFERENCE				FLAVOR PREFERENCE				EATING QUALITY PREFERENCE			
	Red	No Pref.	Green	Neither	No Pref.	Red	Neither	Green	Neither	Green	Red	No Pref.
1												
2												
3												
4												
5												
6												

FIG. 79. Example of ballot used to determine consumer preference for canned cling peaches in a household survey, using paired-preference presentation. Source: Pangborn *et al.* (1958).

the double-hedonic scale. Pilgrim and Wood (1955) asked 20 untrained laboratory panel members to evaluate twelve pairs of foods by a 9-interval hedonic scale and by paired-comparison preference methods and reported that the methods were equally sensitive whether the difference in preference was small or large.

LEMONADE

FAMILY NO. _____

SEX: Male _____   Female _____

AGE: 6 - 12 _____   13 - 20 _____   21 - 40 _____   Over 40 _____

PREFERENCE (check only one)

   I Prefer GREEN over RED

      Extremely   _____

      Very Much   _____

      Moderately   _____

      Slightly   _____

   I Prefer RED over GREEN

      Extremely   _____

      Very Much   _____

      Moderately   _____

      Slightly   _____

   I HAVE NO PREFERENCE _____

Please state reason for preference.

FIG. 80. Example of ballot used to determine consumer preference for frozen lemonade concentrate in a household survey, using paired presentation with scaling of the degree of preference. Source: Pangborn *et al.* (1960).

VIII. Serving Procedures

A. NUMBERS OF SAMPLES

It is generally believed that more than two samples may confuse the consumer (Berg *et al.*, 1955; Crocker *et al.*, 1948; Nair, 1949). However, Bliss *et al.* (1943) reported success with a four-sample ranking method in judging ice cream, and triangle tests have been used by Bell (1956), Carlin *et al.* (1954), and Berg *et al.* (1955) to measure consumer preference for breads, angel cakes, and wines, respectively. With wines, the triangular method was found to be unsuited for use with consumers because of the additional supervision required in conducting the tests, as well as the amount of confusion the method caused. Multiple-sample presentation is used more commonly with laboratory taste panels, and may be used in pilot-scale consumer studies when it is desirable to select one or more samples from a series for presentation to a larger consumer group.

With a completely new food product, single-sample presentation and a quality-rating scale can be used effectively. Hedlund *et al.* (1954) recommended that the "degree of difference" between samples should serve as the guide in deciding between single and paired presentation. As demonstrated by those investigators, the difference in percent preference between two cereals was greater when the samples were presented simultaneously than when presented singly. Filipello (1956) obtained significant differences between wines differing by 1% sucrose by a paired-hedonic methodology, but found no significant differences when the same wines were submitted singly. Preferences for wines differing by 3% sucrose in a consumer survey were the same with paired as with single presentation. The main advantages of the single-sample stimulus are its simplicity of presentation and its resemblance to normal conditions of consumption. With any single product test, however, the evaluation is a memory comparison based on previous experience with similar products. The single-sample presentation is generally considered to be less sensitive than the paired presentation; however, exceptions to this opinion can be found in work reported by Bayton and Bell (1954), and Bell (1955, 1956), who used single-sample presentation with an unstructured hedonic scale for citrus juice and bread. The reliability of this scale had been determined previously (Clements *et al.*, 1954). Using rank order, Bayton and Thomas (1954) found significant preferences based on sweetness and sugar-acid ratio of orange juice. With single-sample procedures only sweetness was significant. Pfaffmann (1935) demonstrated that preferences for brown bread were the same with single presentation as with a constant-stimulus method. In a household consumer survey, Simone *et al.* (1960) obtained significant differences in degree of liking between experimental samples of bread evaluated singly on a seven-point structured hedonic scale, but there was no comparison with paired presentation. In the field of psychometrics and psychophysics, comparable results have been obtained with single- and paired-stimulus techniques (Barnhart, 1936; Newhall, 1954; Wever and Zener, 1928).

A more conscious and discriminating consumer attitude is encouraged by use of the paired stimuli. Simone and Pangborn (1957) solicited consumer opinion of sweetness in canned peaches and found paired-comparison preference to be most sensitive in establishing differences among the samples, followed in order by the single-stimulus hedonic rating and the paired-presentation hedonic rating. Results obtained by the single-stimulus hedonic method approximated that of the paired preference, which is in accord with findings of Pilgrim and Wood (1955), who reported a close agreement between the two methods. In the paired-hedonic design used by Simone and Pangborn (1957), 8% of the ballots were filled out incorrectly and had to be discarded. All samples were rated higher in a single-stimulus hedonic test than in a paired-hedonic presentation.

Ghiselli (1939) pointed out that the number of ways in which respondents are permitted to answer questions may be a factor influencing measurement of their opinion on a given subject, and their willingness to respond. Using the paired presentation, when subjects were limited to making an absolute choice between mutually exclusive alternates rather than being permitted to qualify the strength of their opinion, the expressed opinion was less favorable and fewer subjects were willing to respond. This would cast doubt on the paired method as a representative measure of "average" opinion.

B. ORDER OF PRESENTATION

Most investigators agree that both simultaneous and successive presentation are vulnerable to the influence of order of presentation. Consumers judging paired samples of noodle soup showed a bias for the sample tasted first (Miller et al., 1955). Consumers testing five bread formulas during five successive weeks retested their first sample and indicated no change in degree of liking for some formulas, whereas others received significantly higher ratings in the sixth week than in the first week (Bell, 1956).

Mass survey-testing of wines showed that consumers had a strong bias for the first sample in paired-comparison designs, and for the second sample in the triangular design (Berg et al., 1955). The same effect was reported with green beans (Buck and Weckel, 1956), noodle soup (Miller et al., 1955), and orange juice (Morse, 1952). Filipello (1956) found a bias for the first sample served in paired comparison of wine samples. The results varied with the wine type, the degree of difference in liking between the wines, and the age of the judge (see Chapter 6, Section IV).

C. CODING

Coding of samples can influence responses, as reported by Garnatz (1950), Ishler et al. (1954), and Krum (1955). Coding must be designed to render complete information to the investigator yet not be (or even seem) informative to the respondent. Commodities such as meat, which requires cooking before sampling, have been effectively coded with aluminum rings clamped around the bone portion; consumers expressed preference according to the number of rings in the samples (Naumann et al., 1957). In a study of consumer opinion of five samples of canned pears, Pangborn and Leonard (1958) used randomized two-digit numbers and found that 33% of the 278 families tasted the fruit in increasing numerical order. Combinations of numbers and letters, i.e., X-17, MF-3, have been used effectively, as have color codes (Gould *et al.*, 1957). Morse (1952) labeled two cans of orange juice "O" and "K" and requested householders to taste in "OK" order (see also Chapter 6, Section III,E).

D. Time of Day of Testing

If a food is customarily consumed at a specific meal, the consumer may be instructed to serve the samples at a specified time or to serve at the time of his choice but record the time of day. Orange juice, usually consumed as a breakfast item, did not differ in consumer acceptance between morning, afternoon, and night scoring (Morse, 1952).

IX. Comparison of Laboratory Panels with Consumer Panels

Although members of a laboratory panel are consumers, their opinions and preferences may not be representative of the general population. The laboratory group is carefully selected, highly trained, and hypercritical as compared to the general consumer. Distribution of age, sex, income, and general intelligence will reflect the consuming population only by accident (Nair, 1949). Test-booth conditions, coded containers, and scoring methods are certainly not typical of normal conditions of food consumption. In addition, the opinions of the laboratory panel are not influenced by extraneous factors such as packaging, advertising, ease of preparation, price, or prestige, as the opinions of the consumer may be.

Baker *et al.* (1960, 1961) correctly concluded that a point of prime importance in all general consumer-acceptance testing, as opposed to laboratory testing, is that the direction of preference is not specific and that many consumers are indifferent to the characteristic being tested.

In general, consumers agree with laboratory panel findings in direction but not in magnitude (Miller *et al.*, 1955; Kiehl and Rhodes, 1956; Simone *et al.*, 1956). In a comparison of panel and consumer acceptance of sardines, ranking methods more nearly predicted consumer preference than did paired presentation (Murphy *et al.*, 1958). Calvin and Sather (1959) used a hedonic scale of nine descriptive terms to establish degree of liking for pickles, jam, cheese, crackers, and various fruits and vegetables by a student laboratory panel and by a household consumer panel. Agreement in results between the two panels was very good. The same conclusion was reached by Peryam and Haynes (1957), who compared laboratory-panel and soldier consumer-panel ratings of 12 food items.

X. Limitations of the Consumer Survey

Consumer surveys are expensive, time-consuming, and subject to numerous uncontrollable variables. Although most surveys yield valuable information, investigators experience many problems and should recognize the limitations of their methods. Careful consideration must be given to the manner in which participation is solicited, since the way by which rapport is established with the consumer not only influences the cooperative attitude of the respondent but may influence the answers given. Prospective participants may react differently depending upon whether the survey is being conducted by a near-by university, a commercial processing firm, or an advertising agency (Morse, 1951; Filipello et al., 1958a). In addition, answers are biased by methods of sampling, techniques of sample presentation, amount and type of instruction provided, and the construction of the questionnaire, as previously indicated.

Consumer opinion, as individuals or as a group, can easily be underestimated or overestimated. The following consumer characteristics are encountered in many surveys:

1. Inability to remember, to generalize, or to identify motives.
2. Inability to describe likes, dislikes, and attitudes.
3. Inability to weigh the numerous alternatives.
4. Unawareness of what influenced their behavior.
5. Awareness of more factors than the impact of the influence warrants.
6. Desire to please the interrogator.
7. Desire for social status, prestige, and "keeping up with the Joneses."

Morse (1951) carefully described how most of the above traits can be avoided or compensated for by correct wording of the questionnaire. Skillfully constructed questions can measure the magnitude of these influencing traits so that their effect on the total response can be calculated.

Most surveys do not reveal why people buy, i.e., the conscious and unconscious factors that control behavior. In most surveys it is impossible to duplicate market conditions, so responses are not obtained under normal buying conditions. What consumers say they do may not represent actual behavior. It is extremely difficult to estimate potential patterns of behavior on the basis of past purchases, just as it is to predict whether the item will have short-time or long-time acceptance.

Surveys seldom identify the "leaders" and the "followers," i.e., the consumers with definite preferences who set the styles, tastes, and trends, versus those who are easily swayed and merely "follow the crowd."

The failure of consumers to provide answers to the above-mentioned questions does not mean that surveys should be discontinued. On the contrary, increased efforts should be made to develop techniques for adequately measuring these variables. The areas of needed research, described by Morse in 1951, still apply today: (1) vigorous and systematic studies on methods, techniques, and analysis of data; (2) designing of surveys to include evaluation of research methods as well as of the commodity; and (3) active use of new and improved methods and publication of methodology data to benefit others in the field. Progress could be faster if there were more collaborative studies between food technologists, economists, psychologists, and statisticians.

REFERENCES

Ac'cent International. 1963. Personal communication. Food and Flavor Laboratory, Skokie, Illinois.

Alevizos, J. P. 1959. "Marketing Research-Applications, Procedures, and Cases," 676 pp. Prentice-Hall, Englewood Cliffs, New Jersey.

Alexander, R. S. 1947. Some aspects of sex differences in relation to marketing. *J. Marketing* **12**, 158–172.

Anonymous. 1949. Marketing research notes from national workshops. Report on consumer reactions to banner buy programs. *U. S. Dept. Agr. Bur. Agr. Econ.* pp. 81–85.

Anonymous. 1952. Consumer demand for ripeness of peaches, 1950–1951. *Colorado Agr. Expt. Sta. Tech. Bull.* **48**, 1–24.

Arnold, C. L. 1941. Do consumers have good taste? *Food Inds.* **13**(3), 45–47.

Baker, G. A., M. A. Amerine, E. B. Roessler, and F. Filipello. 1960. The nonspecificity of differences in taste testing for preference. *Food Research* **25**, 810–816.

Baker, G. A., M. A. Amerine, and D. E. Kester. 1961. Dependency of almond preference on consumer category and type of experiment. *J. Food Sci.* **26**, 377–385.

Baker, G. A., M. A. Amerine, and D. E. Kester. 1962. Consumer preference on a rating basis for almond selections with allowance for environmental and subject-induced correlations. *Food Technol.* **16**, 121–123.

Barnhart, E. N. 1936. A comparison of scaling methods for affective judgments. *Psychol. Rev.* **43**, 387–395.

Bayton, J. A., and H. P. Bell. 1954. Preferences for canned orange juices that vary in Brix-acid ratio. *U. S. Dept. Agr. AMS Rept.* **76**, 1–29.

Bayton, J. A., and C. M. Thomas. 1954. Comparative and single stimulus methods in determining taste preferences. *J. Appl. Psychol.* **38**, 443–445.

Bell, H. P. 1955. Preferences for canned grapefruit juices. *U. S. Dept. Agr., AMS Rept.* **108**, 1–31.

Bell, H. P. 1956. Consumers' preferences among bakers' white breads of different formulas. *U. S. Dept. Agr. AMS Rept.* **118**, 1–53.

Benson, P. H. 1955. A model for the analysis of consumer preference and an exploratory test. *J. Appl. Psychol.* **39**, 375–381.

Benson, P. H., and D. R. Peryam. 1958. Preference for foods in relation to cost. *J. Appl. Psychol.* **42**, 171–174.

Berg, H. W., F. Filipello, E. Hinreiner, and F. M. Sawyer. 1955. Consumer wine-preference methodology studies at California fairs. *Food Technol.* **9**, 90–93.

Bliss, C. I., E. O. Anderson, and R. E. Marland. 1943. A technique for testing consumer preferences, with special reference to the constituents of ice cream. *Conn. Agr. Expt. Sta. Bull.* **251**, 1–20.

Bogert, J. L. 1941. A method of consumer product testing. *Food Inds.* **13**(3), 47–49.

Bradley, J. E., C. T. Walliker, and D. R. Peryam. 1954. Influence of continued testing on preference ratings. *In* "Food Acceptance Testing Methodology," 115 pp. (see pp. 92–100). Advisory Board on Quartermaster Research and Development, Committee on Foods, Natl. Acad. Sci., Natl. Research Council, Chicago, Illinois.

Brady, D. E. 1957. Results of consumer preference studies. *J. Animal Sci.* **16**, 233–240.

Branson, R. E., M. Jacobs, and R. Hall. 1955. Frozen grapefruit sections: Evaluating a new product by retail sales audit and household survey. *U. S. Dept. Agr. AMS Rept.* **110**, 1–62.

Breckenridge, M. E. 1959. Food attitudes of five-to-twelve-year-old children. *J. Am. Dietet. Assoc.* **35**, 704–709.

Buck, P. A., and K. G. Weckel. 1956. Study of consumer preference of salt and sugar levels in canned green beans. *Food Technol.* **10**, 421–423.

Burgess, A., and R. F. A. Dean. 1962. "Malnutrition and Food Habits," 210 pp. Macmillan, New York.

Calvin, L. D., and L. A. Sather. 1959. A comparison of student preference panels with a household consumer panel. *Food Technol.* **13**, 469–472.

Carlin, A. F., J. C. Ayres, and P. G. Homeyer. 1954. Consumer evaluation of the flavor of angel cakes prepared from yeast-fermented and enzyme-treated dried albumen. *Food Technol.* **8**, 580–583.

Caul, J. F. 1958. Pilot consumer product testing. *In* "Flavor Research and Food Acceptance" (A. D. Little, Inc., ed.), 391 pp. (see pp. 150–161). Reinhold, New York.

Caul, J. F., and L. B. Sjöström. 1959. Consumer food product acceptance. *Perfumery and Essent. Oil Record* **50**, 916–919.

Clements, F. E., J. A. Bayton, and H. P. Bell. 1954. Method of single stimulus determinations of taste preference. *J. Appl. Psychol.* **38**, 446–451.

Cochran, W. G. 1953. "Sampling Techniques," 330 pp. Wiley, New York.

Coffee Brewing Inst. 1956. Survey of beverage coffee. Preferences of consumers patronizing public eating places. *New York, Coffee Brewing Inst. Publ.* No. 5, 1–25.

Coleman, J. A. 1964. Measuring consumer acceptance of foods and beverages. *Food Technol.* **18**(11), 53–54.

Cowan, D. R. G. 1941. Developing and improving foods by consumer testing. *Food Inds.* **13**(3), 41–44.

Crocker, E. C., L. B. Sjöström, and G. B. Tallman. 1948. Measurement of food acceptance. *Ind. Eng. Chem.* **40**, 2254–2257.

Deming, W. E. 1950. "Some Theories of Sampling," 602 pp. (see pp. 1–352). Wiley, New York.

Dryden, E. C., and C. H. Hills. 1957. Consumer preference studies on applesauce: sugar-acid relations. *Food Technol.* **11**, 489–559.

Dunsing, M. 1959a. Visual and eating preferences of consumer household panel for beef of different grades. *Food Research* **24**, 434–444.

Dunsing, M. 1959b. Visual and eating preferences of consumer household panel for beef from animals of different age. *Food Technol.* **13**, 332–336.

Dunsing, M. 1959c. Visual and eating preferences of consumer household panel for beef from Brahman-Hereford crossbreds and from Herefords. *Food Technol.* **13**, 451–456.

Dunsing, M. 1959d. Consumer preference for beef of different breeds related to carcass and to quality grades. *Food Technol.* **13**, 516–520.

Eberhard, M. F., and P. A. Eke. 1951. Consumer preference for sized Idaho Russet Burbank potatoes. *Idaho Univ. Agr. Expt. Sta. Bull.* **282**, 1–19.

Eindhoven, J., and J. Kamenetzky. 1956. The stability of food preferences. *Quartermaster Food & Container Inst. Rept.* **9**, 1–24.

Elder, L. W. 1954. "Flavor Perception by Consumers," Mimeo report. 9 pp. Central Lab., General Foods Corp., Hoboken, New Jersey.

Eppright, E. S. 1950. Food habits and preferences. A study of Iowa people of two age groups. *Iowa State Coll. Agr. Expt. Sta. Bull.* **376**, 873–976.

Ferris, G. E. 1958. The K-visit method of consumer testing. *Biometrics* **14**, 39–49.

Filipello, F. 1956. Factors in the analysis of mass panel wine preference data. *Food Technol.* **10**, 321–326.

Filipello, F., H. W. Berg, E. Hinreiner, and A. D. Webb. 1955. Reproducibility of results in consumer wine-preference surveys. *Food Technol.* **9**, 431–432.

Filipello, F., H. W. Berg, and A. D. Webb. 1958a. A sampling method for household surveys. I. Panel recruitment for testing wines. *Food Technol.* **12**, 387–390.

Filipello, F., H. W. Berg, and A. D. Webb. 1958b. A sampling method for household surveys. II. Panel characteristics and their relation to usage of wine. *Food Technol.* **12**, 508–510.

Fleishman, E. A. 1951. An experimental consumer panel technique. *J. Appl. Psychol.* **35**, 323–326.

Foster, D. 1956. "Psychological Aspects of Food Colors from the Consumer's Standpoint," Mimeo report. 14 pp. U. S. Testing Co., Hoboken, New Jersey.

Garnatz, G. 1950. But what do the consumers say? *Food Inds.* **22**, 1333–1336.

Garnatz, G. 1952. Consumer acceptance testing at the Kroger Food Foundation. *Proc. Research Conf. Am. Meat Inst., Chicago* **4**, 67–72.

Ghiselli, E. E. 1939. All or none versus graded response questionnaires. *J. Appl. Psychol.* **23**, 405–413.

Gottlieb, D., and P. H. Rossi. 1961. A bibliography and bibliographic review of food and food habit research. *Quartermaster Food and Container Inst., Lib. Bull.* **4**, 1–112.

Gould, W. A., J. A. Stephens, G. DuVernay, J. Feil, J. R. Geisman, I. Prudent, and R. Sherman. 1957. Establishment and use of a consumer panel for the evaluation of quality of foods. *Ohio Agr. Expt. Sta. Research Circ.* **40**, 1–36.

Gridgeman, N. T. 1959. Pair comparison, with and without ties. *Biometrics* **15**, 382–388.

Gustafson, E. 1953. Exploratory methods for the study of children's taste preferences and discrimination. Unpubl. M.S. thesis. 43 pp. Florida State Univ., Tallahassee, Florida.

Hall, I. S., and C. S. Hall. 1939. A study of disliked and unfamiliar foods. *J. Am. Dietet. Assoc.* **15**, 540–548.

Hansen, M. H., W. N. Hurwitz, and W. G. Madow. 1953. "Sampling Survey Methods and Theory," 2 vols., 638 pp; 332 pp. John Wiley, New York.

Hansen, W. P. 1958. Consumer taste testing. *Mfg. Confectioner* **38**, 43, 45, 46, 48.

Hansen, W. P. 1960. New testing technique tells what consumers think of products. *Biscuit and Cracker Baker* **49**, 23–25.

Hanson, H. L., J. G. Davis, A. A. Campbell, J. H. Anderson, and H. Lineweaver. 1955. Sensory test methods. II. Effects of previous tests on consumer response to foods. *Food Technol.* **9**, 56–59.

Harries, J. M. 1953. Sensory tests and consumer acceptance. *J. Sci. Food Agr.* **10**, 477–482.

Hedlund, G. J., B. Albrecht, and R. L. Wyatt. 1954. Single product or paired comparison consumer tests; which should you use? 9 pp. Mimeo of paper presented at 14th Inst. Food Technologists Meeting, Los Angeles, Calif.

Hibbs, R. A. 1960. Butter customers—a study in consumer preferences. *Milk Prods. J.* **51**, 10–12.

Hicks, E. W. 1948. Tasting tests. *Food Preserv. Quart.* **8**, 1–5.

Hillman, J. S., J. W. Stull, and R. C. Angus. 1962. Consumer preference and acceptance for milk varying in fat and solids-not-fat. *Ariz. Univ. Agr. Expt. Sta. Tech. Bull.* **153**, 1–38.

Hobson, A., and M. A. Schaars. 1935. Consumer preferences for cheese. *Wisconsin Univ. Agr. Expt. Sta. Research Bull.* **128**, 1–48.

Home Makers Guild of America. 1958. "A Consumer Study on Pickles," 18 pp. Owens-Illinois Glass Co., Toledo, Ohio.

Ishler, N. H., E. A. Laue, and A. J. Janisch. 1954. Reliability of taste testing and consumer testing methods. II. Code bias in consumer testing. *Food Technol.* **8**, 389–391.

Jasper, W. A. 1953. Some highlights from consumer egg studies. *U. S. Dept. Agr., Inform. Bull.* **110**, 1–25.

Johnson, C. E. 1960. Consumer purchases of citrus and other juices. *U. S. Dept. Agr. AMS* **CPFJ–110**, 1–23.

Kennedy, B. M. 1952. Food preferences of pre-army age California boys. *Food Technol.* **6**, 92–97.

Kiehl, E. R., and V. J. Rhodes. 1956. New techniques in consumer preference research. *J. Farm. Econ.* **38**, 1335–1345.

Kramer, A., F. W. Cooler, J. Cooler, M. Modery, and B. A. Twigg. 1963. Numbers of tasters required to determine consumer preferences for fruit drinks. *Food Technol.* **17**, 86–91.

Krum, J. K. 1955. Truest evaluations in sensory panel testing. *Food Eng.* **27**, 74–83.

Laird, D. A., and W. J. Breen. 1939. Sex and age alterations in taste preference. *J. Am. Dietet. Assoc.* **15**, 549–550.

Langwill, K. E. 1949. Taste perceptions and taste preferences of the consumer. *Food Technol.* **3**, 136–139.

Lepkovsky, S. 1959. Potential pathways in nutritional progress. *Food Technol.* **13**, 421–424.

Liebmann, A. J., and B. R. Panettiere. 1957. Quality control and consumer testing for distilled alcoholic beverages. *Wallerstein Labs. Communs.* **20**, 27–39.

Miller, P. G., J. H. Nair, and A. J. Harriman. 1955. A household and a laboratory type of panel for testing consumer preference. *Food Technol.* **9**, 445–449.

Morse, R. L. D. 1951. Rationale for studies of consumer food preferences. *Advances in Food Research* **3**, 385–427.

Morse, R. L. D. 1952. Selected studies of consumer preferences for canned orange juices. *Proc. Florida State Hort. Soc.* **65**, 230–234.

Morse, R. L. D. 1954. Exploratory studies of preschool children's taste discrimination and preference for selected citrus juices. *Proc. Florida State Hort. Soc.* **66**, 292–301.

Mrak, V., M. A. Amerine, C. S. Ough, and G. A. Baker. 1959. Odor difference test with applications to consumer preferences. *Food Research* **24**, 574–578.

Murphy, E. F., B. S. Clark, and R. M. Berglund. 1958. A consumer survey versus panel testing for acceptance evaluation of Maine sardines. *Food Technol.* **12**, 222–226.

Nair, J. H. 1949. Mass taste panels. *Food Technol.* **3**, 131–136.

Naumann, H. D., V. J. Rhodes, D. E. Brady, and E. R. Kiehl. 1957. Discrimination techniques in meat acceptance studies. *Food Technol.* **11**, 123–125.

Newhall, S. H. 1954. Comparability of the method of single stimuli and the method of paired comparisons. *Am. J. Psychol.* **67**, 96–103.

Nicosia, F. M. 1962. "Consumer Decision Making," 292 pp. Unpubl. mimeo. Univ. of California, Berkeley.

Packard, V. 1957. "The Hidden Persuaders," 273 pp. David McKay, New York.

Pangborn, R. M., and S. J. Leonard. 1958. Factors influencing consumer opinion of canned Bartlett pears. *Food Technol.* **12**, 284–290.

Pangborn, R. M., and T. A. Nickerson. 1959. The influence of sugar in ice cream. II. Consumer preference for strawberry ice cream. *Food Technol.* **13**, 107–109.

Pangborn, R. M., M. Simone, and T. A. Nickerson. 1957. The influence of sugar in ice cream. I. Consumer preferences for vanilla ice cream. *Food Technol.* **11**, 679–682.

Pangborn, R. M., M. J. Simone, S. J. Leonard, and G. Garnatz. 1958. Comparison of mass panel and household consumer responses to canned cling peaches. *Food Technol.* **12**, 693–698.

Pangborn, R. M., G. L. Marsh, W. R. Channell, and H. Campbell. 1960. Consumer opinion of sweeteners in frozen concentrated lemonade and orange juice drink. *Food Technol.* **14**, 515–520.

Payne, S. L. 1951. "The Art of Asking Questions," 249 pp. Princeton Univ. Press, Princeton, New Jersey.

Peryam, D. R., and J. G. Haynes. 1957. Prediction of soldiers' food preferences by laboratory methods. *J. Appl. Psychol.* **41**, 2–6.

Peryam, D. R., and R. W. Seaton. 1962. Food consumption and preferences under conditions of restricted and non-restricted feeding. *Quartermaster Food & Container Interim Rept.* **40–62**, 1–31.

Peryam, D. R., B. W. Polemis, J. M. Kamen, J. Eindhoven, and F. J. Pilgrim. 1960. "Food Preferences of Men in the U. S. Armed Forces," 160 pp. Quartermaster Food & Container Inst., Chicago, Illinois.

Pettersen, E. A. 1958. Market testing and analysis. *In* "Flavor Research and Food Acceptance" (A. D. Little, Inc., ed.), 391 pp. (see pp. 175–187). Reinhold, New York.

Pfaffmann, C. 1935. An experimental comparison of the method of single stimuli and the method of constant stimuli in gustation. *Am. J. Psychol.* **47**, 470–476.

Pilgrim, F. J. 1961. What foods do people accept or reject? *J. Am. Dietet. Assoc.* **38**, 439–443.

Pilgrim, F. J., and J. M. Kamen. 1963. Predictors of human food consumption. *Science* **139**, 501–502.

Pilgrim, F. J., and K. R. Wood. 1955. Comparative sensitivity of rating scale and paired comparison methods for measuring consumer preference. *Food Technol.* **9**, 385–387.

Platt, W. 1941. Why consumer-preference tests? *Food Inds.* **13**(3), 40–41, 50.

Quackenbush, G. G., and J. D. Shaffer. 1955. Factors affecting purchases of ice cream for home use. *Mich. State Univ. Agr. Expt. Sta. Tech. Bull.* No. **249**, 1–28.

Schaal, A. A. 1952. Consumer trends in new food products for homemakers. *Food Technol.* **6**, 13–15.

Simone, M., and R. M. Pangborn. 1957. Consumer acceptance methodology: one vs. two samples. *Food Technol.* **11**, 25–29 (supplement).

Simone, M., S. Leonard, E. Hinreiner, and R. M. Valdés. 1956. Consumer studies on sweetness of canned cling peaches. *Food Technol.* **10**, 279–282.

Simone, M., N. Sharrah, and C. O. Chichester. 1960. Instant bread mix: consumer evaluation of prepared bread. *Food Technol.* **14**, 657–661.

Spector, H., and M. S. Peterson. 1954. "Nutrition Under Climatic Stress, a Symposium," 204 pp. Quartermaster Food and Container Inst., Chicago.

Strom, L. S. 1960. "Consumer Acceptance," 15 pp. Research and Development Associates, Food and Container Inst., Chicago.

Sukhatone, P. V. 1954. "Sampling Theory of Surveys with Applications," 491 pp. Iowa State College Press, Ames, Iowa.

Szczesniak, A. S., and D. H. Kleyn. 1963. Consumer awareness of texture and other food attributes. *Food Technol.* **17**, 74–77.

Twedt, D. K. 1965. Consumer psychology. *Am. Rev. Psychol.* **16**, 265–294.

University of California. 1957. "Wine Consumer Analysis," 50 pp. Davis, California.

U. S. Dept. of Agriculture. 1955. Food consumption of households in the United States. *U. S. Dept. Agr. Rept.* **1**, 1–196.

Valdés, R. M., and E. B. Roessler. 1956. Consumer survey on the dessert quality on canned apricots. *Food Technol.* **10**, 481–486.

Weckel, K. G., P. Buck, W. Beyer, and J. Birdsall. 1959. Consumer preference of sweetness in syrup packed red sour pitted Montmorency cherries. *Food Technol.* **13**, 300–302.

Weckel, K. G., B. Strong, G. F. Garnatz, and M. Lyle. 1960. The effect of added levels of sugar on consumer acceptance of whole kernel corn. *Food Technol.* **14**, 369–371.

Weckel, K. G., W. D. Mathias, G. F. Garnatz, and M. Lyle. 1961. Effect of added sugar on consumer acceptance of canned peas. *Food Technol.* **15**, 241–242.

Wever, E. G., and K. E. Zener. 1928. The method of absolute judgment in psychophysics. *Psychol. Rev.* **35**, 466–493.

Wood, K. R., and D. R. Peryam. 1953. Preliminary analysis of five army food preference surveys. *Food Technol.* **7**, 248–249.

Chapter 10

Statistical Procedures

Although statistical principles have been applied in agricultural research for over 30 years, it is only in the last 15 years that experimental designs have been extensively used in the evaluation of foods and beverages. Today many of the basic designs originally constructed for agricultural experiments are used by workers in the food industry in selecting members of taste panels, in evaluating the ability and consistency of such panels, in determining and controlling the quality of foods, and in ascertaining consumer preference.

Fundamental to sensory analysis of foods are problems in the selection of taste panels and the choice of experimental designs and scoring techniques. Knowledge of the decisions involved in hypothesis testing is essential to an understanding of the statistical procedures discussed in this chapter.

I. Hypothesis Testing

In evaluating a proposed decision procedure, one first defines an empirical population and then formulates a hypothesis about some measurable characteristic, or parameter, of the population. This is the hypothesis to be tested, or "null" hypothesis. A test of a statistical hypothesis directs attention to two possible values of the parameter—one value, the null hypothesis, and the other, the alternative hypothesis. For example, in testing for differences between two products, one of which is supposedly sweeter, the null hypothesis states that there is no difference and sets the probability in a single trial of specifying properly the sweeter one by chance alone as $\frac{1}{2}$.

In testing the null hypothesis against an alternative hypothesis, one assumes the null hypothesis to be true and formulates an appropriate statistic whose probability distribution for all possible samples is determined. A random sample of elements from the population is drawn, and the value of the statistic is observed in the sample. The hypothesis is tested by comparing the value of the observed statistic with values of the probability distribution for all possible samples. If the observed value has little chance of occurring, the hypothesis is rejected; otherwise it is accepted. The probability that a sample will result in rejection of the null hypothesis, under the assumption that it is true, is called the level of significance.

The alternative hypothesis is called a one-sided alternative if it specifies values only to one side of (either above or below) that designated by the null hypothesis. In this case, sample values which lead to rejection of the null hypothesis and acceptance of the alternative hypothesis are all in one tail of the distribution, and, therefore, a test of significance based on a one-sided alternative is called a one-tailed test. If, however, both high and low values tend to support the alternative hypothesis and thus lead to rejection of the null hypothesis, the alternative hypothesis is called a two-sided alternative, and the test is called a two-tailed test.

In Chapters 5, 7, and 9 it was noted that in testing hypotheses, two kinds of error are possible. The rejection of a hypothesis when it is true is an error different from the error committed in accepting a hypothesis when it is false. The two errors are not of the same importance, and the difference in importance must be taken into consideration in selecting an appropriate test.

Rejecting a hypothesis when it is true is called an error of the first kind, or type I error, and its probability is denoted by α. The level of significance is the probability of making an error of this kind. The error made in accepting a hypothesis when it is false is called an error of the second kind, or type II error, and this is usually denoted by β. If a type I error would lead to serious practical consequences while a type II error would not be so serious, which is usually the case, α would be taken to be much smaller than β. Therefore, to choose an appropriate level of significance one should consider carefully and balance the importance of the consequences of the two kinds of errors. For a fixed number of observations, n, the value of α may be chosen by the investigator, but β will thereby be determined. Both α and β can be decreased by increasing n. If a reduction in sample size results in savings without too great an increase in the risks of error, then a reduction in sample size is justifiable. If, however, the cost of an increase in the number of observations is small and is warranted by the resulting reduction in the risks of error, then a larger sample is appropriate. The experimenter must decide on permissible costs and on how large a difference between the null hypothesis and alternative hypothesis is practical or important.

If we assume that the sample proportion, p, is binomially distributed and that the sample size, n, is large enough to justify use of the normal approximation, with mean np and standard error $\sqrt{npq}$, then Fig. 81 shows for the one- and two-tailed cases the relationships between the

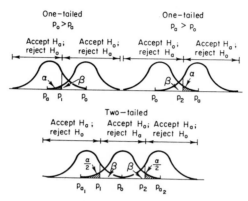

F<small>IG</small>. 81. Diagrams showing the risks involved in testing the null hypothesis, H_o, against the alternative hypothesis, H_a.

various probabilities where p_0 and p_a are the probabilities of the null and alternative hypotheses, and p_1 and p_2 are the proportions of decisions which bound the regions of acceptance and rejection. The corresponding normal curve equations for the one-tailed test are

$$\frac{p_1 - p_0}{\sigma_0} = -z_\alpha, \qquad \frac{p_1 - p_a}{\sigma_a} = z_\beta$$

or

$$\frac{p_2 - p_0}{\sigma_0} = z_\alpha, \qquad \frac{p_2 - p_a}{\sigma_a} = -z_\beta$$

and for the two-tailed test

$$\frac{p'_1 - p_0}{\sigma_0} = -z_{\alpha/2}, \qquad \frac{p'_1 - p_a}{\sigma_a} = z_\beta, \qquad \frac{p'_2 - p_0}{\sigma_0} = z_{\alpha/2},$$

$$\frac{p'_2 - p_a}{\sigma_a} = -z_\beta$$

where

$$\sigma_0 = \sqrt{\frac{p_0(1 - p_0)}{n}}, \qquad \sigma_a = \sqrt{\frac{p_a(1 - p_a)}{n}}$$

and numerical values for $z_{\alpha/2}$, z_α, and z_β can be found from Table A in the Appendix.

From the above equations it follows for the one-tailed test that

$$n = \left[\frac{z_\alpha \sqrt{p_0(1 - p_0)} + z_\beta \sqrt{p_a(1 - p_a)}}{p_a - p_0} \right]^2$$

$$p_1 = p_0 - z_\alpha\sigma_0, \quad \text{and} \quad p_2 = p_0 + z_\alpha\sigma_0$$

Similar expressions exist for the two-tailed test when z_α is replaced by $z_{\alpha/2}$ and p_1 and p_2 by p'_1 and p'_2.

For example, a paired test is used to determine taste preference between two similar products A and B. The null hypothesis, that there is no difference, is to be tested. This may be expressed as $p_0 = 0.50$. The alternative hypothesis, $p_a \neq 0.50$, has an infinite number of possible values. To arrive at a definite value for the alternative hypothesis, the experimenter must decide what difference between the null hypothesis and alternative hypothesis is practical or important. Suppose he selects $p_a = 0.60$, $\alpha = 0.05$, and $\beta = 0.10$. A two-tailed test is appropriate since there is interest in preference for product A over B and also for B over A.

$$\text{Then } n = \left[\frac{1.96 \sqrt{(0.50)(0.50)} + 1.28 \sqrt{(0.60)(0.40)}}{0.60 - 0.50} \right]^2$$

$$= \left[\frac{0.98 + 0.63}{0.10} \right]^2 = 259$$

$$p'_1 = 0.50 - 1.96 \sqrt{\frac{(0.50)(0.50)}{259}} = 0.50 - 0.06 = 0.44$$

$$p'_2 = 0.50 + 0.06 = 0.56$$

Of the 259 preferences expressed, if for both products the number is between $259(0.44) = 114$ and $259(0.56) = 145$, the null hypothesis is accepted and no difference between products is indicated. Preferences in excess of 145 for either product indicate rejection of the null hypothesis. Using these critical values, we can be sure that the probability of rejecting the null hypothesis $p_0 = 0.50$, when in fact it is true, will be equal to or less than 0.05. If the null hypothesis is accepted, the probability of accepting it falsely will be equal to or less than 0.10 if the true value is as large as or larger than $p_a = 0.60$ or as small as or smaller than 0.40.

The effect of type II errors in taste testing has been discussed in more detail by Baker et al. (1954, 1958) and Radkins (1957).

II. Difference Tests

In difference testing, the chi-square (χ^2) distribution is used to test approximately how well an observed frequency distribution compares with a theoretical distribution. If the observed frequency in a class of the distribution is f_o and the theoretical or expected frequency is f_e, then

$$\chi^2 = \Sigma \frac{(f_o - f_e)^2}{f_e}$$

where the corresponding number of degrees of freedom is the number of classes less the number of parameters which have been estimated. Significance can be established by comparing the calculated value of χ^2 with values shown in Table C in the Appendix. If the calculated value exceeds the tabular value at any significance level, then at this level we conclude that the observed and theoretical distributions do not agree. The χ^2 distribution as well as the normal distribution may be used to establish significance in the paired-sample, duo-trio, and triangular difference tests. In these tests, however, involving one degree of freedom, χ^2 should be adjusted as follows:

$$\text{Adj. } \chi^2 = \Sigma \frac{(|f_o - f_e| - \frac{1}{2})^2}{f_e}$$

A. PAIRED-SAMPLE TEST

In this test the taster is given two samples and is asked to pick out the sample higher in some constituent or is asked to state which he prefers. This procedure may be carried out by one taster several times or by a panel of tasters one or more times. On the basis of the null hypothesis—that is, that there is no difference between the samples—the probability, p, of a taster identifying by chance a particular sample in each of the several trials is $\frac{1}{2}$.

In n trials of a paired-sample test the exact probabilities of all possible numbers of correct identifications or agreeing preferences can be found from the expansion of $(\frac{1}{2} + \frac{1}{2})^n$. Approximate probabilities for evaluating differences between samples or for selecting the most reliable judges for a panel can be determined with values of the normal deviate, z, together with Table A, areas under the normal curve, or adjusted χ^2 together with Table C, values of χ^2. To analyze the results of such a test, let n represent the total number of trials, X_1 be the number of opinions favorable to sample 1, and X_2 be the number of opinions favorable to sample 2. Then

$$\chi^2 = \frac{(|X_1 - X_2| - 1)^2}{n} = z^2$$

where $|X_1 - X_2|$ indicates the absolute or positive value of the difference, and χ^2 is based on one degree of freedom.

When only difference (one-tailed) identification is requested, the calculated value of χ^2 must exceed 2.71 for significance at the 5% level, 5.41 for significance at the 1% level, and 9.55 for significance at the 0.1% level. Comparable values for z are 1.64, 2.33, and 3.09. If, instead of merely determining significance at some level, one desires the actual probability of obtaining by chance alone X_1 or more correct identifications in n trials, for small n ($n < 5$) the probability should be calculated directly from the binomial expansion $(\frac{1}{2} + \frac{1}{2})^n$. For large n the binomial probability may be approximated by interpolation from the calculated value of χ^2 or more simply by use of the normal-curve approximation, obtaining from Table A a shaded area similar to those shown under the curves at the top of Fig. 81. It corresponds to the continuity-corrected normal deviate

$$z = \frac{(X_1 - 0.5) - m}{\sigma}$$

where $m = np = n/2$ and $\sigma = \sqrt{npq} = \sqrt{n}/2$.

For example, a taster is given a sample of tomato juice and a second sample of the same juice with a detectable amount of salt added. That is, it was differentiated from the other sample by other tasters. Twenty-two times in 36 trials he identifies correctly the sample to which the salt has been added. In this case $\chi^2 = [(|22 - 14| - 1)^2]/36 = 1.36$. Since this value is less than 2.71, the taster, at the 5% level of significance, would not be an acceptable judge for detecting salt at this level in tomato juice. To evaluate the probability, calculate $m = np = 36(1/2) = 18$, $\sigma = \sqrt{npq} = \sqrt{9} = 3$; and $z = (21.5 - 18)/3 = 1.17$. From Table A, the required probability is 0.1210. Therefore, by chance alone a taster would perform this well more than 12% of the time even if he had no ability for detecting salt at this level.

When comparisons are made on the basis of quality preference (two-tailed), the calculated values of χ^2 necessary for significance at the three levels must exceed 3.84, 6.64, and 10.83, respectively. Corresponding values of z are 1.96, 2.58, and 3.29. For example, if a taster compared two samples 20 times and preferred sample 1 in 15 of the trials, then $\chi^2 = [(|15 - 5| - 1)^2]/20 = 4.0$. This indicates that, on the basis of the taster's performance, sample 1 is, at the 5% level, significantly better than sample 2. The probability may be approximated by calculating $z = (14.5 - 10)/\sqrt{5} = 2.01$. As shown in Fig. 82, the probability of this occurring by chance alone is

$$p = 2(0.0222) = 0.0444.$$

On the basis of the type I error, the number of correct identifications (one-tailed) or agreeing judgments (two-tailed) necessary for significance in each case can be determined directly from Table D in the Appendix. For example, from the table the number of agreeing quality judgments (two-tailed) in 40 trials for significance at the 5% level is

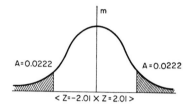

FIG. 82. Probability of exceeding a calculated normal deviate.

found to be 27. This means that if, in 40 trials, a particular product is preferred 27 times, one may state on the basis of this series of trials that the preferred product is better, and the chances of being wrong in this conclusion are only 1 in 20. In the acuity taste test involving identification of salt in tomato juice (one-tailed), 24 correct identifications in 36 trials are necessary for significance at the 5% level.

B. DUO-TRIO TEST

In the duo-trio test the taster is asked to select from two samples the one which is different from the reference sample, and, as in the paired-sample test, the probability is $\frac{1}{2}$ that the odd sample will be chosen by chance in a single trial. The procedures indicated for directional difference testing in the paired-sample tests are applicable after the taster has demonstrated an ability to distinguish correctly between samples.

C. TRIANGULAR TEST

In the triangular procedure, where of three samples, two are known to be alike and the third different, the probability is $\frac{1}{3}$ that the odd sample will be chosen by chance alone, and the value of χ^2 may be calculated from the expression $\chi^2 = [(|4X_1 - 2X_2| - 3)^2]/8n$. As before, the normal curve approximation with $p = \frac{1}{3}$ may be used to obtain approximate probabilities. Considering type I errors for various numbers of trials, Table E gives the number of correct identifications of the odd sample necessary to establish ability in distinguishing between products.

For example, in a triangular test involving 25 trials, a taster selects the odd sample correctly 18 times. From Table E in the Appendix, at the 5% level of significance, only 13 correct identifications are required, so the taster does have ability in detecting a difference.

In applying the foregoing methods one assumes that, throughout the test, the probability of a correct decision by chance alone remains constant. If, however, a peculiar pattern of correct or incorrect answers appears, it is natural to ask if this might not be a warning of some confusing bias in the experiment and a violation of the assumptions on which the procedure is based. Neyman (1950) discussed the case in which an unduly large proportion of incorrect classifications occurred indicating significant recognition but consistently misclassed identification. Periodic or symmetrical arrangements or runs of correct or incorrect identifications as warnings of possible bias are discussed by Bennett and Franklin (1954) and Byer (1964). In these discussions it is pointed out that the classification of permutations of results into combinations regarded as significant or nonsignificant is not enough; the permutations themselves must be subclassified as to whether or not they appear significantly nonrandom.

Duo-trio and triangular tests should be used only as difference tests. Sometimes an attempt is made to combine one of these with a preference or quality-judgment determination. When quality or preference is the prime consideration, the inclusion of a difference test at the same time tends to divert the taster's attention from the question of real interest. There is evidence also that such a procedure will bias the results. Schutz and Bradley (1954) showed that when a preference judgment in addition to a difference determination is required in a triangular test on the same samples, tasters tend to prefer the paired samples. The appropriate procedure, therefore, is first to determine by means of some test the taster's ability to distinguish differences and then to follow this with a paired test to establish preference or quality.

Gridgeman (1955) found that paired tests and triangular tests are normally about equally powerful and appreciably superior to duo-trio tests. However in these tests the question of positional bias has been observed and discussed by many writers, including Harries (1956) and Berg et al. (1955). In sensory assessments the first sample in paired comparisons and the second sample in the triangular design appear to be most often selected. Sawyer et al. (1962) applied repeatability estimates to panel selection in order to predict the proportion of judges whose sensitivity can satisfy established specifications. Repeatability estimates of different test designs indicated paired comparison to be more sensitive than the triangular procedure.

For triangular tests requiring intensity designation, Davis and Hanson (1954) suggested using a triangle-intensity test in which all judgments, whether partially or completely correct, are evaluated. This procedure increases efficiency. However, many statisticians and the authors are reluctant to include in an analysis the opinions of tasters for whom the odd-sample selection was incorrect. Ura (1960a) found that in detecting differences between two samples the paired test had a statistical advantage while in testing the ability of judges the triangular test was preferable.

In paired, duo-trio, and triangular tests, tasters are usually required to make a decision and are not permitted to indicate a tie. Some investigators, however, permit ties and either ignore them in the analysis or assign half their number to one product and half to the other. Gridgeman (1959b), for the paired case, tabulated all relevant probabilities and concluded that when discrimination is the objective it is better to prohibit ties, but that when preference is the objective, ties should be admitted since they form a neutral class and add information.

III. Sequential Analysis

In using paired, duo-trio, and triangular tests to determine an individual's ability as a taster, the candidate judge is required to repeat the experiment successfully a considerable number of times. There is some question regarding the quality of judges so obtained since, in general, too little testing is done—because of limitations in time and suitable experimental material. This can lead to large type II errors.

Sequential methods may afford a saving of time and material over most other selective procedures; they are equally reliable and are well suited to the selection of judges. In a sequential tasting plan the number of observations is not predetermined, and the decision to terminate the experiment depends, at any stage, on the results of previous observations. In taste testing, a small number of trials is desirable since a certain amount of taste and olfactory fatigue accompanies repetition, and only a relatively few trials can be performed at one sitting. Methods which minimize the time interval for an individual to demonstrate discriminating ability and which reduce the cost of preparation and performance of the experiment are to be desired.

Systems of sequential analysis have been developed by Wald (1947) and Rao (1950). Such systems involve the formulation of a rule by which one of the following decisions can be made at any stage of the experiment: (1) accept the taster as a judge, (2) reject him, or (3) continue the experiment by taking an additional observation.

The procedure which follows, developed by Wald, has been applied by Lombardi (1951) and Bradley (1953) to the selection of judges. Let p be the true proportion of correct decisions in paired, duo-trio, or triangular tests if the taster were to continue testing indefinitely. This is his inherent ability under the test administered. Values p_0 and p_1 can be specified so that individuals having abilities equal to or greater than p_1

will be selected as judges and those with abilities equal to or less than p_0 will be considered unacceptable.

Potential judges are accepted or rejected on the basis of their performance as related to two parallel straight lines, L_0 and L_1, which are uniquely determined by assigned values of p_0, p_1, α, and β, where α is the probability of rejecting an acceptable judge and β is the probability of selecting an unacceptable one. These are, as before, the errors of the first and second kind. If potential judges are in good supply, α may be selected large and β small. The lines L_0 and L_1 divide the plane into three regions, one of acceptance, one of rejection, and one of indecision. The equations of these lines may be written

$$d_0 = a_0 + bn \qquad \text{(lower line } L_0\text{)}$$
$$d_1 = a_1 + bn \qquad \text{(upper line } L_1\text{)}$$

where n represents the total number of trials, d the accumulated number of correct decisions, b the slope of the lines, and a the intercept on the vertical axis.

The slope and intercepts are given by the following formulas:

$$b = -\frac{k_2}{k_1 - k_2}$$

$$a_0 = \frac{e_1}{k_1 - k_2}$$

$$a_1 = \frac{e_2}{k_1 - k_2}$$

where
$$k_1 = \log p_1 - \log p_0$$
$$k_2 = \log (1 - p_1) - \log (1 - p_0) = \log q_1 - \log q_0$$
$$e_1 = \log \beta - \log (1 - \alpha)$$
$$e_2 = \log (1 - \beta) - \log \alpha$$

The way in which the plane is divided by the lines L_0 and L_1 is shown in the test chart of Fig. 83.

After each taste trial, the experimenter plots on the graph the point representing the total number of correct decisions against the total number of trials. Each plotted point is therefore one space to the right of the preceding point; it is either one space higher than or on the same level as the preceding point, depending on whether in the last trial the taster made a correct or an incorrect decision. Testing continues until a plotted point falls on or above the upper line, or on or below the lower line. In the former case the taster is accepted as a judge, and in the latter case he is rejected.

Before a definite decision is reached on the specification of values for p_0, p_1, α, and β, it is desirable to compute the average number of tests required to establish the qualifications of judges. Such information is

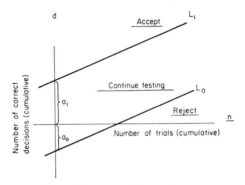

FIG. 83. Sequential test chart.

of value in estimating the time and materials necessary for the test. Obviously the number of tests required depends upon the ability of the taster and the test specification. Usually the approximate numbers of tests, $\bar{n}$, are determined for special values of p, namely 0, p_0, p_1, and 1.

For $p = 0$ (no ability)

$$\bar{n}_0 = \frac{e_1}{k_2}$$

$p = p_0$ (maximum unacceptable ability)

$$\bar{n}_{p0} = \frac{(1 - \alpha)e_1 + \alpha e_2}{p_0 k_1 + q_0 k_2}$$

$p = p_1$ (minimum acceptable ability)

$$\bar{n}_{p1} = \frac{\beta e_1 + (1 - \beta)e_2}{p_1 k_1 + q_1 k_2}$$

$p = 1$ (infallible ability)

$$\bar{n}_1 = \frac{e_2}{k_1}$$

For example, suppose that a triangular test is being used as a basis for selecting judges in a sequential procedure. Reasonable ability limits are $p_0 = 0.45$ and $p_1 = 0.70$. That is, individuals with abilities of 0.70 or greater will be accepted as judges, and those with abilities of 0.45 or less will be rejected. If the probabilities of rejecting a satisfactory judge and accepting an unsatisfactory one are each selected as 0.05, that is, $\alpha = \beta$ = 0.05, then

$$k_1 = \log 0.70 - \log 0.45 = 0.1919$$
$$k_2 = \log 0.30 - \log 0.55 = -0.2632$$
$$e_1 = \log 0.05 - \log 0.95 = -1.2788$$
$$e_2 = \log 0.95 - \log 0.05 = 1.2788$$

and

$$\bar{n}_0 = 5, \qquad \bar{n}_{p_0} = 20,$$
$$\bar{n}_{p_1} = 21, \qquad \bar{n}_1 = 7$$

Therefore, approximately 21 tests will be needed. On the basis of this number the specification of p_0, p_1, α, and β as indicated will be accepted. Substituting these values in the equations for b, a_0, and a_1, one finds

$$b = 0.578, \qquad a_0 = -2.81, \qquad a_1 = 2.81$$

The equations of L_0 and L_1 are

$$L_0: d_0 = -2.81 + 0.578\, n$$
$$L_1: d_1 = 2.81 + 0.578\, n$$

TABLE 58

Sequential Sampling Patterns for Two Tasters, A and B

n no. of trials	A		B	
	Correct decisions	Cumulative correct decisions	Correct decisions	Cumulative correct decisions
1	1	1	0	0
2	0	1	1	1
3	1	2	0	1
4	0	2	1	2
5	0	2	1	3
6	0	2	1	4
7	1	3	0	4
8	0	3	1	5
9	0	3	1	6
10	1	4	1	7
11	1	5	0	7
12	1	6	1	8
13	0	6	1	9
14	0	6	0	9
15	1	7	1	10
16	0	7	1	11
17	1	8	1	12
18	0	8	1	13
19	1	9	1	14

The results of two tasters are given in Table 58, where 1 indicates a correct judgment and 0 denotes a wrong one.

Figure 84 plots the number of trials and the cumulative number of correct decisions. After 19 trials, taster B may be accepted as a judge, but all the points representing taster A up to this number of trials are still in the region of indecision. He will have to continue tasting to qualify as a judge or if the tasting is discontinued he would be eliminated.

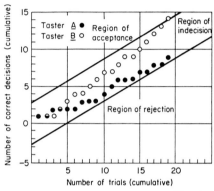

Fig. 84. Test chart for data of Table 58.

Various values of p_0, p_1, α, and β may be used in selecting judges for an experimental panel. As p_0 approaches p_1, the number of required trials increases. One means of reducing the number is to increase α, accepting a greater risk of rejecting a capable judge. This may be done, for example, if large numbers of individuals are available as prospective judges, so that the rejection of an able one is not regarded as serious.

IV. Differences between Two Means

A. INDEPENDENT SAMPLES

Statistical tests for differences between food products are based on the assumption that no differences exist in the populations from which random samples are drawn. This assumption applies not only to population mean scores but also to population standard deviations. If, when two samples $X_1, X_2, X_3, \ldots, X_{n_1}$, and $Y_1, Y_2, Y_3, \ldots, Y_{n_2}$ are randomly selected from possibly two different populations, it may be assumed that both populations are normal, with equal variances, and that the samples are independent and consist of independent observations. The t test may be used to test the null hypothesis that the population means, m_1 and m_2, are equal. The t statistic is

$$t = \frac{\bar{X} - \bar{Y}}{s_{\bar{x}-\bar{y}}} \text{ with } (n_1 - 1) + (n_2 - 1) \text{ degrees of freedom}$$

where

$$s_{\bar{x}-\bar{y}} = \sqrt{\frac{s^2}{n_1} + \frac{s^2}{n_2}}$$

and

$$s^2 = \frac{\Sigma(X - \bar{X})^2 + \Sigma(Y - \bar{Y})^2}{(n_1 - 1) + (n_2 - 1)} = \frac{\Sigma X^2 - [(\Sigma X)^2/n_1] + \Sigma Y^2 - [(\Sigma Y)^2/n_2]}{(n_1 - 1) + (n_2 - 1)}$$

and

$$\bar{X} = \frac{\Sigma X}{n_1}, \qquad \bar{Y} = \frac{\Sigma Y}{n_2}.$$

If the calculated value of t exceeds the tabular value (Table B) at any significance level α for $(n_1 - 1) + (n_2 - 1)$ degrees of freedom, the means are considered significantly different. Instead of comparing calculated and tabular values of t, significance between means may be determined by comparing the actual difference, $\bar{X} - \bar{Y}$, between sample means with the least significant difference (LSD) as calculated from $t_\alpha s_{\bar{x}-\bar{y}}$ where t_α is the tabular value of t, for $(n_1 - 1) + (n_2 - 1)$ degrees of freedom, at the required level of significance. For example, if from two samples of 10 and 15 observations $\bar{X} = 40.1$, $\bar{Y} = 41.7$ and $s_{\bar{x}-\bar{y}} = 0.53$, then at the 5% level for 23 degrees of freedom the difference between means required for significance is $t_{.05}\, s_{\bar{x}-\bar{y}} = 2.069\,(0.53) = 1.10$. Since the difference $\bar{X} - \bar{Y} = 1.6$ exceeds 1.10, the means are significantly different at the 5% level and could not, at this level, have come from populations having equal mean values.

B. PAIRED OBSERVATIONS

Many experiments are performed in such a way that each item of one sample is logically paired with a particular item of another sample. For example, if a taster, in comparing two food products at several tastings, scores a sample of each, these scores are paired; or if members of a panel of tasters score a sample of each of two similar foods, a set of paired scores results. In such a situation the t-distribution for paired samples furnishes a test of significance of the mean differences in scores between the two products. With n pairs of scores, X and Y, the differences, $D = X - Y$ for each pair, are analyzed. To determine whether two sample means, $\bar{X}$ and $\bar{Y}$, from two normal and paired populations differ significantly, one asks whether these samples are likely to have come from two populations with identical means, that is, $m_x = m_y$, and calculates $t = \bar{D}/s_{\bar{d}}$, with $n - 1$ degrees of freedom where $\bar{D} = \bar{X} - \bar{Y}$, and $s_{\bar{d}}$, the best estimate of the standard error of the population of differences between the means of scores, is calculated from the expression $s_{\bar{d}} = s/\sqrt{n}$, where

$$s = \sqrt{\frac{\Sigma(D - \bar{D})^2}{n - 1}} = \sqrt{\frac{\Sigma D^2 - [(\Sigma D)^2/n]}{n - 1}}$$

As before, the significance of the result is determined by comparing the calculated value of t with the tabular value (Table B) for the appropriate number of degrees of freedom, or the actual difference between means may be compared with the difference required for significance as calculated from $t_\alpha s_{\bar{d}}$, where, as before, t_α is the tabular value of t at the appropriate level of significance. The use of the t-distribution is so well known that no illustration is necessary.

V. Analysis of Variance

In the usual tasting design, a panel of tasters scores each of several food products or one taster scores the same products at several different times. Either procedure leads to the same mathematical treatment, and results in an average score for each product. Significance between these average scores might appear to be easily determined by applying the t-test to all possible pairs. Such a procedure, however, can easily lead to false conclusions. For example, with 6 products the resulting 6 mean scores can be paired in 15 different ways. If the t-tests are independent, at the 5% level of significance the probability of arriving at the correct conclusion for all 15 pairs is $(0.95)^{15}$, and the probability of obtaining at least one incorrect conclusion is $1 - (0.95)^{15} = 0.537$. This means that in approximately 54% of the cases at least one wrong conclusion will be obtained by using the t-test to compare pairs of means. For larger numbers of samples this probability would be even higher.

A method, the analysis of variance, which considers all the sample means together is a generalization of the t-test in which the variates are not paired.

The analysis of variance is based upon two principles—partitioning of the total sum of squares and degrees of freedom, and estimation of the standard deviation of the population by two or more methods and a comparison of these estimates.

A. EQUAL SAMPLE SIZES

Suppose there are n samples with k observations each. The experimental pattern is shown in Table 59. The entry X_{ij} represents the ith

TABLE 59

Experimental Pattern of n *Samples with* k *Observations Each*

	Samples				
	1	2	3	. . .	n
	X_{11}	X_{12}	X_{13}		X_{1n}
	X_{21}	X_{22}	X_{23}		X_{2n}
	X_{31}	X_{32}	X_{33}		X_{3n}
	.	.	.		.
	.	.	.		.
	.	.	.		.
	X_{k1}	X_{k2}	X_{k3}	. . .	X_{kn}
Totals	T_1	T_2	T_3	. . .	T_n
Means	$\bar{X}_1$	$\bar{X}_2$	$\bar{X}_3$	. . .	$\bar{X}_n$

Grand total $= T$
Grand mean $= \bar{X}$

item in the *j*th sample. The following sums of squares of deviations from means are calculated, and the corresponding number of degrees of freedom are indicated:

$$\text{Total} = \sum_{i=1}^{k}\sum_{j=1}^{n}(X_{ij} - \bar{X})^2 = \sum_{i=1}^{k}\sum_{j=1}^{n}X_{ij}^2 - \frac{T^2}{kn}$$

with $nk - 1$ d.f.

$$\text{Between samples} = k\sum_{j=1}^{n}(\bar{X}_j - \bar{X})^2 = \frac{\Sigma T_j^2}{k} - \frac{T^2}{kn}$$

with $n - 1$ d.f.

$$\text{Within samples} = \sum_{i=1}^{k}(X_{i1} - \bar{X}_1)^2 + \sum_{i=1}^{k}(X_{i2} - \bar{X}_2)^2 + \dots$$

$$+ \sum_{i=1}^{k}(X_{in} - \bar{X}_n)^2$$

$$= \sum_{i=1}^{k}\sum_{j=1}^{k}X_{ij}^2 - \frac{T_1^2}{k} - \frac{T^2}{k}\dots - \frac{T_n^2}{k}$$

$$= \sum_{i=1}^{k}\sum_{j=1}^{n}X_{ij}^2 - \frac{\Sigma T_i^2}{k}$$

with $n(k - 1)$ d.f.

From these expressions one sees that the total sum of squares is equal to the sum of squares between samples plus the sum of squares within samples. The same relationship applies to the numbers of degrees of freedom. Because of this additive relationship, the sum of squares and degrees of freedom within samples are frequently obtained by subtracting those between samples from the totals.

The term T^2/kn, appearing in the expressions for the sum of squares for the total and between samples, is called the correction term (c.t.) since, when subtracted from the sum of squares of a set of observations, it converts this sum into the required sum of squares of deviations from the grand mean, $\bar{X}$.

On the basis of the hypothesis that all of the n samples belong to the same population, we can obtain two independent estimates of this population variance, σ^2, one estimate from the sum of squares and degrees of freedom between samples, and the other from those within samples. The within-sample mean square is called the error variance and measures the uncontrolled variation between objects treated alike.

On the assumption that the groups making up the total set of measurements are random samples from a homogeneous population, the two estimates of the population variance may be expected to differ only within the limits of chance fluctuations. This hypothesis is tested by comparing the variance between samples with the error variance. The comparison consists of calculating a variance ratio

$$F = \frac{\text{between-samples variance}}{\text{error variance}}$$

Since both variances represent the same population value, their ratio should not differ significantly from 1. If we assume the error variance to represent the variability of the experiment, then we wish to test whether the other variance is significantly larger, and this calls for a one-tailed test. Values of F to be expected at the 5 and 1% levels of significance are given in Table F in the Appendix. If the calculated value of F exceeds the tabular value for the level of significance adopted, the hypothesis of no differences among the populations from which the samples have been drawn is untenable.

If our hypothesis fails to be true, i.e., if the n samples are in fact taken from populations with different means, then the between-samples variance will be considerably greater than the error variance owing to the wider dispersion of the sample means about the grand mean. If their ratio yields a significant F-value, we consider the sample means to be significantly different and conclude that there must be at least one pair of samples whose means differ significantly. Whenever the between-samples variance is less than the error variance, it is not necessary to calculate an F-value, since under these conditions it obviously would not be significant.

The F-distribution provides an over-all test of significance among the different means. If the F-test indicates differences, then specific comparisons may be made using the least significant difference:

$$t_\alpha \sqrt{\frac{2 \times \text{error variance}}{\text{no. of replications}}}$$

based on the t-distribution or by applying one of the newer tests in which protection levels for sets of means are kept at or above preselected values.

The Newman-Keuls (Newman, 1939; Keuls, 1952) method keeps all levels at 95%. The multiple-range test proposed by Duncan (1955), with tabular corrections by Harter (1960, 1961), establishes the level for sets of two means at 95%; for sets of three means at $(0.95)^2$, or 90.25%; for sets of four means at $(0.95)^3$, or 85.7%; and so on. At the expense of lowered protection, the Duncan test is more sensitive in detecting real differences and is frequently used in difference testing to set up a series of shortest significant ranges with which to compare differences between mean scores. The shortest significant range, R_p, for comparing the largest and smallest of p mean scores is given by $Q_p s_{\bar{x}}$; with $(n-1)(k-1)$ degrees of freedom, where the appropriate value of Q_p can be obtained from Table G in the Appendix. The standard error of any mean score, $s_{\bar{x}}$, can be calculated from

$$s_{\bar{x}} = \sqrt{\frac{\text{error variance}}{k}}.$$

B. UNEQUAL SAMPLE SIZES

If there are available unequal numbers of scores for each of n samples, the above procedure is applicable with modifications. Suppose that there are k_1 scores for sample 1, k_2 for sample 2, k_3 for sample 3, . . . , and k_n for sample n. In the analysis of variance the correction term and the total sum of squares (s.s.) are calculated as before. The rest of the calculations follow.

$$\text{Between-sample s.s.} = \frac{T_1^2}{k_1} + \frac{T_2^2}{k_2} + \frac{T_3^2}{k_3} + \ldots + \frac{T_n^2}{k_n} - \text{c.t.}$$

Error (within-sample) s.s. = total s.s. — between-sample s.s.
Degrees of freedom for error = $\Sigma k - n$.

If the k's are not all the same, pairs of sample means may be compared by calculating the least significant difference

$$t_\alpha \sqrt{s^2 \left(\frac{1}{k_i} + \frac{1}{k_j} \right)}$$

where t_α is Student's t for the chosen significance level and error degrees of freedom, s^2 is the error variance, and k_i and k_j are the number of scores in the two means being compared.

When Duncan's method of comparison is used, Kramer (1956) has suggested that the significant studentized ranges be multiplied by s rather than by $s_{\bar{x}}$, to give a set of intermediate significant ranges. In any desired comparison the appropriate intermediate value is then multiplied by

$$\sqrt{\frac{1}{2} \left(\frac{1}{k_i} + \frac{1}{k_j} \right)}$$

If the k's are not all the same, many investigators (see Snedecor, 1956) calculate an effective number of replications applicable to all mean scores. Such an effective number of replications may be obtained from the formula

$$k_0 = \frac{1}{n-1} \left(\Sigma k - \frac{\Sigma k^2}{\Sigma k} \right)$$

from which

$$s_{\bar{x}} = \sqrt{\frac{\text{error variance}}{k_0}}$$

For example, Table 60 shows four samples for which there are unequal numbers of scores. The analysis of variance for the results is summarized in Table 61.

Since the calculated value of F (3.86) exceeds the value 2.88, significant differences between mean scores of samples are indicated at the 5% level of significance. The t-test can be used to compare pairs of mean scores, or Duncan's multiple-range test can be used after calculating the effective number of replications, k_0. This latter procedure will be followed. Then

$$k_0 = \frac{1}{n-1} \left(\Sigma k - \frac{\Sigma k^2}{\Sigma k} \right) = \frac{1}{3} \left(38 - \frac{374}{38} \right) = 9.39$$

and

$$s_{\bar{x}} = \sqrt{\frac{3.07}{9.39}} = \sqrt{0.327} = 0.572$$

TABLE 60
Scores for Four Samples

	Samples				
	A	B	C	D	
	16	17	15	14	
	12	14	11	12	
	11	12	13	17	
	13	17	12	15	
	11	15	13	14	
	15	14	15	13	
	14	17	13	15	
	15	16	10		
	11	15	16		
	13	17			
	14				
	13				
Totals	158	154	118	100	530
Means	13.2	15.4	13.1	14.3	

Correction term (c.t.) $= \dfrac{(530)^2}{38} = 7392.11$

Total s.s. $= (16)^2 + (12)^2 + \ldots + (15)^2 - $ c.t. $= 7532 - 7392.11 = 139.89$

Between-sample s.s. $= \dfrac{(158)^2}{12} + \dfrac{(154)^2}{10} + \dfrac{(118)^2}{9} + \dfrac{(100)^2}{7} - $ c.t.

$\qquad = 7427.62 - 7392.11 = 35.51$

Remainder (error) s.s. $= 139.89 - 35.51 = 104.38$

To determine which mean scores are significantly different at the 5% level, the tabular values of Q_p for 34 degrees of freedom to be used in comparing the largest and smallest values of sets of two ($p = 2$), three ($p = 3$), and four ($p = 4$) means are selected from Table G. They are 2.88, 3.03, and 3.11, respectively, and each is multiplied by the standard

TABLE 61
Analysis of Variance for Data of Table 60

Source of variation	Degrees of freedom	Sum of squares	Mean square (variance)	F value Calculated	F value Tabular (5%)
Total	37	139.89			
Samples	3	35.51	11.84	3.86	2.88
Error	34	104.38	3.07		

error, 0.572, to form the shortest significant ranges, R_p. Adjacent means having a difference greater than R_2 are considered significantly different. Differences between the largest and smallest of three means arranged in order of size are significant if they exceed R_3, or, in general, R_p represents the dividing line between significance and nonsignificance for the smallest and largest of p means arranged in order of size. The results are summarized in Table 62. In the comparisons below, any two means

TABLE 62

Multiple-Range Test for Data of Table 60

	Shortest significant ranges 5% level							
	$p = 2$	$p = 3$	$p = 4$	Comparisons				
Q_p	2.88	3.03	3.11	Samples	C	A	D	B
R_p	1.65	1.73	1.78	Mean scores	13.1	13.2	14.3	15.4

underscored by the same line are not significantly different. Any two means not underscored by the same line are significantly different. Differences between mean scores are compared with R_p as follows:

$$B - D = 1.1 < 1.65 \qquad D - A = 1.1 < 1.65$$
$$B - A = 2.2 > 1.73 \qquad D - C = 1.2 < 1.73$$
$$B - C = 2.3 > 1.78 \qquad A - C = 0.1 < 1.65$$

Therefore, at the 5% level of significance, the mean score of B is significantly better than those of A and C. No other significant differences exist. Comparisons are indicated by underscoring as shown in Table 62. The results would have been the same if Kramer's procedure (p. 455) had been followed.

If a hedonic scale is used in scoring, the hedonic ratings can be converted to point scores and analyzed in the same manner. Harries (1956) has shown that there is a positional bias (differing between tasters) when samples are scored 0 to 7 and are coded 1 to 6. The tendency is to treat the end samples higher or lower according to their position. This is different from the well-known phenomenon of scoring a sample low if it follows a better one, or high if it follows a poorer one. Harries suggested treating the code sample as a factor, and including its effect in the main table of variance and disregarding it in the tests of significance of the main treatment effects. Filipello (1956) reported positional bias in consumer-acceptance tests as well.

C. HOMOGENEITY OF VARIANCE

In the analysis of variance procedure, one assumes that the variations within samples are homogeneous, that is, that the variances within the several samples do not differ significantly among themselves. This is the usual case with experimental data. It may happen, however, that the variances within the various samples are so dissimilar that it is doubtful that they could have come from samples of the same population. Such a situation requires a supplementary test of the hypothesis that the samples are random samples from the same population or from populations with the same variance. Bartlett (1937) developed a procedure for testing the homogeneity of n-estimated population variances $v_1, v_2, v_3, \ldots, v_n$ based on $k_1, k_2, k_3, \ldots, k_n$ degrees of freedom, respectively. Under the hypothesis that the variances are homogeneous, the quantity Q satisfies approximately a χ^2 distribution with $n - 1$ degrees of freedom, where

$$Q = \frac{2.3026}{C} \left[(\Sigma k_i) \log v - \Sigma (k_i \log v_i) \right]$$

and

$$C = 1 + \frac{1}{3(n-1)} \left(\Sigma \frac{1}{k_i} - \frac{1}{\Sigma k_i} \right) \quad \text{and} \quad v = \frac{\Sigma k_i v_i}{\Sigma k_i}.$$

If, at any adopted level of significance, α, the calculated value of Q exceeds the tabular value of χ^2, the hypothesis of homogeneous variances is rejected. If, in a particular case, assuming $C = 1$, Q does not show significance, then there is no need to calculate the actual value of C, since it is always larger than 1 and will only reduce the value of Q.

If n samples all have the same number of variates, k, and if n is fairly large, then an excellent approximation of Q is given by

$$Q' = 2.3026 \left(k - \frac{4}{3} \right) (n \log v - \Sigma \log v_i)$$

where

$$v = \frac{\Sigma v_i}{n}.$$

D. TRANSFORMATIONS

If Bartlett's test does indicate significant differences in the within-sample variances, the analysis-of-variance procedure is invalidated as it applies to the original data. Sometimes the original data can be transformed into others, the variances of which are homogeneous.

The presence of correlation between the variances and means within the various samples is an indication of departure from normality and is likely to be associated with heterogeneity of variance. If the data indicate the existence of correlation between means and variances of the separate samples, then a transformation of the original data to a new scale may correct the difficulty of nonhomogeneous variance and non-normality of the variable.

If the data consist of the numbers of correct or incorrect responses in a limited number of trials, and if the counts are small, the distribution may be such that the means and variances within the various experimental conditions tend to be proportional to one another. The transformation recommended by Bartlett (1936, 1947) in this situation is the square-root transformation, in which the recorded values of X are replaced by $\sqrt{X}$. Sometimes the replacement of each recorded X by log $(1 + X)$ will correct the situation. The analysis of variance is then applied to these transformed values. When the means of the various groups are small, in the range of 2 to 10, Bartlett (1947) suggests the transformation $\sqrt{X + 0.5}$, and for means smaller than 2.0 the transformation and subsequent analysis of variance should not be used.

For data recorded in terms of percentage, especially when large and small values are present, the inverse sine (arcsin) or angular transformation often proves useful. The angles corresponding to various percentages have been tabled by Bliss (1937) and reproduced by Snedecor (1956).

VI. Experimental Designs

A. Randomized Complete-Block

In the preceding discussions each measurement has been classified only according to the sample to which it belonged. Frequently measurements are also classified according to a second criterion. In sensory comparisons where several judges at a single sitting taste and score each of various samples of a food product, the arrangement of scores is known as a randomized complete-block design. Each score (measurement) is fixed in the design; it belongs to one of the samples (treatments) and to one of the judges (blocks). It is therefore classified according to two criteria. The analysis of such a design is similar to that for the one-criterion case. The only modification necessary is to take account of the variations between the (means of scores of) judges. This sum of squares as well as that between samples must be subtracted from the total to obtain the error (sometimes called interaction) sum of squares. The design is indicated in Table 63, where k judges scored n products.

The mathematical model applicable to this design is $X_{ij} = m + \beta_i + t_j + \epsilon_{ij}$, where X_{ij} is the score of the ith judge (block) assigned to

TABLE 63
Randomized Complete-Block Design

Judges (blocks)	Products (treatments)					Totals
	1	2	3	. . .	n	
1	X_{11}	X_{12}	X_{13}		X_{1n}	B_1
2	X_{21}	X_{22}	X_{23}		X_{2n}	B_2
3	X_{31}	X_{32}	X_{33}		X_{3n}	B_3
.	.	.	.		.	.
.	.	.	.		.	.
.	.	.	.		.	.
k	X_{k1}	X_{k2}	X_{k3}	. . .	X_{kn}	B_k
Totals	T_1	T_2	T_3	. . .	T_n	$G = \Sigma T = \Sigma B$

the jth product (treatment); m is the over-all mean; β_i is the judge effect; t_j is the product effect; and ϵ_{ij} is the residual error.

In such an analysis the total sum of squares based upon variation of all scores is broken down into three parts—a sum of squares based upon the variation between judges; a sum of squares based upon the variation between products; and a residual sum of squares which is not the result of variation between judges or products. This last sum of squares is the remainder, or error, sum of squares. It is a measure of the unexplained variation in the experiment. The number of degrees of freedom is broken down in the same way. The computations for this design are as follows:

	Sum of squares[a]	Degrees of freedom
(a) Total	$\displaystyle\sum_{i=1}^{k} \sum_{j=1}^{n} X_{ij}^2 - \text{c.t.}$	$nk - 1$
(b) Judges	$\dfrac{\displaystyle\sum_{i=1}^{k} B_i^2}{n} - \text{c.t.}$	$k - 1$
(c) Products	$\dfrac{\displaystyle\sum_{j=1}^{n} T_j^2}{k} - \text{c.t.}$	$n - 1$
(d) Remainder (error) (Interaction: judges $\times$ products)	$(a) - (b) - (c)$	$(k - 1)(n - 1)$

[a] Correction term (c.t.) $= G^2/nk$

From these sums of squares and degrees of freedom, three estimates of the population variance can be computed and the F-test applied.

TABLE 64
Scores Assigned to Three Products by Five Judges

| Judges | Products | | | Totals |
	X	Y	Z	
A	79	83	76	238
B	74	79	73	226
C	77	81	76	234
D	80	88	79	247
E	80	82	81	243
Totals	390	413	385	1188
Mean	78.0	82.6	77.0	

Computations:

Correction term $= \dfrac{(1188)^2}{15} = 94{,}089.60$

Total s.s. $= (79)^2 + (74)^2 + \ldots + (81)^2 -$ c.t. $= 94{,}288.00 - 94{,}089.60$
$= 198.40$

Judges s.s. $= \dfrac{(238)^2 + (226)^2 + \ldots + (243)^2}{3} -$ c.t.

$= 94{,}178.00 - 94{,}089.60 = 88.40$

Products s.s. $= \dfrac{(390)^2 + (413)^2 + (385)^2}{5} -$ c.t. $= 94{,}178.80 - 94{,}089.60$

$= 89.20$

Error s.s. $= 198.40 - 88.40 - 89.20 = 20.80$

The procedure will be illustrated by using data adapted from a paper by Papakyriakopoulos and Amerine (1956) in which 5 judges scored each of 3 wines shown in Table 64. The results are given in Table 65.

Since, for products and judges, the calculated values of F exceed the

TABLE 65
Analysis of Variance Table for the Data of Table 64

| Source of variation | Degrees of freedom | Sum of squares | Mean square (variance) | F value | | |
| | | | | | Tabular | |
				Calculated	5%	1%
Total	14	198.40				
Judges	4	88.40	22.10	8.50	3.84	7.01
Products	2	89.20	44.60	17.15	4.46	8.65
Error	8	20.80	2.60			

tabular values, the analysis indicates, at both the 5 and 1% levels, significant differences between mean scores of products and mean scores of judges.

To determine which product mean scores are significantly different, the tabular values of Q_p, for 8 degrees of freedom, are each multiplied by the standard error, $\sqrt{2.60/5} = 0.721$, to form the shortest significant ranges, R_p. The results are summarized in Table 66. In the comparisons,

TABLE 66
Multiple-Range Test for Data of Table 64

	\multicolumn{4}{c}{Shortest significant ranges}					
	5% level		1% level					
	$p = 2$	$p = 3$	$p = 2$	$p = 3$	Comparisons			
Q_p	3.26	3.40	4.75	4.94	Products	Z	X	Y
R_p	2.35	2.45	3.42	3.56	Mean scores	77.0	78.0	82.6

any two mean scores underscored by the same line are not significantly different. At both the 5 and 1% level the mean score of product Y is significantly better than those of X and Z, and X and Z are not significantly different.

B. RANGE METHOD FOR MULTIPLE COMPARISONS

Tukey (1953) suggested a rapid, but less critical, method of detecting significant differences between products scored in a simple one-way classification or in a randomized complete block design. It is based upon a comparison of the ranges in scores, and total scores, for the products. The method for a one-way classification will be illustrated by applying it to the data of Table 64 where judges are disregarded. For each product there are, then, five scores. The total score and range in scores for each product are shown below.

Product	X	Y	Z	
Total score	390	413	385	Range 28
Range (R) in scores	6	9	8	$\Sigma R = 23$

In Table H-1 in the Appendix for 3 products with 5 scores each there appear two entries 1.19 and 1.60, the first of which is for the 5% level and the second for the 1% level. These values when multiplied by ΣR give 27.4 and 36.8. At the 5% level the value 27.4 must be exceeded by the range of the product totals to indicate significant differences. Since the range of the total scores is 28, which exceeds 27.4, significant differences are indicated. Expressed in another way, 95% confidence limits for the differences in product totals between Y and Z are $(413 - 385) \pm 27.4$ $= 28 \pm 27.4$. Confidence limits for differences between other product totals may be expressed in the same way.

Actually the data of Table 64 represent a two-way classification. To analyze them as such, the differences between adjacent product scores are determined and the analysis proceeds as indicated.

	$Y - X$	$Z - Y$	$X - Z$		Total Scores				
	4	−7	3						
	5	−6	1		Products	X		Y	Z
	4	−5	1			390		413	385
	8	−9	1		Judges	A	B	C	D	E
	2	−1	−1			238	226	234	247	243
Range	6	8	4	$R = 18$					

From Table H-2 the entries 0.89 (for 3 columns) and 0.84 (for 5 rows) when multiplied by ΣR give 16.02 and 15.12. Products, the difference in whose total scores exceed 16.02, are significantly different at the 5% level, and the same is true of judges the differences of whose total scores exceed 15.12. As before, these values may be used in setting up 95% confidence limits for differences in total scores.

C. FACTORIAL DESIGNS

Many experiments involve two or more variables, each of which may be varied in several ways. When the variables are studied in all possible combinations in the same experiment, it is known as a factorial design. We shall start by discussing the analysis of a randomized complete-block design in which there is an interaction effect present, that is, in which there is at least one treatment for which the effects are not constant in all blocks. Detecting whether such interaction effects are present in a randomized complete-block requires that each treatment be repeated more than once in each block. Otherwise it would be impossible to determine whether or not some treatments have an interaction effect with the blocks. We shall start by assuming that the replications are made under identical conditions so that there is no possibility of interactions of the replications with either blocks or treatments or both. The analysis will be illustrated by means of a simple experiment in which 3 judges (blocks) score 4 products (treatments) in duplicate. This is done at the same sitting, so the replications occur under identical conditions and no interactions related to replications can exist. The mathematical model applicable to this situation is

$$X_{ij} = m + \beta_i + t_j + (\beta t)_{ij} + \epsilon_{ij}$$

where $(\beta t)_{ij}$ is the effect due to the interaction of blocks with treatments. The pattern and calculations for the analysis are shown in Table 67. In Table 68 the data for products and judges are combined in a complete block in which replications are disregarded.

TABLE 67

Pattern in Which Three Judges Score Four Products in Duplicate

Judges (blocks)	Products (treatments)								Totals	
	A		B		C		D			
	(1)	(2)	(1)	(2)	(1)	(2)	(1)	(2)	(1)	(2)
1	6	6	9	7	9	8	9	9	33	30
2	5	8	9	8	10	9	10	8	34	33
3	7	8	8	7	8	8	6	7	29	30
Totals	18	22	26	22	27	25	25	24	96	93
	40		48		52		49		189	

Correction term = $189^2/24$ = 1488.38

Total s.s. = $6^2 + 5^2 + \cdots + 7^2$ − c.t. = 1527.00 − 1488.38 = 38.62 (23 d.f.)

If the interaction is not significant, as in this case, and if there is some reason why a large number of degrees of freedom for error is desirable, then the sum of squares and degrees of freedom for interaction may be combined with those for error to give a new error variance, which may be used in the denominator of the F-ratio to determine significance for products and judges. In this case the new error variance would be 21.5/18 = 1.19 (Table 69). Whichever error variance is used, the analysis indicates significant differences between means of products but not between means of judges.

The preceding analysis was based on the assumption that the two replications occurred under identical conditions. Suppose, now, that this is not the case, but that the replications represent repetitions of the experiment under different conditions. Instead of scoring the products in duplicate at the same sitting, the judges might have scored them at two different times or under quite different circumstances. In this case interactions between replications and products and replications and judges would have to be considered, although in the particular case there might

TABLE 68

Data for Products and Judges Combined from Table 67 (Replications Disregarded)

| Judges | Products | | | | Totals |
	A	B	C	D	
1	12	16	17	18	63
2	13	17	19	18	67
3	15	15	16	13	59
Totals	40	48	52	49	189

Total s.s. $= \dfrac{(12)^2 + (13)^2 + \ldots + (13)^2}{2} - $ c.t. $= 1515.50 - 1488.38$

$= 27.12$ (11 d.f.)

Product s.s. $= \dfrac{(40)^2 + (48)^2 + (52)^2 + (49)^2}{6} - $ c.t. $= 1501.50 - 1488.38$

$= 13.12$ (3 d.f.)

Judge s.s. $= \dfrac{(63)^2 + (67)^2 + (59)^2}{8} - $ c.t. $= 1492.38 - 1488.38 = 4.00$ (2 d.f.)

Remainder s.s. $= 27.12 - 13.12 - 4.00 = 10.00$ ($11 - 3 - 2 = 6$ d.f.)
 (Interaction: products $\times$ judges)

Error s.s. $= 38.62 - 27.12 = 11.50$ ($23 - 11 = 12$ d.f.)

be some doubt as to the meaning of an interaction between replications and products. The preceding analysis will be extended to account for these interactions (Tables 70, 71, 72).

Since none of the interaction variances are significant, as in the preceding case the combined interaction-error variance is used as the denominator in the F-ratios for testing products and judges for significant differences.

TABLE 69

Analysis of Variance for Data of Tables 67 and 68

| Source of variation | Degrees of freedom | Sum of squares | Mean square (variance) | F-value | |
				Calculated	Tabular
Total	23	38.62			
Products	3	13.12	4.37	3.67[a]	3.16
Judges	2	4.00	2.00	1.68[a]	3.55
Interaction (products $\times$ judges)	6	10.00	1.67		3.00
Error (remainder)	12	11.50	0.96		

[a] Calculated using combined error variance 1.19 with 18 degrees of freedom.

TABLE 70

Data for Products and Replications Combined from Table 67 (Judges Disregarded)

Replications	Products				Totals
	A	B	C	D	
I	18	26	27	25	96
II	22	22	25	24	93
Totals	40	48	52	49	189

Total s.s. $= \dfrac{(18)^2 + (22)^2 + \ldots + (24)^2}{3}$ $-$ c.t. $= 1507.67 - 1488.38 = 19.29$ (7 d.f.)

Replication s.s. $= \dfrac{(96)^2 + (93)^2}{12}$ $-$ c.t. $= 1488.75 - 1488.38 = 0.37$ (1 d.f.)

Product s.s. $= 13.12$ (3 d.f.)

Remainder s.s. $= 19.29 - 0.37 - 13.12 = 5.80$ (7 $-$ 1 $-$ 3 $=$ 3 d.f.)
　　　　　(Interaction: products $\times$ replications)

If one or more of the interactions had been significant, the problem would have been more complicated, and for proper evaluation of the data the model being used must be specifically stated. Three models are in common use—the fixed effects, the random effects, and the mixed model, in which at least one criterion of classification involves fixed effects and another random effects.

In randomized complete-block design problems where the fixed-effects model is appropriate, two or more products are selected for testing.

TABLE 71

Data for Judges and Replications Combined from Table 67 (Products Disregarded)

Replications	Judges			Totals
	1	2	3	
I	33	34	29	96
II	30	33	30	93
Totals	63	67	59	189

Total s.s. $= \dfrac{(33)^2 + (30)^2 + \ldots + (30)^2}{4}$ $-$ c.t. $= 1493.75 - 1488.38 = 5.37$ (5 d.f.)

Replication s.s. $= 0.37$ (1 d.f.)

Judge s.s. $= 4.00$ (2 d.f.)

Remainder s.s. $= 5.37 - 4.00 - 0.37 = 1.00$ (5 $-$ 2 $-$ 1 $=$ 2 d.f.)
　　　　　(Interaction: judges $\times$ replications)

These are not randomly drawn from a population of possible products but are selected specially for testing. All products about which inferences are to be drawn are included in the experiment. Block or taster effects are also fixed; tasters are a selected group and do not represent a random sample from all possible tasters. For the fixed model with no interaction, both tasters and products can be tested by the error mean square.

When large significant interactions are present and effects are then subtracted out, resulting in an extremely small error variance, its use in testing main effects may be questioned. Certainly if large interactions exist, care must be used in drawing any conclusions about main effects.

TABLE 72

Analysis of Variance for Data of Table 67

Source of variation	Degrees of freedom	Sum of squares	Mean square (variance)	F value	
				Calculated	Tabular (5%)
Total	23	38.62			
Products	3	13.12	4.37	3.52[a]	4.76
Judges	2	4.00	2.00	1.61[a]	5.14
Replications	1	0.37	0.37		
Interactions:					
P × J	6	10.00	1.67	2.32	4.28
P × R	3	5.80	1.93	2.68	4.76
J × R	2	1.00	0.50		
Error (remainder)	6	4.33	0.72		

[a] Calculated using combined error variance 1.24 with 17 degrees of freedom.

For the random model, both products and judges are considered to be drawn at random from populations of products and judges. Inferences are drawn about the populations of products and judges rather than about the particular ones used in the experiment. The interaction mean square is the appropriate one for testing products and judges.

In some situations, judges are considered to be representative of a population of judges since inferences are desired for a range of persons wider than that of the particular judges used. If judges are assumed random and products fixed, we have a mixed model, and the error mean square is appropriate for testing judges whereas interaction mean square is appropriate for testing products.

Where rather broad inferences are to be drawn from an experiment, care should be taken that the judges used are really representative of the population about which inferences are to be made.

If both interactions involving judges are significant, the problem becomes complicated. One calculates an estimated variance

$$s_a^2 = s_{pj}^2 + s_{jr}^2 - s^2.$$

This estimate, s_a^2, is used in the denominator of the F-value to test for significant differences between judges. The number of degrees of freedom corresponding to s_a^2 can be approximated from the formula

$$k_a = \frac{s_a^4}{\dfrac{s_{pj}^4}{k_{pj}} + \dfrac{s_{jr}^4}{k_{jr}} + \dfrac{s^4}{k}}$$

where k_{pj}, k_{jr}, and k are respectively the numbers of degrees of freedom corresponding to s_{pj}, s_{jr}, and s.

D. INCOMPLETE-BLOCK DESIGNS

In tasting experiments, if each judge scores all samples at the same session, a randomized complete-block design is appropriate. However, the number of samples which a judge can reliably score at any one time depends upon numerous factors which have been discussed in previous chapters. When the number of samples is large and exceeds the number which a taster can differentiate in a single trial, then the balanced incomplete block design, introduced by Yates (1936), is useful, where the block represents all scores for a single trial by an individual taster, and the score for a given sample replaces the plot yield. Use of this design permits equal precision in sample comparisons even for small block size. For most foods there is a block size beyond which fatigue of the taster causes the heterogeneity of scores to be so great that any comparisons are practically useless. Incomplete-block designs reduce the need for the judge to have long-term memory retention since he need be consistent in his level of judgment only within the incomplete-block limit.

An incomplete-block design in which each block contains the same number of units and every pair of treatments occurs together in the same block the same number of times is called a balanced incomplete-block design. The term "balanced" is used since in such designs all pairs of treatments are compared with approximately the same precision even though the differences among blocks may be large.

Since only part of the total number of samples are judged at the same time (that is, only part of the samples appear in any block), and since each sample is compared with every other sample equally often, only certain arrangements of plots, blocks, and replications are possible. These are discussed and have been tabulated by Fisher and Yates (1953) and by Cochran and Cox (1957).

Consider the plan shown in Table 73, in which nine products are compared in incomplete blocks of three units, each with four replications. Every pair of products occurs once, and only once, in the same block. Product 1 occupies the same block with products 2 and 3 in the first replication, with products 4 and 7 in the second replication, with products 5 and 9 in the third replication, and with products 6 and 8 in the

TABLE 73

Balanced Design for Nine Products in Blocks of Three Units

Replication I		Replication II		Replication III		Replication IV	
Block	Products	Block	Products	Block	Products	Block	Products
1	1-2-3	4	1-4-7	7	1-5-9	10	3-5-7
2	4-5-6	5	2-5-8	8	4-8-3	11	6-8-1
3	7-8-9	6	3-6-9	9	7-6-2	12	9-4-2

fourth replication. This design belongs to the group known as balanced lattices, since the plan is conveniently written down by drawing a square lattice, with the product numbers at the intersections of the lines. In the balanced lattice there are k^2 products in blocks of k units, with $(k+1)$ replications.

In analyzing the results of such a design, one calculates for each product an estimated mean score, adjusted for the incomplete design. The value of t_j, the deviation of the estimated mean score of the jth product from the mean score of all products, is

$$t_j = \frac{kT_j - B_j}{k^2}$$

where T_j is the total score for the jth product, and B_j is the total of scores of all blocks containing the jth product.

The estimated mean score for the jth product is then

$$m + t_j$$

where m is the mean score for all products.

The steps in the analysis will be indicated for the balanced-lattice design of Table 73, in which 9 different brands of the same kind of canned fruit are being judged. Four judges score, on a 10-point scale, three brands at each of three sessions. In Table 74, the different brands are identified by the numbers in parentheses, and the other numbers represent assigned scores. Table 75 gives analysis of variance for Table

TABLE 74
Balanced Incomplete Block Design for Nine Brands in Blocks of Three

Block									Block total
				Replication I					
1		(1)	9	(2)	3	(3)	9		21
2		(4)	5	(5)	3	(6)	7		15
3		(7)	9	(8)	7	(9)	2		18
									54
				Replication II					
4		(1)	8	(4)	7	(7)	8		23
5		(2)	4	(5)	1	(8)	5		10
6		(3)	8	(6)	4	(9)	3		15
									48
				Replication III					
7		(1)	5	(5)	2	(9)	1		8
8		(4)	4	(8)	8	(3)	9		21
9		(7)	9	(6)	6	(2)	5		20
									49
				Replication IV					
10		(3)	7	(5)	3	(7)	9		19
11		(6)	8	(8)	7	(1)	7		22
12		(9)	2	(4)	2	(2)	2		6
									47

Brands	I	II	III	IV	$(1)^a$ T_j	$(2)^a$ B_j	$(3)^a$ $k^2 t_j$	$(4)^a$ t_j	$(5)^a$ $m + t_j$
1	9	8	5	7	29	74	13	1.44	6.94
2	3	4	5	2	14	57	−15	−1.67	3.83
3	9	8	9	7	33	76	23	2.56	8.06
4	5	7	4	2	18	65	−11	−1.22	4.28
5	3	1	2	3	9	52	−25	−2.78	2.72
6	7	4	6	8	25	72	3	0.33	5.83
7	9	8	9	9	35	80	25	2.78	8.28
8	7	5	8	7	27	71	10	1.11	6.61
9	2	3	1	2	8	47	−23	−2.56	2.94
Totals	54	48	49	47	198 = G	594 = $3G$	0	−0.01	
					$m = 198/36 = 5.50$				

[a] (1) = Total score for each brand.

(2) = Total of scores for all blocks containing brand j.

(3) = $k^2 t_j = k T_j - B_j$ or $9 t_j = 3 T_j - B_j$.

(4) = Adjustment t_j to general mean to give estimated mean score for each brand

(5) = Estimated mean score $(m + t_j)$ for each brand.

B_j for Brand 1: $B_j = 21 + 23 + 8 + 22 = 74$

Correction term $= 198^2/36 = 1089$

Total s.s. $= 9^2 + 3^2 + \ldots + 2^2 -$ c.t. $= 1342 - 1089 = 253$

Block s.s. $= (21^2 + 15^2 + \ldots + 6^2)/3 -$ c.t. $= 1210 - 1089 = 121$

Replication s.s. $= (54^2 + 48^2 + 49^2 + 47^2)/9 -$ c.t. $= 1092.22 - 1089 = 3.22$

Block in replication s.s. $= 121 - 3.22 = 117.78$

Brand s.s. (adj. for blocks) $= \dfrac{\Sigma(k^2 t_j)^2}{k^3} = \dfrac{13^2 + (-15)^2 + \ldots + (-23)^2}{3^3}$

$$= 2932/27 = 108.59$$

Error s.s. $= 253.00 - 121.00 - 108.59 = 253.00 - 229.59 = 23.41$

TABLE 75

Analysis of Variance for Data of Table 74

Source of variation	Degrees of freedom	Sum of squares	Mean square (variance)	F-value Calculated	F-value Tabular (5%)
Total	35	253.00			
Replications	3	3.22			
Blocks (in repl.)	8	117.78	14.72	10.1	2.59
Brands (adj.)	8	108.59	13.57	9.3	2.59
Error	16	23.41	1.46		

74. The efficiency factor $E = k/(k+1) = \frac{3}{4}$, and the standard error of an estimated brand mean is

$$s_{\bar{x}} = \sqrt{\frac{s_e^2}{(k+1)E}}$$
$$= \sqrt{0.49}$$
$$= 0.70$$

Using Duncan's multiple-range test, the shortest significant ranges at the 5% level are

p:	2	3	4	5	6	7	8	9
R_p:	2.10	2.20	2.26	2.31	2.34	2.36	2.37	2.39

Significant differences between means of brands are as indicated below, where means underlined by the same line are not significantly different.

2.72 2.94 3.83 4.28 5.83 6.61 6.94 8.06 8.28

The variance of the difference between two estimated mean scores is $2\,s_e^2/k$. If the data had been analyzed as a randomized complete-block design with $k+1$ replications (that is, $k+1$ complete blocks in which each brand appeared once), the corresponding variance would have been $2\,s^2/(k+1)$, where s^2 is the error variance in the randomized-block analysis. Therefore, the incomplete-block design provides a more accurate experiment than that for randomized blocks if, and only if,

$$\frac{s_e^2}{s^2} < \frac{k}{k+1} = E$$

the efficiency factor for the design.

The procedure for analyzing incomplete-block designs as described is based on the assumption that the blocks are fixed. If the block effects are assumed to be random, more efficient estimates of the treatment means can be obtained by utilizing the so-called recovery of inter-block information. This estimation procedure was first introduced by Yates (1940). For experiments with fewer than 15 degrees of freedom for estimating the block-effects variance, the method outlined is preferable.

One of the assumptions underlying the analysis of variance is that there be no correlation among the observations within a block other than that introduced by block and treatment effects. In tasting experiments, in which scores are assigned to the samples, there is indication that this assumption is not always met (Dove, 1943; Harrison and Elder, 1950; Hopkins, 1950; Boggs, 1951; Hanson et al., 1951). The score or rating assigned to a particular sample tends to depend upon the relative ratings of the other samples in the block. This effect of dependence on or correlation with other samples in the same block invalidates one of the assumptions underlying the analysis, and one would like some method of removing or accounting for this effect. Calvin (1954) has suggested an appropriate procedure, which, however, is applicable only to a special type of design known as a doubly balanced incomplete-block design. Such designs have balance for triplets as well as pairs of treatments. The mathematical model is similar to that for the ordinary incomplete-block design except for the addition of a correlation term.

Ferris (1957) recommended the use of a modified Latin square where it was desired to find differences between 5 or 6 samples by some form of scoring. His model permitted determination not only of the effect of treatment (or variety) but also as to differences in the effect of the after-taste. He found it particularly applicable to flavor and mouthfeel scoring. Calvin's procedure was better for color, uniformity, and characteristics that can be found by simultaneous inspection of all of the samples.

VII. Ranking Methods

Sometimes judges are required to rank products in order of merit instead of assigning to each a numerical measure of intrinsic worth. Ranking obviously does not supply as much information as scoring, since it gives no indication of the judge's opinion of the degree by which two products differ. On the other hand, in some experiments, ranking not only simplifies the procedure for the judges but in many cases furnishes as satisfactory an evaluation of differences as is needed. Judges may be selected on the basis of ability to rank correctly a given set of samples. Ura (1960b) discusses in detail a procedure for the selection of judges.

With n products ranked by two judges, Spearman's Rank Correlation Coefficient, defined as

$$R = 1 - \frac{6\Sigma d^2}{n^3 - n}$$

where Σd^2 is the sum of squares of the differences in rank, measures the agreement between the rankings assigned by the two judges. R may vary from a value of -1, indicating a complete reversal of ranking between the judges, to $+1$ representing perfect agreement. $R = 0$ indicates the ranks to be totally unrelated. Little reliability can be placed in a value of R determined from fewer than ten pairs of rankings. This places a limitation on the usefulness of the ranking procedure. Significance of a calculated R may be determined by comparing the value of t computed from

$$t = R\sqrt{\frac{n-2}{1-R^2}}$$

with $(n-2)$ d.f. with the required value from Table B in the Appendix. For example, suppose that two judges rank ten products as follows:

					Products					
	J	K	L	M	N	O	P	Q	R	S
Ranked by A	2	1	8	7	10	3	9	4	6	5
Ranked by B	3	2	5	9	10	1	8	4	6	7
Diff. in ranks										
d	1	1	-3	2	0	-2	-1	0	0	2
d^2	1	1	9	4	0	4	1	0	0	4	$\Sigma d^2 = 24$

Then
$$R = 1 - \frac{6(24)}{1000 - 10} = 0.854$$

and
$$t = 0.854\sqrt{\frac{8}{1 - 0.729}} = 4.64 \text{ (with 8 d.f.)}.$$

The tabular value of t for 8 degrees of freedom at the 1% level of significance is 3.36. Therefore, the agreement in ranking by the two judges is highly significant.

If the correct ranking is known according to some characteristic, this method may be employed to test whether an individual is really discriminating and would make an acceptable judge.

If the proper ranking is known, then the number of inversions of rank may be used as a criterion for determining the ability of a panel of judges to discriminate. If the series 1, 2, 3, . . . , n represents the proper order of ranking, then the number of inversions for any other series of rank orders is obtained by starting at the left, or beginning of the series, and proceeding to the right, taking each rank in turn and counting to the right of it the number of ranks that are smaller. For example, if the assigned order of ranking is 2, 1, 5, 3, 4, the number of inversions based on the order 1, 2, 3, 4, 5 is $1 + 0 + 2 + 0 + 0 = 3$, where the terms making up the total represent for each rank in order the number of ranks to the right which are smaller. If n objects can be arranged in all possible orders from 1 to n, and if the order 1, 2, 3, . . . , n is considered a standard order, then the frequency distribution of the number of inversions, X, of rank as measured from the standard order is a discrete, single-peaked, symmetrical distribution with mean $m = [n(n-1)]/4$ and variance $v = [n(n-1)(2n+5)]/72$. The value of

$$\chi^2 = \left[\Sigma X^2 - \frac{(\Sigma X)^2}{n} \right]/v$$

may be used to compare the consistency of the inversions with that of the population.

For example, ten persons are asked to arrange, in ascending order of sweetness, six glasses of orange juice to which various amounts of sugar have been added. Performance is to be measured by the number of inversions in order compared with the correct order. The ten inversion values are: 5, 4, 10, 1, 4, 6, 2, 3, 6, 4. Are these data consistent with the variance of the population, and is there any evidence of ability to discriminate?

The population mean and standard deviation are $m = 6(5)/4 = 7.5$ and $\sigma = \sqrt{6(5)(17)/72} = \sqrt{7.08} = 2.66$. Since $\Sigma X = 5 + 4 \ldots + 4 = 45$ and $\Sigma X^2 = (5)^2 + (4)^2 + \ldots + (4)^2 = 259$, $\chi^2 = [259 - (45)^2/10]/7.08 = 7.98$. For nine degrees of freedom, the tabular value of χ^2 at the 5% level of significance is 16.92. Therefore, the variance of the inversions is consistent with that of the population.

The distribution of inversions approximates a normal curve, and the probability of obtaining a sample mean as small as or smaller than

$\bar{X} = \Sigma X/n = 45/10 = 4.5$ from a population with mean 7.5 may be found by calculating the normal deviate $z = (\bar{X} - m)/\sigma_{\bar{x}} = (4.5 - 7.5)\ 0.84 = -3.57$. From Table A, areas under the normal curve, the probability of obtaining by chance a mean as small as or smaller than 4.5 is 0.0002, and one can infer that the ten judges are exhibiting an ability to discriminate between the sweetness of the samples.

In testing for significant agreement between the rankings assigned to n products by k judges, the data are arranged in an analysis-of-variance pattern, and a statistic, W, the coefficient of concordance, is calculated. The sampling distribution of W under the null hypothesis was investigated by Kendall (1948), who showed that W may be tested for significance by use of the F-distribution. For small values of k, continuity corrections are appropriate. The value of the coefficient of concordance, corrected for continuity, is given by

$$W = \frac{\text{product s.s.} - (1/k)}{\text{total s.s.} + (2/k)}$$

and

$$F = \frac{(k-1)W}{1-W}$$

with the appropriate degrees of freedom estimated from the expressions

degrees of freedom for numerator $= (n-1) - (2/k)$

degrees of freedom for denominator $= (k-1)[(n-1) - (2/k)]$.

For example, consider five wines ($n = 5$) ranked by four judges ($k = 4$). The results are shown in Table 76.

In Table F the value of F at the 5% level is estimated as 3.54. The calculated value is therefore not significant, and it may be concluded that the judges do not exhibit a noticeable degree of agreement in their ranking of the wines. It is not appropriate, therefore, to estimate an overall ranking for the wines based on the combined estimates of the judges.

For n greater than 7, an even simpler test, due to Friedman (1937), may be employed, since then the quantity $k(n-1)W$ is approximately distributed as χ^2 with $n-1$ degrees of freedom.

If a set of n samples has been ranked by a panel of k judges, Reimer (1957) has presented non-parametric methods for testing a subset of n' sample means selected from the n samples. In certain cases these may avoid incorrect applications of the t-test.

Although rank-order methods usually lead to simple calculations, they are frequently limited to tests of two treatments and can often be used to replace the t-test in sensory testing. A test of this type developed by Terry (1952) is a most powerful rank-order test where a t-test would have been appropriate if quantitative measures could have been obtained. His test depends upon order statistics resulting from the transformation of ranks by the use of tables by Fisher and Yates (1953). The same transformation is used in taste-testing problems when ranks are employed in analysis of variance.

Kramer (1960) presents a simple and rapid method of determining whether a product being tested is significantly different from a group of

TABLE 76

Data for Five Wines Ranked by Four Judges

| Judges | Rank of wines | | | | | |
	X	Y	Z	U	V	
A	4	2	3	5	1	
B	3	4	1	5	2	
C	1	2	4	5	3	
D	5	3	2	4	1	
Totals	13	11	10	19	7	60

Correction term $= 60^2/20 = 180$
Products s.s. $= (13^2 + 11^2 + \ldots + 7^2)/4 - $ c.t. $= 200 - 180 = 20$
Total s.s. $= 4(1^2 + 2^2 + 3^2 + 4^2 + 5^2) - $ c.t. $= 220 - 180 = 40$
Then　　$W = (20 - 1/4)/(40 + 2/4) = 19.75/40.5 = 0.488$
and　　$F = 3(0.488)/(1 - 0.488) = 1.464/0.512 = 2.86$
with　　$[(5 - 1) - 2/4 = 3.5]$ degrees of freedom for numerator,
and　　$[3(3.5) = 10.5]$ degrees of freedom for denominator.

similar products on the basis of rankings assigned by a group of panelists. His method also permits detection of interactions between products and panelists.

The original tables provided are in error, but Kramer (1963) has supplied corrected tables, which are reproduced in the Appendix as Table I. Applying Kramer's procedure to the data of Table 76, for 4 judges (replications) and 5 products, we find from Table I at the 5% level, the entries 6–18 and 7–17. The first pair of numbers indicates the limits outside of which rank totals must fall to indicate significant differences. Since the rank total 19 for wine U exceeds 18, significant differences are indicated. The second entry pair is used to determine significance between individual wines. The high rank total of wine U indicates that it is ranked significantly inferior to the other wines. This rapid method has led to slightly different conclusions than the longer, more accurate method, which indicated no significant differences. The method does provide, however, a fast and fairly accurate procedure of comparison.

A. PAIRED COMPARISONS

The method of paired comparisons may be considered as a special rank-order technique. In this procedure, only two treatments need be considered at one time, and only quantitative decisions are required. The design becomes somewhat cumbersome if many items are compared. Bradley and Terry (1952), Terry *et al.* (1952), Bradley (1954a,b, 1955), Mosteller (1951a,b), and Bock and Jones (1963) have presented flexible methods of analysis for the detection of treatment differences, and the results of several judges may be combined without the requirement of uniformity of ranking judgments for the judges. Bradley and Terry (1952) and Bradley (1954b) have supplied extensive tables for easy application of the method.

Scheffé (1952) used a scoring method and the analysis of variance. The effect of order of presentation of paired samples is taken into account. Main effects are defined for the brands under consideration. The method uses the hypothesis of subtractivity, which states, roughly, that the results for any pair, after order effects are eliminated, can be attributed entirely to the difference of the main effects of the two brands in the pair. Significance tests are given for the main effects, for the order effects, and for the hypothesis of subtractivity, as well as estimates of various parameters and their standard errors. The main effects are analyzed by considering all possible comparisons.

Gridgeman (1959a) has described a probabilistic model for dichotomous sensory sorting, covering many experimental designs including the simplest pair comparison.

A number of nonparametric tests based on ranks have been proposed for the comparison of treatments in a completely random design. The Wilcoxin-Mann-Whitney test, developed by Wilcoxin (1945) and Mann and Whitney (1947), is basically a two-sample test with a per-comparison error rate. Kruskal and Wallis (1952) proposed a rank test which is an analog of Snedecor's *F*-test. This test provides evidence concerning the presence of real differences but is of limited use in locating them. Steel (1959, 1960) presented rank tests for comparing treatments with a control for all pairwise comparisons. Both of these tests use experimentwise error rates. Pfanzagl (1959), as part of a more general theory, has devised a two-step nonparametric decision process, based on ranks, for testing the null hypothesis that k samples come from the same population and, if this is rejected, for deciding which one of the samples comes from a different population. No tables are given, but it is suggested that they might be obtained by random sampling.

Steel (1961) discussed rank tests and presented tables for an all-pairs-of-treatments test with an experiment-wise error rate. He explained use of the tables for a fixed-rank sum test, an analog of Tukey's W-procedure, and for two multiple-rank sum tests, analogs of the Newman-Keuls procedure.

Gridgeman (1959b) provided a probabilistic model for pair comparisons, in various experimental settings, and with and without admission of ties. When discrimination is the objective, they should be admitted. Glenn and David (1960) discussed the question of ties in paired-comparison experiments. They included a good discussion of the whole question of paired comparisons.

Where paired comparisons between several products are made, instead of comparing each pair by use of χ^2 and then examining all the data simultaneously to arrive at general conclusions for the entire set, Terry et al. (1952) developed an improved method which takes into account indirect as well as direct comparisons. Their procedure is limited to equal numbers of judgments for each pair. More recently, Dykstra (1960a,b) improved the method to apply to paired comparisons that use unequal repetitions on pairs.

Pendergrass and Bradley (1960) developed a method of triple-comparison testing. Park (1961) evaluated this procedure by contrasting with it the results obtained with paired comparisons. From the results he has concluded that the model on which the triple-comparison analysis is based will prove appropriate to at least a proportion of sensory tests. In those cases where sensory fatigue is not a factor, the method may afford a valuable gain in efficiency over paired comparisons.

VIII. Consumer Preference

Baker et al. (1961a) and Nelson et al. (1963) noted wide variations in the responses of individuals in sensory tests and concluded that preference depends not only on the particular character examined but also on every circumstance surrounding and involved in the evaluation. Sometimes consumer preference testing is conducted in the laboratory under rigidly controlled conditions with trained observers who frequently prefer the same differences. Such testing may bear little relation to general consumer reaction.

Ough and Baker (1961), using a small panel for wine tasting, found that the scores of some tasters had error variances not homogeneous with those of the rest of the taste panel and that the preference patterns of some tasters were distinctly different from those of the main group of qualified tasters.

To obtain a measure of consumer reaction or preference for one sample over another, a large number of panelists is therefore desirable. These panelists not only need not, but should not, be trained, and should be selected at random from the population to be sampled. Sometimes the panelist is asked merely to indicate the sample which he prefers or to state whether he considers it acceptable or not acceptable. In other cases he is asked to indicate intensity of preference for various samples. Such surveys are frequently designed to include more than one criterion of classification, such as men and women evaluating two different products, scoring the same products at different times, or men and women indicating preferences for several products at different times. When two criteria of classification are involved, the data can be arranged in a table with two rows and two columns, known as a 2×2 contingency table. If the table has j rows and k columns, it is known as a $j \times k$ contingency table. The χ^2 distribution with $(j - 1)(k - 1)$ degrees of freedom may be used to investigate whether a relationship exists between the criteria of classification or whether they are independent. As previously indicated, when χ^2 involves only one degree of freedom, an adjusted value should be used. It is calculated from

$$\text{Adj. } \chi^2 = \Sigma \frac{(|f_o - f_e| - \frac{1}{2})^2}{f_e}$$

where $|f_o - f_e|$ is the absolute or positive value of the difference.

For example, 109 people are given paired samples of two brands, A and B, of peanut brittle, and are asked to indicate which brand they prefer. Of the 109, 41 taste the samples in the morning and 68 in the afternoon. Does the time of day affect the indicated preferences? Distribution of preferences for brand and time of day are shown in the following 2×2 contingency table.

Time of day	Preferences		Totals
	Brand A	Brand B	
Morning	11 (6.0)	30 (35.0)	41
Afternoon	5 (10.0)	63 (58.0)	68
Totals	16	93	109

On the basis of the hypothesis that preference and time of day are independent, one would expect the ratio of preferences for Brand A in

TABLE 77

Two Brands of Peanut Brittle Scored by Men and Women at Two Different Times and in Different Orders of Presentation

		Frequency of response																		
		Morning								Afternoon								Totals		
		Male				Female				Male				Female						
		A		B		A		B		A		B		A		B				
	X	f_A	f_B	f_B	f_A	f_A	f_B	f_B	f_A	f_A	f_B	f_B	f_A	f_A	f_B	f_B	f_A	f_A	f_B	f_{A+B}
Like extremely	9	3	8	3	0	2	14	7	0	1	4	4	0	0	15	24	1	7	79	86
Like very much	8	4	7	10	5	4	7	10	8	3	12	8	2	10	18	18	12	48	90	138
Like moderately	7	9	0	6	2	9	1	6	4	9	3	5	5	9	3	3	16	69	22	91
Like slightly	6	1	4	1	0	4	1	2	2	1	0	1	6	14	2	7	7	35	11	46
Neither like nor dislike	5	0	0	3	1	3	0	0	3	2	0	0	0	5	1	0	4	18	1	19
Dislike slightly	4	2	1	2	2	2	1	0	4	2	0	0	0	3	2	0	7	22	5	27
Dislike moderately	3	0	0	0	0	0	0	0	0	2	0	0	0	0	0	0	2	6	0	6
Dislike very much	2	1	0	0	1	0	0	0	0	0	0	0	0	0	0	1	0	1	0	1
Dislike extremely	1	2	0	0	2	0	0	0	0	0	0	0	0	0	0	0	0	2	0	2
Totals		19	19	17	17	24	24	23	23	20	20	15	15	41	41	49	49	208	208	416

the morning to all preferences in the morning to be the same as the ratio of preferences for Brand A in the afternoon to all preferences in the afternoon, and also the same as the ratio of all preferences for Brand A to the total of all preferences for A and B. The same types of ratio would apply to Brand B. On this basis, if a is the number of preferences for Brand A in the morning, then

$$a:41 = 16:109$$

from which $a = 6.0$. After the expected value in one cell of a 2×2 table has been determined, the remaining cell frequencies may be found most easily by subtracting the calculated value from the marginal totals. In the foregoing table, the expected cell frequencies are shown in parentheses. Then

$$\begin{aligned}
\text{Adj. } \chi^2 &= \frac{(4.5)^2}{6.0} + \frac{(4.5)^2}{35.0} + \frac{(4.5)^2}{10.0} + \frac{(4.5)^2}{58.0} \\
&= 3.38 + 0.58 + 2.02 + 0.35 \\
&= 6.33
\end{aligned}$$

Since for a 2×2 table the number of degrees of freedom is one, at the 5% level the tabular value of χ^2 is 3.84. Since the calculated value of χ^2 exceeds the expected value, one concludes that time of day and preference are not independent. It would appear that the preference for Brand B is relatively greater in the afternoon.

In consumer surveys where several factors are being studied and hedonic scoring has been used, consecutive integral scores are usually assigned to increasing hedonic categories. Analysis of variance is then applied to the numerical scores in determining significance of differences.

For example, 36 male and 47 female students scored each of two brands, A and B, of peanut brittle in different orders in both morning and afternoon. The scoring was done on a hedonic scale ranging from "dislike extremely" to "like extremely." This hedonic scale is converted to numerical scores by assigning a score of 1 to the category "dislike extremely" and increasing integral values with, finally, a score of 9 assigned to the category "like extremely." Table 77 records the data, and Table 78 shows the frequencies of response when all four criteria— brand, order, sex, and time—are paired in all possible ways. In each case, all but the paired criteria are disregarded. Table 79 gives analysis of variance for Table 78.

Only the F-values for the time $\times$ order interaction and for brands are significant. Therefore, the average score for Brand B is significantly better than that for Brand A.

TABLE 78

Frequencies of Response for Paired Criteria of Classification in Pairs

Score X	Brand and sex				Brand and time				Brand and order			
	Male		Female		A.M.		P.M.		A–B		B–A	
	A	B	A	B	A	B	A	B	A	B	A	B
9	4	19	3	60	5	32	2	47	6	41	1	38
8	14	37	34	53	21	34	27	56	21	44	27	46
7	29	7	40	15	30	7	39	15	36	7	33	15
6	8	6	27	5	7	8	28	3	20	7	15	4
5	3	0	15	1	7	0	11	1	10	1	8	0
4	6	2	16	3	10	2	12	3	9	4	13	1
3	4	0	2	0	0	0	6	0	2	0	4	0
2	1	0	0	0	1	0	0	0	0	0	1	0
1	2	0	0	0	2	0	0	0	0	0	2	0
Σf	71	71	137	137	83	83	125	125	104	104	104	104
	142		274		166		250		208		208	
ΣfX	454	560	886	1116	544	665	796	1011	686	833	654	843
	1014		2002		1209		1807		1519		1497	

Score X	Sex and time				Sex and order				Time and order			
	Male		Female		Male		Female		A.M.		P.M.	
	A.M.	P.M.	A.M.	P.M.	A–B	B–A	A–B	B–A	A–B	B–A	A–B	B–A
9	14	9	23	40	16	7	31	32	27	10	20	29
8	26	25	29	58	26	25	39	48	22	33	43	40
7	17	19	20	35	21	15	22	33	19	18	24	30
6	6	8	9	23	6	8	21	11	10	5	17	14
5	1	2	6	10	2	1	9	7	3	4	8	4
4	5	3	7	12	5	3	8	11	5	7	8	7
3	0	4	0	2	2	2	0	2	0	0	2	4
2	1	0	0	0	0	1	0	0	0	1	0	0
1	2	0	0	0	0	2	0	0	0	2	0	0
Σf	72	70	94	180	78	64	130	144	86	80	122	128
	142		274		142		274		166		250	
ΣfX	518	496	691	1311	571	443	948	1054	647	562	872	935
	1014		2002		1014		2002		1209		1807	

Correction term $= \dfrac{(f\Sigma_{A+B}X)^2}{\Sigma f_{A+B}} = \dfrac{86(9) + 138(8) + \ldots + 2(1)^2}{416} = \dfrac{(3016)^2}{416} = 21{,}866.00$

Total s.s. $= \Sigma f_{A+B}X^2 - $ c.t. $= 22{,}880.00 - 21{,}866.00 = 1014.00$

Brand s.s. $= \dfrac{(1340)^2 + (1676)^2}{208} - $ c.t. $= 22{,}137.38 - 21{,}866.00 = 271.38$

TABLE 78 (*continued*)

Sex s.s. $= \dfrac{(1014)^2}{142} + \dfrac{(2002)^2}{274} - $ c.t. $= 7,240.82 + 14,627.75 - 21,866.00 = 2.57$

Time s.s. $= \dfrac{(1209)^2}{166} + \dfrac{(1807)^2}{250} - $ c.t. $= 8,805.31 + 13,061.00 - 21,866.00 = 0.31$

Order s.s. $= \dfrac{(1519)^2 + (1497)^2}{208} - $ c.t. $= 21,867.16 - 21,866.00 = 1.16$

Interactions:

Brand $\times$ sex s.s. $= \dfrac{(454)^2 + (560)^2}{71} + \dfrac{(886)^2 + (1116)^2}{137} - $ c.t. $-$ Brand s.s. $-$ Sex s.s.
$$= 7,319.94 + 14,820.82 - 21,866.00 - 271.38 - 2.57 = 0.81$$

Brand $\times$ time s.s. $= \dfrac{(544)^2 + (665)^2}{83} + \dfrac{(796)^2 + (1011)^2}{125} - $ c.t. $-$ Brand s.s. $-$ Time s.s.
$$= 8,893.51 + 13,245.90 - 21,866.00 - 271.38 - 0.31 = 1.72$$

Brand $\times$ order s.s. $= \dfrac{(686)^2 + (833)^2}{104} + \dfrac{(654)^2 + (843)^2}{104} - $ c.t. $-$ Brand s.s. $-$ Order s.s.
$$= 22,142.79 - 21,866.00 - 271.38 - 1.16 = 4.25$$

Sex $\times$ time s.s. $= \dfrac{(518)^2}{72} + \dfrac{(496)^2}{70} + \dfrac{(691)^2}{94} + \dfrac{(1311)^2}{180} - $ c.t. $-$ Sex s.s. $-$ Time s.s.
$$= 21,869.27 - 21,866.00 - 2.57 - 0.31 = 0.39$$

Sex $\times$ order s.s. $= \dfrac{(571)^2}{78} + \dfrac{(443)^2}{64} + \dfrac{(948)^2}{130} + \dfrac{(1054)^2}{144} - $ c.t. $-$ Sex s.s. $-$ Order s.s.
$$= 21,874.20 - 21,866.00 - 2.57 - 1.16 = 4.47$$

Time $\times$ order s.s. $= \dfrac{(647)^2}{86} + \dfrac{(562)^2}{80} + \dfrac{(872)^2}{122} + \dfrac{(935)^2}{128} - $ c.t. $-$ Time s.s. $-$ Order s.s.
$$= 21,878.14 - 21,866.00 - 0.31 - 1.16 = 10.67$$

Remainder (error) s.s. $= $ Total s.s. $-$ all other s.s.
$$= 1014.00 - 297.73 = 716.27$$

TABLE 79
Analysis of Variance for Data of Table 78

Source of variation	Degrees of freedom	Sum of squares	Mean square (variance)	F-value Calculated	F-value Tabular (5%)
Total	415	1014.00			
Brand	1	271.38	271.38	153.32	3.86
Sex	1	2.57	2.57	1.45	
Time of day	1	0.31	0.31		
Order of presentation	1	1.16	1.16		
Brand $\times$ sex	1	0.81	0.81		
Brand $\times$ time	1	1.72	1.72		
Brand $\times$ order	1	4.25	4.25	2.40	3.86
Sex $\times$ time	1	0.39	0.39		
Sex $\times$ order	1	4.47	4.47	2.53	3.86
Time $\times$ order	1	10.67	10.67	6.03	3.86
Remainder (error)	405	716.27	1.77		

Pilgrim and Wood (1955), employing the paired-comparison method and rating by a 9-interval hedonic scale, tested consumer preference for 12 pairs of foods. They found both methods equally sensitive whether the difference in preference was small or large.

Anderson (1959) used a test for the case of r varieties ranked by n consumers. The numbers of consumers ranking each variety were recorded in an $r \times r$ contingency table, with ranks as one classification and varieties as the other. This is not the usual contingency table, with fixed border totals, since repeated sampling is not a random arrangement of rn items, subject to the border restrictions. Each of the n consumers acts independently, with a limited number of preference sequences.

IX. Correlation and Regression

Suppose that X and Y represent two related variables for which n pairs of values are known. These n pairs of values X and Y can be plotted as points on a rectangular coordinate system. If the points of the resulting scatter diagram appear to follow a linear trend, a straight line, $Y' = a + bX$, can be fitted to the points, where b is the slope of the line and a is the Y-intercept. Values of a and b uniquely determine a line, and the problem, then, is to find values for them such that the line will "fit" the points. One such line of "best fit" has values a and b determined by the method of least squares, so that the sum of the squares of the vertical distances from the line to the given points is smaller than for any other straight line for which the slope is not equal to b, that is, $\Sigma(Y - Y')^2 = $ a minimum, where for any value of X, Y represents the observed value, and Y' is the corresponding value on the line. This minimizing process results in a pair of normal equations,

$$an + b\Sigma X = \Sigma Y$$
$$a\Sigma X + b\Sigma X^2 = \Sigma XY$$

from which

$$b = \frac{\Sigma XY - (\Sigma X \Sigma Y/n)}{\Sigma X^2 - [(\Sigma X)^2/n]} = \frac{\Sigma xy}{\Sigma x^2}$$

and

$$a = \bar{Y} - b\bar{X}$$

where $x = X - \bar{X}$ and $y = Y - \bar{Y}$.

For any value of X the corresponding value of Y can be estimated from the regression equation.

An unbiased estimate of the true variance about a regression line is given by the ratio $\Sigma(Y - Y')^2/(n - 2)$. Its square root is called the standard error of estimate, or the standard deviation of Y for fixed X, and has the value S.E. $= \sqrt{[\Sigma(Y - Y')^2/(n - 2)]}$.

The calculations involved in finding the equation of the regression line and the standard error of estimate will be illustrated with data collected by Baker *et al.* (1958). In a paired test to establish the difference for ten different concentrations of tartaric acid, 24 tasters participated, and the percent of correct classifications in 15 trials is shown in Table 80, together with the corresponding concentration numbers, which

TABLE 80

Concentration and Corresponding Number of Correct Identifications

| Concentration no. | % Correct identifications | | X^2 | Y^2 | XY | Y' | $(Y - Y')$ | $(Y - Y')^2$ |
	X	Y						
1/8	1	58	1	3364	58	59.18	−1.18	1.3924
1/4	2	69	4	4761	138	67.24	1.76	3.0976
1/2	3	76	9	5776	228	75.30	0.70	0.4900
1	4	81	16	6561	324	83.36	−2.36	5.5696
2	5	93	25	8649	465	91.42	1.58	2.4964
4	6	99	36	9801	594	99.48	−0.48	0.2304
	21	476	91	38912	1807			13.2764

are logarithmic and are proportional to the logarithms of the concentrations and constitute a linear scale. All values necessary in the calculations are shown in the table. From the table

$$b = \frac{1807 - [(21)(476)/6]}{91 - [(21)(21)/6]} = 8.06$$

and

$$a = \frac{476}{6} - (8.06)\frac{21}{6} = 51.12$$

and the equation expressing the percent of correct identifications in terms of X which is related to the logarithm of the concentration is

$$Y' = 51.12 + 8.06\,X.$$

The regression line and scatter diagram are shown in Fig. 85.

The closeness of fit of the regression line to the points is indicated by the small value of the standard error of estimate, S.E. $= \sqrt{13.2764/4}$ $= 1.82$. Approximately ⅔ of the points are within 1.82 units vertically of the regression line.

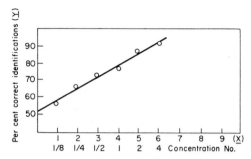

FIG. 85. Line of regression and scatter diagram for percent identifications and concentration of tartaric acid related to a logarithmic scale.

The coefficient of correlation r is also a measure of the linear relationship between pairs of values X and Y, and is written

$$r = \frac{\Sigma xy}{\sqrt{\Sigma x^2 \Sigma y^2}} = \frac{\Sigma XY - [(\Sigma X)(\Sigma Y)/n]}{\sqrt{\left[\Sigma X^2 - \frac{(\Sigma X)^2}{n}\right]\left[\Sigma Y^2 - \frac{(\Sigma Y)^2}{n}\right]}}.$$

The correlation coefficient ranges in value between -1 and $+1$. The value $r = 0$ indicates no correlation, or independence as far as a linear relationship existing between the values of X and Y, and $r = \pm 1$ represents perfect correlation with all points on a straight line.

From the data of Table 80,

$$r = \frac{1807 - [21(476)/6]}{\sqrt{\left[91 - \frac{(21)^2}{6}\right]\left[38912 - \frac{(476)^2}{6}\right]}} = 0.994.$$

This calculated value is very near 1 and indicates that the pairs of values when plotted fall very close to the regression line shown in Fig. 85, indicating that the number of correct identifications increased linearly with increasing concentration.

The significance of any value of r may be determined by calculating

$$t = \frac{r}{\sqrt{(1 - r^2)/(n - 2)}}$$

and comparing the calculated value with the tabular value based on $n - 2$ degrees of freedom.

The coefficient of determination, r^2, represents the proportion of the total variation in Y which is due to the linear relationship existing between X and Y. Then, $r = 0.70$ indicates that only 49% of the variation of $\Sigma(Y - \bar{Y})^2$ is accounted for in terms of the regression of Y on X.

This leaves 51% as the proportion of $\Sigma(Y - \bar{Y})^2$ that is independent of the regression. Usually little or no meaning should be attached to values of r that are less than 0.60 unless determined from an extremely large number of pairs of values. Conclusions based on coefficients of correlation determined from only a few pairs of points may also prove unreliable.

If the value of r indicates no linear relationship between the variables X and Y, the possibility remains that some other type of relation may exist. The scatter diagram might, for example, indicate a polynomial relation of the form

$$Y' = a + bX + cX^2.$$

The normal equations for determining the numerical values of a, b, and c are

$$an + b\Sigma X + c\Sigma X^2 = \Sigma Y$$
$$a\Sigma X + b\Sigma X^2 + c\Sigma X^3 = \Sigma XY$$
$$a\Sigma X^2 + b\Sigma X^3 + c\Sigma X^4 = \Sigma X^2 Y.$$

It is evident how normal equations for polynomials of higher order may be built up. Ezekiel and Fox (1959) listed equations for various types of curves and discussed all phases of curvilinear correlation.

If Y depends upon two independent variables, X_1 and X_2, and the relationship is linear, it may be written

$$Y' = a + b_1 X_1 + b_2 X_2$$

and the resulting normal equations are

$$na + b_1\Sigma X_1 + b_2\Sigma X_2 = \Sigma Y$$
$$a\Sigma X_1 + b_1\Sigma X_1^2 + b_2\Sigma X_1 X_2 = \Sigma X_1 y$$
$$a\Sigma X_2 + b_1\Sigma X_1 X_2 + b_2\Sigma X_2^2 = \Sigma X_2 y.$$

It is evident how the procedure may be extended to more independent variables.

The degree of linear relationship between a dependent variable and two independent variables may be measured by the coefficient of linear multiple correlation, R, where

$$R = \sqrt{\frac{r_{y1}^2 + r_{y2}^2 - 2r_{y1}r_{y2}r_{12}}{1 - r_{12}^2}}$$

and the small r's represent the linear coefficients of correlation of pairs of variables as indicated by the subscripts. The closer R is to 1, the better the linear relationship and the closer the points are to a plane. $R = 0$, as before, indicates no linear relationship.

Kramer and Twigg (1962) note the value of regression equations between visual and objective readings. Simple or multiple correlations may be calculated between the visual score and various objective scores. The relative importance of each objective score on the subjective judgment may be determined. Furthermore, simple and multiple linear or curvilinear equations can be computed and used to construct nomograms for routine calculations.

A. FACTOR ANALYSIS

Systematically planned studies require some knowledge of the main variables of importance. Frequently, in an exploratory stage, this state of affairs has not been reached, and a procedure known as factor analysis may sometimes be employed to isolate the main variables. In applying the procedure to a multivariate complex of variables, $X_1, X_2, X_3, \ldots,$ X_k, an underlying set of variables, $Z_1, Z_2, Z_3, \ldots, Z_p$, with $p < k$, is assumed such that each X is a linear function of the Z's, together with a part, S, specific to itself, that is,

$$X_i = a_{i1}Z_1 + a_{i2}Z_2 + \ldots + a_{ip}Z_p + S_i.$$

Factor analysis is the name given to the technique for estimating the various parameters in a model of this kind. It is a statistical method originally invented and developed primarily by psychologists to study the human mind. The method has been discussed, and the procedure outlined, by Holzinger and Harman (1941), Thurstone (1947), and Cattell (1952). Baker (1954) used the procedure with limited data in an attempt to estimate the quality ratings of wines on the basis of non-sensory tests. Harper (1956) also discussed factor analysis as a technique for examining complex data on foodstuffs, and applied the procedure in a study to Cheshire cheeses. In cases where the distribution of judges' scores are bimodal with different variances, the usual mathematical models for the analysis of data for paired comparisons cannot easily be used. Baker et al. (1961b) illustrated the use of factor analysis in this case.

The method requires assumption of normality of the original measures to justify use of the product-moment correlation technique. Further steps in the analysis are based upon the assumption of a number of linear relationships the effects of which can be added together in a simple manner. Unfortunately, in food evaluation studies the validity of such assumptions is sometimes doubtful. All forms of multivariate analysis tend to be time-consuming, and factor analysis is especially so since the computational procedure involves successive approximations obtained by repeating the entire procedure each time. Electronic computers are proving very useful in carrying out the long and tedious computations required.

B. Response-Surface Procedure

The determination in food products of the proportions of various ingredients which will result in a maximum panel score is important and can be of great value in the food industry. Box and Wilson (1951) developed a response-surface method for exploring functional relationships between variables. Pearson *et al.* (1962) applied the method in determining the optimum levels of various food ingredients (salt and sugar in cured ham) for obtaining maximum panel scores.

Suppose that panel response Y' is related to variable amounts of two ingredients, X_1 and X_2. The data are fitted to the surface equation

$$Y' = a + bX_1 + cX_2 + dX_1^2 + eX_2^2 + fX_1X_2.$$

The coefficients b and c are called linear effects, d and e quadratic effects, and f the interaction effect. The method of least squares is employed in evaluating these coefficients and the constant term. Values of X_1 and X_2 can be found which will lead to a maximum score, Y'. Electronic computers can be of great value in exploring such functional relationships. The method is discussed by Box (1954) and Box and Hunter (1957), besides the references already cited.

X. Summary

The methods and experimental designs discussed so briefly have direct application and frequent use in sensory analysis. They represent, however, only a portion of the various techniques which are available, and many specialized statistical treatments have been developed for use in particular situations. Most of the methods presented are generally simple and basic and require a minimum of computation. Byer (1964) points out possible flaws in sensory testing situations and cautions against over-complicating the statistical procedures.

The great variability displayed by trained as well as untrained participants in sensory testing causes one to question the necessity for elaborate and highly refined statistical procedures, the results of which can be no more reliable than the data upon which they are based.

The statistical procedures adopted in any situation should be those for which the desired standard of accuracy can be attained with the least expenditure of time, effort, and money. An involved experimental plan or a highly refined technique has no special merit if, in some other way, equally valid and accurate results can be obtained with less effort. In general, one should use the simplest experimental design which will assure the desired accuracy. Sometimes, however, no simple procedure exists and one is obliged to use one of the more complex designs.

REFERENCES

Anderson, R. L. 1959. Use of contingency tables in the analysis of consumer preference studies. *Biometrics* 15, 582–590.

Baker, G. A. 1954. Organoleptic ratings and analytical data for wines analyzed into orthogonal factors. *Food Research* 19, 575–580.

Baker, G. A., M. A. Amerine, and E. B. Roessler. 1954. Errors of the second kind in organoleptic difference testing. *Food Research* 19, 206–210.

Baker, G. A., V. Mrak, and M. A. Amerine. 1958. Errors of the second kind in an acid threshold test. *Food Research* 23, 150–154.

Baker, G. A., M. A. Amerine, and D. E. Kester. 1961a. Dependency of almond preference on consumer category and type of experiment. *J. Food Sci.* 26, 377–385.

Baker, G. A., M. A. Amerine, and R. M. Pangborn. 1961b. Factor analysis applied to paired preferences among four grape juices. *J. Food Sci.* 26, 644–647.

Bartlett, M. S. 1936. Square-root transformation in analysis of variance. *J. Roy. Statist. Soc.* B3, 68–78.

Bartlett, M. S. 1937. Some examples of statistical methods of research in agriculture and applied biology. *J. Roy. Statist. Soc. Suppl.* 4, 137–183.

Bartlett, M. S. 1947. The use of transformations. *Biometrics* 3, 39–52.

Bennett, C. A., and N. L. Franklin. 1954. "Statistical Analysis in Chemistry and the Chemical Industry," 724 pp. (see chaps. 10 and 11). Wiley, New York.

Berg, H. W., F. Filipello, E. Hinreiner, and F. M. Sawyer. 1955. Consumer wine-preference methodology studies at California fairs. *Food Technol.* 9, 90–93.

Bliss, C. I. 1937. The analysis of field experimental data expressed in percentages. *Plant Protection (Leningrad)* 12, 67–77.

Bock, R. D., and L. V. Jones. 1963. "The Measurement and Prediction of Judgmental Response: Statistical Methods," 330 pp. The Psychometric Laboratory, University of North Carolina, Chapel Hill, North Carolina.

Boggs, M. 1951. Proceedings of conference on sensory methods for measuring differences in food quality. *U. S. Dept. Agr. Inform. Bull.* 34, 1–134 (see pp. 94–95).

Box, G. E. P. 1954. The exploration and exploitation of response surfaces. *Biometrics* 10, 16–61.

Box, G. E. P., and J. S. Hunter. 1957. Multifactor experimental designs for exploring response surfaces. *Ann. Math. Statistics* 28, 195–241.

Box, G. E. P., and K. P. Wilson. 1951. On the experimental attainment of optimum conditions. *J. Royal Statist. Soc.* B13, 1–45.

Bradley, R. A. 1953. Some statistical methods in taste testing and quality evaluation. *Biometrics* 9, 22–38.

Bradley, R. A. 1954a. Incomplete block rank analysis: On the appropriateness of the model for a method of paired comparisons. *Biometrics* 10, 375–390.

Bradley, R. A. 1954b. Rank analysis of incomplete block designs. II. Additional tables for the method of paired comparisons. *Biometrika* 41, 502–537.

Bradley, R. A. 1955. Rank analysis of incomplete block designs. III. Some large sample results on estimation and power for a method of paired comparisons. *Biometrika* 42, 450–470.

Bradley, R. A., and M. E. Terry. 1952. Rank analysis of incomplete block designs. I. The method of paired comparisons. *Biometrika* 39, 324–345.

Byer, A. J. 1964. Looking askance at statistical sensory testing. *Food Technol.* 18(11), 59–64.

Calvin, L. D. 1954. Doubly balanced incomplete block designs for experiments in which the treatment effects are correlated. *Biometrics* 10, 61–88.

Cattell, R. B. 1952. "Factor Analysis," 462 pp. Harper, New York.

Cochran, W. G., and G. M. Cox. 1957. "Experimental Designs," 2nd ed., 611 pp. Wiley, New York.

Davis, J. G., and H. L. Hanson. 1954. Sensory test methods. The triangle intensity and related test systems for sensory analysis. *Food Technol.* 8, 335–339.

Dove, W. F. 1943. The relative nature of human preference: with an example in the palatability of different varieties of sweet corn. *J. Comp. Psychol.* 35, 219–226.

Duncan, D. B. 1955. Multiple range and multiple F tests. *Biometrics* 11, 1–42.

Dykstra, O., Jr. 1960a. A note on the analysis of consumer preference data. *Food Technol.* 14, 314–315.

Dykstra, O., Jr. 1960b. Rank analysis of incomplete block designs: a method of paired comparisons employing unequal repetitions on pairs. *Biometrics* 16, 176–188.

Ezekiel, M., and K. A. Fox. 1959. "Methods of Correlation and Regression Analysis, Linear and Curvilinear," 3rd ed., 548 pp. Wiley, New York.

Ferris, G. E. 1957. A modified Latin square design for taste testing. *Food Research* 22, 251–258.

Filipello, F. 1956. Factors in the analysis of mass panel wine-preference data. *Food Technol.* 10, 321–326.

Fisher, R. A., and F. Yates. 1953. "Statistical Tables for Biological, Agricultural and Medical Research," 4th ed., 126 pp. Hafner Publ. Co., New York.

Friedman, M. 1937. The use of ranks to avoid the assumption of normality implicit in the analysis of variance. *J. Am. Statist. Assoc.* 32, 675–701.

Glenn, W. A., and H. A. David. 1960. Ties in paired-comparison experiments using a modified Thurstone-Mosteller model. *Biometrics* 16, 86–109.

Gridgeman, N. T. 1955. Taste comparisons: two samples or three? *Food Technol.* 9, 148–150.

Gridgeman, N. T. 1959a. Sensory item sorting. *Biometrics* 15, 298–306.

Gridgeman, N. T. 1959b. Pair comparison, with and without ties. *Biometrics* 15, 382–388.

Hanson, H. L., L. Kline, and H. Lineweaver. 1951. Application of balanced incomplete block design to scoring of ten dried egg samples. *Food Technol.* 5, 9–13.

Harper, R. 1956. Factor analysis as a technique for examining complex data on foodstuffs. *Appl. Statistics* 5, 32–48.

Harries, J. M. 1956. Positional bias in sensory assessments. *Food Technol.* 10, 86–90.

Harrison, S., and L. W. Elder. 1950. Some application of statistics to laboratory taste testing. *Food Technol.* 4, 434–439.

Harter, H. L. 1960. Critical values for Duncan's new multiple range test. *Biometrics* 16, 671–685.

Harter, H. L. 1961. Corrected error rates for Duncan's new multiple range test. *Biometrics* 17, 321–324.

Holzinger, K. J., and H. H. Harman. 1941. "Factor Analysis," 417 pp. Univ. of Chicago Press, Chicago, Illinois.

Hopkins, J. W. 1950. A procedure for quantifying subjective appraisals of odor, flavor and texture of foodstuffs. *Biometrics* 6, 1–16.

Kendall, M. G. 1948. "Rank Correlation Methods." 160 pp. Charles Griffin and Co., London.

Keuls, M. 1952. The use of the "studentized" range in connection with an analysis of variance. *Euphytica* 1, 112–122.

Kramer, A. 1960. A rapid method for determining significance of differences from rank sums. *Food Technol.* 14, 576–581.

Kramer, A. 1963. Revised tables for determining significance of differences. *Food Technol.* 17(12), 124–125.

Kramer, A., and B. A. Twigg. 1962. "Fundamentals of Quality Control in the Food Industry." 512 pp. (see pp. 429–448). Avi Publ. Co., Westport, Connecticut.

Kramer, C. Y. 1956. Extension of multiple range tests to group means with unequal numbers of replications. *Biometrics* 12, 307–310.

Kruskal, W. H., and W. A. Wallis. 1952. Use of ranks in one-criterion variance analysis. *J. Am. Statist. Assoc.* 47, 583–621.

Lombardi, G. J. 1951. The sequential selection of judges for organoleptic testing. Statistical methods for sensory difference tests of food quality. *Virginia Agr. Expt. Sta. Bi-Annual Rept.* 2. Appendix E, 1–37.

Mann, H. B., and D. R. Whitney. 1947. On a test whether one of two random variables is stochastically larger than the other. *Ann. Math. Statistics* 18, 50–60.

Mosteller, F. 1951a. Remarks on the method of paired comparisons. I. The least squares solution assuming equal standard deviation and equal correlations. *Psychometrika* 16, 3–9.

Mosteller, F. 1951b. Remarks on the method of paired comparisons. II. The effect of an aberrant standard deviation when equal standard deviations and equal correlations are assumed. *Psychometrika* 16, 203–218.

Nelson, K. E., G. A. Baker, A. J. Winkler, M. A. Amerine, H. B. Richardson, and F. R. Jones. 1963. Chemical and sensory variability in table grapes. *Hilgardia* 34, 1–42.

Newman, D. 1939. The distribution of the range in samples from a normal population, expressed in terms of an independent estimate of standard deviation. *Biometrika* 31, 20–30.

Neyman, J. 1950. "First Course in Probability and Statistics," 350 pp. (see pp. 273 and 277–278). Henry Holt, New York.

Ough, C. S., and G. A. Baker. 1961. Small panel sensory evaluations of wines by scoring. *Hilgardia* 30, 587–619.

Papakyriakopoulos, V. G., and M. A. Amerine. 1956. Sensory tests on two wine types. *Am. J. Enol.* 7, 98–104.

Park, G. T. 1961. Sensory testing by triple comparisons. *Biometrics* 17, 251–260.

Pearson, A. M., W. D. Baten, A. J. Goembel, and M. E. Spooner. 1962. Application of response-surface methodology to predicting optimum levels of salt and sugar in cured ham. *Food Technol.* 16, 137–138.

Pendergrass, R. N., and R. A. Bradley. 1960. Ranking in triple comparisons. In "Contributions to Probability and Statistics," 517 pp. (see pp. 331–351). Stanford University Press, Stanford, Calif.

Pfanzagl, J. 1959. Ein kombiniertes Test und klassifikations Problem. *Metrika* 2, 11–45.

Pilgrim, F. J., and K. R. Wood. 1955. Comparative sensitivity of rating scale and paired comparison methods for measuring consumer preference. *Food Technol.* 9, 385–387.

Radkins, A. P. 1957. Some statistical considerations in organoleptic research: triangle, paired, duo-trio tests. *Food Research* 22, 259–265.

Rao, C. R. 1950. Sequential tests of null hypotheses. *Sankhya* 10, 361–370.

Reimer, C. 1957. Some applications of rank order statistics in sensory panel testing. *Food Research* **22**, 629–634.

Sawyer, F. M., H. Stone, H. Abplanalp, and G. F. Stewart. 1962. Repeatability estimates in sensory-panel selection. *J. Food Sci.* **27**, 386–393.

Scheffé, H. 1952. An analysis of variance for paired comparisons. *J. Am. Statistical Assoc.* **47**, 381–400.

Schutz, H. G., and J. E. Bradley. 1954. Effect of bias on preference in the difference-preference test. *In* "Food Acceptance Testing Methodology," 115 pp. (see pp. 85–94). Advisory Board on Quartermaster Research and Development, Committee in Foods; and Natl. Acad. Sci., Natl. Research Council. Chicago, Illinois.

Snedecor, G. M. 1956. "Statistical Methods—Applied to Experiments in Agriculture and Biology," 5th ed., 534 pp. (see pp. 269 and 318–319). Iowa State College Press, Ames, Iowa.

Steel, R. G. D. 1959. A multiple comparison rank test: treatments versus control. *Biometrics* **15**, 560–572.

Steel, R. G. D. 1960. A rank sum test for comparing all pairs of treatments. *Technometrics* **2**, 197–207.

Steel, R. G. D. 1961. Some rank sum comparison tests. *Biometrics* **17**, 539–552.

Terry, M. E. 1952. Some rank order tests which are most powerful against specific parametric alternatives. *Ann. Math. Statistics* **23**, 346–366.

Terry, M. E., R. A. Bradley, and L. L. Davis. 1952. New designs and techniques for organoleptic testing. *Food Technol.* **6**, 250–254.

Thurstone, L. L. 1947. "Multiple-Factor Analysis." 535 pp. Univ. of Chicago Press, Chicago, Illinois.

Tukey, J. W. 1953. Some selected quick and easy methods of statistical analysis. *N. Y. Acad. Sci. Trans.* **16**, 88–97.

Ura, S. 1960a. Pair, triangle and duo-trio test. *Rept. Statist. Appl. Res., JUSE* **7**, 107–119.

Ura, S. 1960b. Selection of judges by ranking method. *Rept. Statist. Appl. Res., JUSE* **7**, 120–130.

Wald, A. 1947. "Sequential Analysis," 212 pp. Wiley, New York.

Wilcoxin, F. 1945. Individual comparisons by ranking methods. *Biometrics* **1**, 80–83.

Yates, F. 1936. Incomplete randomized blocks. *Ann. Eugenics* **7**, 121–140.

Yates, F. 1940. The recovery of inter-block information in balanced incomplete block designs. *Ann. Eugenics* **10**, 317–325.

Chapter 11

Physical and Chemical Tests Related to Sensory Properties of Foods

Objective* measurements of food quality are preferable to sensory measurements only if the objective tests can provide a precise measure of a subjective quality. The Fechner relationship (Chapter 5) between objective measurements and subjective response implies that there is a correlation between sensory quality and objective measurement of it. Can responses to taste, odor, tactile, or kinesthetic stimuli be closely correlated with measurements of chemical and physical properties of food? Bartlett (1950) stated that the correlation of objective measurements with subjective responses was possible empirically. A subject may find a minimum perceptible difference in some assigned dimension of a sensation; he may compare different values of the same dimension and conclude that the value or magnitude of one sensation is less or greater than another. Scales relating the stimulus and the sensation were considered "possible and useful" if there was a certain consistency in the assigned relations of measured stimulus differences and sensation dimension differences.

Bartlett noted that "in the case of psychophysical judgments, there seem to be three characters of the internal responding device which are remarkably persistent, though whether they are always in operation and what particular mathematical formulation of relationship they demand are still matters for determination. The first is an element having two positions of equilibrium. This may mean—and in most cases of psychophysical judgment it usually does mean—a nonlinear transformation of

---

* We hope the use of the words *subjective* and *objective* will not be confusing. The subjective response to the sweet taste is an objective fact. In this text when we mention subjective measurements we refer to sensory measurements made by individuals. Objective measurements, on the other hand, are made by instruments. Both may be "objective."

the external variable, for example, to a logarithmic form, and such transformation may involve temporal derivations of the external variable. The second is a shifting standard, structurally built into the response system, and together with the first character, leading to a discontinuous 'all-or-none' expression of continuous change in the external variable. The third is an 'indifference range' which means that there is no apparent change of output or interpretation within experimentally determined limits of 'stimulus' variation, but that outside such limits marked change may suddenly appear."

Can a sensation be truly measured in terms of the functional relations of a physical-stimulus variable with a sequence of step-judgments based upon sensory similarity and/or differences? The answer is not yet established. Some investigators deny categorically that magnitudes of sensation can be measured. Bartlett believes that discrimination data are not applicable, because "the magnitude of a discrimination may be dependent upon any of a number of variables, both external and internal, and nobody can know which are operating. Contrast-qualities cannot be used because all the results of a trial are equally consistent with a number of different assumptions, and we have no crucial way of actually determining which is necessary." Nevertheless, we believe that the commonly accepted correlations of stimulus and sensation variations are of operational value.

The importance of the character of the transforming and conducting processes internal to the responding system needs to be stressed. When subjective judgments have to be made about the effects of a physical variable, it is believed that results are more reliable if a limited number of criteria are used in succession rather than a single criterion. Bartlett noted that the problem of who is to control the physical variables (the subject, the experimenter, or a third person) is important. It is essential that the reliability of the subjective data be established by appropriate statistical analyses.

Harper (1955) is skeptical of objective tests because they do not meet his specifications: (1) that the measurement be based on sound theoretical principles; (2) that control be exercised within specified limits upon all the relevant conditions of testing; and (3) that the "properties" being measured should be largely unaltered by the processes of testing. Harper noted that in order to have satisfactory multidimensional analysis one must be able to: (1) record and, if possible, express in numerical terms, the salient features of a sensory experience; (2) determine the essential objective characteristics underlying this experience; and (3) develop satisfactory methods for relating these. The interpretation may require systematic analysis to assure that the conclusions are not determined partly by the design of the investigation and partly by the techniques of analysis. The relationship between objective and subjective properties may be more complicated than we have indicated. For example, referring specifically to the baking industry, Katz (1938) stated: "The physicist and the psychologist may require different properties, or even a different number of properties, to define the same material in their respective spheres."

Harper (1956, 1962) found three common factors or dimensions were necessary to describe two varieties of cheese. The first factor, which, in some cases, accounted for 58% of the total variance, lay very close to an objective pressure test. Its factor loading varied between 0.74 and 0.96, depending on the variety of cheese. For Cheddar the factorial composition of springiness proved to be distinctly different from that of firmness. For Cheshire cheeses the two were factorially indistinguishable and this confirms to the traditional distinction between the two types.

The disadvantages of subjective measurements compared to objective measurements were noted by Sheppard (1953). Objective assessments *may* be applicable at higher concentrations than subjective assessments without danger of fatigue mechanisms interfering. The objective procedure can be used repeatedly, although with subjective methods the relative discrimination of the subjects can be improved by training. Hopkinson (1952, 1953) supported the use of subjective procedures, noting, however, that "wherever the relation between the subjective reaction and the physical variables is fully understood, and the physical variables can be measured with the necessary degree of absolute and repetitional accuracy, the objective method should be used." The disadvantage of instrumental procedures is that the instrument may "repeat" readings when changes in the material may invalidate the correlation with subjective judgments. This simply means that continuous rechecking against the subjective reaction is necessary. We agree with Ehrenberg and Shewan (1953) that constant relationships between a sensory variable and external variables should be interpreted with caution.

Dawson and Harris (1951) and Kramer and Twigg (1962) summarized a wide variety of instrumental methods for measuring physical and chemical properties related to sensory response. As they clearly stated, however, the final standard of quality is human evaluation—so objective procedures must be judged by their correlation obtained with sensory results. Those researchers consider coefficients of correlation of 0.90 or better desirable, although in some cases correlations as low as 0.80 have been used. For predicting responses, a very high degree of correlation is necessary.

Some of the precautions which need to be considered in comparing subjective and objective measurements are: (1) the samples for both tests must be identical; (2) there must be sufficient replication; (3) the same individual should conduct the objective tests; (4) the same individuals should participate on all panels from which the data are averaged for comparison with the objective test; (5) there should be sufficient range of the test variable; and (6) the degree of variation of the instruments and the sensory panel must be determined. Important limitations of some instruments are that they respond over a period of minutes and measure only one attribute, whereas the human senses respond within seconds and measure the composite "mouthfeel." It is particularly necessary to note that instrumental data which give good correlation with sensory data for fruit of one degree of maturity may fail to show such a correlation with fruit of another degree of maturity. Many instruments can be arranged to operate automatically or semiautomatically, and thus much time is saved. The ideal objective methods should be rapid, accurate, and precise. Methods which isolate or differentiate a single quality factor are most likely to be useful, but several procedures may be needed to express over-all quality adequately.

Plank (1948) considered objective methods to be useful tools "supplementing and controlling, but not replacing the subjective (organoleptic) tests. In estimating the comparative value of the two methods the subjective test based on immediate reactions of our senses must still be given the higher weight." Smith (1955) agreed with this conclusion.

Balavoine (1948) noted that chemical and physical analyses of foods do not replace sensory examination, although for certain foods he approved of chemical or dilution tests to establish quality or authenticity. Wagner (1949) considered that both subjective and objective methods may be used in evaluating food characteristics and quality, and he summarized a variety of data for products as varied as bread, butter, coffee, fish, leeks, tea, etc. In many cases, however, the relationship of objective and sensory measurements was tenuous. It has frequently been noted that one high and one low value may result in a very good mathematical correlation whereas the relationship in the middle range of quality may be slight. The advantages of sensory tests vis-à-vis objective tests have been considered by Amerine (1961) with relation to wines.

Farber and Lerke (1958) established the following criteria for objective tests to be used as a measure of freshness of fishery products: (1) the objective test should correlate well with organoleptic judgment; (2) it should be applicable to all types of spoilage, including fat and protein breakdown; (3) it should be applicable to all varieties of fish, lean and fatty, white and red meat, and to all fish products, including cured, pickled, smoked, and canned fish; (4) there should be as great a difference as possible between fresh and spoiled samples in the content of the material upon which the test depends; (5) the test should be applicable at the beginning of spoilage or at the incipient stage of spoilage; and (6) it should be rapid and carried out relatively easily with equipment as simple and readily available as possible. Farber and Lerke believed that their procedure for the use of volatile reducing substances as a measure of spoilage fitted these criteria better than any other objective test available.

I. Color and Appearance

Mackinney and Little (1962) summarized color measurement problems in a variety of foods. They especially noted that a single plant or region can establish color standards satisfactory for quality control by use of regression lines without converting the data to a standard system. Ultimately, however, comparisons must be made between laboratories. As Mackinney and Little pointed out, color data can be accumulated for two purposes: (1) the identification or characterization of a food type and the permissible color variation before the type is downgraded; and (2) the effect of perceived color on its appreciation by consumers. As already indicated (Chapter 4), very good instrumental measurements are available for the visual characteristics of foods. In the single-category type of correlation, the main problem is the specificity of the objective test and the meaning of the subjective response. In the multiple-category type, the problem is whether the objective tests are sufficiently detailed to provide an adequate basis for correlation with either laboratory panel or consumer quality evaluation. For a review of sensory properties of foods and spectrophotometric analysis of their color, see Mossel (1950).

Scofield (1954) pointed out that the difficulties in improving color grading systems originate in a lack of fundamental knowledge, making it impossible to develop empirical knowledge effectively. He listed four points which are applicable to most problems in foods: (1) the difficulty in relating what is normally seen with what the spectrophotometer measures; (2) the mental processes by which color matches are made; (3) the visual spacing of standards on an empirical basis, without underlying theory; and (4) the mental correction for depth. Where one has a single number system of color grading, it can be done photometrically. However, Scofield believes one has not improved anything except precision by this system. Nothing has been done to improve the correlation between the grade and what the user sees (Mackinney and Little, 1962).

With cauliflower color, Boggs et al. (1961) obtained coefficients of correlation of 0.94 and higher between judges' scores and the Hunter a color value, hue angle, or lightness index. Correlations between these factors were even higher with spinach. Robinson *et al.* (1952) obtained correlation coefficients of 0.95 between U. S. inspector's scores for color in tomato juice and Hunter *a* and *b* values; 0.90 between scores and *a/b* ratios; and 0.94 when compared with hue. However, using a mixture of applesauce and strained raspberries, Little (1964) compared visual redness with reflectance from a Hunterlab color-difference meter. The eye easily distinguished differences the instrument did not, since the eye judges composite visual appearance and does not distinguish between the relative conditions of light scattering and light absorption. No instrument measures composite visual appearance; they only record diffuse reflectance characteristics relative to a standard, and cannot "see" color differences when the same proportion of incident light is returned to the photoelectric detector. For good correlations with wines see Berg *et al.* (1964).

Mackinney and Little (1962) outlined the tools and techniques necessary for adequate visual appraisal of color of foods, including: (1) color aptitudes of panel members; (2) panel size and training; (3) light sources; (4) viewing conditions; (5) standards; and (6) methodology of sample evaluation.

Many appearance factors are best measured by objective tests. Kramer and Twigg (1962) described various methods for measuring size and shape as well as physical defects of several commodities.

II. Taste and Flavor

Refractometry, one of the widely used quality-control methods, is frequently compared with sensory evaluation of sweetness, or density in products such as syrup, honey, fresh and processed fruits, juices, and tomato products. In some cases, refractometry is less sensitive than sensory measurement, as when low levels of sodium chloride are added to tomato juice or vegetable purées. In other cases, small alterations can be detected by refractometric measurement at levels that may be below the sensory difference threshold, i.e., in the adulteration of jams and jellies with commercial glucose, adulteration of milk with water, adulteration of butter with other fats, and impurities of methyl alcohol in distilled spirits. Other optical methods, such as polarimetry, have been used to establish the configuration of optically active compounds whose anomers may vary in taste intensity (see Pangborn and Gee, 1961).

Sensory scores for bitterness in carrots showed good correlation with spectrophotometric measurements of the ultraviolet-absorbing materials in hydrocarbon extracts in tests by Sondheimer *et al.* (1955). Those researchers predicted that if the absorption peak at 265 mμ was small, one could conclude with some assurance that the carrot sample was not very bitter.

A major problem in canning orange juice is the development of a bitter taste, due principally to the presence of limonin (Coote, 1956). A scoring scale devised by Kefford (1962) relates the bitterness intensity of limonin present in the juice from Valencia oranges grown in Australia with the bitterness intensity of caffeine as shown in Table 81.

TABLE 81

Bitterness Intensity of Limonin in Valencia Orange Juice Compared with Caffeine Bitterness

Description	Intensity score	Caffeine (ppm w/v)	Limonin (ppm w/v)
Not bitter	0	0	0
Bitterness doubtful	1	20	4
Very slightly bitter	2	40	7
Slightly bitter	3	70	
	4	100	10
Moderately bitter	5	150	
	6	250	18
Strongly bitter	7	400	
	8	650	35
Extremely bitter	9		
	10		

Source: Kefford (1962).

In general, total titratable acidity of food products correlates more closely with sourness than does pH, because of the various natural buffering agents in foods. With canned fruit products, a common index of palatability is the sugar/acid ratio, or Brix-acid ratio (Kefford, 1957), which is determined by:

$$\frac{\text{Percent total soluble solids by weight}}{\text{Percent total titratable acidity by weight}}$$

For example, the sugar-acid ratio that correlated with optimum consumer acceptance was 38/39 for canned apricots (Valdés and Roessler, 1956); 75/85 for canned cling peaches (Simone *et al.*, 1956; Simone and Pangborn, 1957); 138/170 for canned Bartlett pears (Pangborn and Leonard, 1958); and 65/75 for canned freestone peaches (Pangborn *et al.*, 1959). Although the ratio of soluble solids to total acid is closely related to the over-all palatability of canned fruit, it cannot be used to predict acceptance unless the type, variety, and maturity of the raw fruit are known, composition of the syrup is known, and one member of the ratio is kept constant. Nelson *et al.* (1963) found that the ratio predicted the palatability of table grapes more accurately than did soluble solids content alone. They found, however, that it did not adequately measure the great influence of acid content on palatability. A sliding scale of ratios was suggested to eliminate grapes which were unpalatable because of a low total acidity. They specifically noted that there were no abrupt changes in the chemical-sensory relationship where minimum-standard specifications could be established. In addition they called attention to the striking differences between judges in response to different ratios of soluble solids to acid.

Wiley and Worthington (1955) investigated the relationship between objective tests on fresh Italian prunes and their canned quality as determined by a panel of 14 trained judges. Correlation coefficients between flavor scores and sugar/acid ratios, pressure readings, soluble solids, and Hunter *a* readings were respectively 0.92, 0.91, 0.90, and 0.81. They suggested that two or more tests might be used to establish objective quality standards.

An early report on the correlation of subjective evaluations with physical and chemical measurements was that of Blanchard and Maxwell (1941), who reported that the sugar content of two groups of peas gave correlation coefficients of 0.73 and 0.74 with scores for flavor, texture, appearance, and color as measured by sensory tests.

Hartman (1954) and Hartman and Tolle (1957) reported on an apparatus in which a microammeter responded semiquantitatively to volatile flavor constituents, and predicted (without giving data) that the system would provide "a more promising attack on the practical problem of objective measure of flavor (odor) than mass spectroscopy, infrared and Raman spectroscopy, fractional distillation, well accepted enzyme techniques, and the isolation of individual compounds by chromatographic or more cumbersome techniques and even measurement of effect of volatiles on surface tension." In approaches such as the foregoing, the "human element" is overlooked, i.e., systems are devised to by-pass subjective judgment, without benefit of calibration against the mechanism they are attempting to replace. As pointed out in an editorial by Stewart (1963), "There is no doubt that some important components contributing to the aroma of foods have been isolated and identified—but *what is usually not being done* is to establish *which* of the compounds isolated are responsible for *what* sensory properties! Also, it seems likely that many of the compounds isolated have little or no sensory effect at all. . . . Appropriate (sensory) tests with isolated fractions and compounds will surely help answer such questions as: 1) Does the compound have sensory properties? 2) If so, what is its nature? 3) What combinations of components result in the sensory properties typical of the original product from which they were derived?"

The application of gas-liquid partition chromatography (GLC) to

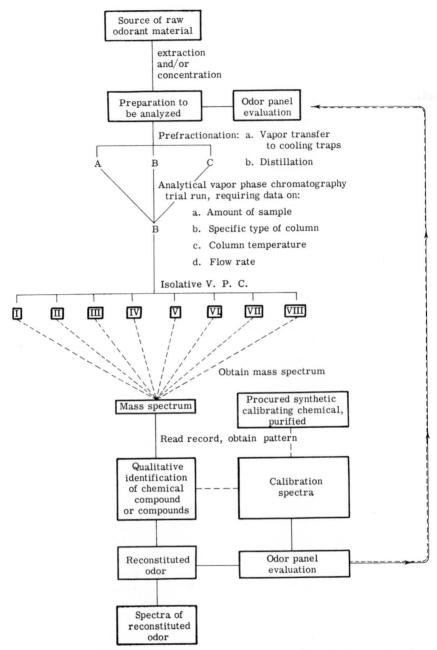

FIG. 86. Scheme for investigation of an unknown odor. V.P.C. = vapor phase chromatography. Source: Stahl (1957).

problems of food science has been rapid and extensive, primarily because of the sensitivity of the instrument to very small amounts of volatile material. Although it will probably be used more in investigations on the composition of foods, we can expect applications in detecting off-odors and of correlations between the amounts of specific compounds and sensory quality. The effluent materials from GLC are frequently further characterized by techniques such as mass spectrometry and/or infrared spectroscopy. Figure 86 shows how separations are combined with sensory evaluation. Gas-liquid chromatography is certainly a powerful tool, but it has certain limitations: (1) the necessity of sample preparation; (2) incomplete resolution of components; (3) creation of artifacts; (4) adsorption losses; and (5) insufficient sensitivity. Nevertheless, data from retention times may lead to identification of components which then may be combined for the creation of imitation flavors or used in quality control. It is even possible to analyze the air space at the surface of the food and to attempt to correlate the results with those obtained by panels (Nawar and Fagerson, 1962). Even when a large number of the components of the volatile material have been identified there usually remain unidentified but important components. Furthermore, according to Nawar and Fagerson (1962), although the chromatogram provides a fairly good analysis for the lower-boiling-point compounds, it does not for the higher-boiling-point compounds, especially those present in trace amounts. They also noted that in some cases it appears that compounds present in subthreshold concentrations exhibit a synergistic effect and thus contribute to the odor of the food.

Odor is, therefore, more than a pattern of peaks on a GLC. The chromatograph achieves separation of individual fractions in the idealized case. The role of these individual fractions, or even combinations of individual fractions, in determining the over-all flavor response may be difficult to determine unless they are present in the same proportion as in the original mixture. Flavor and odor are integrated responses, the taste and olfactory receptors being the integrators. The chromatograph, on the other hand, is a separator, which, though a useful tool for the chemist, must, to have a bearing on flavor, have its response analyzed by and correlated with sensory flavor or odor tests. For sensory examination, the quantities of flavor material necessary to train a panel and to obtain sufficient replication may be greater than the chemist can recover. The problem is further complicated in that some natural flavor materials undergo some degree of change by gas chromatographic separation; rarely are the recombined, recovered fractions identical to the injected mixture. This is, however, more a defect in use rather than in the method when properly used.

GLC equipped with ionization-type detectors was used by Mackay (1961) to demonstrate differences in the composition of unconcentrated vapors from good and deteriorated peppermint oil, real and imitation banana and coffee flavors, various grades of brandy and whiskey, crushed onions before and after treatment with chlorophyllin, and cigar and cigarette smoke. The details of the sensory testing of these constituents is not described.

Jennings *et al.* (1960) collected volatiles, which were trapped as aqueous essences, from Bartlett pears; separated 31 fractions by GLC; and made an odor evaluation of the character and intensity of each diluted fraction. Many fractions contained a pear-like aroma, whereas others were described as "pitch" or "piney." Addition of various fraction-combinations to canned pear nectar did not improve flavor quality but contributed varying degrees of unpleasant flavor character. Further applications of the results of GLC data to sensory quality should be forthcoming, particularly in detecting diluents and adulterants in food products. As Uzzan (1963) has noted, the newer techniques will eventually provide us with the same kind of information regarding taste and odor that colorimetry now provides for color. However, since the number of parameters appear to be so much greater for taste and odor, the correlation of specific components with human response is certain to be difficult. Undoubtedly, computers and new statistical models, as well as advanced psychological theories will help us make such correlations.

Further studies on volatiles in Bartlett pears showed good agreement between sensory aroma intensity and presence of the esters of 2,4-decadienoic acid measured by ultraviolet spectroscopy (Heinz *et al.*, 1964). Using an unusual approach, Ottoson and von Sydow (1964) reported no direct correlation between the amplitude of the gas chromatographic peaks for higher boiling aroma compounds from black currants, and that of the electrical response of the olfactory membrane of a frog.

Andersson and Danielson (1961) reported good correlations of panel results for fish rancidity with the peroxide value or with the malonaldehyde content as determined by the 2-thiobarbituric acid test (TBA test). A close correlation ($r = -0.97$) was found between the amount of enzymatically developed pyruvic acid present and the olfactory threshold of onion juice, according to Schwimmer and Guadagni (1962). In this case, the determination of the pyruvic acid content of freshly prepared onion juice constituted a fairly reliable, simple, and convenient method of estimating at least one aspect of onion odor.

To detect quality changes of orange juice due to microbial activity during concentration, Beisel *et al.* (1954), Byer (1954), Hill *et al.*

(1954), and Hill and Wenzel (1957) measured diacetyl levels in orange juice which were indicative of bacterial growth and spoilage and lowered quality.

A number of studies have been made correlating reduced palatability with excessive use of insecticides. Reynolds *et al.* (1953) showed, for example, that the benzene hexachloride (BHC) content of peanuts generally correlated positively with palatability scores and the quantity of insecticide applied. Harries (1962) compiled a critical review of the literature relating to use of insecticides and their resultant effect on the quality of fruits and vegetables. Mahoney *et al.* (1957a,b) directed uniform sensory evaluations, by 11 laboratories across the United States, of off-flavors in canned foods due to application of pesticides to the growing crop. Wiley *et al.* (1957) summarized the Northeast regional approach to collaborative panel testing of pesticide-treated foods, and listed the advantages and limitations of the sensory methods used in the six laboratories.

III. Texture

Some kinesthetic properties of foods can be determined objectively by instruments which measure compression, cutting, tensile strength, and shear pressure. Kramer and Twigg (1962) summarized objective measurements for viscosity and consistency, some of which are directly related to subjective texture and related tactile sensations. Matz (1962) reviewed a variety of objective measurements of the textural properties of foods. See also the symposium on food texture of the Society of Chemical Industry (1960).

A. LIQUIDS

The texture or mouthfeel of liquid foods, especially those which behave as Newtonian fluids, is closely related to their viscosity. When degree of sliminess of gum solutions was evaluated by a panel trained in descriptive sensory analysis on a 1 (nonslimy) to 7 (extremely slimy) scale, mouthfeel ratings were correlated with viscosity and rate-of-shear behavior (Szczesniak and Farkas, 1962). The mouthfeel characteristics of the gum solutions were highly correlated with their rheological behavior. Surprisingly, gum solutions that were very slimy deviated only slightly from Newtonian viscosity. As the degree of sliminess decreased, the deviation from Newtonian character increased. Gums that exhibited a high degree of shear thinning were nonslimy to the mouth. The reason for the varying behavior of different gums was postulated as being due to: (1) the degree of particle depression; (2) molecular weight; (3) molecular shape; (4) strength of intramolecular bonds; and (5) other characteristics. Harvey (1960) studied gels such as jellies in terms of shear deformation.

B. FRUITS AND VEGETABLES

The texture of fruits and vegetables has been assessed with instruments that measure compression, resistance to penetration, or force required to shear. The Magness pressure tester, wherein a steel plunger of a specified diameter penetrates the flesh, is used widely for determination of the maturity of deciduous fruits. Various penetrometers have been developed for objective evaluation of the texture of cooked, canned, and frozen foods. An apparatus that combines shearing and compression with tearing was developed by Volodkevich (1938) to measure chewing resistance. Candee and Boggs (1941) introduced a penetrometer which measures the toughness of vegetable skins from the relative weights required to penetrate pieces of skin tissue, or the toughness of pieces of vegetable tissue, such as pea cotyledons, by the load required to crush them to $\frac{1}{4}$ their thickness. Strohmaier (1953) used this penetrometer to measure the toughness of the skins and flesh of apricots. Wilder (1948) developed a simple fiberometer for the measurement of fiber content in canned asparagus based on variation of resistance to cutting provided by asparagus stalks varying in degree of fibrousness. A shear press equipped with a special single-bladed attachment was used to measure fibrousness in asparagus by Werner et al. (1963). Pitman (1930) devised an apparatus for measuring the crispness of almonds from the resistance of cut sections to shear.

Smithies (1960) noted that the amounts present of the following chemical constituents were related to texture in peas: phytin, pectins, alcohol-insoluble solids, water-insoluble solids, and starch. For peas, Makower et al. (1953) found good correlations between alcohol-insoluble solids and sensory evaluation of texture. Less reliable were total solids, density, tenderometer values, and two flotation techniques apparently related to density. With potatoes, Cullen (1960) reported that specific gravity and percent dry matter have been used; the latter correlated well with subjective texture. Zaehringer and Le Tourneau (1962) evaluated mealiness of three varieties of potatoes by: (1) mealiness in the mouth; (2) mealiness on continued mashing; and (3) mealiness on mild mashing. They found the last to be the most sensitive measure of subjective quality. There was a highly significant correlation between specific gravity and mealiness. In a subsequent study, Le Tourneau et al. (1962) reported a correlation of —0.77 to —0.92 between cooked potato weight (after sloughing) and subjective appraisal of texture. There was also a high negative correlation between cooked potato weight and the specific gravity of the tubers (−0.88 to −0.95). Sterling and Bettelheim (1955) also noted a correlation between sloughing and subjective appraisals of potato texture. Sloughing is a falling away of the outer layers of the potato tuber on boiling.

According to Isherwood (1960), penetrometer measurements for pears are related to subjective firmness but do not indicate textural properties related to the presence of stone cells in the flesh.

With peaches, a number of investigators have shown that texture is an important aspect of consumer acceptance, and that pectin changes are related to textural changes. Postlmayr *et al.* (1956) reported high protopectin retention to be a major factor responsible for the retention of a firm texture in Halford cling peaches. With the Fay Elberta freestone variety, protopectin was converted to water-soluble pectin during ripening, thus causing softening. Reduction of processing time lowered the retention of protopectin, and hence the firm texture in both cling and freestone peaches. Kramer shear-press measurements of the canned peaches correlated well with sensory tests. However, neither shear nor sensory tests detected significant differences in the texture of cling peaches canned at various raw-fruit pressure tests.

C. Meats

A wide variety of techniques have been used in an attempt to relate objective and subjective measurements of tenderness in meats. For reviews of the literature see Schultz (1957), Cover (1959), Bailey *et al.* (1962), and Sharrah *et al.* (1965). Sale (1960) described instruments for measuring simple shear, shear press, penetration, biting, and mincing. Deatherage and Garnatz (1952) reported that tenderness measured by a sensory panel and shear-strength measurements by the Warner-Bratzler shear press (using broiled steaks from matched pairs of shortloins from 32 steers) were not closely correlated although there was a correlation between some character of the steaks aged at two temperatures and the shear-strength measurements. The Warner-Bratzler shear test has generally been found to give a high correlation between "shear" values and panel scores, although there is some evidence that its sensitivity and reliability could be improved (Hurwicz and Tischer, 1954). Miyada and Tappel (1956) used a simple household food grinder and modified Christel Texturemeter in measuring beef texture, and reported that both were more precise than the Warner-Bratzler shear press. Bockian *et al.* (1958) found a coefficient of correlation of −0.59 and −0.60 between the energy required to grind samples and panel evaluations. The correlation was less if the meat was ground and not tasted for 2–5 hours. Emerson and Palmer (1960), however, found that the Warner-Bratzler shear apparatus gave higher correlations with panel results than the food grinder. Reasonably good agreement between panel tenderness scores and maximum shear force as determined by either the Warner-Bratzler or Kramer shear instruments was reported by Burrill et al. (1962). They noted that the least satisfactory measure of tenderness appeared to be the number of chews to prepare a ½-inch cube of meat for swallowing. Bailey et al. (1962) found significant correlations between mean sensory tenderness scores and mean L. E. E.-Kramer shear (−0.89, $p < 0.001$). Matz (1962) believes the Warner-Bratzler shear apparatus and methods based on the energy required to grind a sample are reasonably satisfactory for estimating the degree of meat tenderness but that panel testing is more accurate. No chemical tests appear to yield sufficiently high correlations with sensory measurements of the tenderness or fibrousness of meats.

A new device for evaluating the tenderness of meat slices was tested by Kulwich et al. (1963). Correlation coefficients with taste panel scores of −0.55 to −0.72 were obtained. The correlations with Warner-Bratzler shear was +0.41 to 0.71. The consistency at which the sample would normally be swallowed was used to determine chew counts and tenderness of pork by Harrington and Pearson (1962). Average chew count was highly correlated with Warner-Bratzler shear values.

Ritchey et al. (1963) did not get good correlations between panel scores for beef tenderness and collagen nitrogen. This, they postulate, is because the panel scores may reflect tenderness of total connective tissue which included not only collagen but elastin and reticulin and also possibly because the judges did not make fine enough distinctions. Similar results were obtained by Fielder et al. (1963) where correlations of subjective and objective methods varied widely with cooking method and/or cut. The problem is also discussed by Cover et al. (1962).

Dassow et al. (1962) recently developed an instrument with devices for measuring shear and tensile strength of fishery products. Shear was reported to have good correlation with sensory ratings.

Recording strain-gage denture tenderometers for foods have been developed by Volodkevich (1938), Krumbholz and Volodkevich (1943), and Proctor et al. (1955, 1956a). The last noted that the following features of the human chewing process are difficult to reproduce with an instrument: the complex movement and variations in force exerted by the lower jaw, the production of saliva and its mixing with food, and the complex movements of the tongue, cheeks, and other fleshy portions of the mouth to move and position the food. Proctor et al. (1956a) obtained a coefficient of correlation of 0.96 between denture tenderometer readings and panel scores. They also found a correlation of 0.99 between

readings on their instrument and those of the Canco tenderometer
(Proctor *et al.*, 1956b). Harper (1962) reported correlation values between firmness of cheese as measured by the thumb and an objective
instrumental procedure of +0.35 to +0.42 with Cheshire cheese. He also
reported correlations of +0.01 to +0.47 with Cheddar and up to +0.78
with Gruyère.

D. OTHER FOODS

For texture in bakery products, Coppock and Cornford (1960) described an instrument for measuring crumb tenderness, a tenderometer
for measuring crumb toughness, and one for crumb stickiness. A com-
pressimeter has been used for bread firmness or softness. For chocolate,
viscosity measurements have been made (Aylward, 1960). Davis (1921)
introduced a shortometer which has been useful in evaluating the shortening quality of lards and oils. Love (1960) measured texture changes in
fish and indicated that soluble protein, viscosity, and degree of cell dis-
ruption were useful in predicting sensory quality.

Viscometers of various types have been used for potatoes, starch
paste, tomato products, oils, heavy cream products, mayonnaise, etc. (see
Kramer and Twigg, 1962). For non-Newtonian materials the rotation of
a spindle or cylinder in the test material may be used to measure viscosity. Measuring the distance a material flows on a level surface under
its own weight during a given time interval has been used as a measure
of the viscosity of jams, pumpkin, cream-style corn, milk puddings, etc.
Penetration into a test material can be used to determine viscosity or
strength—as for jellies, baked custards, tomato products, etc. A new
recording instrument for measuring hardness, cohesiveness, viscosity,
elasticity, adhesiveness, brittleness, chewiness, and gumminess was developed by Friedman *et al.* (1963). A summary of instrumental methods
for measuring the parameters of texture is given by Szczesniak (1963).
Using their standard rating scales for hardness, brittleness, chewiness,
gumminess, viscosity and adhesiveness (Chapter 4, Section III,A),
Szczesniak *et al.* (1963) found good correlation between the sensory and
instrumental methods of texture evaluation. The correlation between
texturometer units and sensory rating for hardness is shown in Fig. 87,
and between texturometer units and sensory rating for chewiness in
Fig. 88. For the special case of almonds Sterling and Simone (1954)
measured crispness (brittleness) as the amount of deformation before
fracture. Fragmentability, the ability to break into many small pieces
under pressure, hardness, the resistance to penetration, and cohesiveness,
the requiring of deep penetration of the teeth before breaking apart, were
determined by sensory tests. Fragmentability in roasted nuts appeared to

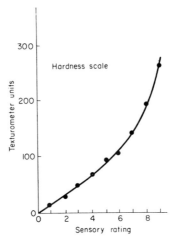

FIG. 87. Correlation between texturometer units and sensory rating for hardness.
Source: Szczesniak *et al.* (1963).

be inversely correlated with brittleness in raw seeds and hardness in
roasted seeds. With the latter there was a general parallelism between
the results of the mechanical tests and those with sensory procedures.

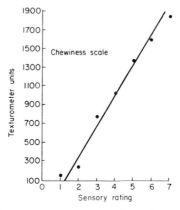

FIG. 88. Correlation between texturometer units and sensory rating for chewiness.
Source: Szczesniak *et al.* (1963).

IV. General Quality

The number of physicochemical methods is so great that only a few
representative examples can be mentioned. Weight, size, moisture content,
alcohol-insoluble solids, fiber content, density, color, acidity, sugar concentration, pH, salt, tannins, volatile reducing substances, peroxide value,
nonprotein nitrogen, and phospho-18-tungstic acid-positive material are

all the basis of one or more procedures which attempt to relate food quality to an objective measurement. Objective methods have been given for determining contamination of foods by biological agents, such as insects, rodents, bacteria, molds, and yeasts.

Federal standards for many food products have been published by the U. S. Department of Agriculture. Table 82 summarizes many of these. Most of these standards are quite arbitrary, and their relation to sensory quality is not clear. Probably, at best, they are related in a general way to product quality as understood by shippers or packers. For a useful summary see Gunderson *et al.* (1963).

Note that "absence of defects" and "color" in many cases are the most important factors in these standards. Kramer and Twigg (1959, 1962) give a useful summary of how grades and standards of quality may be developed, and of statistical procedures for acceptance sampling, inspection, and production control.

In analysis of the data where several variables are to be correlated to quality, some type of multivariate analysis seems indicated. For examples, see Baker and Amerine (1953), Baker (1954), and Harper (1956). Unfortunately, even with the best modern equipment, too few objective tests are available for accurate prediction of sensory results of a given food over a wide range of quality—particularly for different varieties, sources, and methods of production.

V. Summary

The relation of the subjective response to the stimulus is not a simple one. Therefore, objective tests that are not similarly related to the product are difficult to correlate directly with subjective quality. Thus, even though constant relationships are established they cannot be applied without caution. Multidimensional analysis is needed of both the subjective experience and the objective characteristics of the food.

Objective tests have the advantage of being useful at various concentrations, of not being subject to fatigue, and of automatic operation. A major disadvantage is, of course, their tendency to "repeat" a reading when other changes have occurred that clearly influence quality.

Color grading appears to be the most successful of the objective procedures, but still has many problems. Chemical factors influencing taste have been measured for specific foods with some success. Gas-liquid partition chromatography should facilitate identification and quantitative measurement of flavors. Texture has been measured objectively for certain foods with good results.

We believe that factor analysis and other procedures to establish the sensory factors and correlate them with various objective chemical and

TABLE 82

Relative Importance of Factors Involved in U. S. Department of Agriculture Standards for Processed Fruit and Vegetable Products

Product	Absence of defects	Color	Flavor	Character	Consistency	Uniformity	Texture	Tenderness and maturity	Clearness of liquor
Fruit preserves (jam)	20	20	40	—	20	—	—	—	—
Frozen apples	20	20	—	40	—	20	—	—	—
Canned orange juice	40	20	40	—	—	—	—	—	—
Spinach	40	30	—	30	—	—	—	—	—
Canned lima beans	25	35	—	30	—	—	—	—	10
Sliced beets	30	25	—	—	—	15	30	—	—
Cream-style corn	20	10	20	—	20	—	—	30	—
Apple butter	20	20	20	20 fin.	20	—	—	—	—
Apple sauce	20	20	20	20 fin.	20	—	—	—	—
Apricots	30	20	—	35	—	15 siz.	—	—	—
Asparagus	30	20	—	—	—	—	—	40	10
Green and wax beans	35	15	—	—	—	—	—	40	10
Lima beans	25	35	—	30	—	—	—	—	10
Beets	30	25	—	—	—	15	30	—	—
Berries	30	20	—	30	—	20	—	—	—
Blueberries	40	20	—	40	shape	—	—	—	—
Carrots	30	25	—	—	—	15 siz.	30	—	—
Cherries, sweet	30	30	—	20	—	20 siz.	—	—	—
Corn, cream	20	10	20	—	20	—	—	30	—
Corn, whole	20	10	20	—	—	—	—	40	10
Figs, Kadota	30	20	—	35	—	15 siz.	—	—	—
Fruit cocktail	20	20	—	20	—	20	—	—	20
Fruit salad	25	25	—	25	—	25 siz.	—	—	—

Item								
Grapefruit	20	20	—	20	20 siz.	(Drained wt. 20)	—	—
Mushroom	30	20	—	20	20 siz.	—	—	—
Olives, green	30	30	—	20	20	—	—	—
Olives, ripe	10	15	30	25	—	—	—	—
Orange marmalade	20	20	40	20	—	—	—	—
Okra	20	15	15	—	10	—	35	5
Peaches	30	20	35	—	15 siz.	—	—	—
Peanut butter	40	20	40	—	—	—	—	—
Pears	30	20	—	30	20 siz.	—	—	—
Peas	30	10	—	—	20	—	50	10
Cucumber pickles	30	20	—	—	—	30	—	—
Pimientos	40	30	—	10	20 siz.	—	—	—
Pineapples	30	20	—	30	20	—	—	—
Plums	30	20	—	30	20 siz.	—	—	—
Potatoes, peeled	40	20	—	—	20	20	—	—
Prunes, dried	30	20	—	35 fin.	15	—	—	—
Pumpkins and squash	30	20	—	20 fin.	—	—	—	—
Raspberries	20	25	—	35	20 siz.	—	—	—
Sauerkraut	10	15	45	15 crisp	—	—	—	15
Sauerkraut, bulk	10	15	45	15 crisp	—	—	—	15
Sweet potatoes	40	20	—	20	20 siz.	—	—	—
Tomatoes	30	30	40	(wholeness 20)	(drained wt. 20)	—	—	—
Tomato juice	15	30	—	15	—	—	—	—
Tomato paste	40	60	25	—	—	—	—	—
Tomato sauce-catsup	25	25	25	25	—	—	—	—
Chili sauce	20	20	20	20	—	—	—	—

Source: Kramer and Twigg (1962).

physical measurements would be helpful. Simple correlations between a single objective procedure and over-all quality are not adequate.

REFERENCES

Amerine, M. A. 1961. Legal and practical aspects of the sensory examination of wines. *J. Assoc. Offic. Agr. Chemists* **44**, 380–383.

Andersson, K., and C. E. Danielson. 1961. Storage changes in frozen fish: a comparison of objective and subjective tests. *Food Technol.* **15**, 55–57.

Aylward, F. 1960. Chocolate. *In* "Texture in Foods." *Soc. Chem. Ind. (London) Monograph* **7**, 75–88.

Bailey, M. E., H. B. Hedrick, F. C. Parrish, and H. D. Naumann. 1962. L. E. E.-Kramer shear force as a tenderness measure of beef steaks. *Food Technol.* **16** (12), 99–101.

Baker, G. A. 1954. Organoleptic ratings and analytical data for wines analyzed into orthogonal factors. *Food Research* **19**, 575–580.

Baker, G. A., and M. A. Amerine. 1953. Organoleptic ratings of wines estimated from analytical data. *Food Research* **18**, 381–389.

Balavoine, P. 1948. Observations sur les qualités olfactives et gustatives des aliments. *Mitt. Gebiete Lebensm. u. Hyg.* **39**, 342–350.

Bartlett, F. C. 1950. Subjective judgments. *Nature* **166**, 984–985.

Beisel, C. G., D. R. Willard, R. L. Kitchel, K. M. Roswell, C. W. Nagel, and R. H. Vaughn. 1954. Sources and detection of Voges-Proskauer reactants in California Valencia orange juice. *Food Research* **19**, 633–643.

Berg, H. W., C. S. Ough, and C. O. Chichester. 1964. The prediction of perceptibility of luminous-transmittance and dominant wave-length differences among red wines by spectrophotometric measurements. *J. Food Sci.* **29**, 661–667.

Blanchard, E. L., and M. L. Maxwell. 1941. Correlation of subjective scoring with sugar content of frozen peas. *Food Research* **6**, 105–115.

Bockian, A. H., A. F. Anglemier, and L. A. Sather. 1958. A comparison of an objective and subjective measurement of beef tenderness. *Food Technol.* **12**, 483–485.

Boggs, M. M., H. C. Lukens, D. W. Venstrom, J. G. Harris, S. Shenoda, and B. P. Debeau. 1961. Reflectance color measurements and judges' scores for frozen cauliflower and spinach. *J. Food Sci.* **26**, 26–30.

Burrill, L. M., D. Deethardt, and R. L. Saffle. 1962. Two mechanical devices compared with taste-panel evaluation for measuring tenderness. *Food Technol.* **16**(10), 145–166.

Byer, E. M. 1954. Visual detection of either diacetyl or acetylmethylcarbinol in frozen concentrated orange juice. *Food Technol.* **8**, 173–174.

Candee, F. W., and M. M. Boggs. 1941. Apparatus for measuring the texture of cooked peas. *Western Canner and Packer* **33**, 44.

Coote, G. G. 1956. Analysis of scores for bitterness of orange juice. *Food Research* **21**, 1–10.

Coppock, J. B. M., and S. J. Cornford. 1960. Texture in bread and flour confectionery. *In* "Texture in Foods." *Soc. Chem. Ind. (London) Monograph* **7**, 64–74.

Cover, S. 1959. Meat cookery from the scientific viewpoint. *Proc. Research Conf., Amer. Meat Inst. Found.* **11**, 99–111.

Cover, S., S. J. Ritchey, and R. L. Hostetler. 1962. Tenderness of beef. I. The connective tissue component of tenderness. *J. Food Sci.* **27**, 469–475.

Cullen, J. C. 1960. Texture in cooked potatoes. *In* "Texture in Foods." *Soc. Chem. Ind. (London) Monograph* **7**, 128–134.

Dassow, J. A., L. G. McKee, and R. W. Nelson. 1962. Development of an instrument for evaluating texture of fishery products. *Food Technol.* 16(3), 108–110.

Davis, C. E. 1921. Shortening: its definition and measurement. *J. Ind. Eng. Chem.* 13, 797–799.

Dawson, E. H., and B. L. Harris. 1951. Sensory methods for measuring differences in food quality. *U. S. Dept. Agr., Agr. Inform. Bull.* No. 34, 1–134.

Deatherage, F. E., and G. Garnatz. 1952. A comparative study of tenderness determination by sensory panel and by shear strength measurements. *Food Technol.* 6, 260–262.

Ehrenberg, A. S. C., and J. M. Shewan. 1953. The objective approach to sensory tests of food. *J. Sci. Food Agr.* 10, 482–490.

Emerson, J. A., and A. Z. Palmer. 1960. A food grinder–recording ammeter method for measuring beef tenderness. *Food Technol.* 14, 214–216.

Farber, L., and P. A. Lerke. 1958. A review of the value of volatile reducing substances for the chemical assessment of the freshness of fish and fish products. *Food Technol.* 12, 677–680.

Fielder, M. M., A. M. Mullins, M. M. Skellenger, R. Whitehead, and D. S. Moschette. 1963. Subjective and objective evaluations of prefabricated cuts of beef. *Food Technol.* 17, 213–218.

Friedman, H. H., J. E. Whitney, and A. S. Szczesniak. 1963. The texturometer—a new instrument for objective texture measurement. *J. Food Sci.* 28, 390–396.

Gunderson, F. L., H. W. Gunderson, and E. R. Ferguson, Jr. 1963. "Food Standards and Definitions in the United States," 269 pp. Academic Press, New York.

Harper, R. 1955. Fundamental problems in the subjective appraisal of foodstuffs. *Appl. Statistics* 4, 145–160.

Harper, R. 1956. Factor analysis as a technique for examining complex data on foodstuffs. *Appl. Statistics* 5, 32–48.

Harper, R. 1962. The psychologist's role in food-acceptance research. *Food Technol.* 16(10), 70, 72–73.

Harries, J. M. 1962. Some problems in the assessment of "taint" in fruit and vegetables. Paper presented at the First Intern. Congr. Food Sci. and Technol., London, September 1962. (To be published in July 1965.)

Harrington, G., and A. M. Pearson. 1962. Chew count as a measure of tenderness of pork loins with various degrees of marbling. *J. Food Sci.* 27, 106–110.

Hartman, J. 1954. A possible objective method for the rapid estimation of flavors in vegetables. *Proc. Am. Soc. Hort. Sci.* 64, 335–342.

Hartman, J. D., and W. E. Tolle. 1957. An apparatus for the rapid electrochemical estimation of flavors in vegetables. *Food Technol.* 11, 130–132.

Harvey, H. G. 1960. Gels—with special reference to pectin gels. *In* "Texture in Foods." *Soc. Chem. Ind.* (*London*) *Monograph* 7, 29–63.

Heinz, D. E., R. M. Pangborn, and W. G. Jennings. 1964. Pear aroma: relation of instrumental and sensory techniques. *J. Food Sci.* 29, 756–761.

Hill, E. C., and F. W. Wenzel. 1957. The diacetyl test as an aid for quality control of citrus products. I. Detection of bacterial growth in orange juice during concentration. *Food Technol.* 11, 240–243.

Hill, E. C., F. W. Wenzel, and A. Barreto. 1954. Colorimetric method for detection of microbiological spoilage in citrus juices. *Food Technol.* 8, 168–171.

Hopkinson, R. G. 1952. Factors affecting choice and judgment. *Nature* 170, 555.

Hopkinson, R. G. 1953. Factors affecting choice and judgment. *Nature* 171, 848.

Hurwicz, H., and R. G. Tischer. 1954. Variation in determinations of shear force by means of the Bratzler-Warner shear. *Food Technol.* 8, 391–393.

Isherwood, F. A. 1960. Some factors involved in the texture of plant tissues. *In* "Texture in Foods." *Soc. Chem. Ind. (London) Monograph* **7**, 135–143.

Jennings, W. G., S. Leonard, and R. M. Pangborn. 1960. Volatiles contributing to the flavor of Bartlett pears. *Food Technol.* **14**, 587–590.

Katz, D. 1938. The judgments of test bakers. A psychological study. *Occupational Psychol.* **12**, 139–148.

Kefford, J. F. 1957. Acidity and pH values. *C.S.I.R.O. Food Preserv. Quart.* **17**, 30–35.

Kefford, J. F. 1962. Citrus products research in Australia. Paper presented at the Inst. of Food Technologists, Miami Beach, Florida, June, 1962.

Kramer, A., and B. A. Twigg. 1959. Principles and instrumentation for the physical measurement of food quality with special reference to fruit and vegetable products. *Advances in Food Research* **9**, 153–220.

Kramer, A., and B. A. Twigg. 1962. "Fundamentals of Quality Control for the Food Industry," 512 pp. Avi Publ. Co., Westport, Connecticut.

Krumbholz, G., and N. N. Volodkevich. 1943. Festigkeitmessungen an Früchten und ihre Anwendungsmöglichkeiten. I. Die Bestimmung der Fruchtfleischfestigkeit. *Gartenbauwissenschaft* **17**, 543–590.

Kulwich, R., R. W. Decker, and R. H. Alsmeyer. 1963. Use of a slice-tenderness evaluation device with pork. *Food Technol.* **17**, 201–203.

Le Tourneau, D., M. V. Zaehringer, and A. L. Potter. 1962. Textural quality of potatoes. II. An objective method for evaluating texture. *Food Technol.* **16**(10), 135–138.

Little, A. C. 1964. Color measurement of translucent food samples. *J. Food Sci.* **29**, 782–789.

Love, R. M. 1960. Texture change in fish and its measurement. *In* "Texture in Foods." *Soc. Chem. Ind. (London) Monograph* **7**, 109–118.

Mackay, D. A. M. 1961. Objective measurement of odor. Ionization detection of food volatiles. *Anal. Chem.* **33**, 1369–1374.

Mackinney, G., and A. C. Little. 1962. "Color of Foods," 308 pp. Avi Publ. Co., Westport, Connecticut.

Mahoney, C. H., H. L. Stier, and E. A. Crosby. 1957a. Evaluating flavor differences in canned foods. I. Genesis of the simplified procedure for making flavor difference tests. *Food Technol.* **11**, 29–36 (supplement).

Mahoney, C. H., H. L. Stier, and E. A. Crosby. 1957b. Evaluating flavor differences in canned foods. II. Fundamentals of the simplified procedure. *Food Technol.* **11**, 37–43 (supplement).

Makower, R. U., M. M. Boggs, H. K. Burr, and H. S. Olcott. 1953. Comparison of methods for measuring the maturity factor in frozen peas. *Food Technol.* **7**, 43–48.

Matz, S. A. 1962. "Food Texture," 286 pp. Avi Publ. Co., Westport, Connecticut.

Miyada, D. S., and A. L. Tappel. 1956. Meat tenderization. I. Two mechanical devices for measuring texture. *Food Technol.* **10**, 142–145.

Mossel, D. A. A. 1950. Objectieve bepaling von zintuiglijk waarneembare eigenschappen van levensmiddelen. *Pharm. Weekblad* **85**, 381–387.

Nawar, W. W., and I. S. Fagerson. 1962. Direct gas chromatographic analysis as an objective method of flavor measurement. *Food Technol.* **16**(11), 107–109.

Nelson, K. E., G. A. Baker, A. J. Winkler, M. A. Amerine, H. B. Richardson, and F. R. Jones. 1963. Chemical and sensory variability in table grapes. *Hilgardia* **34**, 1–42.

Ottoson, D., and E. von Sydow. 1964. Electrophysiological measurements of the odor of single components of a mixture separated in a gas chromatograph. *Life Sci.* 3, 1111–1115.

Pangborn, R. M., and S. C. Gee. 1961. Relative sweetness of α- and β-forms of selected sugars. *Nature* 191, 810.

Pangborn, R. M., and S. J. Leonard. 1958. Factors influencing consumer opinion of canned Bartlett pears. *Food Technol.* 12, 284–290.

Pangborn, R. M., S. Leonard, M. Simone, and B. S. Luh. 1959. Freestone peaches. I. Effect of sucrose, citric acid and corn syrup on consumer acceptance. *Food Technol.* 13, 444–447.

Pitman, G. 1930. Further comparison of California and imported almonds. *Ind. Eng. Chem.* 22, 1129–1131.

Plank, R. P. 1948. A rational method of grading food quality. *Food Technol.* 2, 241–251.

Postlmayr, H. L., B. S. Luh, and S. J. Leonard. 1956. Characterization of pectin changes in freestone and clingstone peaches during ripening and harvesting. *Food Technol.* 10, 618–625.

Proctor, B. E., S. Davison, G. J. Molecki, and M. Welch. 1955. A recording strain-gage denture tenderometer for foods. I. Instrument evaluation and initial tests. *Food Technol.* 9, 471–477.

Proctor, B. E., S. Davison, and A. L. Brody. 1956a. A recording strain-gage denture tenderometer for foods. II. Studies on the masticating force and motion, and the force-penetration relationship. *Food Technol.* 10, 327–331.

Proctor, B. E., S. Davison, and A. L. Brody. 1956b. A recording strain-gage denture tenderometer for foods. III. Correlation with subjective tests and the Canco tenderometer. *Food Technol.* 10, 344–346.

Reynolds, H., G. L. Gilpin, and I. Hornstein. 1953. Palatability and chemical studies on peanuts grown in rotation with cotton dusted with insecticides containing benzene hexachloride. *Agr. Food Chem.* 1, 772–776.

Ritchey, S. J., S. Cover, and R. L. Hostetler. 1963. Collagen content and its relation to tenderness of connective tissue in two beef muscles. *Food Technol.* 17, 194–197.

Robinson, W. B., T. Wishnetsky, J. R. Ransford, W. L. Clark, and D. B. Hand. 1952. A study of methods for the measurement of tomato juice color. *Food Technol.* 6, 269–275.

Sale, A. J. H. 1960. Measurement of meat tenderness. *In* "Texture in Foods." *Soc. Chem. Ind. (London) Monograph* 7, 103–108.

Schultz, H. W. 1957. Mechanical methods of measuring tenderness of meat. *Proc. Ann. Reciprocal Meat Conf.* 10, 1–25. Natl. Livestock and Meat Board, Chicago, Illinois.

Schwimmer, S., and D. G. Guadagni. 1962. Relation between olfactory threshold concentration and pyruvic acid content of onion juice. *J. Food Sci.* 27, 94–97.

Scofield, R. 1954. Colors of transparent liquids for surface coatings. Symposium on color of transparent and translucent products. *ASTM Bull.* 202, 68–69.

Sharrah, N., M. S. Kunze, and R. M. Pangborn. 1965. Beef tenderness: comparison of sensory methods with the Warner-Bratzler and L. E. E., Kramer shear presses. *Food Technol.* 19(2), 238–245.

Sheppard, D. 1953. Factors affecting choice and judgment. *Nature* 171, 847–848.

Simone, M., and R. M. Pangborn. 1957. Consumer acceptance methodology: one vs. two samples. *Food Technol.* 11, 25–29 (supplement).

Simone, M., S. Leonard, E. Hinreiner, and R. M. Valdés. 1956. Consumer studies on sweetness of canned cling peaches. *Food Technol.* 10, 279–282.

Smith, H. R. 1955. Evaluating the quality of processed foods. *Food Technol.* **9,** 453–455.

Smithies, R. H. 1960. Effect of chemical constitution on texture of peas. *Soc. Chem. Ind.* (*London*) *Monograph* **7,** 119–127.

Society of Chemical Industry (London). 1960. Texture in foods. *Soc. Chem. Ind.* (*London*) *Monograph* **7,** 1–184.

Sondheimer, E., W. F. Phillips, and J. D. Atkin. 1955. Bitter flavor in carrots. I. A tentative spectrophometric method for the estimation of bitterness. *Food Research* **20,** 659–665.

Stahl, W. H. 1957. Gas chromatography and mass spectrometry in the study of flavor. *In* "Chemistry of Natural Food Flavors," 200 pp. (*see* pp. 58–75). Advisory Board on Quartermaster Research and Development, Committee on Foods, Chicago.

Sterling, C., and F. A. Bettelheim. 1955. Factors associated with potato texture. III. Physical attributes and general conclusions. *Food Research* **20,** 130–137.

Sterling, C., and M. J. Simone. 1954. Crispness in almonds. *Food Research* **19,** 276–281.

Stewart, G. F. 1963. The challenge in flavor research. *Food Technol.* **17**(1), 5.

Strohmaier, L. H. 1953. Studies on the toughness and histology of frozen apricot skins. *Food Technol.* **7,** 469–473.

Szczesniak, A. S. 1963. Objective measurements of food texture. *J. Food Sci.* **28,** 410–420.

Szczesniak, A. S., and E. Farkas. 1962. Objective characterization of the mouthfeel of gum solutions. *J. Food Sci.* **27,** 381–385.

Szczesniak, A. S., M. A. Brandt, and H. H. Friedman. 1963. Development of standard rating scales for mechanical parameters of texture and correlation between the objective and the sensory methods of texture evaluation. *J. Food Sci.* **28,** 397–403.

Uzzan, A. 1963. Rôle des essais organoleptiques dans la formulation et l'expertise des produits alimentaires: exemples d'application. *Ann. fals. expert. chim.* **56,** 30–37.

Valdés, R. M., and E. B. Roessler. 1956. Consumer survey on the dessert quality of canned apricots. *Food Technol.* **10,** 481–486.

Volodkevich, N. N. 1938. Apparatus for measurements of chewing resistance or tenderness of foodstuffs. *Food Research* **3,** 221–225.

Wagner, K. G. 1949. Ueber einige Zusammenhänge zwischen organileptischer und analytischen Befund bei Nahrungsmittel. *Z. Lebensmittel-Untersuch. u. Forsch.* **90,** 36–46.

Werner, G., E. E. Meschler, H. Lacey, and A. Kramer. 1963. Use of the shear press in determining fibrousness of raw and canned green asparagus. *Food Technol.* **17**(1), 81–86.

Wilder, H. K. 1948. Instructions for the use of the fibrometer in the measurement of fiber content in canned asparagus. *Natl. Canners Assoc. Research Lab. Rept.* **12312-C,** 1–3. Western Lab., San Francisco, California.

Wiley, R. C., and O. J. Worthington. 1955. The use of fresh fruit objective test to predict the quality of canned Italian prunes. *Food Technol.* **9,** 381–384.

Wiley, R. C., A. M. Briant, I. S. Fagerson, E. F. Murphy, and J. H. Sabry. 1957. Northeast regional approach to collaborative panel testing. *Food Technol.* **11**(9), 43–48 (supplement).

Zaehringer, M. V., and D. Le Tourneau. 1962. Textural quality of potatoes. I. Comparison of three organoleptic methods. *Food Technol.* **16**(10), 131–134.

Appendix: Tables A to I

TABLE A

Areas under the Normal Probability Curve
Area to the right of z (or to the left of $-z$), or the
probability of a random value of z exceeding
the marginal value

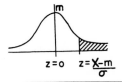

z	.00	.01	.02	.03	.04	.05	.06	.07	.08	.09
.0	.5000	.4960	.4920	.4880	.4840	.4801	.4761	.4721	.4681	.4641
.1	.4602	.4562	.4522	.4483	.4443	.4404	.4364	.4325	.4286	.4247
.2	.4207	.4168	.4129	.4090	.4052	.4013	.3974	.3936	.3897	.3859
.3	.3821	.3783	.3745	.3707	.3669	.3632	.3594	.3557	.3520	.3483
.4	.3446	.3409	.3372	.3336	.3300	.3264	.3228	.3192	.3156	.3121
.5	.3085	.3050	.3015	.2981	.2946	.2912	.2877	.2843	.2810	.2776
.6	.2743	.2709	.2676	.2643	.2611	.2578	.2546	.2514	.2483	.2451
.7	.2420	.2389	.2358	.2327	.2296	.2266	.2236	.2206	.2177	.2148
.8	.2119	.2090	.2061	.2033	.2005	.1977	.1949	.1922	.1894	.1867
.9	.1841	.1814	.1788	.1762	.1736	.1711	.1685	.1660	.1635	.1611
1.0	.1587	.1562	.1539	.1515	.1492	.1469	.1446	.1423	.1401	.1379
1.1	.1357	.1335	.1314	.1292	.1271	.1251	.1230	.1210	.1190	.1170
1.2	.1151	.1131	.1112	.1093	.1075	.1056	.1038	.1020	.1003	.0985
1.3	.0968	.0951	.0934	.0918	.0901	.0885	.0869	.0853	.0838	.0823
1.4	.0808	.0793	.0778	.0764	.0749	.0735	.0721	.0708	.0694	.0681
1.5	.0668	.0655	.0643	.0630	.0618	.0606	.0594	.0582	.0571	.0559
1.6	.0548	.0537	.0526	.0516	.0505	.0495	.0485	.0475	.0465	.0455
1.7	.0446	.0436	.0427	.0418	.0409	.0401	.0392	.0384	.0375	.0367
1.8	.0359	.0351	.0344	.0336	.0329	.0322	.0314	.0307	.0301	.0294
1.9	.0287	.0281	.0274	.0268	.0262	.0256	.0250	.0244	.0239	.0233
2.0	.0228	.0222	.0217	.0212	.0207	.0202	.0197	.0192	.0188	.0183
2.1	.0179	.0174	.0170	.0166	.0162	.0158	.0154	.0150	.0146	.0143
2.2	.0139	.0136	.0132	.0129	.0125	.0122	.0119	.0116	.0113	.0110
2.3	.0107	.0104	.0102	.0099	.0096	.0094	.0091	.0089	.0087	.0084
2.4	.0082	.0080	.0078	.0075	.0073	.0071	.0069	.0068	.0066	.0064
2.5	.0062	.0060	.0059	.0057	.0055	.0054	.0052	.0051	.0049	.0048
2.6	.0047	.0045	.0044	.0043	.0041	.0040	.0039	.0038	.0037	.0036
2.7	.0035	.0034	.0033	.0032	.0031	.0030	.0029	.0028	.0027	.0026
2.8	.0026	.0025	.0024	.0023	.0023	.0022	.0021	.0021	.0020	.0019
2.9	.0019	.0018	.0018	.0017	.0016	.0016	.0015	.0015	.0014	.0014
3.0	.0013	.0013	.0013	.0012	.0012	.0011	.0011	.0011	.0010	.0010
3.1	.0010	.0009	.0009	.0009	.0008	.0008	.0008	.0008	.0007	.0007
3.2	.0007	.0007	.0006	.0006	.0006	.0006	.0006	.0005	.0005	.0005
3.3	.0005	.0005	.0005	.0004	.0004	.0004	.0004	.0004	.0004	.0003
3.4	.0003	.0003	.0003	.0003	.0003	.0003	.0003	.0003	.0003	.0002
3.6	.0002	.0002	.0001	.0001	.0001	.0001	.0001	.0001	.0001	.0001
3.9	.0000									

TABLE B[a]
Student's t-Distribution
A denotes the sum of the two tail areas for the values of t

Degrees of freedom	$A = .1$	$A = .05$	$A = .02$	$A = .01$	$A = .001$
1	6.314	12.706	31.821	63.657	636.619
2	2.920	4.303	6.965	9.925	31.598
3	2.353	3.182	4.541	5.841	12.941
4	2.132	2.776	3.747	4.604	8.610
5	2.015	2.571	3.365	4.032	6.859
6	1.943	2.447	3.143	3.707	5.959
7	1.895	2.365	2.998	3.499	5.405
8	1.860	2.306	2.896	3.355	5.041
9	1.833	2.262	2.821	3.250	4.781
10	1.812	2.228	2.764	3.169	4.587
11	1.796	2.201	2.718	3.106	4.437
12	1.782	2.179	2.681	3.055	4.318
13	1.771	2.160	2.650	3.012	4.221
14	1.761	2.145	2.624	2.977	4.140
15	1.753	2.131	2.602	2.947	4.073
16	1.746	2.120	2.583	2.921	4.015
17	1.740	2.110	2.567	2.898	3.965
18	1.734	2.101	2.552	2.878	3.922
19	1.729	2.093	2.539	2.861	3.883
20	1.725	2.086	2.528	2.845	3.850
21	1.721	2.080	2.518	2.831	3.819
22	1.717	2.074	2.508	2.819	3.792
23	1.714	2.069	2.500	2.807	3.767
24	1.711	2.064	2.492	2.797	3.745
25	1.708	2.060	2.485	2.787	3.725
26	1.706	2.056	2.479	2.779	3.707
27	1.703	2.052	2.473	2.771	3.690
28	1.701	2.048	2.467	2.763	3.674
29	1.699	2.045	2.462	2.756	3.659
30	1.697	2.042	2.457	2.750	3.646
40	1.684	2.021	2.423	2.704	3.551
60	1.671	2.000	2.390	2.660	3.460
120	1.658	1.980	2.358	2.617	3.373
∞	1.645	1.960	2.326	2.576	3.291

[a] Table B is abridged from Table III of R. A. Fisher and F. Yates: "Statistical Tables for Biological, Agricultural, and Medical Research," 146 pp. Oliver & Boyd Ltd., Edinburgh, by permission of the authors and publishers (1963).

TABLE C-1[a]

Chi-Square Distribution
A denotes the right tail area for the values of χ^2
given below. ν is the number of degrees
of freedom

Degrees of freedom	$A = .99$	$A = .98$	$A = .95$	$A = .90$	$A = .80$	$A = .70$	$A = .50$
1	.00016	.00063	.0039	.016	.064	.15	.46
2	.02	.04	.10	.21	.45	.71	1.39
3	.12	.18	.35	.58	1.00	1.42	2.37
4	.30	.43	.71	1.06	1.65	2.20	3.36
5	.55	.75	1.14	1.61	2.34	3.00	4.35
6	.87	1.13	1.64	2.20	3.07	3.83	5.35
7	1.24	1.56	2.17	2.83	3.82	4.67	6.35
8	1.65	2.03	2.73	3.49	4.59	5.53	7.34
9	2.09	2.53	3.32	4.17	5.38	6.39	8.34
10	2.56	3.06	3.94	4.86	6.18	7.27	9.34
11	3.05	3.61	4.58	5.58	6.99	8.15	10.34
12	3.57	4.18	5.23	6.30	7.81	9.03	11.34
13	4.11	4.76	5.89	7.04	8.63	9.93	12.34
14	4.66	5.37	6.57	7.79	9.47	10.82	13.34
15	5.23	5.98	7.26	8.55	10.31	11.72	14.34
16	5.81	6.61	7.96	9.31	11.15	12.62	15.34
17	6.41	7.26	8.67	10.08	12.00	13.53	16.34
18	7.02	7.91	9.39	10.86	12.86	14.44	17.34
19	7.63	8.57	10.12	11.65	13.72	15.35	18.34
20	8.26	9.24	10.85	12.44	14.58	16.27	19.34
21	8.90	9.92	11.59	13.24	15.44	17.18	20.34
22	9.54	10.60	12.34	14.04	16.31	18.10	21.34
23	10.20	11.29	13.09	14.85	17.19	19.02	22.34
24	10.86	11.99	13.85	15.66	18.06	19.94	23.34
25	11.52	12.70	14.61	16.47	18.94	20.87	24.34
26	12.20	13.41	15.38	17.29	19.82	21.79	25.34
27	12.88	14.12	16.15	18.11	20.70	22.72	26.34
28	13.56	14.85	16.93	18.94	21.59	23.65	27.34
29	14.26	15.57	17.71	19.77	22.48	24.58	28.34
30	14.95	16.31	18.49	20.60	23.36	25.51	29.34

TABLE C-2[a]
Chi-Square Distribution
(continued)

Degrees of freedom	$A = .30$	$A = .20$	$A = .10$	$A = .05$	$A = .02$	$A = .01$	$A = .001$
1	1.07	1.64	2.71	3.84	5.41	6.64	10.83
2	2.41	3.22	4.60	5.99	7.82	9.21	13.82
3	3.66	4.64	6.25	7.82	9.84	11.34	16.27
4	4.88	5.99	7.78	9.49	11.67	13.28	18.46
5	6.06	7.29	9.24	11.07	13.39	15.09	20.52
6	7.23	8.56	10.64	12.59	15.03	16.81	22.46
7	8.38	9.80	12.02	14.07	16.62	18.48	24.32
8	9.52	11.03	13.36	15.51	18.17	20.09	26.12
9	10.66	12.24	14.68	16.92	19.68	21.67	27.88
10	11.78	13.44	15.99	18.31	21.16	23.21	29.59
11	12.90	14.63	17.28	19.68	22.62	24.72	31.26
12	14.01	15.81	18.55	21.03	24.05	26.22	32.91
13	15.12	16.98	19.81	22.36	25.47	27.69	34.53
14	16.22	18.15	21.06	23.68	26.87	29.14	36.12
15	17.32	19.31	22.31	25.00	28.26	30.58	37.70
16	18.42	20.46	23.54	26.30	29.63	32.00	39.25
17	19.51	21.62	24.77	27.59	31.00	33.41	40.79
18	20.60	22.76	25.99	28.87	32.35	34.80	42.31
19	21.69	23.90	27.20	30.14	33.69	36.19	43.82
20	22.78	25.04	28.41	31.41	35.02	37.57	45.32
21	23.86	26.17	29.62	32.67	36.34	38.93	46.80
22	24.94	27.30	30.81	33.92	37.66	30.29	48.27
23	26.02	28.43	32.01	35.17	38.97	41.64	49.73
24	27.10	29.55	33.20	36.42	40.27	42.98	51.18
25	28.17	30.68	34.38	37.65	41.57	44.31	52.62
26	29.25	31.80	35.56	38.88	42.86	45.64	54.05
27	30.32	32.91	36.74	40.11	44.14	46.96	55.48
28	31.39	34.03	37.92	41.34	45.42	48.28	56.89
29	32.46	35.14	39.09	42.56	46.69	49.59	58.30
30	33.53	36.25	40.26	43.77	47.96	50.89	59.70

[a] Tables C-1 and C-2 are abridged from Table IV of R. A. Fisher and F. Yates: "Statistical Tables for Fiological, Agricultural, Medical Research," 146 pp. Oliver & Eoyd Ltd., Edinburgh, by permission of the authors and publishers (1963).

For larger values of d.f., the expression $\sqrt{2\chi^2} - \sqrt{2(\text{d.f.}) - 1}$ may be used as a normal deviate with unit standard error.

TABLE D[a]
Significance in Paired Tests $(p = \frac{1}{2})$

Number of judges or judgments	Minimum correct judgments to establish significant differentiation (one-tailed test)			Minimum agreeing judgments necessary to establish significant preference (two-tailed test)		
	Probability level*					
	.05	.01	.001	.05	.01	.001
7	7	7	—	7	—	—
8	7	8	—	8	8	—
9	8	9	—	8	9	—
10	9	10	10	9	10	—
11	9	10	11	10	11	11
12	10	11	12	10	11	12
13	10	12	13	11	12	13
14	11	12	13	12	13	14
15	12	13	14	12	13	14
16	12	14	15	13	14	15
17	13	14	16	13	15	16
18	13	15	16	14	15	17
19	14	15	17	15	16	17
20	15	16	18	15	17	18
21	15	17	18	16	17	19
22	16	17	19	17	18	19
23	16	18	20	17	19	20
24	17	19	20	18	19	21
25	18	19	21	18	20	21
30	20	22	24	21	23	25
35	23	25	27	24	26	28
40	26	28	31	27	29	31
45	29	31	34	30	32	34
50	32	34	37	33	35	37
60	37	40	43	39	41	44
70	43	46	49	44	47	50
80	48	51	55	50	52	56
90	54	57	61	55	58	61
100	59	63	66	61	64	67

[a] Table D is adapted from a table by E. B. Roessler, G. A. Baker, and M. A. Amerine. *Food Research* **21**, 117–121 (1956).

* $p = .05$ indicates that the odds are only 1 in 20 that this result is due to chance; $p = .01$ indicates a chance of only 1 in 100; and $p = .001$, 1 in 1000.

TABLE E[a]

Significance in Triangular Tests $(p = \frac{1}{3})$

No. of judges or judgments	Minimum correct judgments to establish significant differentiation			No. of tasters or tastings	Minimum correct judgments to establish significant differentiation		
	$p = .05$	$p = .01$	$p = .001$		$p = .05$	$p = .01$	$p = .001$
5	4	5	5	46	22	24	26
6	5	6	6	47	23	25	27
7	5	6	7	48	23	25	27
8	6	7	8	49	23	25	28
9	6	7	8	50	24	26	28
10	7	8	9	51	24	26	29
11	7	8	9	52	25	27	29
12	8	9	10	53	25	27	29
13	8	9	10	54	25	27	30
14	9	10	11	55	26	28	30
15	9	10	12	56	26	28	31
16	10	11	12	57	27	29	31
17	10	11	13	58	27	29	32
18	10	12	13	59	27	30	32
19	11	12	14	60	28	30	33
20	11	13	14	61	28	30	33
21	12	13	15	62	28	31	33
22	12	14	15	63	29	31	34
23	13	14	16	64	29	32	34
24	13	14	16	65	30	32	35
25	13	15	17	66	30	32	35
26	14	15	17	67	30	33	36
27	14	16	18	68	31	33	36
28	15	16	18	69	31	34	36
29	15	17	19	70	32	34	37
30	16	17	19	71	32	34	37
31	16	18	19	72	32	35	38
32	16	18	20	73	33	35	38
33	17	19	20	74	33	36	39
34	17	19	21	75	34	36	39
35	18	19	21	76	34	36	39
36	18	20	22	77	34	37	40
37	18	20	22	78	35	37	40
38	19	21	23	79	35	38	41
39	19	21	23	80	35	38	41
40	20	22	24	81	36	38	41
41	20	22	24	82	36	39	42
42	21	22	25	83	37	39	42
43	21	23	25	84	37	40	43
44	21	23	25	85	37	40	43
45	22	24	26	86	38	40	44

TABLE E (*continued*)

No. of judges or judgments	Minimum correct judgments to establish significant differentiation			No. of tasters or tastings	Minimum correct judgments to establish significant differentiation		
	$p = .05$	$p = .01$	$p = .001$		$p = .05$	$p = .01$	$p = .001$
87	38	41	44	98	42	45	49
88	39	41	44	99	43	46	49
89	39	42	45	100	43	46	49
90	39	42	45	200	80	84	89
91	40	42	46	300	117	122	127
92	40	43	46	400	152	158	165
93	40	43	46	500	188	194	202
94	41	44	47	1,000	363	372	383
95	41	44	47	2,000	709	722	737
96	42	44	48				
97	42	45	48				

[a] Table E is reproduced from a table by E. B. Roessler, J. Warren, and J. F. Guymon. *Food Research* **13,** 503–505 (1948).

TABLE F-1
F-Distribution $(F_{.95})$

(The numbers given in this table are the values of F for which the area to the left equals 0.95 for tables F-1 and F-2, and 0.99 for tables F-3 and F-4 for the indicated numerator and denominator degrees of freedom)

Deg. of freedom for denom.	Degrees of freedom for numerator									
	1	2	3	4	5	6	7	8	9	10
1	161	200	216	225	230	234	237	239	241	242
2	18.5	19.0	19.2	19.2	19.3	19.3	19.4	19.4	19.4	19.4
3	10.1	9.55	9.28	9.12	9.01	8.94	8.89	8.85	8.81	8.79
4	7.71	6.94	6.59	6.39	6.26	6.16	6.09	6.04	6.00	5.96
5	6.61	5.79	5.41	5.19	5.05	4.95	4.88	4.82	4.77	4.74
6	5.99	5.14	4.76	4.53	4.39	4.28	4.21	4.15	4.10	4.06
7	5.59	4.74	4.35	4.12	3.97	3.87	3.79	3.73	3.68	3.64
8	5.32	4.46	4.07	3.84	3.69	3.58	3.50	3.44	3.39	3.35
9	5.12	4.26	3.86	3.63	3.48	3.37	3.29	3.23	3.18	3.14
10	4.96	4.10	3.71	3.48	3.33	3.22	3.14	3.07	3.02	2.98
11	4.84	3.98	3.59	3.36	3.20	3.09	3.01	2.95	2.90	2.85
12	4.75	3.89	3.49	3.26	3.11	3.00	2.91	2.85	2.80	2.75
13	4.67	3.81	3.41	3.18	3.03	2.92	2.83	2.77	2.71	2.67
14	4.60	3.74	3.34	3.11	2.96	2.85	2.76	2.70	2.65	2.60
15	4.54	3.68	3.29	3.06	2.90	2.79	2.71	2.64	2.59	2.54
16	4.49	3.63	3.24	3.01	2.85	2.74	2.66	2.59	2.54	2.49
17	4.45	3.59	3.20	2.96	2.81	2.70	2.61	2.55	2.49	2.45
18	4.41	3.55	3.16	2.93	2.77	2.66	2.58	2.51	2.46	2.41
19	4.38	3.52	3.13	2.90	2.74	2.63	2.54	2.48	2.42	2.38
20	4.35	3.49	3.10	2.87	2.71	2.60	2.51	2.45	2.39	2.35
21	4.32	3.47	3.07	2.84	2.68	2.57	2.49	2.42	2.37	2.32
22	4.30	3.44	3.05	2.82	2.66	2.55	2.46	2.40	2.34	2.30
23	4.28	3.42	3.03	2.80	2.64	2.53	2.44	2.37	2.32	2.27
24	4.26	3.40	3.01	2.78	2.62	2.51	2.42	2.36	2.30	2.25
25	4.24	3.39	2.99	2.76	2.60	2.49	2.40	2.34	2.28	2.24
30	4.17	3.32	2.92	2.69	2.53	2.42	2.33	2.27	2.21	2.16
40	4.08	3.23	2.84	2.61	2.45	2.34	2.25	2.18	2.12	2.08
60	4.00	3.15	2.76	2.53	2.37	2.25	2.17	2.10	2.04	1.99
120	3.92	3.07	2.68	2.45	2.29	2.18	2.09	2.02	1.96	1.91
∞	3.84	3.00	2.60	2.37	2.21	2.10	2.01	1.94	1.88	1.83

TABLE F-2
F-Distribution $(F_{.95})$
(*continued*)

Deg. of freedom for denom.	Degrees for freedom for numerator								
	12	15	20	24	30	40	60	120	∞
1	244	246	248	249	250	251	252	253	254
2	19.4	19.4	19.4	19.5	19.5	19.5	19.5	19.5	19.5
3	8.74	8.70	8.66	8.64	8.62	8.59	8.57	8.55	8.53
4	5.91	5.86	5.80	5.77	5.75	5.72	5.69	5.66	5.63
5	4.68	4.62	4.56	4.53	4.50	4.46	4.43	4.40	4.37
6	4.00	3.94	3.87	3.84	3.81	3.77	3.74	3.70	3.67
7	3.57	3.51	3.44	3.41	3.38	3.34	3.30	3.27	3.23
8	3.28	3.22	3.15	3.12	3.08	3.04	3.01	2.97	2.93
9	3.07	3.01	2.94	2.90	2.86	2.83	2.79	2.75	2.71
10	2.91	2.85	2.77	2.74	2.70	2.66	2.62	2.58	2.54
11	2.79	2.72	2.65	2.61	2.57	2.53	2.49	2.45	2.40
12	2.69	2.62	2.54	2.51	2.47	2.43	2.38	2.34	2.30
13	2.60	2.53	2.46	2.42	2.38	2.34	2.30	2.25	2.21
14	2.53	2.46	2.39	2.35	2.31	2.27	2.22	2.18	2.13
15	2.48	2.40	2.33	2.29	2.25	2.20	2.16	2.11	2.07
16	2.42	2.35	2.28	2.24	2.19	2.15	2.11	2.06	2.01
17	2.38	2.31	2.23	2.19	2.15	2.10	2.06	2.01	1.96
18	2.34	2.27	2.19	2.15	2.11	2.06	2.02	1.97	1.92
19	2.31	2.23	2.16	2.11	2.07	2.03	1.98	1.93	1.88
20	2.28	2.20	2.12	2.08	2.04	1.99	1.95	1.90	1.84
21	2.25	2.18	2.10	2.05	2.01	1.96	1.92	1.87	1.81
22	2.23	2.15	2.07	2.03	1.98	1.94	1.89	1.84	1.78
23	2.20	2.13	2.05	2.01	1.96	1.91	1.86	1.81	1.76
24	2.18	2.11	2.03	1.98	1.94	1.89	1.84	1.79	1.73
25	2.16	2.09	2.01	1.96	1.92	1.87	1.82	1.77	1.71
26	2.09	2.01	1.93	1.89	1.84	1.79	1.74	1.68	1.62
27	2.00	1.92	1.84	1.79	1.74	1.69	1.64	1.58	1.51
28	1.92	1.84	1.75	1.70	1.65	1.59	1.53	1.47	1.39
29	1.83	1.75	1.66	1.61	1.55	1.50	1.43	1.35	1.25
30	1.75	1.67	1.57	1.52	1.46	1.39	1.32	1.22	1.00

TABLE F-3
F-Distribution $(F_{.99})$

Deg. of freedom for denom.	Degrees of freedom for numerator									
	1	2	3	4	5	6	7	8	9	10
1	4,052	5,000	5,403	5,625	5,764	5,859	5,928	5,982	6,023	6,056
2	98.5	99.0	99.2	99.2	99.3	99.3	99.4	99.4	99.4	99.4
3	34.1	30.8	29.5	28.7	28.2	27.9	27.7	27.5	27.3	27.2
4	21.2	18.0	16.7	16.0	15.5	15.2	15.0	14.8	14.7	14.5
5	16.3	13.3	12.1	11.4	11.0	10.7	10.5	10.3	10.2	10.1
6	13.7	10.9	9.78	9.15	8.75	8.47	8.26	8.10	7.98	7.87
7	12.2	9.55	8.45	7.85	7.46	7.19	6.99	6.84	6.72	6.62
8	11.3	8.65	7.59	7.01	6.63	6.37	6.18	6.03	5.91	5.81
9	10.6	8.02	6.99	6.42	6.06	5.80	5.61	5.47	5.35	5.26
10	10.0	7.56	6.55	5.99	5.64	5.39	5.20	5.06	4.94	4.85
11	9.65	7.21	6.22	5.67	5.32	5.07	4.89	4.74	4.63	4.54
12	9.33	6.93	5.95	5.41	5.06	4.82	4.64	4.50	4.39	4.30
13	9.07	6.70	5.74	5.21	4.86	4.62	4.44	4.30	4.19	4.10
14	8.86	6.51	5.56	5.04	4.70	4.46	4.28	4.14	4.03	3.94
15	8.68	6.36	5.42	4.89	4.56	4.32	4.14	4.00	3.89	3.80
16	8.53	6.23	5.29	4.77	4.44	4.20	4.03	3.89	3.78	3.69
17	8.40	6.11	5.19	4.67	4.34	4.10	3.93	3.79	3.68	3.59
18	8.29	6.01	5.09	4.58	4.25	4.01	3.84	3.71	3.60	3.51
19	8.19	5.93	5.01	4.50	4.17	3.94	3.77	3.63	3.52	3.43
20	8.10	5.85	4.94	4.43	4.10	3.87	3.70	3.56	3.46	3.37
21	8.02	5.78	4.87	4.37	4.04	3.81	3.64	3.51	3.40	3.31
22	7.95	5.72	4.82	4.31	3.99	3.76	3.59	3.45	3.35	3.26
23	7.88	5.66	4.76	4.26	3.94	3.71	3.54	3.41	3.30	3.21
24	7.82	5.61	4.72	4.22	3.90	3.67	3.50	3.36	3.26	3.17
25	7.77	5.57	4.68	4.18	3.86	3.63	3.46	3.32	3.22	3.13
30	7.56	5.39	4.51	4.02	3.70	3.47	3.30	3.17	3.07	2.98
40	7.31	5.18	4.31	3.83	3.51	3.29	3.12	2.99	2.89	2.80
60	7.08	4.98	4.13	3.65	3.34	3.12	2.95	2.82	2.72	2.63
120	6.85	4.79	3.95	3.48	3.17	2.96	2.79	2.66	2.56	2.47
∞	6.63	4.61	3.78	3.32	3.02	2.80	2.64	2.51	2.41	2.32

TABLE F-4[a]
F-Distribution $(F_{.99})$
(*continued*)

Deg. of freedom for denom.	Degrees of freedom for numerator								
	12	15	20	24	30	40	60	120	∞
1	6,106	6,157	6,209	6,235	6,261	6,287	6,313	6,339	6,366
2	99.4	99.4	99.4	99.5	99.5	99.5	99.5	99.5	99.5
3	27.1	26.9	26.7	26.6	26.5	26.4	26.3	26.2	26.1
4	14.4	14.2	14.0	13.9	13.8	13.7	13.7	13.6	13.5
5	9.89	9.72	9.55	9.47	9.38	9.29	9.20	9.11	9.02
6	7.72	7.56	7.40	7.31	7.23	7.14	7.06	6.97	6.88
7	6.47	6.31	6.16	6.07	5.99	5.91	5.82	5.74	5.65
8	5.67	5.52	5.36	5.28	5.20	5.12	5.03	4.95	4.86
9	5.11	4.96	4.81	4.73	4.65	4.57	4.48	4.40	4.31
10	4.71	4.56	4.41	4.33	4.25	4.17	4.08	4.00	3.91
11	4.40	4.25	4.10	4.02	3.94	3.86	3.78	3.69	3.60
12	4.16	4.01	3.86	3.78	3.70	3.62	3.54	3.45	3.36
13	3.96	3.82	3.66	3.59	3.51	3.43	3.34	3.25	3.17
14	3.80	3.66	3.51	3.43	3.35	3.27	3.18	3.09	3.00
15	3.67	3.52	3.37	3.29	3.21	3.13	3.05	2.96	2.87
16	3.55	3.41	3.26	3.18	3.10	3.02	2.93	2.84	2.75
17	3.46	3.31	3.16	3.08	3.00	2.92	2.83	2.75	2.65
18	3.37	3.23	3.08	3.00	2.92	2.84	2.75	2.66	2.57
19	3.30	3.15	3.00	2.92	2.84	2.76	2.67	2.58	2.49
20	3.23	3.09	2.94	2.86	2.78	2.69	2.61	2.52	2.42
21	3.17	3.03	2.88	2.80	2.72	2.64	2.55	2.46	2.36
22	3.12	2.98	2.83	2.75	2.67	2.58	2.50	2.40	2.31
23	3.07	2.93	2.78	2.70	2.62	2.54	2.45	2.35	2.26
24	3.03	2.89	2.74	2.66	2.58	2.49	2.40	2.31	2.21
25	2.99	2.85	2.70	2.62	2.53	2.45	2.36	2.27	2.17
30	2.84	2.70	2.55	2.47	2.39	2.30	2.21	2.11	2.01
40	2.66	2.52	2.37	2.29	2.20	2.11	2.02	1.92	1.80
60	2.50	2.35	2.20	2.12	2.03	1.94	1.84	1.73	1.60
120	2.34	2.19	2.03	1.95	1.86	1.76	1.66	1.53	1.38
∞	2.18	2.04	1.88	1.79	1.70	1.59	1.47	1.32	1.00

[a] Tables F-1 to F-4 are reproduced with the permission of Professor E. S. Pearson from M. Merrington, C. M. Thompson, Tables of percentage points of the inverted beta (F) distribution. *Biometrika* **33**, 73–99 (1943).

TABLE G-1

Significant Studentized Ranges, Multiple Range Test (5% level)

Degrees of freedom	p											
	2	3	4	5	6	7	8	9	10	20	50	100
1	18.00	18.00	18.00	18.00	18.00	18.00	18.00	18.00	18.00	18.00	18.00	18.00
2	6.08	6.08	6.08	6.08	6.08	6.08	6.08	6.08	6.08	6.08	6.08	6.08
3	4.50	4.52	4.52	4.52	4.52	4.52	4.52	4.52	4.52	4.52	4.52	4.52
4	3.93	4.01	4.03	4.03	4.03	4.03	4.03	4.03	4.03	4.03	4.03	4.03
5	3.64	3.75	3.80	3.81	3.81	3.81	3.81	3.81	3.81	3.81	3.81	3.81
6	3.46	3.59	3.65	3.68	3.69	3.70	3.70	3.70	3.70	3.70	3.70	3.70
7	3.34	3.48	3.55	3.59	3.61	3.62	3.63	3.63	3.63	3.63	3.63	3.63
8	3.26	3.40	3.48	3.52	3.55	3.57	3.58	3.58	3.58	3.58	3.58	3.58
9	3.20	3.34	3.42	3.47	3.50	3.52	3.54	3.54	3.55	3.55	3.55	3.55
10	3.15	3.29	3.38	3.43	3.46	3.49	3.50	3.52	3.52	3.53	3.53	3.53
11	3.11	3.26	3.34	3.40	3.44	3.46	3.48	3.49	3.50	3.51	3.51	3.51
12	3.08	3.22	3.31	3.37	3.41	3.44	3.46	3.47	3.48	3.50	3.50	3.50
13	3.06	3.20	3.29	3.35	3.39	3.42	3.44	3.46	3.47	3.49	3.49	3.49
14	3.03	3.18	3.27	3.33	3.37	3.40	3.43	3.44	3.46	3.48	3.48	3.48
15	3.01	3.16	3.25	3.31	3.36	3.39	3.41	3.43	3.45	3.48	3.48	3.48
16	3.00	3.14	3.24	3.30	3.34	3.38	3.40	3.42	3.44	3.48	3.48	3.48
17	2.98	3.13	3.22	3.28	3.33	3.37	3.39	3.41	3.43	3.48	3.48	3.48
18	2.97	3.12	3.21	3.27	3.32	3.36	3.38	3.40	3.42	3.47	3.47	3.47
19	2.96	3.11	3.20	3.26	3.31	3.35	3.38	3.40	3.42	3.47	3.47	3.47
20	2.95	3.10	3.19	3.26	3.30	3.34	3.37	3.39	3.41	3.47	3.47	3.47
30	2.89	3.04	3.13	3.20	3.25	3.29	3.32	3.35	3.37	3.47	3.49	3.49
40	2.86	3.01	3.10	3.17	3.22	3.27	3.30	3.33	3.35	3.47	3.50	3.50
60	2.83	2.98	3.07	3.14	3.20	3.24	3.28	3.31	3.33	3.47	3.54	3.54
120	2.80	2.95	3.04	3.12	3.17	3.22	3.25	3.29	3.31	3.47	3.58	3.60
∞	2.77	2.92	3.02	3.09	3.15	3.19	3.23	3.26	3.29	3.47	3.64	3.74

TABLE G-2[a]

Significant Studentized Ranges, Multiple Range Test (1% level)

Degrees of freedom	\(p \)											
	2	3	4	5	6	7	8	9	10	20	50	100
1	90.00	90.00	90.00	90.00	90.00	90.00	90.00	90.00	90.00	90.00	90.00	90.00
2	14.00	14.00	14.00	14.00	14.00	14.00	14.00	14.00	14.00	14.00	14.00	14.00
3	8.26	8.32	8.32	8.32	8.32	8.32	8.32	8.32	8.32	8.32	8.32	8.32
4	6.51	6.68	6.74	6.76	6.76	6.76	6.76	6.76	6.76	6.76	6.76	6.76
5	5.70	5.89	6.00	6.04	6.06	6.07	6.07	6.07	6.07	6.07	6.07	6.07
6	5.25	5.44	5.55	5.61	5.66	5.68	5.69	5.70	5.70	5.70	5.70	5.70
7	4.95	5.14	5.26	5.33	5.38	5.42	5.44	5.45	5.46	5.47	5.47	5.47
8	4.75	4.94	5.06	5.14	5.19	5.23	5.26	5.28	5.29	5.32	5.32	5.32
9	4.60	4.79	4.91	4.99	5.04	5.09	5.12	5.14	5.16	5.21	5.21	5.21
10	4.48	4.67	4.79	4.87	4.93	4.98	5.01	5.04	5.06	5.12	5.12	5.12
11	4.39	4.58	4.70	4.78	4.84	4.89	4.92	4.95	4.98	5.06	5.06	5.06
12	4.32	4.50	4.62	4.71	4.77	4.82	4.85	4.88	4.91	5.01	5.01	5.01
13	4.26	4.44	4.56	4.64	4.71	4.76	4.79	4.82	4.85	4.96	4.97	4.97
14	4.21	4.39	4.51	4.59	4.65	4.70	4.74	4.78	4.80	4.92	4.94	4.94
15	4.17	4.35	4.46	4.55	4.61	4.66	4.70	4.73	4.76	4.89	4.91	4.91
16	4.13	4.31	4.42	4.51	4.57	4.62	4.66	4.70	4.72	4.86	4.89	4.89
17	4.10	4.28	4.39	4.48	4.54	4.59	4.63	4.66	4.69	4.83	4.87	4.87
18	4.07	4.25	4.36	4.44	4.51	4.56	4.60	4.64	4.66	4.81	4.86	4.86
19	4.05	4.22	4.34	4.42	4.48	4.53	4.58	4.61	4.64	4.79	4.84	4.84
20	4.02	4.20	4.31	4.40	4.46	4.51	4.55	4.59	4.62	4.77	4.83	4.83
30	3.89	4.06	4.17	4.25	4.31	4.37	4.41	4.44	4.48	4.65	4.77	4.78
40	3.82	3.99	4.10	4.18	4.24	4.30	4.34	4.38	4.41	4.59	4.74	4.76
60	3.76	3.92	4.03	4.11	4.17	4.23	4.27	4.31	4.34	4.53	4.71	4.76
120	3.70	3.86	3.96	4.04	4.11	4.16	4.20	4.24	4.27	4.47	4.67	4.77
∞	3.64	3.80	3.90	3.98	4.04	4.09	4.14	4.17	4.20	4.41	4.64	4.78

[a] Tables G-1 and G-2 are abridged from those compiled by D. B. Duncan, *Biometrics* 11, 1–42 (1955) and modified and corrected by H. L. Harter, *Biometrics* 16, 671–685 (1960) and *Biometrics* 17, 321–324 (1961) and are used by permission of the authors and editors.

TABLE H-1[a]

Multipliers for Estimating Significance of Difference by Range
(One-way classification)

Number in group = number per range = number of scores per product	Number of groups = number of ranges = number of products								
	2	3	4	5	6	7	8	9	10
2	3.43[b]	2.35	1.74	1.39	1.15	.99	.87	.77	.70
	7.92[c]	4.32	2.84	2.10	1.66	1.38	1.17	1.02	.91
3	1.90	1.44	1.14	.94	.80	.70	.62	.56	.51
	3.14	2.12	1.57	1.25	1.04	.89	.78	.69	.62
4	1.62	1.25	1.01	.84	.72	.63	.57	.51	.47
	2.48	1.74	1.33	1.08	.91	.78	.69	.62	.56
5	1.53	1.19	.96	.81	.70	.61	.55	.50	.45
	2.24	1.60	1.24	1.02	.86	.75	.66	.59	.54
6	1.50	1.17	.95	.80	.69	.61	.55	.49	.45
	2.14	1.55	1.21	.99	.85	.74	.65	.59	.53
7	1.49	1.17	.95	.80	.69	.61	.55	.50	.45
	2.10	1.53	1.20	.99	.84	.73	.65	.59	.53
8	1.49	1.18	.96	.81	.70	.62	.55	.50	.46
	2.09	1.53	1.20	.99	.85	.74	.66	.59	.54
9	1.50	1.19	.97	.82	.71	.62	.56	.51	.47
	2.09	1.54	1.21	1.00	.85	.75	.66	.60	.54
10	1.52	1.20	.98	.83	.72	.63	.57	.52	.47
	2.10	1.55	1.22	1.01	.86	.76	.67	.61	.55
11	1.54	1.22	.99	.84	.73	.64	.58	.52	.48
	2.11	1.56	1.23	1.02	.87	.76	.68	.61	.56
12	1.56	1.23	1.01	.85	.74	.65	.58	.53	.49
	2.13	1.58	1.25	1.04	.89	.78	.69	.62	.57
13	1.58	1.25	1.02	.86	.75	.66	.59	.54	.49
	2.15	1.60	1.26	1.05	.90	.79	.70	.63	.58
14	1.60	1.26	1.03	.87	.76	.67	.60	.55	.50
	2.18	1.62	1.28	1.06	.91	.80	.71	.64	.58
15	1.62	1.28	1.05	.89	.77	.68	.61	.55	.51
	2.20	1.63	1.30	1.08	.92	.81	.72	.65	.59
16	1.64	1.30	1.06	.90	.78	.69	.62	.56	.52
	2.22	1.65	1.31	1.09	.93	.82	.73	.66	.60

[a] Table H-1 is adapted from unpublished tables by T. E. Kurtz, R. F. Link, J. W. Tukey, and D. L. Wallace, reproduced by permission of J. W. Tukey and D. L. Wallace.

[b,c] The upper and lower entries are for the 5 and 1% error rates, respectively, and are to be multiplied by the sum of ranges within groups to obtain the difference between group totals required for significance.

TABLE H-2[a]

Multipliers for Estimating Significance of Difference by Range[b]
(Two-way classification—5% error rate)

Number per range = number of rows	Number of ranges = number of columns								
	2	3	4	5	6	7	8	9	10
2	6.35	2.19	1.52	1.16	.94	.79	.69	.60	.54
	6.35	1.96	1.39	1.12	.95	.84	.76	.70	.65
3	1.96	1.14	.88	.72	.61	.53	.47	.42	.38
	2.19	1.14	.90	.76	.67	.61	.56	.52	.49
4	1.43	.96	.76	.63	.54	.47	.42	.38	.34
	1.54	.93	.76	.65	.58	.53	.49	.45	.43
5	1.27	.89	.71	.60	.51	.45	.40	.36	.33
	1.28	.84	.69	.60	.53	.49	.45	.42	.40
6	1.19	.87	.70	.58	.50	.44	.39	.36	.33
	1.14	.78	.64	.56	.50	.46	.43	.40	.38
7	1.16	.86	.69	.58	.50	.44	.40	.36	.33
	1.06	.74	.62	.54	.48	.44	.41	.38	.36
8	1.15	.86	.69	.58	.50	.44	.40	.36	.33
	1.01	.71	.59	.52	.47	.43	.40	.37	.35
9	1.15	.86	.70	.59	.51	.45	.40	.36	.33
	.97	.69	.58	.51	.46	.42	.39	.36	.34
10	1.15	.87	.71	.60	.51	.45	.41	.37	.34
	.93	.67	.56	.50	.45	.41	.38	.36	.34
11	1.16	.88	.71	.60	.52	.46	.41	.37	.34
	.91	.66	.55	.49	.44	.40	.38	.35	.33
12	1.16	.89	.72	.61	.53	.47	.42	.38	.35
	.89	.65	.55	.48	.43	.40	.37	.35	.33
13	1.17	.90	.73	.62	.54	.47	.42	.38	.35
	.87	.64	.54	.47	.43	.39	.37	.34	.32
14	1.19	.91	.74	.63	.54	.48	.43	.39	.36
	.85	.63	.53	.47	.42	.39	.36	.34	.32
15	1.20	.92	.75	.63	.55	.49	.44	.40	.36
	.84	.62	.53	.46	.42	.39	.36	.34	.32
16	1.21	.93	.76	.64	.56	.49	.44	.40	.37
	.83	.61	.52	.46	.42	.38	.36	.33	.32

[a] Table H-2 is adapted from unpublished tables by T. E. Kurtz, R. F. Link, J. W. Tukey, and D. L. Wallace, reproduced by permission of J. W. Tukey and D. L. Wallace.

[b] Entries are to be multiplied by the sum of ranges of differences between adjacent observations to obtain difference required for significance for column totals (use upper entry) and row totals (use lower entry). Differences are to be taken horizontally, their ranges vertically.

TABLE I-1

Rank Totals Required for Significance at the 5% Level $(p < .05)$[a]

No. of reps.	2	3	4	5	6	7	8	9	10	11	12
						No. of treatments, or samples ranked					
2	—	—	—	—	—	—	—	4-16	4-18	—	—
	—	—	—	3-9	3-11	3-13	4-14			5-19	5-21
3	—	—	—	4-14	4-17	4-20	4-23	5-25	5-28	5-31	5-34
	—	4-8	4-11	5-13	6-15	6-18	7-20	8-22	8-25	9-27	10-29
4	—	5-11	5-15	6-18	6-22	7-25	7-29	8-32	8-36	8-39	9-43
	—	5-11	6-14	7-17	8-20	9-23	10-26	11-29	13-31	14-34	15-37
5	—	6-14	7-18	8-22	9-26	9-31	10-35	11-39	12-43	12-48	13-52
	6-9	7-13	8-17	10-20	11-24	13-27	14-31	15-35	17-38	18-42	20-45
6	7-11	8-16	9-21	10-26	11-31	12-36	13-41	14-46	15-51	17-55	18-60
	7-11	9-15	11-19	12-24	14-28	16-32	18-36	20-40	21-45	23-49	25-53
7	8-13	10-18	11-24	12-30	14-35	15-41	17-46	18-52	19-58	21-63	22-69
	8-13	10-18	13-22	15-27	17-32	19-37	22-41	24-46	26-51	28-56	30-61
8	9-15	11-21	13-27	15-33	17-39	18-46	20-52	22-58	24-64	25-71	27-77
	10-14	12-20	15-25	17-31	20-36	23-41	25-47	28-52	31-57	33-63	36-68
9	11-16	13-23	15-30	17-37	19-44	22-50	24-57	26-64	28-71	30-78	32-85
	11-16	14-22	17-28	20-34	23-44	26-46	29-52	32-58	35-64	38-70	41-76
10	12-18	15-25	17-33	20-40	22-48	25-25	27-63	30-70	32-78	35-85	37-93
	12-18	16-24	19-31	23-37	26-44	30-50	34-56	37-63	40-70	44-76	47-83

11	13-20 14-19	16-28 18-26	19-36 21-34	22-44 25-41	25-52 29-48	28-60 33-55	31-68 37-62	34-76 41-69	36-85 45-76	39-93 49-83	42-101 53-90
12	15-21 15-21	18-30 19-29	21-39 24-36	25-47 28-44	28-56 32-52	31-65 37-59	34-74 41-67	38-82 45-75	41-91 50-82	44-100 54-90	47-109 58-98
13	16-23 17-22	20-32 21-31	24-41 26-39	27-51 31-47	31-60 35-56	35-69 40-64	38-79 45-72	42-88 50-80	45-98 54-89	49-107 59-97	52-117 64-105
14	17-25 18-24	22-34 23-35	26-44 28-42	30-54 33-51	34-64 38-60	38-74 44-68	42-84 49-77	46-94 54-86	50-104 59-95	54-114 65-103	57-125 70-112
15	19-26 19-26	23-37 25-35	28-47 30-45	32-58 36-54	37-68 42-63	41-79 47-73	46-89 53-82	50-100 59-91	54-111 64-101	58-122 70-110	63-132 75-120
16	20-28 21-27	25-39 27-37	30-50 33-47	35-61 39-57	40-72 45-67	45-83 51-77	49-95 57-87	54-106 62-98	59-117 69-107	63-129 75-117	68-140 81-127
17	22-29 22-29	27-41 28-40	32-53 35-50	38-64 41-61	43-76 48-71	48-88 54-82	53-100 61-92	58-112 67-103	63-124 74-113	68-136 81-123	73-148 87-134
18	23-31 24-30	29-43 30-42	34-56 37-53	40-68 44-64	46-80 51-75	52-92 58-86	57-105 65-97	61-118 72-108	68-130 79-119	73-143 86-130	79-155 93-141
19	24-33 25-32	30-46 32-44	37-58 39-56	43-71 47-67	49-84 54-79	55-97 62-90	61-110 69-102	67-123 76-114	73-136 84-125	78-150 91-137	84-163 99-148
20	26-34 26-34	32-48 34-46	39-61 42-58	45-95 50-70	52-88 57-83	58-102 65-95	65-115 73-107	71-129 81-119	77-143 89-131	83-157 97-143	90-170 105-155

a The four-figure blocks represent: Lowest insignificant rank sum, any treatment—highest insignificant rank sum, any treatment; lowest insignificant rank sum, predetermined treatment—highest insignificant rank sum, predetermined treatment.

TABLE I-2[a]

Rank Totals Required for Significance at the 1% Level $(p < .01)$[b]

No. of reps.	Number of treatments, or samples ranked										
	2	3	4	5	6	7	8	9	10	11	12
2	—	—	—	—	—	—	—	—	—	—	—
	—	—	—	—	—	—	—	—	3-19	3-21	3-23
3	—	—	—	4-14	4-17	4-20	—	—	4-29	4-32	4-35
	—	—	—	—	—	—	5-22	5-25	6-27	6-30	6-33
4	—	—	—	5-19	5-23	5-27	6-30	6-34	6-38	6-42	7-45
	—	—	5-15	6-18	6-22	7-25	8-28	8-32	9-35	10-38	10-42
5	—	—	6-19	7-23	7-28	8-32	8-37	9-41	9-46	10-50	10-55
	—	6-14	7-18	8-22	9-26	10-30	11-34	12-38	13-42	14-46	15-50
6	—	7-17	8-22	9-27	9-33	10-38	11-43	12-48	13-53	13-59	14-64
	—	8-16	9-21	10-26	12-30	13-35	14-40	16-44	17-49	18-54	20-58
7	—	8-20	10-25	11-31	12-37	13-43	14-49	15-55	16-61	17-67	18-73
	8-13	9-19	11-24	12-30	14-35	16-40	18-45	19-51	21-56	23-61	25-66
8	9-15	10-22	11-29	13-35	14-42	16-48	17-55	19-61	20-68	21-75	23-81
	9-15	11-21	13-27	15-33	17-39	19-45	21-51	23-57	25-63	28-68	30-74
9	10-17	12-24	13-32	15-39	17-46	19-53	21-60	22-68	24-75	26-82	27-90
	10-17	12-24	15-30	17-37	20-43	22-50	25-56	27-63	30-69	32-76	35-82
10	11-19	13-27	15-35	18-42	20-50	22-58	24-66	26-74	28-82	30-90	32-98
	11-19	14-26	17-33	20-40	23-47	25-55	28-62	31-69	34-76	37-83	40-90

11	12-21	15-29	17-38	20-46	22-55	25-63	27-72	30-80	32-89	34-98	37-106
	13-20	16-28	19-36	22-44	25-52	29-59	32-67	35-75	39-82	42-90	45-98
12	14-22	17-31	19-41	22-50	25-59	28-68	31-77	33-87	36-96	39-105	42-114
	14-22	18-30	21-39	25-47	28-56	32-64	36-72	39-81	43-89	47-97	50-106
13	15-24	18-34	21-44	25-53	28-63	31-73	34-83	37-93	40-103	43-113	46-123
	15-24	19-33	23-42	27-51	31-60	35-69	39-78	44-86	48-95	52-104	56-113
14	16-26	20-36	24-46	27-57	31-67	34-78	38-88	41-98	45-109	48-120	51-131
	17-25	21-35	25-45	30-54	34-64	39-73	43-83	48-92	52-102	57-121	61-121
15	18-27	22-38	26-49	30-60	34-71	37-83	41-94	45-105	49-116	53-127	56-139
	18-27	23-37	28-47	32-58	37-68	42-78	47-88	52-98	57-108	62-118	67-128
16	19-29	23-41	28-52	32-64	36-76	41-87	45-99	49-111	53-123	57-135	62-146
	19-29	25-39	30-50	35-61	40-72	46-82	51-93	56-104	61-115	67-125	72-136
17	20-31	25-43	30-55	35-67	39-80	44-92	49-104	53-117	58-129	62-142	67-154
	21-30	26-42	32-53	38-64	43-76	49-87	55-98	60-110	66-121	72-132	78-143
18	22-32	27-45	32-58	37-71	42-84	47-97	52-110	57-123	62-136	67-149	72-162
	22-32	28-44	34-56	40-68	46-80	52-92	57-105	62-118	68-130	73-143	79-155
19	23-34	29-47	34-61	40-74	45-88	50-102	56-115	61-129	67-142	72-156	77-170
	24-33	30-46	36-59	43-71	49-84	56-96	62-109	69-121	76-133	82-146	89-158
20	24-36	30-50	36-64	42-78	48-92	54-106	60-120	65-135	71-149	77-163	82-178
	25-35	32-48	38-62	45-75	52-88	59-101	66-114	73-127	80-140	87-153	94-166

[a] Tables I-1 and I-2 are reproduced from a table compiled by A. Kramer and published in revised form in *Food Technol.* **17** (12), 124–125 (1963) and are used by permission of the author.
[b] The four figure blocks represent: Lowest insignificant rank sum, any treatment–highest insignificant rank sum, any treatment; lowest insignificant rank sum, predetermined treatment–highest insignificant rank sum, predetermined treatment.

Glossary of Terms*

A

Absolute judgment—Psychophysical method permitting no external standard stimulus, requiring instead an estimate of the absolute intensity of a stimulus or a categorical judgment based on the observer's experience.

Absolute scaling—Transforming the obtained values of a set of observations into a scale that permits direct comparison with a set of observations on a different scale.

Absolute threshold—See **Threshold**.

Acceptance—(1) An experience, or feature of experience, characterized by a positive (approach in a pleasant) attitude. (2) Actual utilization (purchase, eating). May be measured by preference or liking for specific food item. The two definitions are often highly correlated, but they are not necessarily the same.

Acid—(1) Any chemical compound containing hydrogen capable of giving off protons (hydrogen ions). (2) Refers to the acid content of a stimulus; use in place of the word "sour" is erroneous.

Acrid—Sharp and harsh odor; pungent.

Acuity—Fineness of sensory recognition or discrimination; ability to discern small absolute or relative differences in stimuli; sharpness or acuteness.

---

* Among the glossaries consulted were:

American Society for Testing and Materials. 1963. Nomenclature and Definitions. 11-page mimeo. report compiled by Subcommittee 1, ASTM Committee E-18 on Sensory Evaluation of Materials and Products.

Kramer, A. 1959. Glossary of some terms used in the sensory (panel) evaluation of foods and beverages. *Food Technol.* **13**, 733–736.

Kramer, A., and B. A. Twigg. 1962. "Fundamentals of Quality Control for the Food Industry," 512 pp. (see pp. 489–501). Avi Publ. Co., Westport, Connecticut.

Le Magnen, J. 1962. Vocabulaire technique des caractères organoleptiques et de la dégustation des produits alimentaires. *Bull. Centre Natl. Recherche Sci.* **11**, 86 pp.

Moncrieff, R. W. 1951. "The Chemical Senses," 538 pp. (see pp. 469–480). Leonard Hill, London.

Wenger, M. A., F. N. Jones, and M. H. Jones. 1956. "Physiological Psychology," 472 pp. (see pp. 449–464). Holt, New York.

Adaptation—Loss of or change in sensitivity to a given stimulus as a result of continuous exposure to that stimulus or a similar one. Also known as **Fatigue** (*q.v.*).

Adaptation level—Momentary state resulting in a neutral or indifferent response.

Adequate stimulus—Normal stimulus sufficient to elicit a response from a given sense.

Adhesive—Textural property perceived by tongue and teeth; sticky, tenacious, as glutinous substance.

Affective responses—Acceptance or avoidance responses. Hedonic scales measure affective responses, *i.e.*, degree of pleasantness.

After-sensation, negative—After-image or aftertaste in which the qualities are complements of those originally and normally induced by the stimulus.

After-sensation, positive—After-image or aftertaste in which the qualities are the same as those originally and normally induced by the stimulus.

Aftertaste—The experience that, under certain conditions, follows removal of the taste stimulus; it may be continuous with the primary experience or may follow as a different quality after a period during which swallowing, saliva, dilution, and other influences may have affected the stimulus substance.

Aged—Refers to flavors and other sensory properties that develop in foods as a result of time and conditions of storage; may be desirable or undesirable.

Ageusia—Lack or impairment of sensitivity to taste stimuli.

Agnosia—Inability to recognize sensations; may be primarily in one sense, e.g., olfactory agnosia.

Alkaline—A taste sensation usually attributed to a combination of sourness and bitterness (and possibly tactile) stimuli.

Alliaceous—Of or pertaining to the genus *Allium* or the family Alliaceae, containing the garlic, onion, and leek; having the smell of garlic or onions.

Amarogen—Bitter-producing groups, e.g., $-SH^-$.

Ambrosial—Exquisitely pleasing in taste or smell; Gr. & Rom. myth.—worthy of the gods; delicious.

Amplitude—In the flavor-profile method, a combination of qualitative and quantitative evaluation of a product; over-all judgment.

Analysis of variance—An arithmetical procedure for segregating the sources of variability affecting a set of observations.

Anchoring point—A reference point from which other items in a series are judged.

Anosmia—Inability to smell, either totally or a particular substance or group of substances.

Antetaste—A prior taste, or foretaste, usually of short duration, preceding the main taste or flavor characteristic.

Anticipation error—In serial presentation of increasing or decreasing stimuli, making a response before the stimulus is actually perceived.

Appearance—The visual properties of a food, including size, shape, color, and conformation.

Appetite—Learned or unlearned positive orientation toward an object, such as food, not necessarily accompanied by gross physiologic deficit. Appetite for food can exist without hunger, and in civilized man often does.

Appetizing—Appealing to the appetite; tempting.

Aroma—The fragrance or odor of food, perceived by the nose by sniffing. In wines, aroma refers to odors derived from the variety of grape, *e.g.*, muscat aroma.

Aromatic—Possessing a fragrant, slightly pungent, aroma, usually pleasant.

Assessment—A judgment or an evaluation.

Astringent—Quality perceived through the complex of sensations caused by shrinking, drawing, or puckering of the skin surfaces of the oral cavity; dry feeling in the mouth.

Autosmia—Disorder of the sense of smell in which odors are perceived even when none are present.

Auxogluc—Chemical group that, if present with a glucophore (*q.v.*) group, confers sweetness.

Aversion—Dislike and avoidance of a stimulus; repugnance; antipathy.

B

Bakey—In tea, an unpleasant taste in the brew, usually caused by too high a temperature during firing of the leaves and/or the driving off of too much moisture.

Balanced lattice design—A lattice design in which every pair of samples occurs once in the same incomplete block and all pairs are therefore compared with the same degree of accuracy.

Barny flavor (cowy, unclean)—An unpleasant flavor of milk that is associated with poor ventilation of the stable, with improper feeding routine, with physical contamination, or with a combination of these.

Basic tastes—Sweet, sour, salty, and bitter sensations, which may respectively be characterized by sucrose, tartaric acid, sodium chloride, and quinine.

Bias—A propensity, prepossession, or prejudiced judgment.

Binary test—See **Paired comparison.**

Biting—A physical sensation perceived on the tongue, independent of temperature, taste, and odor; can be caused by substances such as pepper and ginger. Distinct from burning, which is of greater intensity and/or longer duration.

Bitter—One of the basic tastes characterized by solution of caffeine, quinine, and certain alkaloids, perceived primarily by the circumvallate papillae at the back of the tongue.

Bland—Having no distinctive taste or odor property.

Blast-injection test—Method of measuring minimum identifiable odors. Used extensively by Elsberg and Levy (1935).*

Blended—With reference to flavor, a smooth flavor having good balance of character notes, perceived in the proper order, with no unpleasant aftertaste. With reference to coffee, tea, whiskey, and wine, a mixture of individual types to achieve a desired commercial product.

"Blind" test—Evaluation of coded samples whose identity is known only to the investigator.

Bloom—With reference to fats, the whitish appearance on the surface of chocolate that sometimes occurs on storage, due to a change in the form of the fat at the surface or to fat diffusing outward and being deposited on the surface. May also refer to surface appearance of grapes, peaches, etc.

Body—The quality of a food or beverage relating variously to its consistency, compactness of texture, fullness, or richness. In dry table wines, body is related to alcohol content.

Boredom—Psychological fatigue in the absence of meaningful previous stimuli.

Bouquet—The distinctive odor of a perfume, wine, beer, or distilled spirit.

Brackish—Salty, alkaline taste, such as that of water from a saline soil.

Briny—A taste sensation consisting of a complex of saltiness and sourness.

Brisk—In tea, a live taste in the brew, as opposed to flat or soft.

Brittle—Textural property characterized by breaking easily and leaving sharp edges.

Burning—The oral sensation of heat caused by pepper, mustard, or other strong spices. It arises from the skin's senses, including pain as well as temperature.

Burnt—A smoky or tarry odor or flavor; empyreumatic (*q.v.*).

C

Cacogeusia—Persistent or intermittent unpleasant taste in the mouth.

Cacosmia—Perception of persistent or intermittent unpleasant odor.

Caramelized—Color and flavor produced when sugars are heated or treated with acid. The effect is distinct from the Maillard reaction between sugar and proteins, which develops on storage.

Cardboardy (cappy)— Flavor defect characteristic of oxidized milk.

Chalky—A texture property characterized by a dry, powdery oral sensation.

Character notes—In the flavor profile method, the separate taste and aroma properties perceived by an individual or a panel in a single substance.

Chemoreceptors—The organs of reception responding to chemical stimuli, *e.g.*, the taste buds and the nerve endings in the olfactory mucosa.

---

* Elsberg, C. A., and I. Levy. 1935. The sense of smell. I. A new and simple method of quantitative olfactometry. *Bull. Neurol. Inst. New York* 4, 5–19.

Chewy—Tending to remain in the mouth without readily breaking up or dissolving; requiring mastication.

Chi-square distribution—The ratio $(n-1)s^2/\sigma^2$ where s^2 is the best estimate of σ^2 obtained from a sample of n observations. The quantity

$$\sum \frac{(f_o - f_e)^2}{f_e}, \qquad (f_e > 5)$$

closely approximates the χ^2 distribution, when f_o represents observed frequencies and f_e the corresponding expected frequencies.

Choking—Unpleasant sensation of suffocating irritation of the throat produced by compounds such as aldehyde C-8 and aldehyde C-11.

Chorda tympani—One of the cranial nerves given off from the facial nerve crossing over the tympanic membrane of the ear to join the lingual branch of the mandibular nerve. It conveys taste sensation from the anterior two-thirds of the tongue and extends via parasympathetic preganglionic fibers to the submaxillary and sublingual salivary glands.

Circumvallate—Large papillae forming a chevron near the back of the tongue, containing many taste buds.

Clear—With reference to visual properties of a liquid or beverage, free of turbidity; unclouded.

Cloudy—Having turbidity; not clear.

Cloying—A taste sensation that stimulates beyond the point of satiation. Frequently used to describe overly sweet products.

Coarse—Composed of large particles, as opposed to fine. Also used to denote a harsh, unpleasant flavor in wines.

Coating—Forming of a film on the tongue and/or teeth, sometimes caused by combination of tannins of a food with proteins of saliva.

Coding—Assignment of symbols, usually letters and/or numbers, to test samples so that they may be presented to a subject without identification.

Coefficient of concordance (W)—A measure $(0 \leqslant W \leqslant 1)$ of the degree of agreement between the rankings assigned a number of products by a group of judges.

Coefficient of correlation—A measure of the intensity of association.

Coefficient of determination—The square of the coefficient of correlation (r^2); or, in regression analysis r^2 is the proportion of a total sum of squares that is attributable to another source of variation, the independent variable.

Coefficient of linear multiple correlation—A measure of the closeness of association between the observed values and a function of the independent values.

Cohesiveness—A textural property perceived by the tongue and teeth related to the strength of the internal bonds of the molecular structure of the stimuli.

Common chemical sense—Sensibility to chemical irritants perceived in various places on the animal body.

Comparative judgment—Direct evaluation of one stimulus with another relative to a specified dimension, such as intensity or degree of liking.

Comparison stimulus—One of a set of stimuli each one of which is to be compared with an invariant, or standard, stimulus.

Compensation—The result of interaction of the components in a mixture of stimuli each component of which is perceived as less intense than it would be alone.

Condiment—An additive, such as pepper or mustard, used to enhance or add a flavor to foods; a seasoning.

Conditioned response—A response which comes to be elicited by an originally neutral stimulus, as a result of previous learning.

Consistency—(1) An oral tactile sensation, a degree of firmness, density, or viscosity. (2) Agreement or harmony of parts; congruity; uniformity.

Constant stimulus—Presentation of a stimulus of a constant quality and intensity, whether presented as a single stimulus, as a member of a pair, or in a multiple presentation.

Consumer—An individual who obtains and uses a commodity.

Consumer panel—A group of individuals representative of a specific population whose behavior is measured. Distinct from a laboratory panel, which is not necessarily representative of any specific consumer population.

Continuum—Anything in which a fundamental common character can be perceived amid a series of insensible or indefinite variations; as in a sensation continuum.

Contrast—Juxtaposition of two different sensations so as to intensify or emphasize the contrary characteristics. Contrast may be of two types: (a) simultaneous or (b) successive, depending on the temporal characteristics of the stimuli presented.

Contrast effect—A judgmental phenomenon that appears in the evaluation of food samples of different preference (or quality) levels, wherein the presentation of one sample tends to make a following sample of the opposite quality rate either higher or lower than it would have if rated independently.

Convergence—Tendency of a test sample, regardless of quality, to be perceived as similar to prior sample(s); sometimes called the halo effect.

Cooked—A flavor that develops in milk upon exposure to heat; often identifiable by a characteristic odor and/or a sweet taste.

Cooling—A physical sensation in the mouth resulting from a cold liquid or solid; also a result of chemical action sensed by the skin, such as that produced by menthol.

Corky—(1) Textural property similar to the tough, elastic cortical tissue of the cork oak. (2) Having a peculiar, unpleasant flavor or odor attributable to the cork; said especially of wines when the bottle cork is defective.

Correction for continuity—A correction to be applied for improving a probability approximation in evaluating a discrete frequency in terms of continuous distribution.

Cowy flavor—See **Barny.**

Creamy—(1) Textural property of liquids and soft semisolids resembling the smooth, oily consistency of an emulsion of fat or cream. (2) Creamy flavors refer to apparent fat content, or richness.

Crisp—Textural property characterized by a brittle, friable nature.

Critical flicker frequency—The frequency at which a flickering light appears to fuse into a continuous light. Can be considered a measure of the activity of the central nervous system.

Crumbly—Textural property characterized by ease with which a substance can be separated into smaller particles.

Crunchy—Textural property that produces a characteristic grinding or crushing sound during mastication of a substance.

Crusty—Having a dry, hard, or coarse surface.

Cryptosmia—Impairment of olfaction by obstruction of the nasal passages.

Crystalline—Textural property resembling the surface conformation of a crystal; clear, transparent.

Cue—An item or feature acting as an indication of the nature of the object or situation perceived.

Curdy—Textural property resembling the thickened, coagulated part of milk.

Cutaneous—Sensory system consisting of cells in skin and free nerve endings responding to warmth, cold, pressure, and pain.

D

Deodorize—To remove odors from air or materials.

Descriptive analysis—The use of descriptive terms in evaluating the sensory properties of a substance.

Difference test—A comparison of quantitative or qualitative variations without indication of preference.

Dilute—To make thinner or more liquid by admixture, especially with water; to diminish strength, flavor, or brilliancy by thinning, hence, to attenuate.

Dilution test—Serial evaluation of changes in the intensity or character of various attributes as a material is given stepwise dilution in water or some other standard substance.

Discrimination—(1) Perception of difference between two or more objects in respect to certain characteristics. (2) A differential response to stimuli that differ quantitatively or qualitatively.

Disguising potential—A testing method wherein various increments of a flavoring compound are added to a substance (usually distasteful) to mask or disguise its sensory properties.

Doubly balanced incomplete-block design—A design having balance for triplets as well as for pairs of treatments (samples).

Doughy—Textural property resembling an unbaked water and flour mixture; pasty, soft and heavy.

Dry—No impression of sweetness on tasting. Wines with less than 0.4% reducing sugar are dry.

Drying—See **Astringent**.

Duo-standard—(Method of difference testing.) Two samples are identified and presented first as knowns, and then they are given again as unknowns for the observer to identify.

Duo-trio—(Method of difference testing.) One of a pair of samples is identified and presented first. Then the observer receives two differing samples as unknowns in random order. The time interval can be varied as desired. Permutations can be A-AB, A-BA, B-AB, B-BA, with the question: which member of the pair matches the standard (*i.e.*, the first item)?

Dusty—An odor of flavor property suggesting the drying, choking sensations of finely divided particles.

Dysosmia—Difficulty in ability to smell.

E

Earthy—Having the odor of earth or soil; see **Musty**.

Effervescent—Containing gas bubbles induced by fermentation or carbonation, as champagne, beer, or soda water.

Elasticity—Textural property reflecting rate of recovery of a material from deformation, such as measured or perceived by tongue and teeth.

Electrophysiology—Study of the function of organs and physiological systems with instruments designed to record bioelectrical concomitants of physiological events.

Emotional expression—Overt muscular activity elicited either by emotion or by emotional ideation.

Empyreumatic—Smoky or tarlike in character. See **Burnt**.

Enhancement—The effect of increasing the total apparent quality of a substance.

Epicure—One who displays fastidiousness in his tastes or enjoyments; a connoisseur.

Error of first kind (α)—The error committed when the experimentor rejects the null hypothesis and it is true.

Error of second kind (β)—The error committed when the experimentor accepts the null hypothesis and it is not true.

Essential oils—Volatile odorous liquids, found in plants, which bear no relation to the edible oils since they are not glycerol esters. They are inflammable, and soluble in alcohol and in ether but not in water; they are used for adding flavor and odor to foods and other materials. Examples: oil of peppermint, oil of spearmint, oil of bitter almonds, oil of citronella, spirits of turpentine.

Excitation—Refers to the process of arousing or irritating a cell to heightened activity; the opposite of **Inhibition.**

Exocrinology—Term suggested by Parkes and Bruce (1961)[*] for study of the effects of odorous materials on endocrine function.

Expectation, error of—A psychological error caused by a preconceived impression arising from the nature of the stimuli being presented or the techniques of presentation.

Expert—Generally an individual acknowledged to be experienced and skillful in a special practice; in the food and beverage field a specialist who usually confines his diagnostic judgments to a specific product under specific conditions, even though others may attribute to him special powers of discrimination, sensitivity, and perspicacity applying to other products and conditions.

F

Factor analysis—A procedure for estimating the various parameters in a model of the form $X_i = a_{i1}z_1 + a_{i2}z_2 + \ldots + a_{ip}z_p + s_i$ where X_i $(i = 1, 2, \ldots, k)$ is a multivariate complex of variables, and the set of variables $z_1, z_2, \ldots, z_p$, with $p < k$, are assumed such that each X is a linear function of the z's together with a part s_i specific to itself.

Factorial design—A design whose treatments are made up of combinations of the variants (qualitative or quantitative) of several factors.

Fatigue, physiological—Reduction in an organism's ability to do work as a result of previous activity. See **Adaptation.**

Fatigue, psychological—A feeling or perception of tiredness that usually increases with work output and with time elapsed after rest and sleep.

Fechner-Weber law—A psychophysical law which states that the strength of the sensory process is proportional to the logarithm of the stimulus.

Feed flavor—A flavor defect of milk and cottage cheese that is characterized by its aromatic, not necessarily unpleasant, readily detectable odor. The flavor occurs in milk from cows fed feeds containing weeds or weed seeds.

Feeling factors—Usually refers to tactile sensations in the mouth. See **Tactile.**

Fibrous—Stringy textural property.

Filiform—Small papillae on surface of tongue; they are devoid of taste buds.

Finish—Term used in grading raw meat, referring to quality, color, and distribution of the fat. In wines, refers to aftertaste.

Firm—Solid, compact textural property.

---

[*] Parkes, A. S., and H. M. Bruce. 1961. Olfactory stimuli in mammalian reproduction. *Science* **134**, 1049–1054.

Fishy—Having a flavor or odor resembling fish, such as trimethylamine.

Fizzy—Effervescent; having hissing sounds, as champagne.

Flaky—Textural property consisting of loose layers that separate easily.

Flat—(1) Having little or no flavor. In milk, this flavor defect can be simulated by adding water. (2) A term applied to wines of low acidity. (3) Loss of carbonation in sparkling beverages.

Flavor—(1) A mingled but unitary experience which includes sensations of taste, smell, pressure, and other cutaneous sensations such as warmth, cold, mild pain. (2) An attribute of foods, beverages, and seasonings resulting from stimulation of the sense ends that are grouped together at the entrance of the alimentary and respiratory tracts—especially odor and taste.

Flavor memory—As used in descriptive sensory analysis, an ability to recognize and identify many individual odors and flavors.

Flavoring—Any substance, such as an essence or extract, employed to give a particular flavor.

Flavor profile technique—A method of qualitative descriptive analysis of aroma and flavor. The method makes it possible to indicate degrees of difference between two samples on the basis of individual character notes, degree of blending, and over-all impression of the product (amplitude).

Floral—Having a flowerlike odor.

Fluffy—Soft and downy textural property; light and airy.

Foamy—Textural property consisting of a mass of bubbles formed on liquids, or in the mouth by agitation or by fermentation; frothy.

Foliate—Papillae derived from a series of grooves or folds in the midlateral border of the tongue; they contain taste buds.

Forced-choice judgment—A response that must be given in terms of one or more clearly defined categories, *i.e.*, does not permit "don't know" or other indeterminate answers.

Foreign flavor—Containing a flavor not normally associated with the product.

Foxy—Aroma and taste (due to methyl anthranilate) found in wines made from Concord or other Labrusca-type grapes.

Fragrant—A pleasing olfactory quality; odors which are distinctly pleasant smelling.

Friable—Easily pulverized.

Fruity flavor—An aromatic or fruitlike flavor. In milk or cottage cheese, a flavor defect resulting from microbial activity.

F-test—A test involving the ratio of two variances, usually used to determine whether two independent estimates of variance can be assumed to be two estimates of the variance of a single normally distributed population.

Fungiform papillae—Small, mushroomlike raised areas scattered over the anterior surface of the tongue, containing taste buds and innervated by the chorda tympani.

G

Gastronomy—The art of good eating.

Gel—A sol or colloidal suspension that has set to a jelly. Agar and pectin make elastic gels, and gum arabic and silicic acid make inelastic gels.

Gelatinous—A sticky, jellylike consistency.

Glitter—A bright, sparkling surface.

Gloss—A smooth shiny surface; brightness or luster; polish.

Glucophore—Main sweet-producing group. Operative only if accompanied by an auxogluc (*q.v.*).

Gourmet—A connoisseur in eating and drinking.

Grainy—Granular texture.

Grassy—A flavor defect suggesting the bitterness or astringency of green grass.

Greasy—Textural property suggesting a covering of oil or fat.

Gristly—Having cartilaginouslike properties.

Gritty—A hard, coarse, stonelike sensation, usually caused by the presence of sand particles or stone cells.

Gummy—Textural property of a semisolid perceived by the tongue.

Gust—A unit of gustatory intensity relating to the threshold of a given substance.

Gustation—The taste sense whose receptors lie in the mucous membrane covering the tongue and whose stimuli consist of certain soluble chemicals, e.g., salts, acids, sugar.

Gymnemic acid—An acid that abolishes the sensation of sweetness and restricts that of bitterness, but leaves salty and sour tastes more or less unchanged.

H

Halo effect—See **Convergence.**

Haptic—Pertaining to the skin or to the sense of touch in its broadest sense.

Hardness—A textural property; force necessary to attain deformation.

Harsh—Lacking harmony or smoothness; rasping, coarse, rough, grating, discordant, astringent.

Hedonic—Pertaining to feeling; hedonic tone is the pleasurable or unpleasurable accompaniment or characteristics of conscious experiences.

Hedonic scale—A calibrated continuum upon which degree of like and dislike is recorded.

Hemianosmia—Loss of the sense of smell on one side.

Herby—Pertaining to or resembling the odor or flavor of herbs.

Hircine—A goatlike odor.

Hue—One dimension of visual sensation (or color), correlated with the wavelength of light falling on the receptors, i.e., redness, blueness, or greeness of a substance.

Hunger—A desire for food sometimes accompanied by strong contractions of the stomach.

"Hungry"—Descriptive term applied to the brew of a tea that lacks the characteristics generally associated with that particular tea.

Hyperosmia—Unusually keen olfactory sensitivity.

Hyperphagia—Consumption of abnormally large amounts of food.

Hypesthesia—Impaired power of sensation.

Hypogeusia—Diminished sense of taste.

Hyposmia—Diminished sense of smell; olfactory hypesthesia (*q.v.*).

Hypostyptic—Mildly styptic or astringent.

I

Inadequate stimulus—Application to a sense system, of energy not "normal" to that system (such as an electrical current applied to the tongue) and thereby producing a sensation appropriate to a normal stimulus. Besides "inadequate," also termed "insipid," "tasteless."

Incentive—An external goal-object toward which an organism is motivated.

Incomplete block design—A design which permits judging more products than can be evaluated at one sitting. Such a design is said to be balanced if the same number of products are judged at each sitting and every pair of products occurs together in the same number of sittings.

Induction—Enhanced sensitivity of the receptor resulting from fatigue of an adjacent receptor.

Inhibition—In general, the opposite of excitation (*q.v.*); usually the reduction in or prevention of response to a stimulation.

Innervated—Provision of a given effector cell, tissue, or organ with one or more neurons that can excite or inhibit it.

Insipid—Tasteless, flat, vapid.

Instinctive behavior—A complex pattern of activity that is common to a given species and that occurs without opportunity for learning.

Intensity—A quantitative attribute of a sensation approximately proportional to the intensity of physical energy of the stimulus, such as brightness of colors, loudness of sounds, and concentration of taste or odor compounds.

Intensity scale—Scaling method consisting of numbers or terms used to denote the strength of a stimulus.

Interaction—A measure of the extent to which the effect of changing the level of one factor depends on the level(s) of another or others.

Introspective technique—Psychological method in which the observer (subject) describes his awareness of the stimuli to the experimenter.

Ipsative scaling—A method of assigning scale values that takes the individual's own characteristic behavior as the standard of comparison.

Irritability—The property of responding to one or more kinds of energy change.

Isohedonic—Equality in degree of pleasantness and unpleasantness.

J

Jnd—Just-noticeable difference, or difference limen (DL); the smallest detectible difference between two stimuli. See also **Limen.**

Jnnd—Just-not-noticeable difference.

Judge—One who participates in a test by providing data which generally are verbal reports of his experience. The term connotes that the person has some special qualifications.

Juicy—Containing moisture; succulent.

K

Kinesthesis—The sense whose end organs lie in the muscles, tendons, and joints and are stimulated by bodily tensions.

L

Lattice design—An incomplete block experimental design in which the number of samples is a perfect square and the number of samples scored at one sitting is the square root of this number.

Limen—Threshold (*q.v.*).

Liminal—The lowest value of any given form of energy that will arouse a receptor to cause a sensation.

Line of regression—A straight line which "best fits" a set of points; its equation is known as the regression equation.

Liquor—Any liquid substance; an alcoholic beverage; a solution of a substance in water such as brewed tea.

Logical error—Errors resulting from assigning similar ratings to characteristics because they "appear" to the observer to be logically associated with other unrelated characteristics.

M

Macrosmatic—Abnormally keen olfactory sense.

Malty—A flavor defect suggestive of malt, and sometimes resembling the flavor of Grape-nuts, walnuts, or maple. In milk, malty flavor is generally caused by the growth of *Streptococcus lactis* var. *maltigenes*.

Marbling—The intermingling of fat with lean on the cut surface of meat.

Masking—Term used when two odors or flavors neutralize each other. In taste, odor, or flavor applications, it is a component quality within a mixture which dominates or overrides another quality or other qualities present, thus changing the quality of the perceived result without benefit of chemical interaction of the components themselves.

Mastication—The act of chewing; grinding and comminuting with the teeth.

Matching—Process of equating or relating, pair by pair, for experimental purposes, usually to determine the degree of similarity between a standard and unknown or two unknowns.

Mealy—A quality of mouthfeel imparting a starchlike or cornmeal-like sensation. See **Friable.**

Medicinal—Olfactory and/or gustatory sensation denoting a medicinelike flavor or odor (usually unpleasant); the smell and taste of disinfectant, chlorine, iodine, or some phenolic compounds.

Merosmia—A condition analogous to color blindness, in which certain odors are not perceived.

Metallic—Flavor defect suggesting iron or copper contamination. In fat-containing foods, related to oxidative changes.

Microsmatic—Having a poorly developed sense of smell.

Microvilli—Submicroscopic projections of cell membranes greatly increasing surface area. Taste buds have numerous microvilli which are thought to facilitate rapid absorption of taste substances.

MID—Minimum identifiable difference; difference threshold.

MIO—Minimum identifiable odor; recognition threshold.

Modality—Differentiation of a sense, partly or fully emerged. The taste modalities are sweet, sour, salty, and bitter.

Moldy—An odor or flavor suggestive of mold.

Monadic—Consisting of units along one continuum.

Monosodium glutamate (MSG)—The sodium salt of glutamic acid.

Mono stimulus—See **Single stimulus.**

Motivation—A term employed to account for behavior initiated or controlled by conditions within an organism; inducement, incentive.

Motive—An internal organismic state that initiates or otherwise determines behavior.

Mouthfeel—A mingled experience deriving from the sensations of the skin in the mouth during and after ingestion of a food or beverage that relates to density, viscosity, surface tension, and other physical and chemical properties of the material being sampled.

Multiple comparison—An unlimited number (usually more than three) of samples is presented to the observer simultaneously in random arrangement or in accordance with a predetermined statistical design. Significance of results is usually calculated by the variance method, or a rapid approximation thereof.

Multiple-range test—A test employing different significance values depending upon the number of means being compared.

Mushy—A soft, thick, pulpy consistency.

Musty—Flavor similar to the odor of a damp, poorly ventilated cellar.

N

Narcotic—A drug that induces stupor, drowsiness, or insensibility.

Nares—Exterior opening to the nose.

Nasal mucosa—Mucous membranes lining the upper nasal regions.

Neutral stimulus—A sensation that is perceived but which elicits little or no measurable response.

Neutralize—To obliterate or subdue a taste or olfactory sensation with another stimuli. Also, chemically, a reaction of acids and bases.

Nippy—Sharp, biting oral sensation.

Nose—The aroma of tea liquor or wines.

Nose-filling—Highly aromatic, pungent material.

Null hypothesis—A hypothesis, applicable to a population or distribution, for which it is possible to compute a statistic and the corresponding probability of a more extreme value.

Numbing—Anesthetic property of compounds such as eugenol.

O

Objective—(1) Capable of being recorded by physical instruments or as a consequence of the repeatable operation. (2) Not totally dependent upon the observations and reports of an individual, but verifiable by others. Usually the opposite of subjective (*q.v.*).

Observer—One who participates in a test by providing data that generally are verbal reports of his own experience. This term, in contrast to *judge*, connotes a situation where the primary attention is directed toward the person's response rather than the test material.

Odor—That which is smelled. Odor may refer to the stimulus or to the sensation resulting from the stimulation of olfactory receptors in the nasal cavity by gaseous material.

Odorimetry—Measurement of the odor properties of various compounds, with emphasis on the stimulus rather than the subject.

Odorphore—Odor-producing group.

Odor prism—A schematic representation of relations between postulated basic classes of odors and of transitional or mixed odors.

Oily—Slick, greasy oral sensation.

Olfactie—Unit of odor stimulus used by Zwaardemaker, consisting of the ratio of the true concentration divided by the threshold concentration of an odorous material.

Olfaction—The sense of smell.

Olfactometer—An instrument for controlled (volume, temperature, humidity, flow rate) presentation of odor stimuli, used for measuring thresholds and other quantitative values.

Olfactometry—The measurement of olfactory sensitivity in human subjects, with emphasis on the subject rather than the stimulus.

Olfactorium—A room or large chamber in which odorous materials are tested by a subject.

Olfactory apparatus—The olfactory cells, hairs, nerves.

Olfactory bulb—Part of the brain into which the olfactory nerve leads.

Olfactory cells—Long, narrow cells furnished with hairlike processes which are smell receptors.

Olfactory cleft—Posterior part of the nasal cavity in which the olfactory cells are situated.

Olfactory coefficient—The smallest volume of vapor of a substance necessary for identification of its odor.

Olfactory epithelium—Pigmented layer in the nose containing the receptor cells for olfaction.

Olfactory hairs—Fragile, protoplasmic filaments on the olfactory cells.

Olfactory-negative—That which reduces odor, e.g., an electro-positive element in a compound.

Olfactory pit—The elementary olfactory organ found in invertebrates and lower vertebrates.

Olfactory prism—A method devised by Henning to represent six fundamental odors as the corners of a prism.

Olfactory region—Seat of the smell receptors.

One-tailed (or one-sided) test—A test of significance based upon one tail (side) of the distribution, *e.g.*, as in a paired difference test.

Organoleptic—(1) Affecting or making an impression on an organ or the whole organism; (2) Capable of receiving an impression; (3) Sometimes used as a synonym for "sensory" when referring to examination by taste and smell. The word is obsolete in food analysis, replaced by "sensory evaluation" or "psychophysics."

Osmics—The science of smell.

Osmoceptor—Smell receptor.

Osmophore—A smell-inducing chemical group.

Osmoscope—Instrument for measuring odor intensity.

Osmyl—An odorous substance.

Oxidized—Flavor defect—in dairy products resembling cardboard flavor, and in wines an aldehyde odor.

P

Paired comparison (method of)—A psychometric or psychophysical method in which stimuli (samples) are presented in pairs for comparison on the basis of some defined criterion such as preference, intensity, or degree of a defined quality. (1) Presentation of permutations of AA, AB, BA, BB under code, with the question: Do the members of the pair differ? (2) Presentation of permutations of AB, BA, under code, with the question: Which member is stronger, sweeter, etc.?, or which do you prefer?

Paired preference—Paired comparison method with preference the criterion.

Palatable—Agreeable to the taste; savory, hence pleasing.

Palate—The roof of the mouth; also individual subjective preference patterns.

Panel—A group of people (observers, subjects, judges) comprising a test population which has been specially selected or designated in some manner, *e.g.*, they may be trained or have spécial knowledge or skills or may merely be available and predesignated.

Panel leader—In the flavor profile method, the person responsible for organizing, conducting, and directing a panel.

Papillae (papilla)—Structures of various shapes on the tongue which contain taste buds. Four kinds are found on the human tongue: foliate, circumvallate, fungiform, and filiform.

Parageusia—Gustatory disturbance resulting in erroneous identification of taste stimuli.

Parosmia—A disturbance to the sense of smell resulting in smelling the "wrong" odors, usually perceived as repulsive.

Pasty—Textural property characterized by flour-water paste.

Perception—The process of becoming aware of objects, qualities, or relations by way of the sense organs.

Phenomenology—A method of observation admitting subjective experience as a legitimate object of scientific investigation, *i.e.* no analysis is made of the description of the immediate experience.

Physiological psychology—The study of relationships between bodily processes and behavior.

Piquant—Agreeably stimulating to the palate; pleasantly tart, sharp, or biting; pungent.

Pithy—A textural property resembling the loose, spongy tissue occupying the center of the stem in dicotyledonous plants; soft and spongy.

Plastic—A property of texture; capable of being deformed continuously and permanently in any direction without rupture.

Pleasant—That which is agreeable; in harmony with one's tastes or likings.

Preference—(1) Expression of higher degree of liking. (2) Choice of one object over others. (3) Psychological continuum of affectivity (pleasantness—unpleasantness) on which such choices are based. This continuum is also referred to as that of degree of liking or disliking.

Pretest—A practical exercise intended to familiarize a subject with a procedure; a test administered before instruction to determine a subject's information or prejudices prior to testing.

Primary qualities—Within a specific sense, the qualities that are basic and from which all other qualities can be compounded. The four primary taste qualities are generally believed to be sweet, sour, salty, and bitter. See **Modality**.

Probability model—A useful and convenient representation of the essentially important aspects of a situation based on probability theory.

Proprioception—Senses having receptors in muscles, tendons, joints, and the nonauditory inner ear.

Protection level—The probability, in testing the significance of a difference between two measures, that a significant difference between means will not be found if the population means are equal.

Psychology—Study of the behavior of animal organisms.

Psychometrics—Study of the application of quantitative measures to behavior.

Psychophysics—Study of the relation between physical-stimulus variables and psychological measures of sensory variables.

Puckery—A sensation which causes the mouth to contract or to draw up into folds or wrinkles; astringent.

Pulpy—Consisting of a moist, slightly cohering mass; fleshy; succulent.

Pungent—A sharp, stinging, or painful sensation of a flavor or odor, such as that of aldehyde C-9 and aldehyde C-10.

Pure odors (or true odors)—Olfactory experience unaffected by the action of the other senses of the skin in the mouth, especially the trigeminal and taste receptors.

Putrid—Unpleasant flavor and odor associated with proteolytic spoilage.

Q

Quality—(1) (Psychological) An aspect, attribute, characteristic, or fundamental dimension of experience involving variation in kind rather than in degree. (2) The composite of the characteristics that differentiate among individual units of the product and have significance in determining the degree of acceptability of that unit by the user. (3) an esthetic standard for a product, usually set by experienced users.

Quality control—Application of sensory, physical, and chemical tests in industrial production to prevent undue variation in quality attributes, such as color, viscosity, flavor, etc.

R

Rancid—Having a rank odor or taste, as that of old oil; characterized by aldehyde C-9 or aldehyde C-10.

Randomized block design—A design in which each judge at one sitting scores all samples presented in a randomized order.

Rank order—(1) A psychometric method that may be used in multiple comparisons where the subject considers all of the samples in a series at the same time and is required to rank them in order on some designated dimension such as preference, intensity, quality, etc. (2) A procedure of arranging food products in order according to some criterion and assigning consecutive integers (ranks) corresponding to the order.

Rating method—A method for securing and recording a judgment concerning the degree to which a stimulus material possesses a specified attribute, usually by placing a mark at an appropriate position between the two extremes of a line that represents the possible range of degrees of that attribute. Allocation of samples to defined categories which are recognized by training.

Rating scale—A continuum created for quantification of judgments.

Reaction—In the behaviorial sciences, action in response to known or inferred stimulation.

Reaction time—The time that elapses between application of stimulus and response.

Receptor—A cell differentiated from others in terms of its increased irritability to certain stimuli.

Redolent—Emitting a scent or suggesting an odor.

Reference sample—In a multisample test, the sample with which all others are to be compared.

Region of acceptance—The region for which the null hypothesis is accepted.

Region of rejection—The region for which the null hypothesis is rejected.

Response-surface procedure—A method for exploring functional relationships between variables which permits the determination of optimum proportions of various ingredients to give a maximum score.

Rhinitis—Inflammation of the nasal membranes.

RL—Absolute threshold (from the German *Reiz Limen*)—See **Threshold.**

Rough—Term used to describe degree of astringency, particularly in wine.

Rubbery—(1) Odor of natural or synthetic rubber, characterized by paratertiary butyl phenol. (2) Resilient, rubberlike texture.

S

Saliva—A clear, alkaline, somewhat viscous secretion from the parotid, submandibular and submaxillary glands in the mouth.

Salty (saline)—A quality of taste sensation of which the taste of sodium chloride is a typical example.

Sample—A specimen or aliquot presented for inspection.

Sandy—A textural property resembling small, loose, dry, granular particles.

Sapid—Having the power of affecting the taste receptors.

Sapophores—Sweet-producing chemical groups.

Satiety—State of being replete, satisfied, not hungry or lacking appetite.

Savory—Appetizing; having an agreeable flavor.

Scaling—Location of points, characteristic of the sample, on a sensory continuum relative to fixed standard points. Differs from scoring where numerical ratings are used.

Scent—A characteristic odor, often subtle.

Score—(1) (*noun*) A value assigned to a specific response made to a test item; (2) (*verb*) to score a food is to rate its properties on a scale or according to some numerically defined sense of criteria.

Screening—Pretesting of possible samples, techniques, or judges.

Seasoning—A condiment used to supplement or enhance the flavor of food, such as spices, flavorings.

Sensation—The uninterrupted experience accompanying afferent activity which reaches the cortical level; the immediate awareness when a receptor is stimulated.

Sensitivity—Acuity; ability to perceive quantitative and/or qualitative differences.

Sensitizer—Essentially a motive; an internal factor that predisposes an organism to respond selectively to external stimuli.

Sequential analysis—A procedure in which the sample number is not fixed in advance but depends to some extent on the outcome of the sampling as it proceeds.

Series effect—A tendency to over- or underestimate a stimulus according to its magnitude in relation to the series as a whole.

Set—A readiness to respond to certain situations and not others; a preparation for selection of certain stimuli and for a particular type of response.

Sharp—Characterizing an intense or painful, well-localized reaction to a substance being eaten or smelled, e.g., various acids and alcohols.

Shear—The type of force exerted on foods by chewing, in which the food is first compressed and then shorn.

Sheen—Luster, shine, glistening.

Short—In pastry, easily broken, friable, or crisp.

Single stimulus—Refers to any psychophysical or phychometric method in which a judgment follows a presentation of one stimulus only.

Skunky—A characteristic odor and flavor in beer and ale resulting from exposure to light, causing the development of 3-methyl-2-butene thiol. Also called "sunstruck" or "lightstruck" flavor.

Slimy—A sensation imparted by material which is thick, coats the mouth, is not readily diluted by saliva, and is difficult to swallow.

Smell—To perceive by excitation of the olfactory nerves.

Smoky—Emitting smoke; having a gray, cloudy appearance; having a burntlike odor or flavor.

Smooth—Having an even surface or consistency; devoid of roughness.

Sniff—To evaluate an odor by drawing air audibly and abruptly through the nose.

Soft—(1) Affecting the senses in a gentle and pleasant way; lacking in harshness, stiffness, coarseness, acidity, or like qualities offensive to taste, sight, hearing, or touch. (2) Easily yielding to physical pressure; unresistant to molding, cutting, wear, etc. (3) Water: freedom from calcium and magnesium salts, which prevent the formation of lather with soap. (4) Fruit beverages: having no alcohol. (5) Wheat: having starchy kernels low in gluten.

Soggy—Saturated with moisture; heavy and wet; sodden or soaked.

Somesthesis—Body sensibilities; sense of deep and cutaneous pressure, pain warmth, and cold.

Sorting—Method of presentation of several samples of one variable and several samples of another variable, in randomized order, with instructions to sort into two homogeneous groups.

"Soupy"—Usually refers to undesirable dilution of a semisolid or a suspension.

Sour—The taste sensation caused by acids. May also describe spoiled foods.

Specific smell strength—The reciprocal of the number of grams of a substance per liter that can just be smelled.

Specific tenacity of odor—The number of hours times 100 during which one gram of 1% solution of a substance in absolute alcohol retains its odor under defined conditions.

Spicy—Flavored with, containing, or characteristic of a spice or spice complex; aromatic; piquant; pungent.

Spongy—Having the consistency of a sponge; open, loose, pliable texture; elastic, porous, springy.

Springy—An elastic surface texture, such as that of freshly baked bread.

Stale—Not fresh; vapid or tasteless from age, such as stale beer, stale bread, or stale nonfat milk powder.

Standard sample—A constant sample designated as a reference with which others are compared.

Standards—In the flavor profile method, compounds and mixtures against which descriptive terms are calibrated.

Starchy—Containing a high amount of carbohydrate, as a starchy diet; resembling the flavor or mouthfeel of uncooked starch.

Stimulus—That which incites the receptors, e.g., an odorous substance or a sapid (*q.v.*) solution or an electric current.

Stimulus error—The result of paying attention to the properties of the stimulus rather than to the characteristics of the sensation.

Student's (t) distribution—A distribution representing the ratio x/s, where x is an observation from a normal population with mean zero and s is an efficient estimate of the population standard deviation.

Styptic—See **Astringent.**

Subject—One who participates in a test by providing data. This generic term is appropriate whenever any of the related terms may be used; thus, it embraces not only those who provide subjective or verbal data but also those who respond in any other way. *Subject, judge,* and *observer* are terms whose use is supported by custom and, as such, are distinguished from such casual words as "tester," "taster," "panelist," "sniffer," etc.

Subjective—Pertaining to individual experience which can be observed or reported only by the person involved, and subject to influence of temperament, personal bias, and emotional background. Opposite of objective (*q.v.*).

Subliminal—Below the threshold; applied to stimuli that are not intense enough to arouse definite sensations but that nevertheless have some effect upon the responses of the individual.

Succulent—Having juicy tissues, such as those of melons.

Sunlight flavor—Defect in milk caused when the amino acid methionine is broken down by sunlight or artificial light in the presence of vitamin B_2.

Sunstruck flavor—See **Skunky**.

Supraliminal—Above the threshold—either absolute threshold or difference threshold; see **Subliminal**.

Sweet—A quality of taste sensation of which the taste of sucrose is a typical example.

T

Tacky—Sticky, adhesive.

Tactile—Pertaining to the sense of touch.

Tactometer—An instrument for testing and measuring the acuteness of the sense of touch.

Tainted flavor—A general flavor defect, such as feed flavor in milk.

Tallowy flavor—Flavor defect suggestive of a fatty-waxy complex, as in oxidized or rancid lard.

Tangy—Having a sharp, tart taste.

Tannin—An astringent material present in many natural products, e.g., red wine, tea, and coffee.

Tarry—Suggestive of the odor of tar, such as the odor of carvacrol.

Tart—See **Sour**.

Taste—One of the senses, the receptors for which are located in the mouth and are activated by a large variety of different compounds and solutions. Most investigators usually limit gustatory qualities to four: saline, sweet, sour, and bitter. Distinguish from **Flavor**, the sensation to which taste contributes.

Taste blindness—A deficiency in taste perception. See **Ageusia**.

Taste buds—The end organs of the taste-nerves, located in the folds of the tongue and, to a lesser extent, other areas of the oral cavity. Also "taste-beakers" or "taste-onions."

Tasty—Having a pleasant taste or flavor; savory.

Tender—Easily broken, cut, or masticated. Opposite of tough or hard.

Tenderometer—An instrument for testing and measuring the tenderness of food.

Terpy—Suggestive of the odor of terpenes, such as the odor of linalyl cinnamate.

Texture—Properties of a foodstuff apprehended both by the eyes and by the skin and muscle senses in the mouth, embracing roughness, smoothness, graininess, etc.

Texturometer—An instrument for testing and measuring the texture of food.

Thin—Lacking in substance, richness, strength, or density, relative to flavor or texture.

Threshold—(limen)—A statistically determined point on the stimulus scale at which occurs a transition in a series of sensations or judgments. There are several types of thresholds: (1) absolute threshold, threshold of sensation, detection threshold, or stimulus threshold, often designated as RL, which is that magnitude of stimulus at which a transition occurs from no sensation to sensation; (2) difference threshold is the least amount of change of a given stimulus necessary to produce a change in sensation. It is often designated as the DL, and the interval or unit as the jnd (just-noticeable difference); (3) recognition threshold, or identification threshold, is the minimum concentration at which a substance is correctly identified; (4) terminal threshold is that magnitude of a stimulus above which there is no increase in perceived intensity of the appropriate quality for the stimulus. Above this point, pain often occurs.

Time errors—Errors of judgment in a paired presentation: (1) negative—tendency to overestimate the first stimulus in relation to the second; (2) positive—tendency to overestimate the second stimulus in relation to the first.

Time-intensity test—Measurement of the rate, duration, and intensity of stimulation by a single stimulus.

Tough—Having flexibility without brittleness; yielding to force without breaking; tenacious, such as the ligaments in meat.

Triangle test—A method of difference testing consisting of three coded samples, wherein two are identical and one is different. The task of the observer is to select the *different* sample. Possible permutations are AAB, ABA, BAA, ABB, BAB, and BBA.

Trigeminal—Relating to the Vth cranial nerve, over which pain sensations are transmitted to the central nervous system. Common chemical sense; see Chapter 4.

Tristimulus coefficients—Specification of a color on the basis of three measurements.

Turbid—Cloudy, muddy, unclear.

Turbidimetric—Relating to the method for determining the concentration of a substance suspended in solution by the degree of cloudiness or turbidity that it causes or by the degree of clarification that it induces in a turbid solution.

Turbinates—The conchae of the nasal structure.

Two-tailed (two-sided) test—A test of significance based upon both tails (sides) of the distribution, *e.g.* as in a paired preference test.

U

Unbalanced—Excessive amounts of one constituent or another, causing disharmony of taste or olfactory impression.

Unclean flavor—See **Barny.**

Unconditioned response—A response which occurs to appropriate stimulation without prior conditioning.

Unconditioned stimulus—A stimulus that affects behavior in a way not influenced by prior learning.

Use test—A test aimed at eliciting from the consumer reactions to one or more products after a period of use.

V

Value—Lightness and darkness of a color.

Vapid—Absence of character, spirit, zest; insipid, dull, flat.

Viscous—Thick.

W

"Warm-up" sample—Samples presented to a judge for introduction and orientation prior to evaluation of the test samples.

Watery—Diluted flavor; flat, lacking in intensity of flavor.

Weathery—An unpleasant taste in tea liquors, resembling rain water.

Weber ratio—A psychophysical law stating that the strength of the sensory process is proportional to the logarithm of the stimulus.

Weber's law—A psychophysical law stating that small, equally perceptible increments in a response correspond to proportional increments in the physical stimuli (S), i.e., $\Delta S + KS$, where ΔS is any increment in S corresponding to a defined unitary change in R, and K is the ratio of the increment to S.

Weedy—A flavor defect occurring in milk from cows feeding on weeds prior to milking. The character and intensity of the flavor is dependent on the type and quantity of weeds consumed and the interval between feeding and milking. Some weed flavors are onion, garlic, french weed, and dog fennel.

"Wet dog" odor—Odor of burnt protein, characteristic of some irradiated foods.

Whiffing—A short, quick sniffing procedure.

"White taste"—A taste mixture having no readily identifiable taste, consisting of 0.01 M sucrose, 0.0002 M citric acid, 0.014 M sodium chloride, and 0.000004 M quinine sulfate.

Author Index

Numbers in italics refer to pages on which the complete references are listed.

Subject Index*†

A

Absolute judgments, 198, 264, 355, 540
Absorption theory of odor, *200–204*
Ac'cent, *see* Monosodium glutamate
Acceptability, 124; and color, 220–222; and discrimination, 289
Acceptance, 540; food, 399
Accuracy, *see* Validity
Acetaldehyde, odor threshold, 185, 296
Acetic acid, effect on taste, 123; effect on olfactory acuity, 181; odor, 150, 151, 160, 183, 296; response, 43, 75–81, 121, 122, 124, 269; threshold, 75–77
Acetylcholine, effect on taste, 56, 57; and olfactory acuity, 182; produces anosmia, 170; *see also* Flavor
Acid, adaptation to, 122; effect on salty taste, 123; effect on sweet taste, 123; odor, 184, 197; response, 45, 50, 53, 75–79; *see also* Sour
Acid phosphatase, 37
Acid taste, *see* Sour
Acid odor, 151, 152
Adaptation, 30, 46, 50, 69, *171–174*, 180, 181, *267–271*, 297, 312, 327, 329, 331, 336, 343, 541; "absolute limit of," 122; to color, 225–226; to common chemical sense, 240; effect on food testing, 270; effect of temperature, 63–64; effect on thresholds, 120, 121, 269; olfactory, 150, 154, *190–193*, 194, 206; and pain, 236, 237; to touch, 230
Adaptation-level, defined, 265, 266
Adenosine triphosphate (ATP), 203
Adhesiveness, *see* Texture
Adrenal insufficiency, and taste, 52
Adrenalectomy, and salt intake, 9, 13–16, 19–20, 52
Adsorption, and taste, 71–73
Adsorption theory of odor, *194–196*
Advertising, of food, 400, 408, 411, 429
Afterimages, 226
Aftertaste, 3, 114, 541; of monosodium glutamate, 378; of sulfited foods, 378

Agar, effect on taste, 66
Age, and food preference, 400, *403–404*, 408; effect on odor, 183, 184; effect on taste, 57, 58; of judges, 282, 291
Ageusia, 51, 127, 541
"Aggridants," defined, 21
Air conditioning, *see* Temperature
Alanine, bitter taste, 104; neural response, 67
Alcohol, effect on olfactory acuity, 181; effect on sweetness, 99; odor, 184; odor and taste, 145; sweetness, 86; threshold and preference, 14, 19
Alcohols, aliphatic, odor, 152, 154, 159, 189, 196, 197
Aldehydes, bitter taste, 104; odor, 197; sweetness, 87
Algin, effect on taste, 65
Alkaline taste, 39, 40
Alkaloids, bitter taste, 103
n-Alkanals, threshold, 188
4-Alkoxy-3-aminonitrobenzenes, sweetness, 86, 87
Alliaceous, odor, 150, 541
Allyl isothiocyanate, odor threshold, 186
Allyl mercaptan, odor threshold, 187
Almond, flavor and color, 221; odor, 156
Aluminum acetate, effect on odor, 192
Alveolotubular glands, 163
Ambrosiac odor, 150, 541
Amides, taste, 87, 104
p-Aminoazobenzene sulfonic acid, mixed taste, 104
Amino acids, response, 50; taste, 66–67, 86, 104
Ammonia, odor, 173; and pain, 238
Ammonium chloride, neural response, 87; threshold, 85
Ammonium glutamate, in soya sauce, 115
Ammonium salts, bitter taste, 104
Amoore's steoreochemical theory, *156–158*, 190, 196, 206
Amphetamine, effect on olfactory acuity, 181

* See also the glossary, pp. 540–564.
† Page numbers in italics refer to primary source of information on the subject.